PATHOLOGY OF MELANOCYTIC NEVI AND MALIGNANT MELANOMA

SECOND EDITION

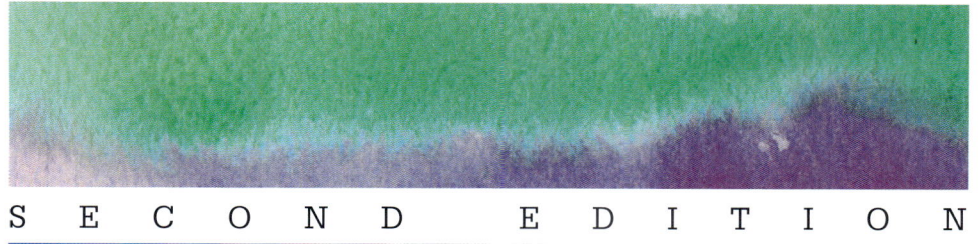

SECOND EDITION

PATHOLOGY OF MELANOCYTIC NEVI AND MALIGNANT MELANOMA

Raymond L. Barnhill, MD

Chair, Professor of Dermatology and Pathology, Department of Dermatology,
George Washington University Medical Center, Washington, DC, USA

EDITOR-IN-CHIEF

Michael Piepkorn, MD, PhD

Clinical Professor, Division of Dermatology and Department of Pathology,
University of Washington School of Medicine, Seattle, Washington, USA

Klaus J. Busam, MD

Associate Professor, Department of Pathology,
Memorial Sloan-Kettering Cancer Center, New York, New York, USA

EDITORS

With 151 Illustrations in 363 Parts, 347 in Full Color

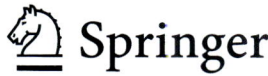

Raymond L. Barnhill, MD
Chair
Professor of Dermatology and Pathology
Department of Dermatology
George Washington University Medical Center
Washington, DC 20037
USA

Michael Piepkorn, MD, PhD
Clinical Professor
Division of Dermatology and
 Department of Pathology
University of Washington School of Medicine
Seattle, WA 98195
USA

Klaus J. Busam, MD
Associate Professor
Department of Pathology
Memorial Sloan-Kettering Cancer Center
New York, NY 10021
USA

Library of Congress Cataloging-in-Publication Data
Barnhill, Raymond L.
 Pathology of melanocytic nevi and malignant melanoma / Raymond Barnhill, Michael Piepkorn, Klaus Busam—2nd ed.
   p. ; cm.
  Includes bibliographical references and index.
  ISBN 0-387-40326-4 (alk. paper)
  1. Melanoma—Pathophysiology. I. Piepkorn, Michael. II. Busam, Klaus J. III. Title.
  [DNLM: 1. Nevus—pathology. 2. Skin Neoplasms—pathology.
 3. Melanocytes—pathology. 4. Melanoma—pathology. QZ 310 B262 2003]
 RC280.M37B37 2003
 616.99′477—dc21   2003052956

ISBN 0-387-40326-4   Printed on acid-free paper.

© 2004 Springer Science+Business Media, Inc.
All rights reserved. This work may not be translated or copied in whole or in part without the written permission of the publisher (Springer Science+Business Media, Inc., 233 Spring Street, New York, NY 10013, USA), except for brief excerpts in connection with reviews or scholarly analysis. Use in connection with any form of information storage and retrieval, electronic adaptation, computer software, or by similar or dissimilar methodology now know or hereafter developed is forbidden.
The use in this publication of trade names, trademarks, service marks and similar terms, even if the are not identified as such, is not to be taken as an expression of opinion as to whether or not they are subject to proprietary rights.

Printed in Canada.

9 8 7 6 5 4 3 2

springeronline.com

FOREWORD

Descriptions of the pathology of melanocytic lesions have been a feature of the histopathology literature from its early beginnings. This is not surprising because these lesions are common (few of us are without the occasional mole) and, of course, they are highly visible on white skin. Furthermore, the rather dramatic and recent rise in incidence of malignant melanoma in Caucasian populations has heightened interest in understanding the pathobiology of the melanocyte, particularly since this is arguably among the most malignant of all tumors.

However, a surprising amount is still unknown about these lesions, including even the developmental route of the nevus cell, which is the integral cell of the commonest melanocytic lesion. Furthermore, among histopathologists and dermatologists, there has been considerable self-inflicted confusion over nomenclature and classification, resulting in a plethora of frequently incongruous names, often for lesions that subsequently turned out to be the same. This confusion has contributed to the pathological reputation of melanocytic lesions being "difficult." However, this reputation is also the result of genuine difficulties in differentiating different types of lesions and, indeed, studies on interobserver variation in possible malignant melanoma have shown that, even among specialists, diagnostic and prognostic reproducibility is, at best, modest.

In the last 30 years or so, a more consistent and standardized approach to the pathology of melanocytic lesions has started to emerge. More recently, this has been supplemented by application of modern clinical research techniques, with large population-based epidemiological studies, rigorous statistical analysis, and incorporation of new methodologies, such as specific antibodies for immunohistology and polymerase chain reaction (PCR) for detection of tiny numbers of melanocytic cells in sentinel lymph nodes and in peripheral blood. Indeed, the progress in understanding melanocytic lesions is a good counter to the oft-lamented disappearance of clinical research.

All of the above has highlighted the need for a single text that can provide a modern reference point. This second edition of Raymond Barnhill's *Pathology of Melanocytic Nevi and Malignant Melanoma* provides this. It incorporates many of the newer advances in morphology, immunohistology, and molecular biology and relates them to the recent insights into diagnosis and prognosis of melanocytic lesions. Several chapters have been expanded from the first edition with pertinent clinical and pathological research findings, and there is a completely new chapter on the recently described and very important genetic abnormalities in malignant melanoma. The section on atypical nevi is significantly rewritten, providing an excellent and comprehensively clear description of these contentious lesions. Similarly, the chapter on malignant melanoma has undergone a significant change by regarding the majority of the various histological forms as part of a continuum, rather than regarding them as different biological types. It also usefully promotes the abandonment of the concept of radial and vertical growth phase patterns as historical background.

Dr. Barnhill's long experience as a practicing pathologist and researcher in melanocytic lesions has provided him with the ideal background to write authoritatively on the subject and to bring together a distinguished group of contributing authors. *Pathology of Melanocytic Nevi and Malignant Melanoma* is an excellent exemplar of the crucially important need to integrate the clinical and pathological sciences and as such will appeal to clinician and pathologist alike. Both groups, and any others interested in melanocytic lesions, will find the content interesting, informative, and stimulating.

Kenneth A. Fleming

PREFACE to the Second Edition

... Quand il s'agit d'écrire, on est scrupuleux, on regarde de très près, on rejette tout ce qui n'est pas vérité [for when it is a question of writing, one is scrupulous, one examines things meticulously, one rejects all that is not true].

—MARCEL PROUST
à *La Recherche du Temps Perdu* (*Le Temps Retrouvé*, La Pléiade, III p. 909)

The authors have been gratified by the enthusiastic response to the first edition and that the monograph has proved useful to so many pathologists and other physicians who encounter melanocytic lesions on a regular basis. Since the publication of the first edition, the challenge of diagnosis and management of melanocytic lesions to physicians has become even more compelling; hence there is a need for as much information as possible on this subject. In writing the second edition the Editor-in-Chief (RLB) has been joined by Co-Editors Michael Piepkorn and Klaus Busam (a contributor to the first edition), both superb melanoma pathologists and writers. As a result, the authors are pleased to offer a thoroughly revised second edition incorporating much new material.

The goal of the second edition remains the same as the first, that is, "to provide a comprehensive [yet practical] description of melanocytic lesions occurring in the skin" *in order to facilitate physicians in providing the best possible care for patients*. Although the format and general content of the book remain unchanged, a major emphasis of the second edition, in the spirit of Marcel Proust, has been to critically examine our current understanding of many entities and concepts in the pathology of melanocytic lesions. In this light the authors have attempted to honestly scrutinize current information and to provide balanced perspectives on controversial subjects such as atypical ('dysplastic") nevi, Spitz nevi, clinical and histopathological variants of melanoma, prognostic factors, etc. It is obvious that this is a work in progress since no one has all the answers and much remains to be learned.

The second edition is larger in order to accommodate both new material and revised, in-depth discussion of many existing entities. A new chapter on the molecular biology of melanoma has been added. This edition includes new information on the immunohistochemistry of melanocytic lesions, greater coverage of childhood melanoma (with the assistance of Dr. Alain Spatz), description of sentinel lymph node biopsy, the new AJCC staging system for melanoma, and new data concerning prognostic factors for melanoma. As in the first edition emphasis has been placed on clinical descriptions, detailed histopathological criteria for diagnosis, and a thorough discussion of differential diagnosis. A synoptic listing of the most pertinent information for all major entities is again presented in tables throughout the book. Many new color photomicrographs have been included in this edition.

The authors are grateful for the kind and generous help from many friends and colleagues at their respective medical institutions both past and present and from many referring physicians around the country and world. Without the referral of pathological material for consultation and the experience resulting from this, the realization of this book would not have been possible. The collective experience of rendering such consultations and writing this monograph is ultimately to assist other physicians and to manage patients most effectively, honestly, and compassionately.

Raymond L. Barnhill, MD

PREFACE
to the First Edition

The histopathologic interpretation of melanocytic lesions of the skin remains one of the most frustrating and difficult areas in dermatopathology and surgical pathology. The continued increase in incidence of cutaneous melanoma coupled with earlier diagnosis will undoubtedly present even greater challenges in histologic diagnosis. Thus, there is an unquestioned need for more information on this subject.

The goal of this book is to provide a comprehensive description of melanocytic lesions occurring in the skin. Considerable effort has also been made to provide detailed clinical descriptions of the lesions in order to assist histopathologists in differential diagnosis. A thorough knowledge of the clinical features of the various melanocytic lesions is essential in histologic diagnosis but is often neglected in textbooks of histopathology. The most important aspects of differential diagnosis are presented, and for most of the entries in the book, a concise description (précis) of the neoplasm has been provided in tables. Much other information useful to the practicing clinician, dermatopathologist, and surgical pathologist has also been summarized in numerous other tables in each of the chapters. Because of the importance of illustrating histopathologic criteria for diagnosis, over 250 color photomicrographs are included in the book.

The author is grateful for the kind and generous help provided by many friends and colleagues. The major sources of material used in this book are from the Dermatopathology Division, Harvard Medical School (the Brigham and Women's Hospital, Children's Hospital, Massachusetts General Hospital, and Harvard Community Health Plan). However, the author also gratefully acknowledges the use of other material from consultations, friends and colleagues, and from the Pigmented Lesion Clinic, Massachusetts General Hospital.

With particular reference to the completion of this book, the author is especially indebted to his secretary, Miss Michelle Wood. Without her highly skilled assistance and dedication to this project, undoubtedly the book would not have been completed. The author also acknowledges the contributions of Klaus J. Busam, M.D. Dr. Busam provided assistance in writing some chapters and advice on the manuscript at a critical time in the evolution of the book. The author is also highly appreciative of the support provided by his chairman, Ramzi Cotran, M.D., in pursuing projects such as this. The author is also grateful to other colleagues for critical analysis of portions of the manuscript.

Raymond L. Barnhill, MD

CONTENTS

Foreword *by Kenneth A. Fleming* v

Preface to the Second Edition vii

Preface to the First Edition ix

Chapter 1   **Melanocytes**   1
Klaus J. Busam and Raymond L. Barnhill

Chapter 2   **Biopsies, Tissue Processing, Immunohistochemistry, and Ancillary Techniques**   11
Klaus J. Busam and Raymond L. Barnhill

Chapter 3   **Genetic and Molecular Pathology of Melanoma**   20
Michael Piepkorn

Chapter 4   **Circumscribed Pigmented Lesions Composed of Basilar Melanocytes**   37
Raymond L. Barnhill

Chapter 5   **Common Acquired and Atypical (Dysplastic) Melanocytic Nevi**   51
Michael Piepkorn and Raymond L. Barnhill

Chapter 6   **Congenital Melanocytic Nevi and Associated Neoplasms, Congenital and Childhood Melanoma**   111
Raymond L. Barnhill

Chapter 7   **Spitz Nevus and Variants**   148
Raymond L. Barnhill and Klaus J. Busam

Chapter 8   **Dermal Melanocytoses, Blue Nevi, and Related Conditions**   199
Klaus J. Busam and Raymond L. Barnhill

Chapter 9   **Melanocytic Nevi with Phenotypic Heterogeneity**   223
Raymond L. Barnhill

Chapter 10   **Malignant Melanoma**   238
Raymond L. Barnhill

Chapter 11   **Metastatic Malignant Melanoma**   357
Klaus J. Busam and Raymond L. Barnhill

Chapter 12   **Prognostic Factors in Cutaneous Malignant Melanoma**   372
Michael Piepkorn and Raymond L. Barnhill

Index   395

PATHOLOGY OF MELANOCYTIC NEVI AND MALIGNANT MELANOMA

SECOND EDITION

CHAPTER 1

Melanocytes

Klaus J. Busam and Raymond L. Barnhill

MELANIN PIGMENT

Melanocytes are cells, whose unique property is the production of melanin pigments (1), which allow a wide range of colors, as seen for example in mammalian hair, which may be black, brown, yellow, reddish brown, or carroty red. The type of pigmentation is under genetic control, involving a number of interacting gene products, some of which have recently been identified (2). While in many animals melanin pigments play an important role in camouflage and mimicry, their major function in humans is the protection against the potentially toxic or carcinogenic effects of sunlight. Their broad spectral absorbance makes them suitable for light-shielding purposes. Melanins have also been suggested to be involved in radiant heat loss and detoxification of oxygen radicals and metals (3–6). In addition to their protective role against UV damage, recent evidence shows that melanocytes also participate in the inflammatory response. Melanocytes have been found to be the source of and responsive to a variety of inflammatory mediators (7).

Two prototypes of melanin have traditionally been described: *eumelanin*, which is brown-black and insoluble, and *pheomelanin*, which is reddish yellow and alkali soluble (8). However, this classification represents an oversimplification of the actual variety of natural melanins, because each of the two groups includes pigments with different physical and chemical properties. Typical eumelanins such as those of dark human hair are a mixture of large molecular weight polymers consisting mainly of 5,6-dihydroxyindole units, which are derived from multiple enzymatic and nonenzymatic reactions (8,9). Pheomelanin is a polymer formed via cysteinyldopas through reactions of dopaquinone with cysteine or glutathione (10). Pheomelanin is more photolabile than eumelanin. Irradiation of pheomelanin may lead to the formation of potentially toxic hydroxyl radicals, which are thought to play a role in carcinogenesis (11,12). They may contribute to the higher incidence of melanoma in red-haired individuals.

The metabolic pathways of both eumelanin and pheomelanin biosynthesis were established by Raper (13), Mason (14), Prota and Nicolaus (10) and their co-workers. L-tyrosine is the initial substrate for the melanin pathway. It is oxidized by the enzyme tyrosinase to 3,4-dihydroxyphenylalanine (L-DOPA), and then dehydrogenized to DOPAchinone. While in the Raper-Mason scheme of melanin synthesis melanogenesis is primarily regulated at the level of the enzyme tyrosinase, recent evidence suggests that additional regulatory sites exist in which the pigmentation gene family may play a role (*pmel 17* gene family) (2,9).

Melanin synthesis is stimulated by melanin-stimulating hormone (MSH) and a variety of other hormones, including ACTH and sex steroids (15) as well as by a number of inflammatory mediators (7). While melanin is produced by many melanocytes during embryonic life, only melanocytes of the epidermis and hair follicles form measurable amounts of melanin in adult life (1). Epidermal melanocytes connect to neighboring keratinocytes, to which they transfer melanin pigment particles, a relationship that has been termed the *epidermal melanin unit* (16). The melanocytes in hair follicles have a similar relationship with cells of the hair matrix (1). They actively synthesize and transfer melanin into matrix cells during the anagen phase of the hair cycle (17). No melanin synthesis, however, is observed in the telogen stage of the hair cycle.

Because epidermal and hair follicle melanocytes transfer melanin to neighboring cells, they have been called *secretory melanocytes* (16). In contrast, other melanocytes such as dermal melanocytes that retain the melanin that they have produced have been called *continent melanocytes* (16).

Melanin pigment is not always apparent in hematoxylin and eosin (H&E) stained sections. It may be present intracellularly within melanocytes, keratinocytes, or macrophages, or it may be found extracellularly. When it is seen within melanocytes, it is usually finely granular or dust like. Within keratinocytes or macrophages or extracellularly, melanin pigment granules appear coarser and more uneven in size and shape (18). When melanin pigment granules assume unusually large dimensions (up to 6 μm), they are called macromelanosomes (19). These giant granules very rarely occur in normal melanocytes. They have been described, however, as an occasional finding in association with a variety of melanocytic lesions, such as simple lentigo and café-au-lait spots, especially in cases of neurofibromatosis (19), and in a number of different types of melanocytic nevi (20).

Melanin needs to be distinguished from other brown pigments. Melanin is the only endogenous brown-black pigment besides *homogentisic acid pigment* that is deposited in various tissues, including the skin in ochronosis (21). *Hemosiderin*, a hemoglobin-derived pigment, usually presents as a golden yellow to brown granular pigment (21) and may occasionally be confused with melanin. Hemosiderin can easily be identified by its iron content (see Chapter 2). *Lipofuscin*, which appears as a yellow-brown, finely granular intracytoplasmic pigment on H&E-stained sections (also referred to as *wear-and-tear* pigment), contains insoluble material of lipids complexed with protein, which is thought to derive from indigestible residues of autophagic vacuoles. Lipofuscin is seen in cells undergoing slow, regressive changes. It may be confused with melanin, since it also stains when silver stains are used to identify melanin (22). However, lipofuscin is positive on fat stains and is resistant to bleaching—unlike melanin (see Chapter 2). Moreover, lipofuscin has a characteristic appearance on electron microscopy. Lipofuscin granules are highly electron dense, often surround membranous structures, and are located typically around the nucleus (21). *Bilirubin*, which appears as green-brown to black deposits, can usually be readily distinguished from melanin by microscopy because of its green color and the amorphous globular composition of the pigment (21). The pigment of *pseudomelanosis coli* is not melanin but rather is related to lipofuscin (23). It is found as fine brown granules of variable size within macrophages of the lamina propria of the large bowel, most often affecting the right colon. It is thought to be due to anthracene-containing laxatives. Similar pigment can also be seen in various storage diseases and in chronic granulomatous disease.

Neuromelanin is a melanin pigment that accumulates in catecholaminergic neurons during aging (24). It is particularly prominent at the substantia nigra and the locus ceruleus. Electron paramagnetic resonance spectroscopy has shown that neuromelanin is indeed a melanin pigment, although with some unusual features in its mode of formation (auto-oxidation rather than enzymatically) and its composition (it has been suggested to be a copolymer derived from dopamine and glutathione). Its function in the brain is still unknown. It is thought to have a cytoprotective role under normal conditions, but it may be involved in neurocytotoxicity at advanced ages and in patients with Parkinson's disease (25).

ANATOMIC DISTRIBUTION OF MELANOCYTES

The majority of melanocytes reside in the skin, in particular within the epidermis and hair follicles (1). Some of them reside in the dermis and may be found around sebaceous glands or near the lactiferous ducts of the nipple (26). Melanocytes have also been identified in visceral organs, the orbital cavity, leptomeninges, and inner ear (27).

Epidermal melanocytes are present in all regions of the body. Estimations of the volume of melanocyte mass in an adult human range between 1 and 1.5 mL (28). Their population density varies, depending on the region (1). The ratio of melanocytes to keratinocytes of the basal layer ranges from approximately 1:4 to 1:10. The population density of melanocytes is highest on the face and genitalia ($> 2000/mm^2$) and lowest on the skin of the trunk and upper arm ($800–1000/mm^2$) (29). Aging results in a decreased number of melanocytes as well as a decline in the activity of melanin synthesis (27). The relative concentration of melanocytes appears to be independent of race and sex (30). Racial differences in skin coloration result primarily from differences in the production and packaging of melanin pigment, not from differences in the number of melanocytes (31,32).

MORPHOLOGY OF MELANOCYTES

Light Microscopy
Melanocytes of the human epidermis exhibit a territorial behavior (33). They are distributed at a distance from each other in a network located along the dermoepidermal junction (28). Melanocytes appear as small round or oval cells with pale cytoplasm in and immediately beneath the basal-cell layer of the epidermis (Fig. 1-1). Their dendrites are usually invisible in H&E-stained paraffin sec-

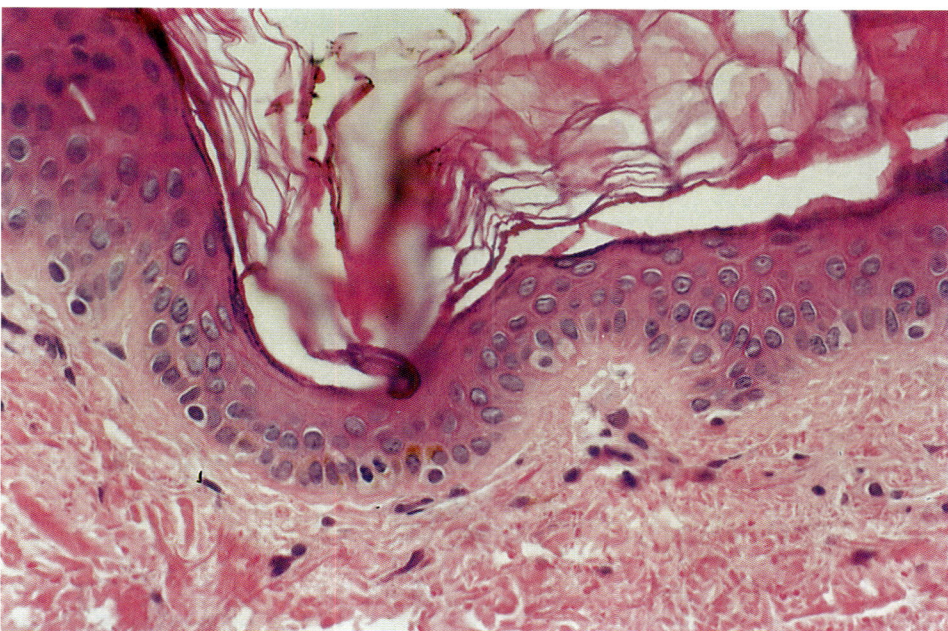

FIGURE 1-1 Epidermal melanocytes. Solitary cells with pale cytoplasm and round or ovoid nuclei are situated at the dermoepidermal junction, just below basal layer keratinocytes.

tions, unless they are packed with melanin. In hair follicles, melanocytes are located at the epithelial side of the basement membrane bordering the central hair papilla.

The nucleus of melanocytes, whose contour often appears polygonal or indented, is somewhat smaller and more hyperchromatic than the nucleus of nearby keratinocytes (34). The chromatin pattern is uniform with no apparent nucleoli. Thin cytoplasmic dendrites project from the cell body and extend in all directions (Fig. 1-2). Their visualization usually requires special histochemical stains (see Chapter 2).

Adult resident epidermal melanocytes may proliferate in response to ultraviolet (UV) light or growth factors released during tissue regeneration (35). Three proliferative patterns have been described (36). *Lentiginous melanocytic hyperplasia* refers to a pattern of single-cell melanocytic proliferation along the dermoepidermal junction. *Nesting* describes a clustered proliferation melanocytes. If single-cell growth is discohesive and seen throughout the entire epidermis, a pattern of *pagetoid proliferation* is present. Lentiginous hyperplasia is often a feature of lentigines or "lentiginous" forms of melanocytic nevi. Nesting is typical of melanocytic nevi. Pagetoid spread, although often associated with melanoma, may also be observed in both acquired and congenital nevi of children, Spitz nevi, pigmented spindle cell nevi, and in common acquired nevi of acral skin. The pattern of benign melanocytic proliferation is typically symmetric and shows in vertical growth a gradient of cytologic development, which is referred to as maturation.

Electron Microscopy

Electron micrographs of melanocytes typically show a prominent Golgi complex and rough endoplasmatic reticulum as well as numerous mitochondria—features characteristic of metabolically active cells. Melanocytes lack tonofilaments and desmosomes. They contain, however, intermediate filaments (vimentin). Where melanocytes appose the epidermal basal lamina, half-desmosome-like structures are seen (18). The nucleus of melanocytes may be smooth or lobulated. Nuclear lobation has been suggested to be a feature of metabolically active melanocytes (37).

The ultrastructural hallmark of melanocytes is a unique organelle, the melanosome (38). Melanosomes originate from the Golgi apparatus and contain enzymes involved in melanogenesis (39).

In the formation of eumelanosomes, four stages have been described (40): Premelanosomes make up stage I and II melanosomes, while stages III and IV represent mature melanosomes. Stage I melanosomes are spherical structures that contain vesicular inclusions with histochemically detectable tyrosinase activity or, occasionally, a few filaments that have a distinct periodicity (Fig. 1-3A). Stage II melanosomes are oval organelles with a characteristic internal lamellar structure (Fig. 1-3B). These

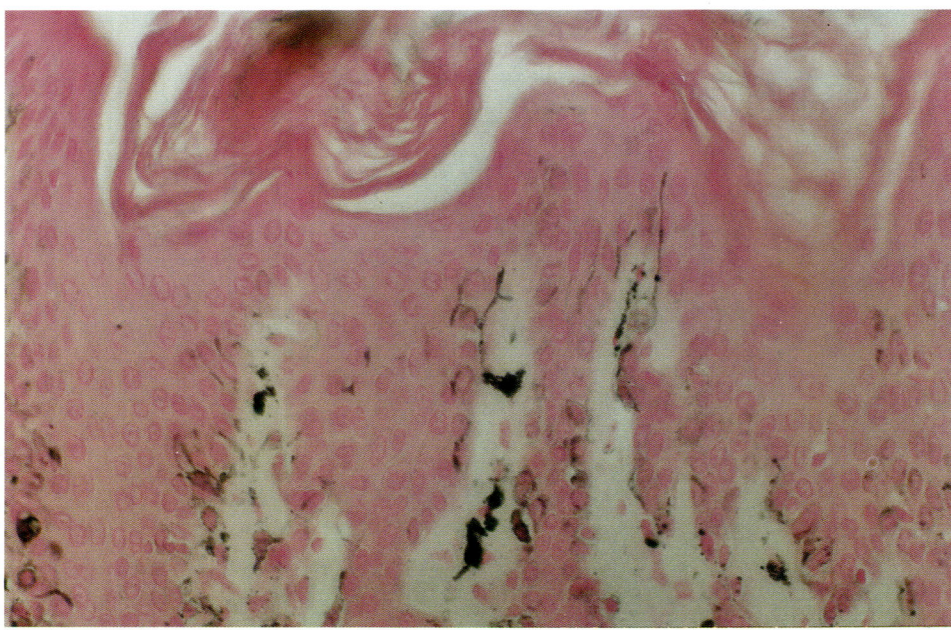

FIGURE 1-2 Silver-stained melanocytes. The dendritic processes of melanocytes become apparent.

membranous filaments have a distinctive periodicity with or without regular cross-striations. They are more extensively developed in stage II than in stage I melanosomes. Granular deposits of melanin pigment appear on early stage III melanosomes (Fig. 1-3C). These pigment granules are more developed in late stage III (Fig. 1-3D) when they partly obliterate the organelle. Stage IV melanosomes are completely melanized (Fig. 1-3E). While stage I melanosomes measure approximately 0.3 μm in length, stage II–IV melanosomes measure 0.4–1.0 μm in the greatest dimension. As melanosomes mature, they gradually move from the cytoplasm of the melanocyte into the dendritic processes. The tip of the dendrites, filled with mature melanosomes, are snipped off (apocopated) and are phagocytosed by neighboring keratinocytes, wherein melanosomes fuse with lysosomes (1).

The development of phaeomelanosomes has also been discerned into four stages (18). Phaeomelanosomes are round rather than oval throughout all stages. In stage I, a vacuole is present, which contains small microvesicles. These microvesicles become more numerous in stage II. Deposition of melanin pigment on microvesicles and in the matrix characterizes stage III. When the matrix is completely filled with melanin, stage IV is reached.

Skin pigmentation depends on the number and maturation of melanosomes as well as their packaging (1). In whites, melanosomes are less numerous than in blacks. While in the former, melanosomes are present mainly in stage I and II, most melanosomes are stage IV in blacks.

Sun-induced darkening of the skin corresponds to an increase in stage III and IV melanosomes in keratinocytes. In blacks, melanosomes lie individually rather than grouped together in melanosome complexes and are degraded more slowly (31,32).

HISTOGENESIS OF MELANOCYTES

Melanocytes are thought to be of neural crest origin based on in vivo studies of ablation and transplants of the neural crest, which produced changes in patterns of cutaneous pigmentation (41,42). This theory is supported also by in vitro studies demonstrating that neural crest cells from various species can directly give rise to melanocytes (43,44).

Much controversy still exists about when and where along the migration of neural crest–derived cells commitment toward melanocytic differentiation occurs (45). In the center of this debate is the concept of a melanoblast, which has been defined as a melanocytic stem cell (1). Although it seems possible that such melanoblasts undergo commitment toward melanocytic differentiation before or during early migration with other primitive cells from the neural crest, to date, no direct evidence for the existence of nonpluripotential stem cells has been provided (45). Alternatively, it has been postulated that melanocytes might derive from pluripotential cells that travel from the neural crest to the skin via the paraspinal ganglia and their peripheral nerves and become commit-

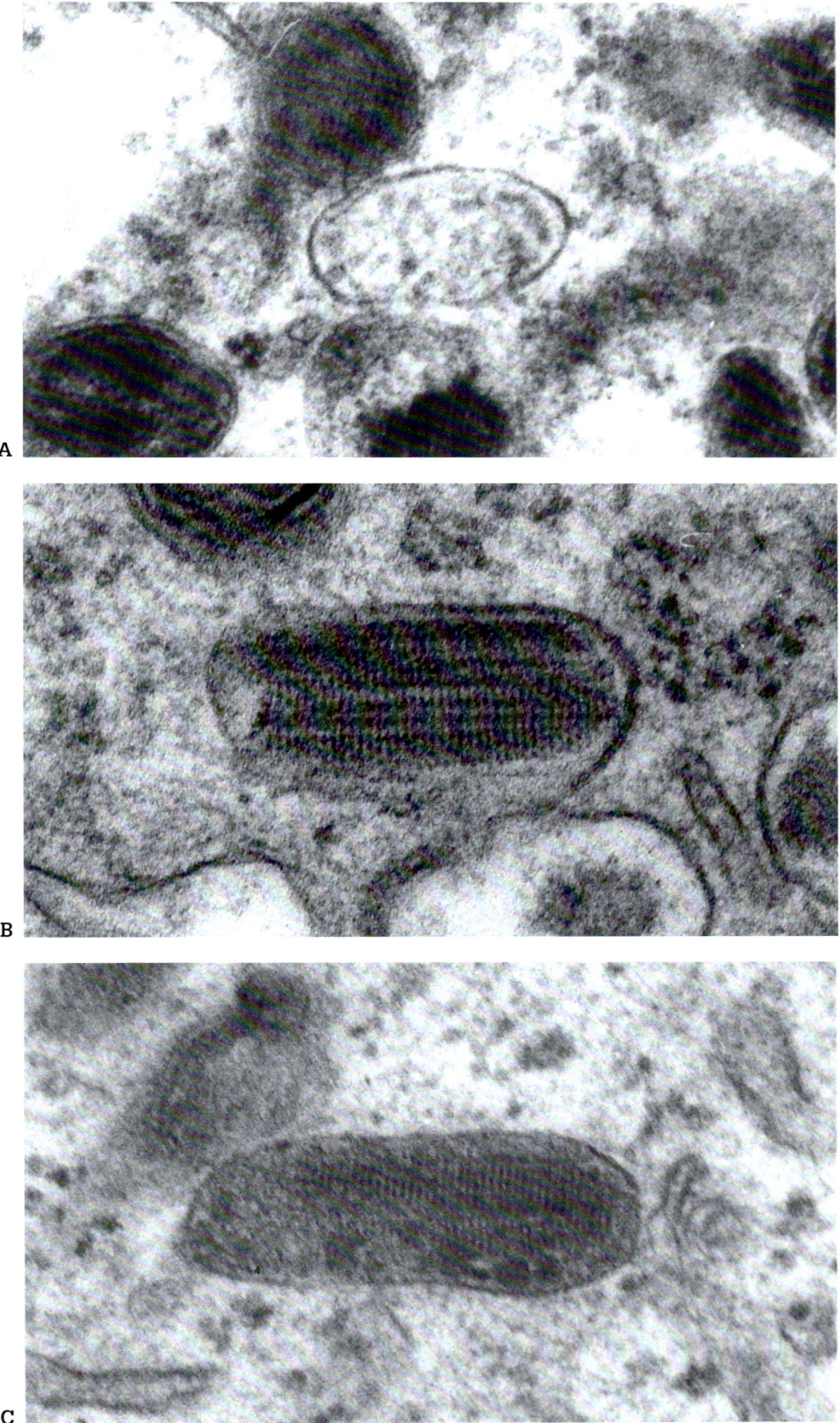

FIGURE 1-3 Ultrastructure of eumelanosomes The four stages of eumelanosome formation are shown in electron micrographs. **A,** Stage I: vesicular inclusions (×100,000). **B,** Stage II: striated inclusions. **C,** Early stage III: granular deposits on striated inclusions.

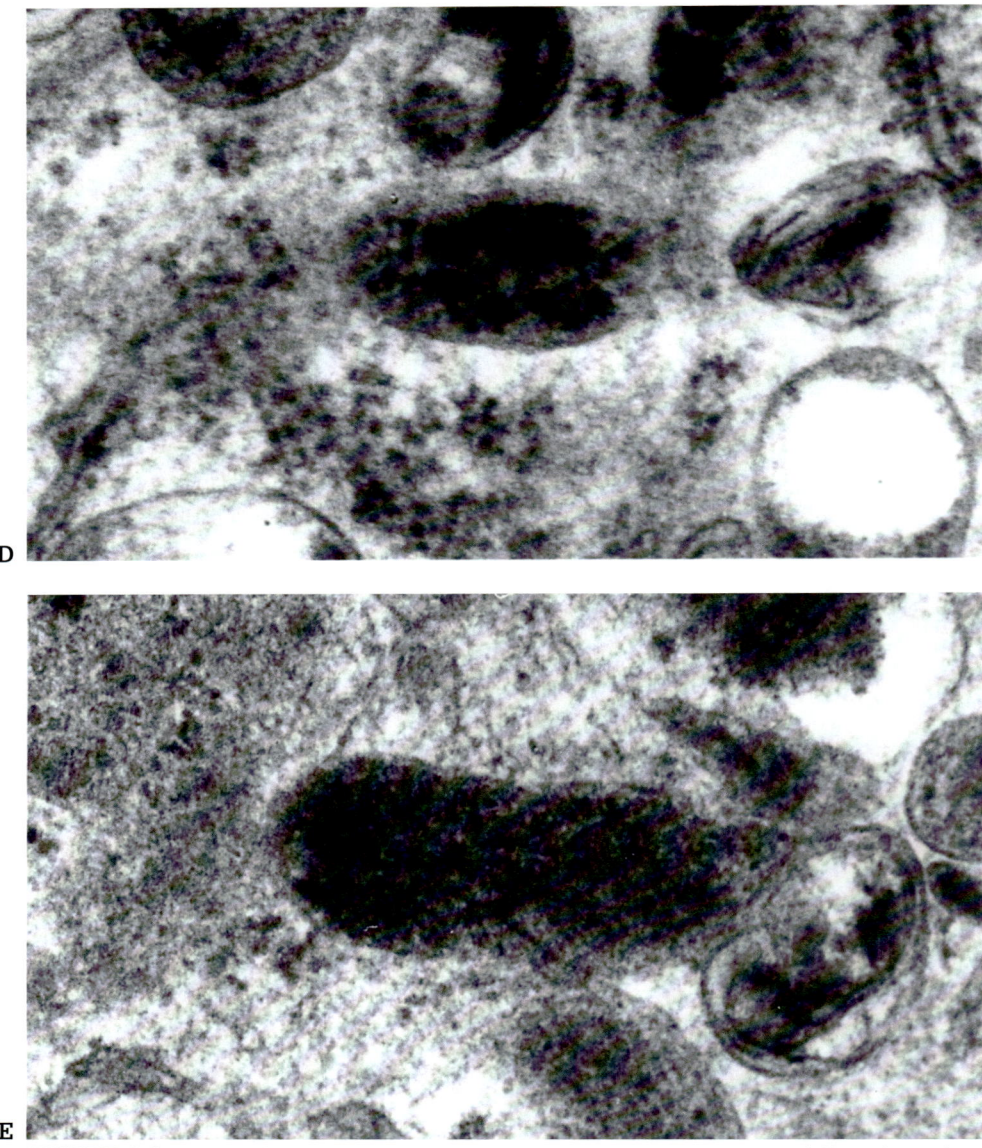

FIGURE 1-3 *Continued.* **D,** Late stage III: more granular deposits. **E,** Stage IV: fully melanized organelles. (Courtesy of Dr. M. Seiler, West Roxbury VA Medical Center, West Roxbury, MA.)

ted only late—that is, after migration to the local microenvironment of dermis and epidermis (44,46,47). This view has been supported by several studies showing that explants of peripheral developing nerves or embryonic paraspinal ganglia can be manipulated to give rise to melanocytes (48,49). It is also interesting to note in this context that embryonic nerves have extended close to the human epidermis by 8 weeks of gestation, which coincides with the earliest time that melanocytes have been identified in human skin (46,50). Commitment late during migration is furthermore suggested by the observation that it is only in the periderm where usually the first characteristic melanocytic features such as dendrites and melanosomes become detectable (36).

Once commitment to melanocytic differentiation has occurred after arrival of the pluripotential cells in the periderm and dermis, immature melanocytes mature as they migrate through the dermis and dermoepidermal junction to become terminally differentiated resident melanocytes in the epidermis (45).

In spite of its migratory potential, the location of mature melanocytes in the basal cell layer of the epidermis is quite stable. Proliferation and migration of melanocytes may be observed in epidermal regeneration and repigmentation after tissue injury. The principal reservoir for melanocytes repopulating reepithelialized epidermis are thought to be melanocytes normally dispersed along the basal layer of hair follicles and/or melanocytes derived from pluripotential perineural stem cells (51).

MORPHOLOGY OF NEVUS CELLS

The cells of nevocellular nevi, which are thought to be melanocytic, are typically grouped in nests with apposition of individual cells to each other (36). Nesting can occur along the dermoepidermal junction (junctional nevus) or within the dermis (dermal nevus). Both patterns are often present simultaneously (compound nevus). The dermal component may extend deep and involve adnexal or neural structures (congenital features).

Three different cytologic variations of melanocytes have been described in nevi (36). The intraepidermal or intradermal melanocytes, which typically have an epithelioid appearance with prominent cytoplasm containing moderate coarse melanin pigment, are also historically referred to as type A cells (Fig. 1-4A). They contain a round to oval nucleus, slightly smaller in size than the nucleus of a keratinocyte, with uniformly dispersed chromatin and occasionally an inconspicuous nucleolus. Type B melanocytes resemble lymphocytes (Fig. 1-4B). Their nuclei are small, are round to oval, and are surrounded by scant cytoplasm. The nuclear chromatin is uniformly dispersed with no apparent nucleoli. Type B cells are usually part of the dermal component or compound nevi. The neural or type C cell is spindle shaped and typically present in the deeper layers of a melanocytic lesion. It resembles fibroblasts or peripheral nerve sheath cells (Fig. 1-4C).

HISTOGENESIS OF NEVUS CELLS

The histogenesis of melanocytes in nevi (nevus cells) is still not entirely resolved (45). It has been suggested that nevocytes represent a distinct cellular entity, which arises from a nevoblast, a pluripotential precursor that migrates from the neural crest (52). However, no such nevoblast with distinctive phenotypic characteristics has ever been identified (45). Alternatively, it is currently widely accepted that nevocytes are melanocytes (53). In this view, their nesting pattern may be interpreted as a melanocytic response to a distinct local microenvironment, a functionally altered state, or injury.

It is contingent to the concept of neural crest origin that precursors of epidermal melanocytes must actually migrate from the dermis to the epidermis during development. With this in mind, there are two ways to explain the dermal presence of melanocytes. Melanocytes may come to reside in the dermis after a process of "dropping off" (*Abtropfung*) from proliferating epidermal melanocytes (54). Alternatively, they may stay in the dermis because they are unable to complete upward migration (*Hochsteigerung*) into the epidermis (45). In this latter view, if incomplete upward migration occurs during development, congenital nevi arise. Acquired nevi result in this interpretation from increasing loss of migratory capability of melanocytes derived from proliferating pluripotential peripheral nerve sheath precursor cells. Both theories, however, remain speculative, since to date no direct evidence for either direction of cell movement exists.

Acquired melanocytic nevi are thought to reflect a melanocytic response to chronic growth stimulation by UV light or inflammatory mediators and may represent an early stage in the process of melanocytic carcinogenesis (35).

FIGURE 1-4 Cytology of melanocytes in nevi. **A,** Epithelioid or type A cells.

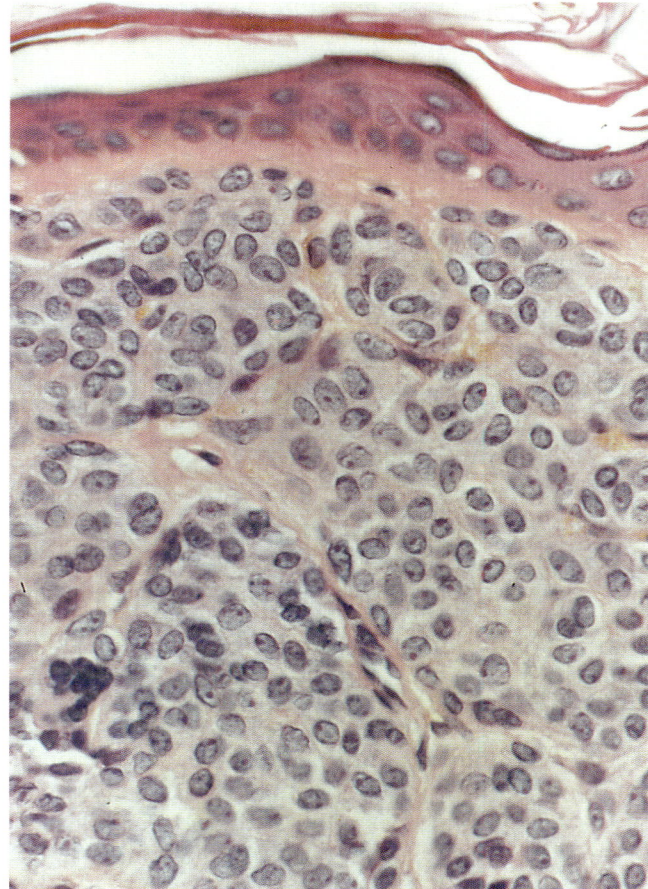

A

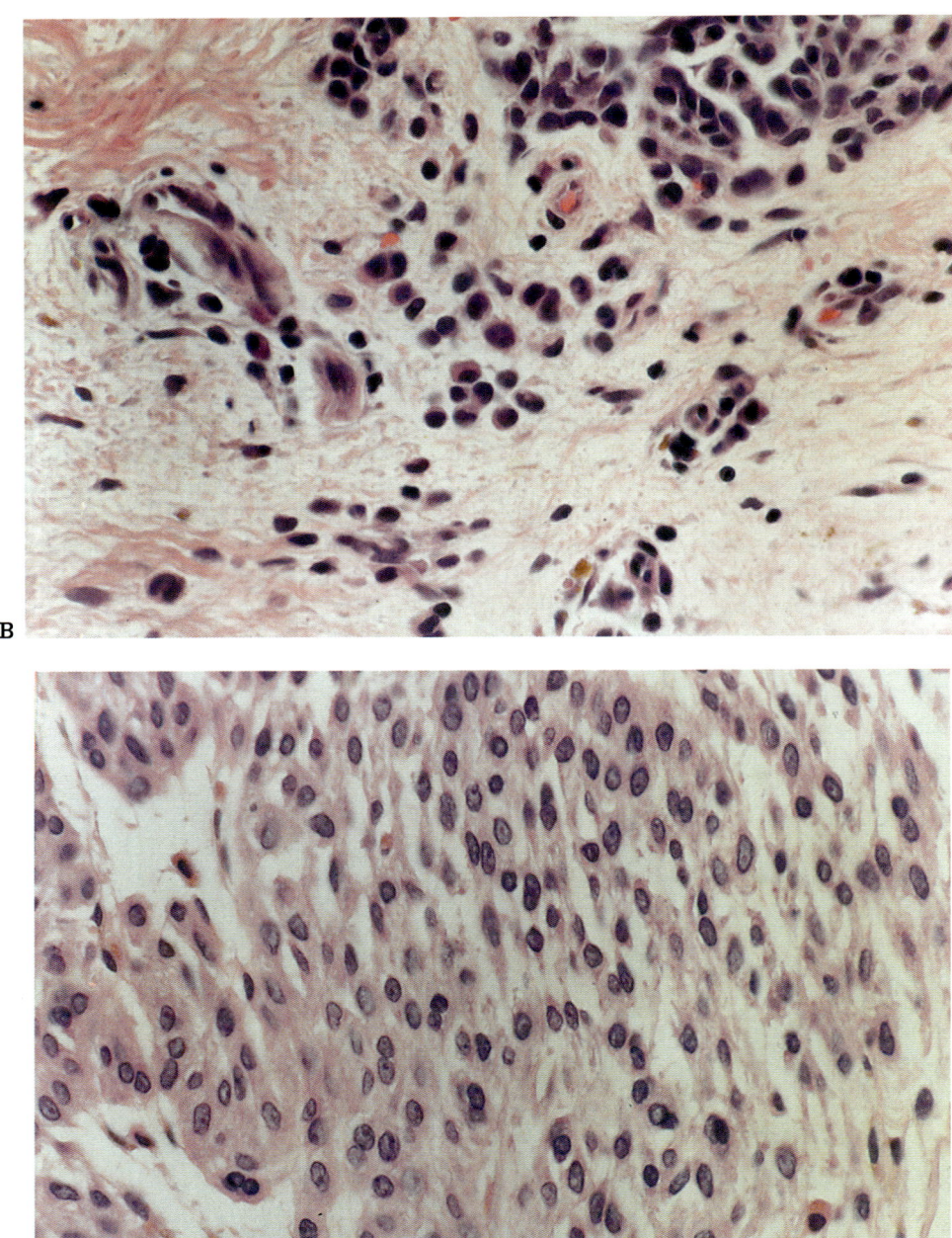

FIGURE 1-4 *Continued.* **B,** Lymphoid or type B cells. **C,** Schwannian or type C cells.

EMBRYOLOGY OF MELANOCYTES

During development of human skin, melanocytes appear first in the vicinity of nerves and blood vessels of the dermis at 4–10-weeks of fetal life (55). They reach the epidermis by the end of the 2nd month of gestational age (56). Production of melanin is first observed in the skin of the eyelids, the external auditory canal, and in the labial mucosa. Pigment synthesis in fetal body skin begins between the 3rd and 5th month, depending on the racial background (56–58). During this period of time, the number of melanocytes increases approximately threefold (59).

While initially melanocytes are randomly distributed throughout all epidermal layers (60,61), a stable population residing near the basal cell layer with bipolar dendritic processes is established by 6 months of gestation

(58). Melanosome transfer to keratinocytes begins at this time. Morphologically, fetal melanocytes are more uniform in size and structure and in number of dendritic processes than adult melanocytes (59).

REFERENCES

1. Quevedo WC Jr, Fitzpatrick TB, Szabo G, Jimbow K. Biology of melanocytes. In: Fitzpatrick TB, Eisen AZ, Wolff K, Freedberg IM, Austen KF, eds. Dermatology in General Medicine. 3rd ed. New York: McGraw-Hill, 1987:224–51.
2. Kwon BS. Pigmentation genes: the tyrosinase gene family and the pmel 17 gene family. J Invest Dermatol 1993;100:134S–40S.
3. Morison WL. What is the function of melanin? Arch Dermatol 1985;121:1160–3.
4. Nordlund JJ, Abdel-Malek ZA, Boissy RE, Rheins CA. Pigment cell biology: a historical review. J Invest Dermatol 1989;92:53S–60S.
5. Proctor PH, McGinnis JE. The function of melanin. Arch Dermatol 1986;122:507–8.
6. Riley PA. Materia melaninca: further dark thoughts. Pigment Cell Res 1990;5(3):101–6.
7. Morelli JG, Norris DA. Influence of inflammatory mediators and cytokines on human melanocyte function. J Invest Dermatol 1993;100:191S–6S.
8. Prota G. Recent advances in the chemistry of melanogenesis in mammals. J Invest Dermatol 1980;75:122–7.
9. Prota G. Regulatory mechanisms of melanogenesis: beyond the tyrosinase concept. J Invest Dermatol 1993;100:156S–61S.
10. Prota G, Nicolaus RA. On the biogenesis of phaeomelanins. In: Montagna W, Hu F, eds. Advances in Biology of Skin. New York: Pergamon, 1966;8:323–8.
11. Chedekel MR, Smith SK, Post PW, et al. Photodestruction of pheomelanin: role of oxygen. Proc Natl Acad Sci USA 1978;75:5395–9.
12. Tomita Y, Hariu A, Kato C, Seiji M. Radical production during tyrosine reaction, dopa-melanin formation, and photo-irradiation of dopa-melanin. J Invest Dermatol 1984;16:573–6.
13. Raper HS. The aerobic oxidases. Physiol Rev 1928;8:245–82.
14. Mason HS. The chemistry of melanin. III. Mechanism of oxidation of dihydroxyphenylalanine by tyrosinase. J Biol Chem 1948;172:83–99.
15. Thody AJ, Smith AG. Hormones and skin pigmentation. Int J Dermatol 1977;16:657–64.
16. Masson P. Pigment cells in man. In: Miner RW, Gordon M, eds. The Biology of Melanomas. New York: New York Academy of Sciences, 1948;8:15–51.
17. Kukita A. Changes in tyrosinase activity during melanocyte proliferation. J Invest Dermatol 1957;28:273–4.
18. Mooi WJ, Krausz T. Melanin and melanocytes. In: Mooi WJ, Krausz T, eds. Biopsy Pathology of Melanocytic Disorders. London: Chapman & Hall, 1991:1–16.
19. Jimbow K, Szabo G, Fitzpatrick TB. Ultrastructure of giant pigment granules (macromelanosomes) in the cutaneous pigmented macules of neurofibromatosis. J Invest Dermatol 1973;61:300–9.
20. Konrad KK, Wolff K, Hoenigsmann H. The giant melanosome: a model of deranged melanosome-morphogenesis. J Ultrastruct Res 1974;48:102–23.
21. Cotran RS, Kumar V, Robbins SL. Pigments. In: Cotran RS, Kumar V, Robbins SL, eds. Pathologic Basis of Disease, 4th ed. Philadelphia: Saunders, 1989:24–6.
22. Burck HC. Pigmentnachweis. In: Burck HC, ed. Histologische Technik. 3rd ed. Stuttgart: Thieme, 1973:141–51.
23. Goldman H. Effects of laxative and enemas. In: Ming SC, Goldman H, eds. Pathology of the Gastrointestinal Tract. Philadelphia: Saunders, 1992:706.
24. Enochs WS, Nilges MJ, Swartz HM. Purified human neuromelanin, synthetic dopamine melanin as a potential model pigment, and the normal human substantia nigra: characterization by electron paramagnetic resonance spectroscopy. J Neurochem 1993;61:68–79.
25. Kastner A, Hirsch EC, Lejeune O, et al. Is the vulnerability of neurons in the substantia nigra of patients with Parkinson's disease related to their neuromelanin content? J Neurochem 1992;59:1080–9.
26. Montagna W. Histology and cytochemistry of human skin. XXXV. The nipple and areola. Br J Dermatol 1970;83:2–13.
27. Nordlund JJ. The lives of pigment cells. Clin Geriatr Med 1989;5(1):91–108.
28. Rosdahl I, Rorsman H. An estimate of the melanocyte mass in humans. J Invest Dermatol 1983;81:278–81.
29. Fitzpatrick TB, Szabo G. The melanocyte: cytology and cytochemistry. J Invest Dermatol 1959;32:197–209.
30. Szabo G. The number of melanocytes in human epidermis. Br Med J 1954;1:1016–7.
31. Szabo G, Gerald AB, Pathak MA, Fitzpatrick TB. Racial differences in human pigmentation at the ultrastructural level. J Cell Biol 1968;39:132–3.
32. Szabo G, Shelburne J, Linder J, Klintworth GK. Racial differences in the fate of melanosomes in human epidermis. Nature 1969;222:1081–2.
33. Cochran AJ. The incidence of melanocytes in normal skin. J Invest Dermatol 1970;57:38–43.
34. Hu F. Melanocyte cytology in normal skin, melanocytic nevi, and malignant melanomas: a review. In: Ackerman AB, ed. Pathology of Malignant Melanoma. New York: Masson, 1981:1–21.
35. Medrano EE, Farooqui JZ, Boissy RE, et al. Chronic growth stimulation of human adult melanocytes by inflammatory mediators in vitro: implications for nevus formation and initial steps in melanocyte oncogenesis. Proc Natl Acad Sci USA 1993;90:1790–4.

36. Imber MJ, Mihm MC. Benign melanocytic tumors. In: Farmer ER, Hood AF, eds. Pathology of the Skin. East Norwalk, CT: Appleton & Lange, 1990:663–83.
37. Szabo G, Flynn E. Morphological aspects of normal human melanocytes. In: Veronesi U, Cascinelli N, Santinami M, eds. Cutaneous Melanoma: Status of Knowledge and Future Perspective. London: Academic Press, 1987:127–38.
38. Seiji M, Fitzpatrick TB, Birbeck MSC. The melanosome: a distinctive subcellular particle of mammalian melanocytes and the site of melanogenesis. J Invest Dermatol 1961;36:243–52.
39. Seiji M, Iwashita S. Intracellular localization of tyrosinase and site of melanin formation in melanocytes. J Invest Dermatol 1965;45:305–14.
40. Jimbow K, Kukita A. Fine structure of pigment granules. In: Kawamura, ed. Biology of Normal and Abnormal Melanocytes. Tokyo: University of Tokyo Press, 1971:171–93.
41. Rawles ME. Origin of melanophores and their role in development of color patterns in vertebrates. Physiol Rev 1948;28:383–408.
42. LeDouarin NM. The Neural Crest. New York: Cambridge University Press, 1982.
43. Barrofino A, Dupin E, LeDouarin NM. Clone forming ability and differentiation potential of migratory (quail) neural crest cells. Proc Natl Acad Sci USA 1988;85:5325–9.
44. Perris von Boxberg Y, Lofberg J. Local embryonic matrices determine region-specific phenotypes in (axolotl) neural crest cells. Science 1988;241:86–9.
45. Cramer SF. The origin of epidermal melanocytes. Arch Pathol Lab Med 1991;115:115–9.
46. Cramer SF. The histogenesis of acquired melanocytic nevi: based on a new concept of melanocytic differentiation. Am J Dermatopathol 1984;6(Suppl 1):289–98.
47. Cramer SF. The melanocytic differentiation pathway in congenital melanocytic nevi: theoretical considerations. Pediatr Pathol 1988;8:253–65.
48. Weston JA. Neural crest cell development. Prog Clin Biol Res 1982;85:359–79.
49. Ciment G, Glimelius B, Nelson DM, Weston JA. Reversal of a developmental restriction in neural crest cells of avian embryos by a phorbol ester drug. Dev Biol 1986;118:392–8.
50. Sagebiel RW, Odland GF. Ultrastructural identification of melanocytes in early human embryos. In: Riley V, ed. Pigmentation: Its Genesis and Biologic Control. East Norwalk, CT: Appleton & Lange, 1969:43–50.
51. Staricco RG. Mechanism of migration of the melanocyte from the hair follicle into the epidermis following dermabrasion. J Invest Dermatol 1961;36:99–104.
52. Mishima Y. Macromolecular changes in pigmentary disorders. Arch Dermatol 1965;91:519–57.
53. Magna-Garcia M, Ackermann B. What are nevus cells? Am J Dermatopathol 1990;12:93–102.
54. Unna PG. Naevi and Naevocarcinome. Berl Klin Wochenschr 1893;30:14–6.
55. Zimmermann AA, Becker SW Jr. Precursors of epidermal melanocytes in the Negro fetus. In: Gordon M, ed. Pigment Cell Biology. Orlando, FL: Academic Press, 1959:159–70.
56. Holbrook KA, Vogel AM, Underwood RA, Foster CA. Melanocytes in human embryonic and fetal skin: A review and new findings. Pig Cell Res 1988;1(Suppl):6–17.
57. Breathnach AS, Wyllie LM. Electron microscopy of melanocytes and Langerhans cells in human fetal epidermis at 14 weeks. J Invest Dermatol 1965;44:51–60.
58. Zimmermann AA, Cornbleet T. The development of epidermal pigmentation in the Negro fetus. J Invest Dermatol 1948;11:383–95.
59. Becker SW, Zimmermann AA. Further studies on melanocytes and melanogenesis in human fetus and newborn. J Invest Dermatol 1955;25:103–12.
60. Mishima Y, Widlan S. Embryonic development of melanocytes in human hair and epidermis. J Invest Dermatol 1966;46:263–77.
61. Barla-Szabo L. Ejection of melanocytes and melanin from fetuses and newborn mammalian animals. Acta Morphol Acad Sci Hung 1970;18:213–25.

CHAPTER 2

Biopsies, Tissue Processing, Immunohistochemistry, and Ancillary Techniques

Klaus J. Busam and Raymond L. Barnhill

TYPES OF BIOPSIES

Excisional Biopsies

The specimen submitted for histopathologic examination needs to provide critical diagnostic and prognostic information, such as symmetry and lateral and deep extension. Therefore, the proper procedure for most pigmented cutaneous lesions is an excisional biopsy. The biopsy should not be too large to avoid unnecessary removal of normal skin, if the lesion is benign, in which case, the biopsy constitutes definitive treatment. Furthermore one must consider if a sentinel lymph node biopsy will be performed, since a large excision usually disrupts lymphatic drainage and may affect the sentinel lymph node mapping and biopsy, if carried out before sentinel lymph node (SLN) biopsy. When the lesion is malignant, excision of the whole lesion becomes necessary, with margins appropriate for tumor thickness.

A skin excision usually provides an ellipse of skin with some subcutaneous fat. The biopsy should be oriented in such a way that a reexcision, when indicated, can be done with minimal skin loss. Generally, the excision is best performed with the long axis in the direction of cutaneous lymphatics. Orientation by the clinician or the pathologist handling the specimen can be accomplished by attaching suture material to a designated margin.

The skin excision is fixed whole. The pathologist should provide a macroscopic description of the lesion itself and give particular attention to the size of the lesion and its proximity to the surgical margins (Table 2-1). The margins should be inked before dissection of the specimen. Orientation of the surgical margins is facilitated by applying two different colors of ink to each half of the lateral and deep margins of the excisional biopsy. Scoring of the specimen for orientation by superficial incisions with razor blades is not recommended because it often leads to separation of fragments from the remainder of the specimen. Sections are taken so that the minimal distance of the lesion to a resection margin, the maximal thickness of the lesion, and any additional relevant features such as ulceration are demonstrated (Fig. 2-1). Small excisional biopsies (< 1 cm in greatest dimension) may be bisected along their longitudinal axes and the two halves processed separately if orientation is important.

Punch Biopsies/Excisions

Punch biopsies of cutaneous pigmented lesions are indicated in two situations: to establish a diagnosis with minimal loss of tissue for large lesions, such as lentigo maligna or congenital nevi, and to excise lesions that are so small that a punch biopsy includes the entire lesion with a rim of surrounding normal skin. Otherwise, small biopsies are not recommended for pigmented lesions because they generally do not provide adequate information on symmetry and extension of the lesion.

The macroscopic description should include the diameter of the specimen, its depth, and the presence of subcutaneous fat. A brief description of the surface should be recorded. A punch biopsy is bisected through its center with a sharp razor blade. Small punch biopsies (diameters ≤ 4 mm) should be embedded intact.

Shave Biopsy

The use of shave biopsy is popular among many dermatologists for the diagnosis of small, flat pigmented lesions. A shave biopsy seems appropriate for small lesions as long as a rim of normal tissue is included. However, it needs to be used judiciously. A reliable distinction between atypical lentiginous melanocytic proliferations, melanoma in situ, and lentiginous junctional nevus of chronically sun-damaged skin, for example, may not be possible on a small shave biopsy that lacks surrounding normal

TABLE 2-1 Routine handling of skin excisions for pigmented lesions.

1. Record dimensions of specimen: length, width, depth
2. Record gross morphologic features of pigmented lesion:
   - Length and width (in millimeters or centimeters) and proximity to surgical margins
   - Symmetry or asymmetry
   - Regularity or irregularity of borders
   - Coloration: uniform or variegated
   - Colors present: flesh, tan, brown, black, blue, gray, white
   - Topography: flat, raised, nodular, ulcerated, presence of crust, hemorrhage
3. In general, specimen is inked for surgical margins
4. Transverse sections should be taken through thickest or darkest area or through the center of lesion
5. Serial sections every 2 to 3 mm may be taken through the remainder of the specimen or the "rule of halves" applied—the subsequent transverse sections are taken to bisect each half of the residual specimen until one has tissue sections 2 to 3 mm in thickness after the initial transverse section

skin. Large shave biopsies may be split along their longitudinal axis in two halves. Biopsies measuring < 4 mm in greatest dimension may best be embedded in toto.

Curettage Biopsy

Curettings of clinically suspected melanocytic lesions are discouraged. Inevitable fragmentation of the lesion compromises diagnostic and prognostic accuracy.

MOHS MICROGRAPHIC SURGERY

The technique of Mohs micrographically controlled surgery is well established for the treatment of basal cell and squamous cell carcinomas and has also been applied to melanocytic tumors (1–4). The goals of Mohs surgery are (a) to achieve complete evaluation of all surgical margins so that there is no residual tumor at any margin and (b) to remove as little normal tissue as is possible to achieve tumor-free margins for optimal cosmetic results.

In general, one should be cautious in applying this methodology to melanocytic lesions. As it is often difficult enough to reliably determine the peripheral margin of a histologically subtle in situ melanoma or to detect focal invasion on routinely processed (formalin-fixed and paraffin-embedded) tissue, histologic assessment is much more difficult using frozen material. Another potential problem is the common practice of many Mohs surgeons to discard the central portion of the tumor (*debulking*). The debulked tissue often contains residual tumor, whose histologic features may be relevant for prognosis and management.

Because of the problems mentioned above, many Mohs surgeons sensitive to quality assurance issues and dedicated to optimal histologic diagnoses have adopted a "slow" Mohs approach, in which tumor is debulked and margins are taken as for Mohs surgery, but the tissue specimens are processed for permanent sections (2). This method allows optimal assessment of tissue sections, achieves complete assessment of all margins, and allows examination of the central tumor for prognostic parameters.

TISSUE PROCESSING

Frozen sections are generally not recommended for melanocytic lesions for a number of reasons: The histologic appearance is inferior, the study of multiple levels is more difficult, and a portion of the tissue is lost in the cutting of sections. Moreover, measurements of tumor thickness on frozen sections are not comparable to those on paraffin-embedded tissue, which has been used for standardization of tumor thickness as a prognostic marker. These considerations do not apply to frozen section diagnoses of metastatic lesions.

On the other hand, frozen sections are appropriate for laboratories capable of providing high-quality frozen sections. The use of frozen sections for assessment of

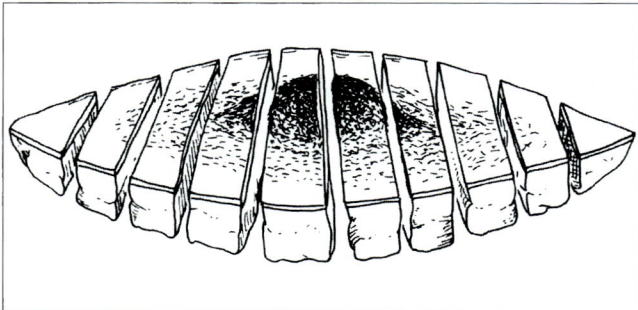

FIGURE 2-1 Handling of excisional specimens. The initial tranverse section should be taken through the thickest or darkest portion of the pigmented lesion. Serial sections should then be taken at 2- to 3-mm intervals through the remainder of the specimen.

margins is particularly relevant for the surgery of facial melanoma involving tissues in the vicinity of the facial nerve. The use of frozen sections minimizes the need for a reexcision, which may be accompanied by increased morbidity due to a higher risk for facial nerve injury.

Tissue for Research

In general, obtaining tissue for research is acceptable only if it is done in the context of an institutional review board (IRB)–approved protocol and consented by the patient. Generally, a lesion suitable for research use should be > 1 cm in greatest dimension. Only a thin slice of lesional tissue should be taken. The thickest part of a tumor and relevant margins need to be spared for routine histologic assessment so that patient care is not compromised. Tissue may be frozen in liquid nitrogen or in another suitable fluid for immediate tissue freezing, such as dry ice–cooled 2-methyl-butane. Tissue for cytogenetic and molecular biologic studies or for experimental therapy using tumor-infiltrating lymphocytes requires handling of the specimen under sterile conditions.

Fixation

Most biopsies of melanocytic lesions are small tissue samples that are fixed in toto by immersion in neutral buffered formalin. Larger (> 1 cm) specimens and lymph nodes should be incised to secure adequate penetration by the fixative. Paraffin sections are adequate for most routine diagnostic purposes. Most antibodies available to distinguish melanocytic from nonmelanocytic lesions are applicable to paraffin-embedded tissue. Frozen tissue and occasionally fresh sterile tissue for cytogenetics should be saved if the diagnosis is uncertain and sarcomas or lymphomas are considered.

ANCILLARY STUDIES IN THE EVALUATION OF MELANOCYTIC LESIONS

Melanin Stains

In the histologic and cytologic diagnosis of melanocytic lesions, the correct identification of melanin is important (Table 2-2). If a pigment cannot readily be identified as melanin on routine histologic sections by morphologic criteria alone, a variety of staining procedures can enable one to confirm the presence of melanin. The most widely used methods are reducing silver stains, such as the Masson-Fontana and Schmorl stains or the more sensitive Warthin-Starry stain (5). These stains, however, are not entirely specific, because they also highlight some lipofuscins and argentaffin endocrine cells. It is prudent to use an iron stain in parallel with a melanin stain, if melanin is to be distinguished from hemosiderin. Bleaching might also be useful for the latter distinction: Melanin pigment can be removed by bleaching, for example, in 0.5% potassium permanganate, whereas hemosiderin and lipofuscin are resistant to bleaching. The brown pigment of pseudomelanosis coli is generally periodic acid-Schiff (PAS) positive, but melanin is negative.

Occasionally, formalin pigment, a hemoglobin-derived pigment, may cause confusion (6). The pigment forms if formalin is not buffered to a neutral pH. It does not stain with silver stains and can rapidly be distinguished by incubating the slide in a picric acid solution.

Enzyme Histochemistry

Tyrosinase activity can be demonstrated by the DOPA oxidase technique, which may be useful in identifying traces of melanin synthesis in hypomelanotic lesions. This reaction can be performed on frozen sections as well as on paraffin sections of adequately fixed tissue (7). False-

TABLE 2-2 Ancillary techniques used in the evaluation of melanoma.[a]

Technique	Comments
Fontana-Masson stain	Detection of melanin pigment
Enzyme chemistry	DOPA reaction to detect melanocytes
Immunohistochemistry	Presence or absence of proteins associated with melanocyte differentiation; proliferation and other biomarkers for diagnosis and/or prognosis
Electron microscopy	Demonstration of premelanosomes, melanosomes; demonstration of nonmelanocytic (e.g., epithelial or Schwannian) features
Molecular studies	
RT-PCR	ATF-1/EWS fusion product to diagnoses clear cell sarcoma/melanoma of soft parts
CGH	Assessment of chromosomal aberrations (investigational)
In situ hybridization	Detection of mRNA expression in melanocytes (investigational)

[a]*DOPA*, dihydroxyphenylalanine; *RT-PCR*, reverse transcriptase polymerase chain reaction; *ATF-1/EWS*, activating transcription factor/Ewing's sarcoma; *CGH*, comparative genomic hybridization.

positive results may be seen in the presence of mast cells, since their granules also stain with this technique. However, because of their metachromatic properties, this should not generate diagnostic problems. With the availability of antibodies to tyrosinase and other melanocyte differentiation markers, most laboratories have switched from enzyme histochemistry to immunohistochemistry for the detection of melanocytes.

Immunohistochemistry

A growing number of immunomarkers has become available over the past decades to identify a cell as melanocytic in differentiation. Their most important application is in the diagnosis of tumors, such as for the distinction of amelanotic metastatic malignant melanoma from lymphoma, metastatic carcinoma, and sarcoma. Whenever the melanocytic origin of a lesion needs to be confirmed, it is critical to apply a panel of markers and to weigh the pattern of immunoreactivities against the clinical and histologic impression. We do not recommend an expensive multimarker approach to each tumor but advise a careful limited choice, focusing on markers likely positive based on morphologic analysis and clinical data. For the diagnosis of epithelioid melanomas, the use of one or more melanocyte differentiation markers, such as Mart-1/Melan-A, gp100, or tyrosinase, usually readily reveals melanocytic differentiation. Of these markers, tyrosinase appears most sensitive, followed by Mart-1/Melan-A and gp100 (Table 2-3). For spindle cell melanomas, S-100 protein remains the most sensitive marker (8–32).

S-100 Protein Antibodies reactive with S-100 protein are useful markers in the diagnosis of melanocytic tumors because of their high sensitivity: The vast majority of melanocytic lesions ($> 95\%$), including amelanotic melanoma and its metastases, are immunoreactive with these antibodies (8–12). Both nuclear and cytoplasmic staining are seen. Usually, the majority of melanocytes stain, although a heterogeneous distribution can be observed. Rare melanomas fail to show positivity with S-100 protein.

S-100 protein comprises a family of acidic calcium-binding proteins forming homodimers and heterodimers of its subunits (11). It was first isolated from brain extract and acquired its name from its solubility in saturated ammonium sulfate at neutral pH (9). The protein is expressed in many cell types, including astrocytes, Schwann cells, melanocytes, Langerhans cells, chondrocytes, adipocytes, sustentacular cells of the adrenal medulla, and myoepithelial cells (11). Accordingly, expression of S-100 protein is seen in a number of nonmelanocytic tumors, such as peripheral nerve sheath tumors, chordoma, granular cell tumor, chondroma, chondrosarcoma, chondroblastoma, osteosarcoma, glioma, benign and malignant myoepithelial tumors, and some carcinomas. However, since the majority of S-100 protein-positive, nonmelanocytic tumors can easily be distinguished from melanocytic tumors on morphologic grounds alone or with a limited panel of additional markers, the lack of specificity of S-100 protein antibodies is usually not a major diagnostic problem. S-100 protein is of particular value for the diagnosis of spindle cell desmoplastic melanomas. Rabbit polyclonal antibody against S-100 protein is commercially available. Recently, monoclonal antibodies against the α and β subunits have been developed and are also commercially available (11).

gp100 HMB-45 is a monoclonal antibody, which was developed against human melanoma cells (13). It recognizes gp100, a premelanosomal glycoprotein (13), which explains its relative specificity for melanin-producing cells. The staining pattern is intracytoplasmic and often heterogeneous. The antibody is commercially available. HMB-45 is particularly helpful in the evaluation of a nonmelanocytic, S-100 protein–positive tumor. While the majority of dermal melanocytes in common nevi do not stain with HMB-45, many nevi may be positive (14), especially blue nevi (15) but also Spitz's nevi, the junctional and superficial dermal components of dysplastic nevi. HMB-45 also stains normal intraepidermal melanocytes, although not all of them. More intraepidermal melanocytes are immunoreactive with HMB-45 in the setting of wound repair. HMB-45 is one of the best markers for blue nevi.

HMB-45 is not entirely specific for melanocytes. HMB-45 positivity has been reported for a number of

TABLE 2-3 Commonly used melanocyte differentiation markers for paraffin-embedded tissue.

Antibody	Antigen	Sensitivity (%)	Specificity
Anti-S100P	S-100 protein	> 95	Low
T311	Tyrosinase	70–90	High
A103/M2-7C10	Melan-A/Mart-1	70–85	High
HMB-45	gp100	60–80	High
D5/C5	MITF	60–80	Intermediate

nonmelanocytic tumors, including some breast carcinomas (16), peripheral nerve sheath tumors (17), adrenal pheo-chromocytomas (18), angiomyolipomas (19), lymphangiomyomatosis of the lung (20), and other tumors of the PEComa family. Almost all (> 95%) desmoplastic and neurotropic melanomas are negative for HMB-45, except for perhaps the intraepidermal or superficial dermal components of some tumors, which generally contain epithelioid melanoma cells (21).

Melan-A/Mart-1 During the course of analyzing melanoma antigens recognized by autologous cytotoxic T lymphocytes, Coulie et al. (22) and Kawakami et al. (23) independently cloned the same gene: *Melan-A* from a melanoma cell line SK-MEL-29 and Mart-1, respectively. Mononclonal antibodies for use on archival material are commercially available. The clone against *Melan-A* has been named A-103 (24–29). The clone against Mart-1 has been named M2-7C10. Antibodies to Melan-A/Mart-1 have been shown to be slightly superior in sensitivity to HMB-45 by many investigators. They stain intraepidermal melanocytes of normal skin and most melanocytic nevi, including ordinary nevi, atypical (dysplastic) nevi, Spitz tumors, and blue nevi (26,28). The only nevi that rarely stain for Melan-A/Mart-1 are neurotized nevi (26). Almost all (> 95%) primary nondesmoplastic melanoma show expression of *Melan-A,* whereas most (~75%) metastatic melanoma specimens are positive for the marker. The pattern of immunostaining is membranous and cytoplasmic.

The monoclonal antibody A-103 cross-reacts with an epitope present on adrenocortical cells and other steroid cells and tumors derived thereof. However, in the area of melanoma pathology, potential confusion with adrenocortical tumors is rarely ever a relevant issue. Thus this cross-reactivity does not limit the diagnostic use of the antibody. Similar to gp100, Melan-A/Mart-1 is also expressed in PEComas (e.g., angioleiomyomas, clear-cell sugar tumors).

Tyrosinase Tyrosinase is a key enzyme for the normal biosynthesis of melanin pigment. It is a prototypical melanocyte differentiation antigen. The antibody T311, which recognizes tyrosinase in archival material has emerged as an excellent marker for melanocytes (30–32). It stains normal melanocytes, nevi, and melanoma. Its sensitivity for epithelioid melanocytic neoplasms and mucosal melanomas approaches S-100 protein. It is highly specific for melanocytes. Only rare nonmelanocytic tumors may express tyrosinase, such as pigmented (melanin-containing) nerve sheath tumors and angiomyolipomas. Although T311 is slightly more sensitive than A-103 and HMB-45 for desmoplastic melanoma, most desmoplastic melanomas are negative for T311. Antibodies to tyrosinase have been found useful not only for cutaneous but also mucosal melanomas (29).

Tyrosinase-Related Protein 1 Tyrosinase-related protein 1 (TRP-1; gp75), a pigmentation-associated, is a melanocyte differentiation marker commonly expressed in normal melanocytes and melanoma (33,34). The antibody Mel-5 (clone TA-99) is an excellent reagent for the demonstration of normal melanocytes. In our experience, it works best on frozen tissue material and is less suitable for paraffin-embedded tissue, although other workers have successfully used it on archival material.

Microphthalmia Transcription Factor Microphthalmia transcription factor (MITF) is necessary for the survival and development of melanocytes. For example, MITF-deficient mice are devoid of all mature pigment cells (35–41). MITF regulates the expression of a number of melanocyte genes, including tyrosinase. Monoclonal antibodies developed against human MITF (C5 and D5) have proved to detect normal basilar melanocytes and both benign and malignant melanocytic tumors in formalin-fixed, paraffin-embedded tissue. The pattern of immunoreactivity is nuclear with MITF. Staining for MITF is less sensitive for melanoma than S-100 protein or tyrosinase, but it is comparable to Melan-A/Mart-1 and gp100 (HMB-45). There are several isoforms of MITF. Only one of them (MITF-M) is melanocyte specific (35). Currently available antibodies (clones D5, C5) to MITF are not MITF-M specific. Accordingly, immunoreactivity using D5/C5 is not restricted to melanocytes. Positive staining is also seen in several nonmelanocytic cells, such as mast cells, osteoclasts, and histioctyes.

P75 Neurotrophin Receptor The p75 neurotrophin receptor (p75NR; nerve growth factor receptor) is a transmembrane glycoprotein of about 75 kDa involved in the development of the nervous system. A monoclonal antibody directed against this receptor has been shown to have high sensititity for spindle cell melanomas (42–44). However, like S-100 protein, expression of p75NR is not specific for melanocytes. Immunoreactivity for p75NR has also been noted in nerve sheath tumors, spindle cell squamous cell carcinoma, atypical fibroxanthoma, and scars, which limits the diagnostic use of this marker.

NKI/C3 NKI/C3, another monoclonal antibody raised against melanomas and found to react with melanocytic lesions in paraffin-embedded tissue (12,45,46). It is currently rarely used because of the development of the novel antibodies mentioned above. It recognizes the lysozomal glycoprotein CD63. While normal adult melanocytes are not immunoreactive with this antibody, the cytoplasm of melanocytic tumor cells is intensely stained. The staining of melanocytes is often heterogeneous. Junctional and subepidermal melanocytes are preferentially stained in melanocytic nevi or primary melanoma. NKI/C3 is not specific for melanocytes. Staining for NKI/C3 may be seen in some carcinomas, neuroendocrine tumors, gastrointestinal autonomic tumors, cellular neurothekeomas, some tumors with fibrohistiocytic differentiation, and in any tumor containing many lysosomes (e.g., granular cell tumors). In paraffin sections of the normal skin, immunoreactivity can be seen in the acinar cells of sweat glands and in mast cells. In frozen sections, its specificity is even lower. NKI/C3 is less sensitive for melanocytic lesions than antibodies against S-100 protein.

Other Miscellaneous Antibodies Other monoclonal antibodies have been developed against melanoma (12), such as KBA-62 and NKIbeteb. They are not discussed here because they lack sufficient sensitivity or specificity for diagnostic purposes or have not been completely evaluated for their diagnostic utility on paraffin-embedded material.

Whenever melanoma is being considered in the differential diagnosis and a panel of immunomarkers is applied, one needs to be aware of the fact that occasionally melanoma may stain for nonmelanocytic markers, such as low molecular weight cytokeratins or smooth muscle actin (Table 2-4). Keratin positivity does not exclude melanoma but can only be accepted if there is other compelling evidence (strong staining for a melanocyte differentiation marker and/or clinical history of melanoma) in favor of melanoma.

Immunohistochemistry has not only been applied to the differential diagnosis of melanocytic lesions from nonmelanocytic tumors but is also being investigated for the distinction of nevus from melanoma and for prognostic purposes (see Chapter 11). Ki-67, for example, a nuclear antigen of 395 and 345 kDa size, which is expressed in late G_1, S, G_2, and M phases but not in early G_1 and G_0 phases of the cell cycle (47,48), has been explored for assessing melanocytic lesions (49–54). Preliminary data indicate that the (MIB-1) labeling index and the pattern of MIB-1 staining may be useful in distinguishing Spitz nevi from melanoma and may also be of value for the recognition of nevoid melanomas (49–52). MIB-1 labeling has also been found useful for the evaluation of nodal nevi and their distinction from metastatic melanoma (53).

In addition to its utility for diagnostic purposes, MIB-1 labeling of melanoma has also been suggested to provide prognostic information (54). Another marker, which may be of prognostic significance, is the oncogene HDM2. Polsky et al. (55) recently showed that HMD2 overexpression in melanoma was significantly associated with improved disease-free survival. However, the use of immunomarkers for prognosis is currently limited to investigational studies and needs validation through prospective studies.

ELECTRON MICROSCOPY

With the advent of melanocytic differentiation markers, immunohistochemistry has become the central aide in solving differential diagnostic problems. At present, electron microscopy is only rarely needed in the diagnosis of melanocytic lesions. It has been used to identify premelanosomes, melanosomes, and atypical melanosomes, such as spherical forms with irregular granular material, which are more likely found in melanoma or atypical nevi and are rarely seen in normal melanocytes or common acquired nevi.

A diagnostic dilemma, in which electron microscopy may still be required is the differential diagnosis of a pigmented HMB-45-positive schwannoma from a melanoma. While melanosomes may be found in both schwannoma and melanoma, schwannomas are distinguished ultrastructurally by the following features: (a) spindle cells with intertwining processes, (b) basal lamina covering processes and cell bodies, and (c) long-spacing collagen (Luse bodies).

TABLE 2-4 Unusual immunostaining results that may occasionally be observed in melanoma.

Finding	Comments
Cytokeratins (CAM5.2, AE1/AE3)	Positivity in up to 10% of melanomas (metastases most frequent); rare scattered positive cells
EMA	Conventional and desmoplastic melanoma (perineurial differentiation)
Desmin	Conventional and desmoplastic melanoma
Smooth muscle actin	Desmoplastic melanoma
Glial fibrillary acid protein	Conventional melanoma
Factor XIIIa	Desmoplastic melanoma
CD68 ("histiocytic" marker)	Conventional melanoma

Electron microscopy may also on rare occasions be useful in the differential diagnosis of an amelanotic melanoma from poorly differentiated carcinoma. If immunohistochemical studies fail to provide an answer, the detection of desmosomes or basal lamina may favor carcinoma.

CYTOGENETICS

Chromosome analyses of human melanocytic tumors have demonstrated a variety of nonrandom abnormalities, involving several chromosomes. While cytogenetic analysis has evolved as an important adjunct in the diagnosis of soft tissue neoplasms and lymphomas (56), it is currently of limited value for the diagnosis melanocytic tumors. The only setting in which cytogentic analysis has been established as a valuable tool for the diagnosis of melanoma is the distinction of cutaneous melanoma from clear-cell sarcoma/melanoma of soft parts (MMSP). MMSP exhibits a recurrent chromosome translocation involving t(12;22) (q13;q12) (57–59). The resulting chimeric protein consists of the N-terminal domain of Ewing sarcoma (EWS) linked to the bZIP domain of activating transcription factor 1 (ATF-1), a transcription factor that may normally be regulated by cyclic adenosine monophosphate (cAMP). This aberration is not seen in cutaneous melanoma.

More recently, comparative genomic hybridization was found to be a technique with some promise for the evaluation of melanocytic neoplasm, but its use at the current time is for investigational purposes only (60,61).

OTHER TECHNIQUES FOR THE DIAGNOSIS OF MELANOMA

A variety of other techniques have been used in tumor pathology to measure parameters that might assist in the evaluation of the malignant potential of a lesion. Such parameters are DNA ploidy, angiogenesis (microvessel density), and in situ hybridization, such as for melastatin mRNA (62). The utility of either parameter for diagnostic or prognostic purposes is still under investigation.

REFERENCES

1. Johnson TM, Headington JT, Baker SR, Lowe L. Usefulness of the staged excision for lentigo maligna and lentigo maligna melanoma: the "square" procedure. J Am Acad Dermatol 1997;37:758–64.
2. Cohen LM, McCall MW, Hodge SJ, et al. Successful treatment of lentigo maligna and lentigo maligna melanoma with Mohs micrographic surgery aided by rush permanent sections. Cancer 1994;37:422–9.
3. Zalla MJ, Lim KK, DiCaudo DJ, Gagnot MM. Mohs micrographic excision of melanoma using immunostains. Dermatol Surg 2000;26:771–84.
4. Dhawan SS, Wolf DJ, Rabinovitz HS, et al. Lentigo maligna: the use of rush permanent sections in therapy. Arch Dermatol 1990;126:928–30.
5. Warkel R, Luna L, Helwig E. A modified Warthin-Starry procedure at low pH for melanin. Am J Clin Pathol 1980; 73:812–5.
6. Ackerman A, Penneys N. Formalin pigment in skin. Arch Dermatol 1970;102:318–21.
7. Rodriguez H, McGavran M. A modified dopa reaction for the diagnosis and investigation of pigmented cells. Am J Clin Pathol 1969;52:219–27.
8. Gatter K, Ralfkaier E, Skinner J, et al. An immunohistochemical study of malignant melanoma and its differential diagnosis from other malignant tumors. J Clin Pathol 1985; 38:7–15.
9. Gaynor RB, Herschman HR, Irie R, et al. S-100 protein: a marker for malignant melanoma. J Clin Pathol 1981;38: 1353–7.
10. Cochran A, Wen DR, Herschman HR, Gaynor RB. Detection of S-100 protein as an aid to the identification of melanocytic tumors. Int J Cancer 1982;30:295–7.
11. McNutt NS. The S-100 family of multipurpose calcium-binding proteins. J Cutan Pathol 1998;25:521–9.
12. Wang R, Dworak LJ, Lacy MJ. A panel immunoblot using co-incubated monoclonal antibodies for identification of melanoma cells. J Immunol Methods 2001;249:167–83.
13. Gown A, Vogel A, Hoak D, et al. Monoclonal antibodies specific for melanocytic tumors distinguish subpopulations of melanocytes. Am J Pathol 1986;123:195–203.
14. Colombari R, Bonetti F, Zambone G, et al. Distribution of melanoma specific antibody (HMB-45) in benign and malignant melanocytic tumors. An immunohistochemical study on paraffin sections. Virchows Arch A Pathol Anat 1988;413:17–24.
15. Wood W, Tron V. Analysis of HMB-45 immunoreactivity in common and cellular blue nevi. J Cutan Pathol 1991; 18:261–3.
16. Bonetti F, Colombari E, Zamboni G, et al. Breast carcinoma positive for melanoma marker (HMB-45). Am J Clin Pathol 1989;22:491–5.
17. Zimmer C, Gottschalk J, Goebel S, Cercos-Navarro J. Melanoma-associated antigens in tumors of the nervous system: an immunohistochemical study with the monoclonal antibody HMB-45. Virchows Arch A Pathol Anat Histopathol 1992;420(2):121–6.
18. Unger P, Hoffman K, Thung S, et al. HMB-45 reactivity in adrenal pheochromocytomas. Arch Pathol Lab Med 1992; 116:151–3

19. Tsui W, Yuen A, Ma K, Tse C. Hepatic angiomyolipomas with a deceptive trabecular pattern and HMB-45 reactivity. Histopathology 1992;21:569–73.
20. Bonetti F, Chiodera P, Pea M, et al. Transbronchial biopsy in lymphangiomatosis of the lung. Am J Surg Pathol 1993;17:1092–102.
21. Pelosi G, Bonetti F, Colombardi R, et al. Use of monoclonal antibody HMB-45 in the cytological diagnosis of melanoma. Acta Cytol 1990;34:382–4.
22. Coulie PG, Brichard V, Van Pel A, et al. A new gene coding for a differentiation antigen recognized by autologous cytolytic T-lymphocytes on HLA-A2 melanomas. J Exp Med 1994;180:35–42.
23. Kawakami Y, Eliyahu S, Delgado CH, et al. Cloning of the gene coding for shared human melanoma antigen recognized by autologous T cells infiltrating into tumor. Proc Natl Acad Sci USA 1994;91:3515–9.
24. Chen YT, Stockert E, Jungbluth A, et al. Serological analysis of Melan-A (Mart-1), a melanocyte-specific protein homogeneously expressed in human melanomas. Proc Natl Acad Sci USA 1996;93:5915–9.
25. Beaty MW, Fetsch P, Wilder AM, et al. Effusion cytology of malignant melanoma. A morphologic and immunocytochemical analysis including application of the MART-1 antibody. Cancer Cytopathol 1997:81:57–63.
26. Busam KJ, Iversen K, Coplan KA, et al. Expression of Melan-A (Mart-1) in benign melanocytic nevi and primary malignant melanoma. Am J Surg Pathol 1998;22:976–82.
27. Jungbluth AA, Busam KJ, Gerald WL, et al. A103, an anti-melan-a monoclonal antibody for the detection of malignant melanoma in paraffin-embedded tissues. Am J Surg Pathol 1998;22(5):595–602.
28. Busam KJ, Junbluth AA. Melan-A, a new melanocytic differentiation marker. Adv Anat Pathol 1999;6:12–8.
29. Prasad ML, Jungbluth AA, Iversen K, et al. Expression of melanocytic differentiation markers in malignant melanomas of the oral and sinonasal mucosa. Am J Surg Pathol 2001;25(6):782–787.
30. Chen YT, Stockert E, Tsang S, et al. Immunophenotyping of melanomas for tyrosinase: Implications for vaccine development. Proc Natl Acad Sci USA 1995;92:8125–9.
31. Jungbluth AA, Iversen K, Coplan K, et al. T311: an anti-tyrosinase monoclonal antibody for the detection of melanocytic lesions in paraffin-embedded tissues. Path Res Pract 2000;196:235–42.
32. Hofbauer GFL, Kamarashev J, Geertsen R, et al. Tyrosinase immunoreactivity in formalin-fixed, paraffin-embedded primary and metastatic melanoma: frequency and distribution. J Cutan Pathol 1998;25:204–9.
33. Dean NR, Brennan J, Haynes J, et al. Immunohistochemical labeling of normal melanocytes. Appl Immunohistochem Mol Morphol 2002;10:199–204.
34. Gross EA, Andersen WK, Rogers GS. Mohs micrographic excision of lentigo maligna using Mel-5 for margin control. Arch Dermatol 1999;135:15–7.
35. Shibahara S, Takeda K, Yasumoto K, et al. Microphthalmia-associated transcription factor (MITF): multiplicity in structure, function and regulation. J Invest Dermatol Symp Proc 2001;6:99–104.
36. King R, Weilbaecher KN, McGill G, et al. Microphthalmia transcription factor. A sensitive and specific melanocyte melanoma diagnosis. Am J Pathol. 1999;155(3):731–8.
37. King R, Googe PB, Weilbaecher KN, et al. Microphthalmia transcription factor expression in cutaneous benign, malig and nonmelanocytic tumors. Am J Surg Pathol. 2001;25(1):51–7.
38. Miettinen M, Fernandez M, Franssila K, et al. Microphthalmia transcription factor in the immunohistochemical diagnosis of metastatic melanoma. Comparison with four other melanoma markers. Am J Surg Pathol 2001;25(2):205–11.
39. Koch MB, Arbiser ZK, Weiss SW, et al. Melanoma cell adhesion molecule (Mel-CAM, CD146) and microphthalmia transcription factor (MiTF) expression distinguish desmoplastic/sarcomatoid melanoma (DM) from morphologic mimics. Mod Pathol 2000;13:63A.
40. Koch MB, Shih IM, Weiss SW, Folpe AL. Microphthalmia transcription factor and melanoma cell adhesion molecule distinguish desmoplastic/spindle cell melanoma from morphologic mimics. Am J Surg Pathol. 2001;25(1):58–64.
41. Busam KJ, Iversen K, Coplan KC, Jungbluth A. Analysis of microphthalmia transcription factor expression in normal tissues and tumors, and comparison of its expression with S-100 protein, gp100, and tyrosinase in desmoplastic malignant melanoma. Am J Surg Path 2001;25(2):197–204.
42. Iwamoto S, Odland PB, Piepkorn M, et al. Evidence that the p75 neurotrophin receptor mediates perineural spread of desmoplastic melanoma. J Am Acad Dermatol 1996;35:725–31.
43. Kanik AB, Yaar M, Bhawan J. p75 nerve growth factor receptor staining helps identify desmoplastic and neurotropic melanoma. J Cutan Pathol 1996;23:205–10.
44. Iwamoto S, Burrows RC, Agorff SN, et al. The p75 neurotrophin receptor, relative to other Schwann cell and melanoma markers, is abunduntly expressed in spindled melanomas Am J Dermatopathol 2001;23:288–94.
45. Vennegoor C, Calafat J, Hageman P, et al. Biochemical characterization and cellular localization of formalin-resistant melanoma-associated antigen reacting with monoclonal antibody NHI/C3. Int J Cancer 1985;35:287–95.
46. MacKie R, Campbell L, Turbitt M. Use of NKI/C3 monoclonal antibody in the assessment of benign and malignant melanocytic lesions. J Clin Path 1984;37:367–72.
47. Kurki P, Vanderlaan M, Dolbeare F, et al. Expression of proliferating cell nuclear antigen (PCNA)/cyclin during the cell cycle. Exp Cell Res 1986;166:209–19.

48. Gerdes J, Lemke H, Baisch H, et al. Cell cycle analysis of a cell proliferation-associated human nuclear antigen defined by the monoclonal antibody Ki-67. J Immunol 1984;133:1710–5.
49. Rieger E, Hofmann-Wellenhof R, Soyer H, et al. Comparison of proliferative activity as assessed by proliferating cell nuclear antigen (PCNA) and Ki-67 monoclonal antibodies in melanocytic lesions. J Cutan Pathol 1993;20:229–36.
50. Li LL, Crotty KA, McCarthy SW, et al. A zonal comparison of MIB1-Ki67 immunoreactivity in benign and malignant melanocytic lesions. Am J Dermatopathol 2000;22(6):489–495.
51. Pereira F, Carey W, Shibata H, et al. Multiple nevoid malignant melanomas in a patient with AIDS: the role of proliferating cell nuclear antigen in the diagnosis. J Am Acad Dermatol 2002;47:S172–4.
52. McNutt NS. "Triggered trap": nevoid malignant melanoma. Semin Diagn Pathol 1998;15:203–9.
53. Lohmann CM, Iversen K, Jungbluth AA, et al. Expression of melanocyte differentiation antigens and ki-67 in nodal nevi and comparison of ki-67 expression with metastatic melanoma. Am J Surg Pathol 2002;26:1351–7.
54. Hazan C, Melzer K, Panageas KS, et al. Evaluation of the proliferation marker MIB-1 in the prognosis of cutaneous malignant melanoma. Cancer 2002;95:634–40.
55. Polsky D, Melzer K, Hazan C, et al. HDM2 protein overexpression and prognosis in primary malignant melanoma. J Natl Cancer Inst 2002;94:1803–6.
56. Fletcher J, Kozakewich H, Hoffer E, et al. Diagnostic relevance of clonal cytogenetic aberrations in malignant soft-tissue tumors. N Engl J Med 1991;324:436–42.
57. Fletcher J. Translocation (12;22) (q13-14;q12) is a nonrandom aberration in soft tissue clear cell sarcoma. Genes Chrom Cancer 1992;5:184.
58. Zucman J, Delattre O, Desmaze C, et al. EWS and ATF-1 gene fusion induced by t(12;22) translocation in malignant melanoma of soft parts. Nature Genet 1993;4:341–5.
59. Antonescu CR, Tschernyavsky SJ, Woodruff JM, et al. Molecular diagnosis of clear cell sarcoma: detection of EWS-ATF1 and MITF-M transcripts and histopathological and ultrastructural analysis of 12 cases. J Mol Diagn 2002;4:44–52.
60. Bastian BC, LeBoit PE, Pinkel D. Mutations and copy number increase of HRAS in Spitz nevi with distinctive histologic features. Am J Pathol 2000;157:967–72.
61. Bastian BC. Molecular cytogenetics as a diagnostic tool for typing melanocytic tumors. Recent Results Cancer Res 2002;160:92–9.
62. Duncan LM, Deeds J, Cronin FE, et al. Melastatin expression and prognosis in cutaneous malignant melanoma. J Clin Oncol 2001;15:568–76.

CHAPTER 3

Genetic and Molecular Pathology of Melanoma

Michael Piepkorn

In so far as neoplastic development and progression involve pathogenic deletions or mutations in critical genes, all cancers are fundamentally genetic. In the specific case of melanoma, the genetic basis of its cause is reflected in the observation that approximately 10% of cases result from the familial transmission of melanoma susceptibility loci in the germline. Whereas most melanomas are sporadic, the genetic basis is reflected in acquired or postzygotic lesions at genomic loci within melanocytes that initiate the pathway of neoplastic progression. Notably, the same genes targeted in the germline in familial melanoma, as well as in other cancer syndromes such as Li-Faumeni syndrome, are involved rather commonly in a broad range of cancer types through the mechanism of random, postzygotic mutations in somatic cells targeted for neoplastic transformation (1,2).

As currently envisioned, the acquisition of the neoplastic phenotype occurs as a stepwise process resulting from the accumulation of activating or deactivating mutations at critical genetic loci that confer a growth advantage of the nascent cancer cells. There are two principal types of cancer genes. Proto-oncogenes acquire gain-in-function mutations that convert them into oncogenes, which then positively contribute to the neoplastic phenotype in a "dominant" fashion—that is, one mutated allele results in a functional effect. In contrast, tumor-suppressor genes, which in the wild type form act to control aberrant cell growth, are targeted for loss-of-function mutation during neoplastic transformation. Mutations in tumor-suppressor genes are "recessive" because both alleles at the genetic locus must sustain inactivating genetic lesions (mutation or deletion) for the gene to lose function. Most genes targeted for activation or inactivation during the development of melanoma are involved in the control of cell proliferation or motility. Some of these genes, as discussed later in this chapter, interact with environmental factors, most specifically ultraviolet radiation, to promote neoplastic development.

Within the last decade, the major advance furthering our understanding of the molecular basis of melanoma was the mapping, cloning, and elucidation of the mechanism of action of CDKN2A, also known as p16. This advance was initiated by an interest in the familial aggregation of melanoma cases and by the clinical association between an atypical nevus phenotype and the susceptibility to melanoma. By the use of genetic linkage analysis, the genomic location of a major susceptibility locus was mapped to the short arm of chromosome 9p. Positional cloning strategies then proved successful in isolating the gene's sequence, and subsequent studies, as discussed later in this section, rapidly led to an elucidation of its mechanism of action. The gene remains the major melanoma locus so far identified and has prompted initial efforts to evaluate the utility of clinical testing for hereditary melanoma susceptibility. From the molecular perspective, targeting of the CDKN2A locus has emerged as an early, potentially initiating, and often critical event in the neoplastic transformation of melanocytes (2,3).

The fields of the genetic and molecular pathology of melanoma are vast and beyond the limited scope of this chapter. The purpose of this overview is to focus on selected molecular genetic mechanisms that illustrate key principles regarding the development and progression of melanoma. Initial focus will be placed on familial melanoma loci, which presumably act proximally in the transformation pathway as initiating events. These loci vary in their penetrance, with major loci being highly penetrant—that is, likely to eventuate in disease in individuals harboring mutations in those genes within the germline. Among the major genes, the tumor-suppressor CDKN2A is by far the most common in prevalence and is also highly penetrant. Other penetrant melanoma loci identified to date are CDK4, a proto-oncogene, and ARF (for alternative reading frame), a tumor-suppressor gene; but those loci are much less commonly targeted for mutation in the setting of familial melanoma. Minor familial melanoma loci can be defined as those that act proximally in the transformation pathway but are much less penetrant when mutated in the germline. Among these, the focus of most recent interest has been the melanocortin 1 receptor. This gene product mediates the epidermal response to ultraviolet (UV) light exposure and has been proposed as a modifier gene in the penetrance of mutations at the CDKN2A locus.

Yet other gene elements act more distally in the neoplastic pathway of melanoma development. These are targeted for deletion or mutation not in the germline of melanoma prone families but as acquired or postzygotic events in people with sporadic melanoma. As such, their inactivation or overexpression relates to growth control, motility, and metastatic functions of the neoplastic cells. Two genes with opposing functions are offered as examples here. One of these, RhoC, promotes neoplastic progression when targeted by gain-in-function mutations. The other, melastatin, is a tumor suppressor that, when inactivated, contributes to melanoma progression and metastasis. Distally acting elements may also include genes whose products are involved in evasion of the host's antitumor immunity by melanoma cells. The example used here is that of the Fas (CD95) and Fas ligand (FasL) pathway.

Some day, the diagnosis, classification, and treatment of melanoma will come to rely on molecular analyses of key genetic elements and their expression patterns as a supplement to the histologic interpretation (4). To this end, this chapter provides an overview of the aforementioned key molecular pathways in the acquisition of the malignant melanoma phenotype and, in so doing, identifies potential genes that may ultimately be exploited for sensitive and specific tests for reliable diagnosis of melanoma or targeted for specific therapy of the disease.

FAMILIAL MELANOMA SUSCEPTIBILITY LOCI

Major Melanoma Genes

Familial melanoma loci can be defined as those genes that, when mutated in the germ cell line and transmitted through successive generations, confer increased susceptibility to melanoma. The importance of these loci outside the setting of familial melanoma is their targeting by sporadic mutations or deletions in acquired melanoma and their position as proximally acting elements in the stepwise process of melanoma development. The relative importance of these genes also varies with the frequency with which they are targeted for mutation or deletion and the penetrance of genetic alterations in the germline at those loci. A penetrant gene is defined by a high probability of developing disease, in this case melanoma, when a mutation is present at the locus.

As noted previously, the major familial melanoma loci thus far identified are CDKN2A, CDK4, and ARF (Table 3-1). Although mutations or deletions at any of the three loci are generally quite penetrant, the relative importance as familial melanoma genes based on frequency of occurrence is CDKN2A >>> CDK4 = ARF. The gene products of each of the three loci act in the same or overlapping biochemical pathways that regulate the control of cell growth. CDKN2A and ARF are tumor-suppressor genes, and CDK4 is an protooncogene. Their isolation and the elucidation of their mechanism of action followed from the original mapping and cloning of the CDKN2A locus (2). Because of the rarity of germline defects in CDK4 and ARF as a basis for familial melanoma, the focus in this section is CDKN2A.

The CDKN2A Locus and Homologs

In familial melanoma kindreds, susceptibility to the cancer is transmitted through successive generations in accordance with Mendelian expectations for a dominant locus (1). Mapping of melanoma genes, which led to the discovery of CDKN2A, involved the use of genetic markers for loci linked to regions of the genome suspected to harbor candidate genes and, in so doing, tested the coinheritance, or co-segregation, of the markers with the occurrence of melanoma (2). Interest from several lines of experimental evidence came to be focused on chromosome 9p as a candidate region for the genomic localization of a major gene for melanoma. The evidence included the observation that a region on that chromosomal arm is a common target for nonrandom deletions in melanoma cells and for karyotypic alterations in melanocytic proliferations and was found to be the site for a stable germline chromosomal translocation in a patient with multiple

TABLE 3-1 Major familial melanoma susceptibility loci.

Genes	Frequency	Mechanism	Penetrance
CDKN2A/p16	Common	Loss of CDK4 inhibition	High
CDK4	Very rare	Resistance to p16 inhibition	High
ARF	Very rare	Loss of p53 guardian	High

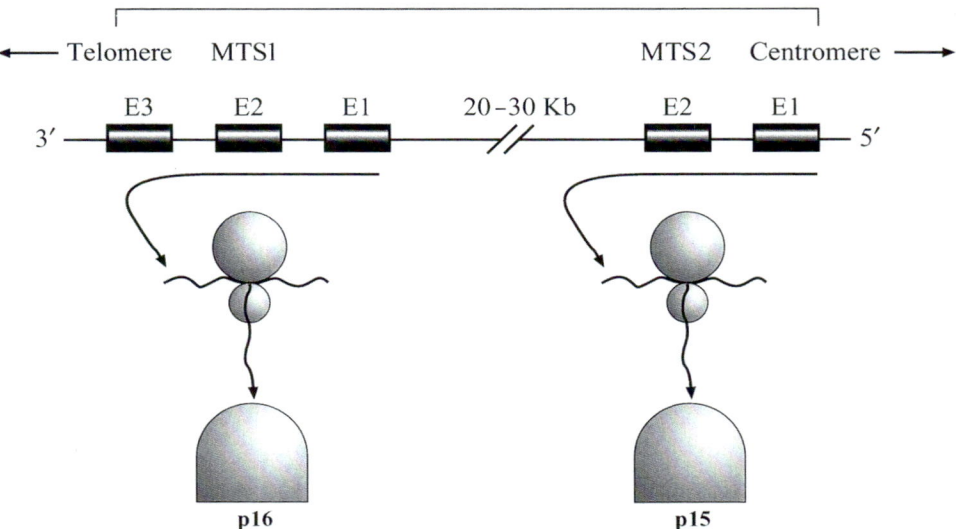

FIGURE 3-1 CDKN2A (MTS1) and its homolog CDKN2B (MTS2) are assigned to the short arm of chromosome 9p. The three exons (E) of CDKN2A and the two of CDKN2B are separated by 20–30 kilobase pairs. Their translation produces proteins of 16 and 15 kDa. (From J Am Acad Dermatol, 42, Piepkorn M., Melanoma genetics: an update with focus on the CDKN2A (p16)/ARF tumor suppressors, 705–22 (2000), with permission from Elsevier Science.)

melanomas (1,2). Genetic linkage analysis of multiple melanoma kindreds thus employed markers for the region of interest on chromosome 9p and placed the candidate locus near the interferon α cluster with a high degree of statistical confidence (5). Rapid confirmation by multiple independent groups worldwide ensued (6–9).

Experimental evidence resulting from genetic linkage analysis converged with independent molecular analyses of regulators of cell-division cycle progression, which together led to the discovery of CDKN2A as a major gene for melanoma and the elucidation of its mechanism of action (2). Pioneering research in the cell-division cycle had previously shown that progression of cells through a checkpoint at the G_1 phase of the cycle depends on molecular complexes formed from the catalytic subunit CDK4 (cyclin-dependent kinase 4) and the regulatory subunit cyclin D1. Investigators observed that CDK4 also associated as a molecular complex with an inhibitory factor of observed mass 16 kDa. Two-hybrid screening was applied to clone this inhibitor of the CDK4–cyclin D1 complexes. The cDNA of the factor (p16) was thereby isolated, permitting a determination of the nucleotide sequence of the 156-amino-acid protein (10).

In the case of melanoma, complementary research of melanoma kindreds led to the cloning and sequence analysis of the CDKN2A gene. The strategy of positional cloning with genetic markers situated along a map of chromosome 9p21 was employed in the determination of the smallest genomic region that was homozygously deleted in melanoma cell lines; candidate genes were thereby isolated from that region and tested for germline mutations in patients with familial melanoma (11). Within the 40-kilobase pair region, a gene originally designated as multiple tumor suppressor 1 (MTS1) was isolated, and the genomic structure determined. The open reading frame of MTS1 proved to be identical to the reported p16 cDNA sequence (11). Presently, the formal name assigned to the gene is CDKN2A, and the protein is designated $p16^{INK4a}$ or INK4a (Fig. 3-1; Table 3-2); for simplicity, the protein is referred to herein as p16. The cloning of the locus prompted a search for homologous genes within the human genome, of which there are three that have sufficiently conserved sequence and structural elements to indicate their evolution from a common ancestral gene. Regardless of the evolutionary relationships among these homologs, however, the evidence thus far is weak that any of them other than CDKN2A plays a significant role in melanoma (Table 3-3) (12).

TABLE 3-2 Nomenclature of p16.

Acronym	Derivation
Gene	
CDKN2A	Cyclin-dependent kinase inhibitor 2A
MTS1	Multiple tumor suppressor 1
Protein	
$p16^{INK4a}$	
INK4a	Inhibitor of kinase 4a
p16	Protein with relative mass of 16 kDa

Source: Adapted from J Am Acad Dermatol, 42, Piepkorn M., Melanoma genetics: an update with focus on the CDKN2A (p16)/ARF tumor suppressors, 705–22 (2000), with permission from Elsevier Science.

TABLE 3-3 The INK4 family.

Gene	Synonym(s)	Chromosome	Role in melanoma[a]	CDK4/6 inhibition[a]
p16	CDKN2A, MTS1, INK4a	9p21	+++	+
p15	CDKN2B, MTS2, INK4b	9p21	+/−	+
p18	INK4c	1p32	−	+
p19	INK4d	19p13	−	+

Source: Adapted from J Am Acad Dermatol, 42, Piepkorn M., Melanoma genetics: an update with focus on the CDKN2A (p16)/ARF tumor suppressors, 705–22 (2000), with permission from Elsevier Science.

[a]−, No role in melanoma development; +/−, questionable role; +++, strong role.

Genomic Structure of CDKN2A/ARF It was apparent soon after the cloning of the CDKN2A locus that the nucleotide sequence encoded not one but two potential transcripts read in staggered or alternative reading frames. Such a dual use of a nucleotide sequence is unique in mammalian genomes. The open reading frame of the CDKN2A gene itself is partitioned into exons E1α, E2, and E3, representing 150, 307, and 11 base pairs (Fig. 3-2). The alternate transcript also uses exons E2 and E3, albeit in a staggered reading frame, and initiates its transcription in unique exon, E1β, upstream from E1α (13,14). The gene, referred to as *ARF*, and its gene product of 14-kDa mass (p14^{ARF}) share no sequence homology with any other known gene.

Mutation/Deletion Analysis of CDKN2A/ARF The frequency with which a candidate gene is mutated or deleted in the germline of familial cancer patients and in sporadic cancers is a reflection of its relative importance as a cancer susceptibility locus. Accordingly, initial efforts after cloning the CDKN2A/ARF locus were focused on evaluating genetic alterations within the coding sequence in malignant cells of primary melanomas and melanoma cell lines as well as in melanoma patients' germlines. In general terms, point mutations constitute the predominant mode of CDKN2A inactivation in familial melanoma, whereas deletion is the major mechanism in sporadic melanoma cells (2). Present evidence suggests that loss or inactivation of one CDKN2A homolog occurs early in the cancer progression and that targeting of the second homolog by genetic alterations either does not occur or occurs late in tumor progression. Thus either complete inactivation of both copies or a dose deficiency, referred to as "haploinsufficiency," appears adequate in many instances to launch melanocytes on a tumorigenic pathway (2,15).

Genetic alterations at the CDKN2A locus are very common in melanoma cell lines, with a rate approximating 70% across many studies (2). Deletions are more

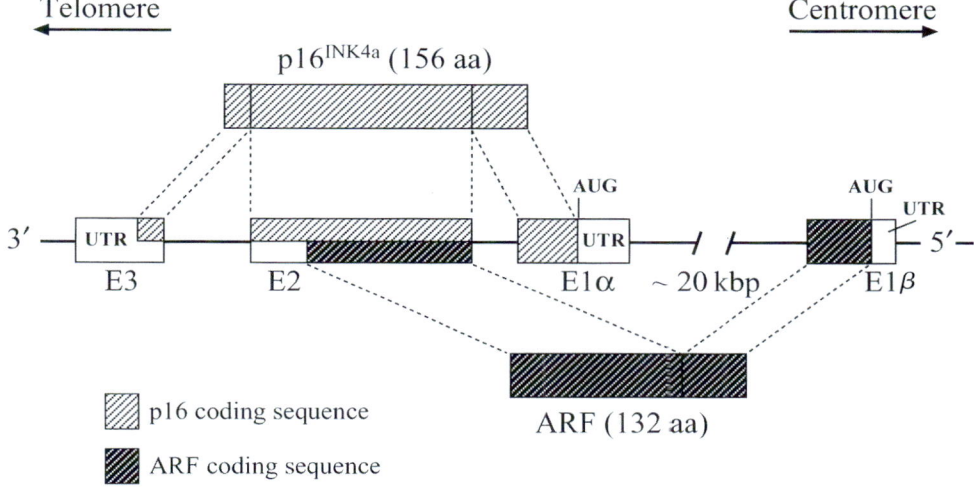

FIGURE 3-2 Genomic structure of CDKN2A and ARF. The CDKN2A locus encodes two gene products involved in cell growth regulation. Transcription from E2 is shared by CDKN2A and ARF, albeit in different reading frames. CDKN2A initiates within unique E1α and ARF within E1β, which is located approximately 20 kilobase pairs upstream of E1α. (Adapted from J Am Acad Dermatol, 42, Piepkorn M., Melanoma genetics: an update with focus on the CDKN2A (p16)/ARF tumor suppressors, 705–22 (2000), with permission from Elsevier Science.)

common in the lines than are point mutations. The latter include a broad range of missense, nonsense, frameshift, and splice junction mutations. Among these, C to T and CC to TT transitions, which are signature mutations of UV irradiation, are common in cell lines established from sporadic melanomas (16). Because melanoma cell lines may show no genetic alterations at the CDKN2A locus, compromise of the function of the gene product is not strictly necessary for neoplastic progression in the melanocytic system (2). Nonetheless, >90% of melanoma cell lines demonstrate genetic aberrations at the CDKN2A, CDKN2B (p15), or CDK4 loci (17).

Genetic alterations in cultured melanoma cell lines may reflect adaptive changes to in vitro conditions and thus may not represent the in vivo situation. Characterization of the CDKN2A gene in uncultured melanoma cells eliminates these potential artifacts. Across numerous studies, the frequency of mutation and/or deletion is approximately 36% (2). The effective rate of transcriptional silencing of CDKN2A could be much higher than this, however, due to epigenetic mechanisms such as methylation of the gene's promoter region, which has the effect of downregulating transcriptional expression of the gene (18).

Loss of CDKN2A expression in melanomas has been correlated with advanced microstage of the primary tumor at the time of diagnosis and with significantly increased risk of relapse by multivariate analysis (19), but the data across independent studies have not been completely consistent (20–22). It has been assumed that, in melanomas displaying genetic alteration(s) at CDKN2A, the targeting of the locus for inactivation is an early or initiating event in melanoma development (2). Empirical data, however, in support of this assertion have been somewhat conflicting, with reduced expression of the CDKN2A gene product in melanomas in situ by immunostaining of the protein or by detection of the corresponding mRNA in the tumor cells in some studies (21,23,24) but not in others (25,26). In melanomas in situ that lack structural lesions in the CDKN2A gene, upregulation of Id1, a transcriptional repressor of the gene, may account for reduced, but potentially reversible, expression of p16 (24). Once invasive disease has occurred, however, multiple independent analyses have confirmed progressive loss of gene expression with advancing stage of disease from primary tumor to metastasis, as a consequence of either epigenetic mechanisms (e.g., promoter methylation) or, more commonly, irreversible structural lesions within the gene (20,23–27).

Germline mutations that co-segregate with melanoma susceptibility have been found in an average of 40% of melanoma-prone families across multiple studies (2). Observed rates are likely to represent minimum estimates due to contamination of familial melanoma with sporadic cases of melanoma (28) or to methodologic insufficiency (i.e., limited sensitivity) in the detection of sequence variations. Moreover, potential mutations outside the open reading frame could account for yet more cases of familial transmission of melanoma susceptibility. Such occult genetic alterations may include, for example, sequence variations within the promoter or enchancer elements that affect transcription rates, in the intronic domains affecting mRNA processing, or in the 3'-UTR sequences that relate to transcript stability or translation efficiency (29). Promoter sequence variations that adversely affect transcription of CDKN2A, however, are apparently quite rare in well-studied populations (30), as are polymorphisms in the enhancer elements of the 3'-UTR region (12). Persons afflicted with multiple melanomas but without an apparent family history of melanoma harbor CDKN2A mutations at a frequency of 10–15% (31–33). Surprisingly, a patient has been reported with biallelic deletion at the locus but with no obvious signs of disease (34), suggesting the existence of compensatory molecular mechanisms that in some instances can circumvent the carcinogenic effect of CDKN2A inactivation.

Outside the setting of melanocytic tumors, postzygotic inactivation of the CDKN2A locus is especially common in pancreatic, esophageal, and non-small-cell lung cancers, and in certain T cell lymphomas such as mycosis fungoides (35,36). An interesting paradox, which has yet to be adequately explained, is that, with the rare exception of pancreatic carcinoma (37–40) and the even rarer exception of glioblastoma, mutant-allele-carrying members of melanoma kindreds are at increased susceptibility only to melanoma (2).

Germline mutations in CDKN2A are as a rule quite penetrant, resulting on average in the expression of melanoma in > 50% of persons inheriting a mutant allele (41). From 55% to virtually 100% of those with the specific mutations listed in Table 3-4 will ultimately acquire melanoma. The range of penetrance correlates with

TABLE 3-4 Penetrance of CDKN2A mutations in melanoma kindreds.

Mutation	Penetrance (%)
V118D	91
G93W	88
R79P	100
R50Stop	66
L24P	83
M45I	88
Q42R	67
G27A	100
Del 40	55

the deleterious effect that the specific mutation has on the ability of the gene product to bind its target molecule, CDK4 (discussed later in this chapter) (2,42–45).

Murine Knockout (Targeted Deletion) Models The CDKN2A locus has been deleted in fertilized mouse ova by the technique of homologous recombination, and the deletion was passed in the germline of these knockout mice. The mice are highly sensitive to carcinogens but tend to develop fibrosarcomas and B cell lymphomas rather than melanomas (46). However, mice bred on the CDKN2A-deficient background and genetically engineered with the activated oncogene Ha-*ras* are susceptible to spontaneous melanomas in a highly penetrant fashion (46,47). More recent studies indicate that the tumorigenic efficiency and susceptibility to exogenous carcinogens of this targeted deletion model apparently require either loss or haploinsufficiency of the ARF gene along with deletion of CDKN2A (48–50). In the genesis of melanoma, therefore, present evidence indicates that loss of function of both CDKN2A loci (p16, ARF) is determinative for disease initiation and/or progression.

The Status of CDKN2A in Melanocytic Nevi The prevailing model posits nevi as intermediate stages in melanocytic tumor progression (51). If the model is valid, genetic alterations within nevi, and more specifically atypical nevi, could represent the earliest molecular events in the development of melanoma. There is as of yet no clear consensus as to whether nevi, typical or otherwise, sustain genetic lesions at the CDKN2A locus. Several studies have evaluated the heterozygous loss (deletion) of molecular markers near the CDKN2A locus under the hypothesis that nascent nevoid tumor cells selectively inactivate that locus as a means of unleashing cell growth. Loss of heterozygosity bracketing the CDKN2A locus on chromosome 9p reportedly occurs in 17–78% of atypical (52–56) but less commonly in banal (55–57), nevi. Other studies have found no allelic loss at the locus (58). The atypical nevus phenotype (i.e., the dysplastic nevus syndrome) does not readily link genetically by the use of polymorphous markers to the CDKN2A locus (59). Data on the integrity of the CDKN2A gene itself within nevi are quite conflicting. Several reports have suggested that in atypical nevi, as in melanoma, there may be point mutations or allelic deletions in the vicinity of that critical locus on chromosome 9p (55,56,60). The reported rates of mutation or deletion at the locus have ranged from none to >30% of atypical nevi (54,58,61). On the other hand, chromosomal loss, sequence mutations in the p16 exonic sequence, and promoter methylation were not found in a detailed genetic analysis of 45 typical nevi, the data being consistent with the hypothesis that variants in the coding and noncoding regions of the p16 gene are not the major genetic determinants of the nevus phenotype (62). Further studies are therefore awaited to reliably quantify the rate of inactivation by deletion or mutation within the gene in precursor nevi.

As noted above, it has been difficult to link the atypical nevus phenotype to alterations or markers at the CDKN2A locus. Within melanoma families linked to mutations in the gene, people with atypical nevi but without histories of melanoma do not commonly carry the mutant allele within the germline (59,63,64). In melanoma families in the UK, there is a broad overlap in numbers, sizes, and clinical atypia of nevi among family members with or without a mutant allele (65,66).

At the level of gene expression, the existing data regarding the CDKN2A gene product are more consistent. Nearly all common and atypical nevi evaluated by immunostaining express p16 protein (20–23,25,26) at normal levels, and mRNA levels for the gene product are indistinguishable between common and atypical nevi (23). In contrast, p16 protein and mRNA levels are reduced in lesions of melanoma in situ (23). The latter finding in conjunction with other lines of prevailing experimental evidence supports the assertion that inactivation of the CDKN2A is an early event in the development of many melanomas. The fact that atypical nevi do not clearly share this genetic alteration may indicate that most such lesions are not formal precursors to melanoma.

Mechanisms of CDKN2A Action The products of the CDKN2A/ARF locus function in the control of cell proliferation. Somatic cells integrate and funnel a large, divergent array of intrinsic and extracellular signals acting on them into a molecular pathway broadly conserved across vertebrate evolution. The pathway regulates progression within the cell-division cycle at two major "restriction points situated at the G_1/S and G_2/M transitions. These checkpoints allow the cell to determine whether to progress through the division cycle or to withdraw to a nonproliferative state (2). Loss of control at the restriction points can lead to cell replication before repair of DNA damage, eventually giving rise to the propagation of genetically flawed cells, genomic instability, and, finally, the uncontrolled proliferation that is a hallmark of neoplasia (2).

Much of the molecular control of cell-cycle progression is integrated into gene products that act in the CDKN2A/RB pathway (Fig. 3-3). RB, the retinoblastoma gene product, is positioned as the key gatekeeper of the G_1/S cell-division cycle checkpoint. Active RB maintains cell arrest at the checkpoint by binding and thereby sequestering members of a group of transcription factors known as E2F (67–69). These factors, when released from their binding to RB, promote the transcription of genes essential for S phase DNA synthesis, such as thymidine kinase, thymidylate synthetase, DNA polymerase α, and dihidrofolate reductase (67,69). Upstream of RB are situated proteins that transmit positive (e.g., the cyclin-dependent kinases, CDK4 and CDK6) and negative (e.g., the CDK inhibitors CDKN2A, p21^{cip-1}, and p27) signals that either promote cell growth by inactivating RB or inhibit cell growth by protecting RB from inactivation, respectively (2). The CDKs are catalytic subunits of serine-threonine kinases that specifically target RB for phosphorylation, but they require for this action the cooperation of a binding partner—namely a member of the D-type cyclin family. D-type cyclins are rate-limiting growth sensors that are undetectable in quiescent cells, increase in early G_1 on stimulation of cell proliferation by growth factors, and then decrease with a short half-life during the G_1/S transition (70,71). The CDK–cyclin complex phosphorylates RB to render it inactive, resulting in the release of the E2F factors, S-phase gene synthesis, and cell-cycle progression (67,68).

CDKN2A (p16) functions in a specific RB pathway along with CDK4 and cyclin D1. It acts as a competitive inhibitor with cyclin D1 for the binding of CDK4 (Fig. 3-3) (71–73). When p16 binds CDK4, it excludes the concurrent binding of cyclin D1 due to the overlapping nature of the binding sites for p16 and cyclin D1 on CDK4 (73). The p16–CDK4 complex is catalytically inactive; RB remains in its active, nonphosphorylated state (68); and the cell is arrested at the restriction point. In cells lacking functional RB, CDKN2A mRNA accumulates owing to the presence of an autoregulatory feedback loop involving the respective proteins (74–76). Germline or acquired mutations in p16 that target the functional domains of the protein result in defective binding to CDK4, thereby shifting the equilibrium in favor of active cyclin D1–CDK4 complexes and cell-cycle progression (77,78). CDKN2A protein and mRNA are transiently upregulated in melanocytes on exposure to UV radiation, which presumably contributes to the brief growth arrest induced by the radiation (79).

Structure and Function of the Tumor Suppressor p14^{ARF}

Alternative reading frame (ARF) (p14^{ARF}), the second product of the CDKN2A locus, is widely expressed throughout somatic tissues (80). Much of its functional domain is encoded by E1β (81). It is a nucleolar and nuclear factor that largely functions outside the RB pathway in a cell-cycle-dependent fashion (Fig. 3-4) (82). Mutagenic agents acting on cells induce the expression of the 14-kDa ARF protein, most notably during S phase and

FIGURE 3-3 CDKN2A negatively regulates the kinase activity of CDK4 in the RB pathway. The retinoblastoma gene product, RB, constitutes the master gatekeeper, regulating cell passage through the G_1/S restriction point of the cell-division cycle. It does so by binding and thereby sequestering the E2F family of transcription factors required for expression of S-phase genes. Release of this blockade is effected by the kinase activity of the holoenzyme complex of cyclin D1–CDK4, which phosphorylates and thus inactivates RB, resulting in the dissociation of the E2F factors. The p16 protein functions upstream in this pathway, competing with cyclin D1 for binding of CDK4. Complexes of CDK4 and p16 are catalytically inactive, shifting the equilibrium in favor of hypophosphorylated RB, sequestration of E2F, and cell-cycle arrest. *DFHR*, dihydrofolate reductase; *TK*, thymidine kinase; *TS*, thymidylate synthetase. (Adapted from J Am Acad Dermatol, 42, Piepkorn M., Melanoma genetics: an update with focus on the CDKN2A (p16)/ARF tumor suppressors, 705–22 (2000), with permission from Elsevier Science.)

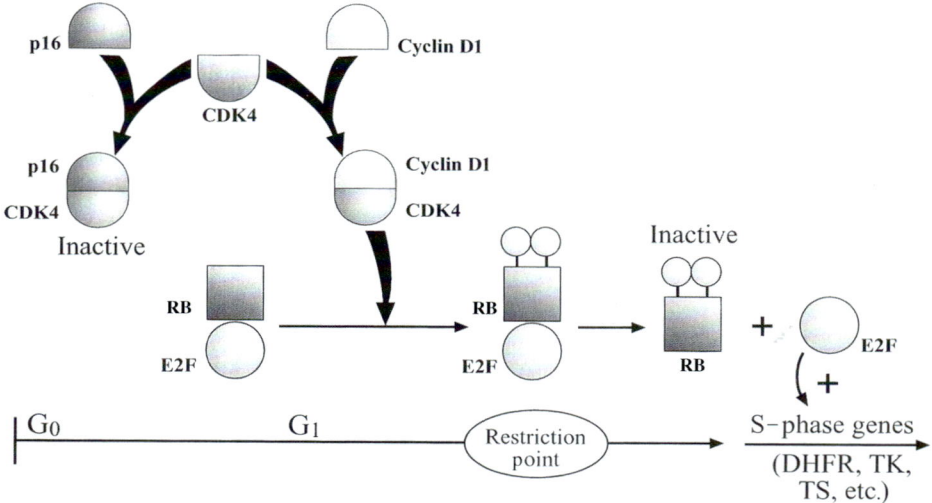

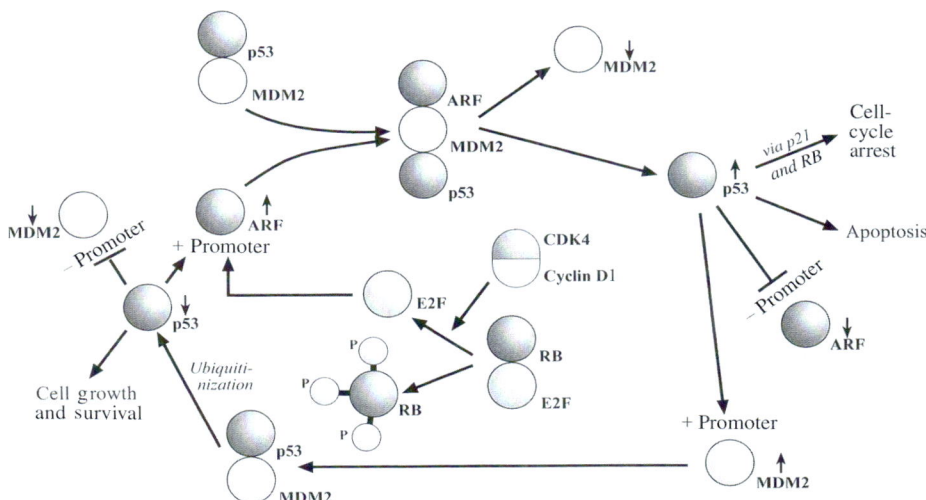

FIGURE 3-4 Multiple autoregulatory feedback loops integrate the p16/RB and ARF/p53 pathways. The pathways are linked via the E2F transcription factors. The action of active cyclin D1–CDK4 complexes dissociates E2F (*center*), which then stimulates transcription of ARF, among other effects. Upregulated ARF blocks the MDM2-mediated degradation of p53, leading to cell-cycle arrest via the intermediary action of p21^{cip-1} in the RB pathway and/or apoptosis (*right*). In an autoregulatory feedback loop, upregulated p53 executes decreased transcription of ARF and increased transcription of MDM2; the actions of the latter cause p53 depletion via the ubiquitin pathway (*left*), which in turn promotes cell growth and downregulation of MDM2. (Adapted from J Am Acad Dermatol, 42, Piepkorn M., Melanoma genetics: an update with focus on the CDKN2A (p16)/ARF tumor suppressors, 705–22 (2000), with permission from Elsevier Science.)

postmitotically, which in turn activates the factor p53 (83), counteracting the oncogenic effects of the agents. ARF exerts this effect through the binding and blockade of a factor known as MDM2, whose function it is to bind p53 and target it for degradation via the ubiquitin pathway (84). The action of ARF is thus to protect and stabilize the p53 protein (Fig. 3-4). There is an inverse correlation between expression of the ARF protein, as detected by immunostaining, and progression of melanoma, so that expression may be completely lost in metastatic tumors by promoter hypermethylation or post-transcriptional mechanisms (85). Two families have now been described in which segregating mutations in E1β of the ARF reading frame accounts for the genetic susceptibility to melanoma; in other families, mutations at the chromosome 9p21 locus outside of E1β perturb, in about 40% of all cases, the expression of both CDKN2A and ARF, thus impairing the nucleolar localization of ARF and diminishing the ability of that protein to activate the p53 pathway (86–88).

A Role for CDK4 in Familial Melanoma

A mutational hot spot in the CDK4 locus at chromosome 12q13 was originally identified in a patient with a relapsing and remitting clinical course attributed to antitumor immunity mediated by cytolytic lymphocytes specifically targeting a Arg24Cys missense mutation (89). The mutation not only created a tumor neoantigen recognized by the sensitized lymphocytes but also rendered the protein insensitive to inhibition by p16 because the amino acid substitution encoded by the mutation occurred at the binding site for the inhibitor (89). Mice genetically engineered to express the Arg24Cys-mutant CDK4 protein proved to be susceptible to the development of melanoma on carcinogenic stimulation (90). Co-segregating germline Arg24Cys and/or Arg24His mutations in CDK4 codon 24 have been identified as the basis for melanoma susceptibility in three melanoma kindreds worldwide; as with mutations in CDKN2A, the codon 24 mutation is highly penetrant, with an estimated penetrance function of 63% (91).

Less Penetrant (Minor) Familial Melanoma Genes

Minor familial genes can be defined as those that are much less penetrant in producing the neoplastic phenotype when transmitted in the germline of melanoma kindreds. The principal example of such a locus is the melanocortin 1 receptor (MC1R), the "red hair and freckle" gene. Although mutant or variant alleles at this locus confer a relatively lower enhancement of melanoma risk compared to, for example, highly penetrant CDKN2A mutants, they are much more common in the general population than are germline CDKN2A mutations (92).

Moreover, it is now apparent that important gene–gene interactions between the two loci promote the development of melanoma, probably in relation to molecular events within melanocytes following UV radiation (93).

Melanocortin 1 Receptor (MC1R) As a molecule functioning at the highest level in cutaneous melanocytes, the MC1R is the key cell membrane receptor for α melanocytic-stimulating hormone (αMSH) and related melanocortins in the skin. Both the receptor and the ligand are substantially overexpressed in melanoma cells, with up to 20-fold higher levels compared to normal melanocytes (94). The gene product is a member of a G-coupled protein family, which enhances activity of adenylate cyclase and increases intracellular concentrations of the second messenger, cyclic adenosine monophosphate (cAMP) (Fig. 3-5). It mediates the skin's pigmentary response to UV radiation, thus stimulating the autocrine and paracrine expression of αMSH by melanocytes and other cell types, augmenting melanocytic differentiation and/or proliferation, and stimulating tyrosinase activity that leads to increased melanin production (94). Expression of MC1R is controlled in part and upregulated by microphthalmia-associated transcription factor (MITF), which is a factor that also regulates the transcription of melanogenesis-related enzyme genes such as tyrosinase and tyrosine-related protein 1 (TRP-1) (95). The melanocortin family of related peptide ligands for the receptor derives from processing of pro-opiomelanocortin within the hypothalamus and at other sites (94,96). These peptides (principally αMSH) are upregulated in the skin on exposure to UV radiation and bind with high affinity to MC1R; the downstream effects of this ligand–receptor interaction determine the melanocyte's proliferative and pigmentary response to sunlight (Fig. 3-5). UV radiation upregulates the in vitro expression of p16 in melanocytes (79,97), and this upregulation is potentiated by αMSH (93); these responses presumably reflect a protective cell-cycle response within melanocytic cells to UV radiation mediated via transcription factors for CDKN2A expression on the one hand, and downstream signaling pathways following ligand engagement of the MC1R on the other (79,93). As shown by the foregoing empirical observations, the two molecular pathways provide a model for the integration of environmental (UV radiation) and genetic factors (CDKN2A, MC1R) in the protection of melanocytes from oncogenic stresses in genotypically normal individuals and in dysfunctional regulation in those persons with aberrant genotypes.

The wild type MC1R enables the high-affinity binding of the receptor with its cognate ligands. The sequence variations that constitute the common allelic variants act in an autosomal recessive fashion by loss of function of the gene product and are associated with lower affinity binding to melanocortin ligands (98). High-affinity binding of αMSH to wild type MC1R effectuates the production of dark (brown to black) eumelanin; lower-affinity binding to allelic variants generates light (yellow to red) pheomelanin, or a combination thereof (Fig. 3-6). Eumelanin is photoprotective, whereas pheomelanin is less so and generates mutagenic intermediaries on interaction with photon energy that increase UV radiation skin sensitivity. Cultured melanocytes homozygous, or in some cases heterozygous, for the allelic variants are not able to

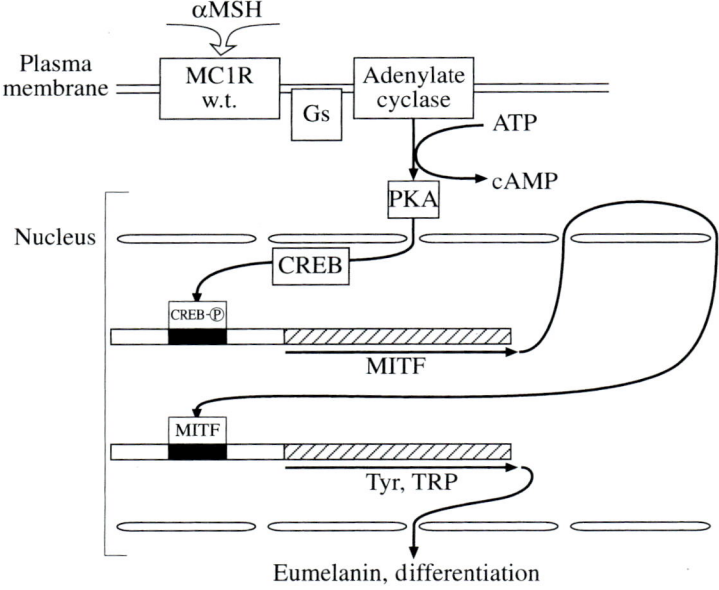

FIGURE 3-5 The MC1R and its signaling pathway. At the plasma membrane of melanocytic cells, MC1R engages αMSH and related ligands that are upregulated by autocrine and/or paracrine mechanisms after UV radiation. Downstream signaling pathways are linked to activation of adenylate cyclase, leading to upregulation of transcription factors such as cAMP-responsive element-binding protein (*CREB*), which in turn promotes the upregulation of MITF. MITF stimulates expression of tyrosinase and TRP, the net effect of which is induction of melanin synthesis. *PKA*, protein kinase A; *w.t.*, wild type. (Data from Wikberg et al., 2000.)

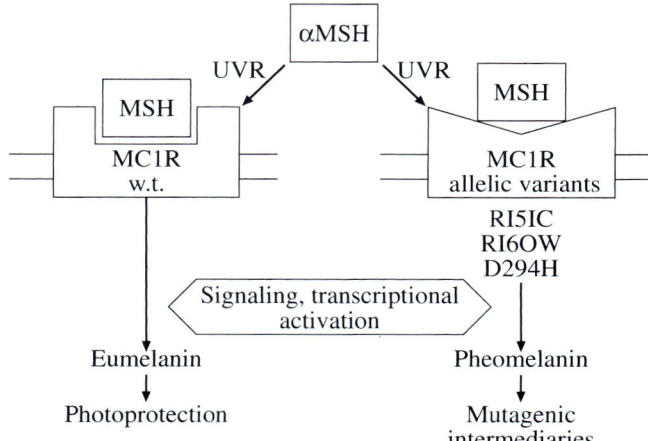

FIGURE 3-6 Generation of melanins by wild type (w.t.) and variant MC1R. Wild type and variant MC1R bind αMSH with high and low affinity, respectively. After the signaling and transcriptional events shown in Figure 3-5, photoprotective eumelanin is predominantly generated via ligand binding of wild type receptor; in contrast, mutagenic pheomelanin may be preferentially generated from ligand activation of variant MC1R receptors.

respond normally to exogenous αMSH with increased production of cAMP and tyrosinase and with increased proliferation and are more susceptible to the cytotoxic effects of UV radiation (99). The relative proportion of eumelanin and pheomelanin influences the relative risk of UV-induced skin cancer. In addition, the link between p16 upregulation by UV radiation that is potentiated by αMSH suggests that signaling upon αMSH binding to MC1R variant receptors could provide a basis for the increased risk of skin cancer associated with MC1R polymorphisms (see below) (93).

The Red Hair and Freckle Gene and the Risk of Melanoma To date, polymorphisms at just one locus, the MC1R, have been linked to physiologic variations in hair and skin color (96). The MC1R is highly polymorphous, with allelic variations from the wild type sequence estimated to be present in up to 50% of population of northern European ancestry. About 45% of the Dutch population has one allelic variant and 26% has two (compound heterozygotes) (100). The most common variants are Arg151Cys, Arg84Glu, Arg160Trp, and Asp294His, which are autosomal recessive and act in a loss-of-function fashion (101). Allelic variants are associated with red hair and freckling. Carriers of one or two variant alleles have been found to have a 3- to 11-fold increased likelihood of developing ephelids in childhood, independent of hair color and skin type; nearly all individual with ephelids are carriers of at least one MC1R gene variant (100). The attributable contribution of the variant alleles for ephelids has been estimated to be 60%. When the common variants are inherited in a homozygous fashion at the MC1R locus, the affected individual almost always has red hair (101). UV radiation sensitivity is increased in people carrying one or more variant alleles (102).

In some studies, the phenotype of red hair and inability to tan is associated with up to a fourfold increased risk of melanoma; case-controlled analyses have linked this increased relative risk to the allelic variants (96,103). For example, the Arg84Glu variant has been associated with a relative melanoma risk of 3.91 (104), and, among all known polymorphisms, the Arg84Glu variant confers the highest risk for melanoma, with an odds ratio of 16.1; this effect is largely independent of skin type and hair color (105). Some of the variant alleles (e.g., Arg151Cys) are expressed more often than expected by chance in melanoma patients harboring germline mutations in CDKN2A, suggesting that the MC1R variants increase the penetrance of the latter in individuals co-inheriting genetic lesions at both loci (106,107). In people with the CDKN2A-Leiden mutation, melanoma risk specifically increases in accordance with the number of MC1R variants in the genotype, with an odds ratio of 2.4 for each additional variant (107). In a corroborating study of a different population base, the penetrance of CDKN2A mutations increased from a mean of 50% in those persons with consensus (wild type) MC1R genotype to 84% with a co-existing MC1R variant allele such as Arg151Cys, Arg160Trp, or Asp294His (108).

Two theories have been evoked to explain the increased susceptibility to melanoma that is associated with pheomelanin production in people heterozygous or homozygous for variant alleles at the MC1R locus (109). One is that pheomelanin is simply an inferior sun block compared to eumelanin, allowing relatively greater transepidermal passage of harmful UV radiation and thus greater carcinogenic burden (109). The other posits that pheomelanin is directly harmful due to its induction of carcinogenic radicals in response to UV radiation (94,109).

DISTALLY ACTING MELANOMA LOCI INVOLVED IN METASTASIS

Oncogenes Promoting Metastasis

Foremost among its phenotypic attributes, melanoma is recognized for its propensity to widespread metastasis via lymphatic and hematogenous routes to major viscera. The genes regulating the metastatic phenotype illustrate the yin and yang paradox of the genetic elements that on the one hand serve to control metastatic spread and on the other to promote the process. In efforts to characterize major genes involved in metastasis so that novel therapies may ultimately be developed that target key control elements in the evolution of metastatic melanoma, researchers have employed the technique of cDNA microarrays. By this method, genes can be identified that are differentially expressed at high levels in tumor cell lines with high metastatic competence but at low levels in cell lines with little metastatic potential, or vice versa.

Microarrays of cDNA from murine melanoma cell lines varying in their metastatic propensity identified RhoC, fibronectin, and thymosin as candidate genes that when pathologically activated promote the process of metastasis (110). Among the three, RhoC exerted the major effect. This was shown by cDNA transection experiments that enforced high levels of expression of the RhoC gene product in cell lines normally underexpressing the gene (110). Such overexpression of RhoC by itself proved to be sufficient to convert transfected cell lines from weakly metastatic lines to ones with high metastatic propensity. Expression of a dominant-negative form of RhoC inhibited metastasis (110).

The metastasis-promoting effects of RhoC overexpression were determined to result not from increased proliferation per se but rather from increased migratory or motility properties of the transected cell lines through the extracellular matrix (110). The gene product is a GTPase. As such, it potentially could regulate many cellular processes. However, its role in controlling assembly of the actin cytoskeleton is considered to be potentially causal in its metastasis-promoting effects.

Tumor-Suppressor Genes Controlling Metastasis

Because metastasis is the most lethal phenotypic trait of a cancer, research efforts have focused on the identification of metastasis-suppressor genes, thereby providing insights into the biologic mechanisms of metastasis (111). Although it takes the coordinated effects of many genes to allow the development of metastatic colonization, it takes only one gene to block metastasis because the inability to complete any step of the metastatic process renders a cell nonmetastatic. A number of metastasis-suppressor genes have been identified to date by micro-cell-mediated chromosomal-transfer methodologies, and many more will undoubtedly be discovered in the near future (111). In the case of melanoma, a differentiation-associated molecule expressed in melanocytic cells has emerged as a potential metastasis-suppressor factor.

Melastatin exemplifies a tumor-suppressor gene that may act to reign in the metastatic spread of melanoma. Studies employing differential DNA displays of mouse melanoma tumors with varying metastatic potential identified this locus as a potential gene of interest in the control of metastatic spread within evolving melanoma lesions (112). It is a member of the tryrosinase-related protein family of calcium channel proteins and is a melanocyte-specific gene that is expressed in a differentiation-dependent fashion. Experimental upregulation of its expression is detrimental to cell proliferation.

The protein product of the gene is expressed at high levels in benign nevi and early melanoma; however, its expression is lost with disease progression in most cases, being absent or barely detectable by immunostaining and by in situ northern hybridization for melastatin mRNA in metastatic melanoma cells (112,113). Not only has the expression level been inversely correlated with tumor thickness (112) and rates of metastasis but also notably reduced levels of expression constitute an independent prognostic indicator by multivariate analysis in predicting worsening of disease-free survival in melanoma patients (114). Both the transcription and the mRNA processing of melastatin, however, can be upregulated in melanoma cells by differentiation-promoting factors (115), suggesting a potential target for novel treatment strategies.

GENES FUNCTIONING IN EVADING THE IMMUNE SYSTEM

Current understanding of melanoma progression holds that evolving melanoma clones must escape immune detection and destruction to succeed in depositing metastatic emboli that grow and develop at distant sites. The complex process of immune recognition of tumor cells and their destruction by effector cells such as T lymphocytes and natural-killer cells is beyond the scope of this chapter. Although melanomas are immunogenic and induce specific cytotoxic T lymphocytes, it is clear that melanoma cells are usually able to evade immunologic destruction. In this context, Fas (CD95) and its ligand illustrate a cellular process involved in cellular homeostasis via induction of apoptosis, which can be exploited by melanoma cells in the acquisition of the metastatic phenotype (116). Whereas nevus cells and melanocytes apparently do not express significant levels of Fas and Fas ligand (117), overexpression of these factors, along with their dysfunctional regulation, is significantly associated with the development and progression of melanoma (118,119).

Fas is a major member of the tumor necrosis factor (TNF) transmembrane family of death receptors (116). This receptor detects the presence of extracellular death signals, principally FasL. Detection occurs on engagement of the ligand by the receptor, which induces multimerization of the latter. The intracellular "death" domain of the receptor cou-

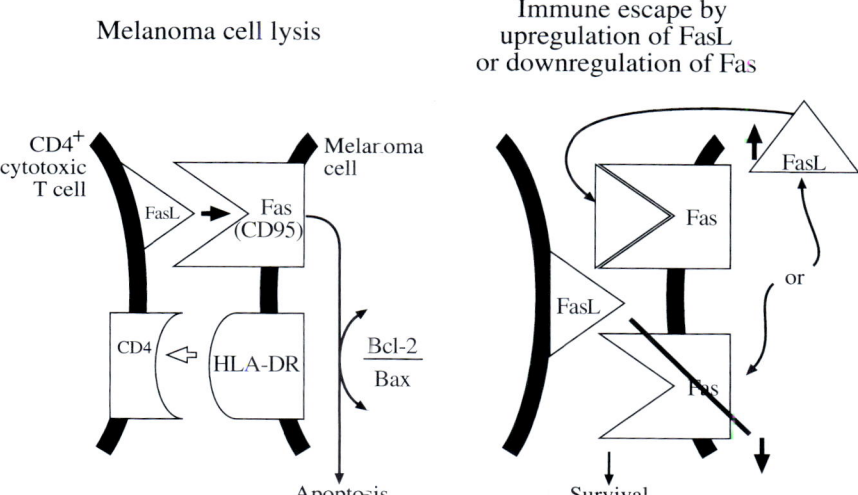

FIGURE 3-7 T cell–mediated antitumor immunity and its evasion by melanoma. Tumor cell killing via sensitized, cytolytic T cells is achieved through the Fas and FasL pathway, involving engagement of membrane-bound FasL on the lymphoid cells with Fas on the target tumor cell, coordinated with binding of MHC-related molecules by lymphocyte CD4 (*left*). Apoptotic pathways mediated by caspase factors are activated on Fas–FasL binding; the efficiency of apoptotic cell death is influenced by the relative ratio of anti-Bcl-2 and pro-Bax apoptotic factors. Melanoma cells may subvert this process either by upregulating soluble FasL as a form of molecular decoy or by downregulating expression of Fas; in either case, effective interaction of the cytolytic cell with the target cell is abrogated (*right*).

ples an adaptor molecule, Fas-associated protein with death domain (FADD), to a caspase-3,8,9 cascade that rapidly leads to cell death via apoptosis (116,120). Dysregulation of the pathway is exploited by melanoma cells for the purpose of evading antitumor immunity (Fig. 3-7) (116).

In the cell-mediated killing of melanoma cells, CD4+ cytotoxic T cells engage their target tumor cells via at least two membrane-based, ligand–receptor interactions (Fig. 3-7). Membrane CD4 on the T cell couples with major histocompatibility complex (MHC) molecules on the target cell. Concurrently, FasL at the membrane of the lymphocyte engages the Fas receptor of the melanoma cell. This coordinate binding initiates the process of receptor multimerization and activation of downstream signaling molecules, leading to apoptosis of the target cell. The efficiency of cell killing by this mechanism is regulated by two factors that function in a diametrically opposing manner. One of these, Bcl-2, acts as an antiapoptotic factor, whereas its counterpart, Bax, promotes the process of cell death; the relative levels of the two factors (i.e., the Bax/Bcl-2 ratio) thus influences the susceptibility of melanoma cells to Fas-mediated apoptosis (116,121). Low Bax/Bcl-2 ratios are characteristic of melanoma cells resistant to Fas-mediated apoptosis, and high ratios are found in melanoma cells sensitive to apoptosis by this mechanism (121).

To escape immune-mediated cell destruction via this mechanism, evolving melanoma cells can perturb the process at one of at least two levels (Fig. 3-7): the receptor, Fas, may be downregulated on the surface of melanoma cells or the cells may upregulate their own expression of soluble FasL (118,119). Fas downregulation can be achieved, in part, by upregulation in the tumor cell of the oncogenic *ras* protein, which is a membrane protein that participates in signal-transduction pathways controlling cell growth and differentiation (120). The reduction in membrane Fas resulting from the effects of oncogenic *ras* and/or other oncogenic stresses leads to less presentation of membrane receptor for engagement of cognate FasL at the cell membrane of cytotoxic cells (118). Upregulation of soluble FasL creates a competitive ligand decoy in the soluble phase that completes with lymphocyte membrane FasL for binding of Fas on the surface of melanoma cells. By either mechanism, the coordinate binding of complementary ligands and receptors on the effector and target cells is mitigated, leading to reduced rates of FasL-mediated tumor cell killing.

In a reversal of the apoptotic pathway, immune cells may also be directly destroyed by the evasive strategies of the melanoma cells to escape Fas-mediated apoptosis (117). Studies have shown that FasL expression is stronger in metastatic than in primary melanoma cells, indicating the successful exploitation of these strategies by melanoma cells. The increased levels of soluble FasL found in the plasma of metastatic melanoma patients correlates with a worsening of prognosis (119).

MOLECULAR PATHWAYS AND THE DEVELOPMENT OF MELANOMA

In this brief overview of the molecular pathology of melanoma, examples were given of molecular pathways that, when perturbed by oncogenic mutations or deletions at key genomic loci, facilitate the clonal evolution and selection of melanoma, leading to the development of the fully evolved malignant phenotype. The pathways illustrated here range from putatively initiating molecular events to mechanisms that facilitate evasion of immune-mediated tumor cell killing to counterbalancing forces that control the process of metastasis. At the level of tumor initiation are situated the familial melanoma susceptibility loci. Of these, CDKN2A (p16), CDK4, and ARF constitute the major melanoma genes because of the high rate of penetrance in individuals harboring mutations at these loci within their germ cell line. CDKN2A is by far the most prevalent target known at present for germline mutation in the setting of familial melanoma; CDK4 and ARF account for very few instances of melanoma kindreds. Minor susceptibility melanoma loci are genes that, although commonly mutated or polymorphous in the population, are much less penetrant in so far as the expression of the malignant phenotype in the individual affected by the variant genotype. Among these loci, MC1R, the red hair and freckle gene, has emerged as a gene frequently harboring sequence polymorphisms that generate proteins with less binding affinity for αMSH and related peptides. This reduction in binding affinity leads to a shift in the pattern of melanins synthesized in melanocytes on exposure to UV radiation, such that mutagenic pheomelanin, rather that photoprotective eumelanin, may preferentially be produced, increasing susceptibility to melanoma.

Other loci are involved more distally in the process of melanoma development. As such, these genes are not generally candidates for familial loci, so far as is known. The Fas/FasL pathway illustrates, on one hand, a mechanism that can lead to efficient killing of tumor cell targets by conditioned CD4 cytotoxic lymphocytes. On the other hand, however, melanomas cells have been shown to possess the ability to modulate the pathway to escape immune-mediated destruction. The cells accomplish this feat on one of at least two levels—namely upregulation of the soluble Fas ligand, which acts as a competitive ligand with the lymphocyte membrane FasL for engagement of Fas on the surface of melanoma cells, or downregulation of the receptor itself, which results in reduced coupling of cytotoxic cells with their target cells.

Other distally acting genetic elements are involved in controlling metastasis, which is the process that so often is effectively exploited by melanoma in its efforts to achieve growth advantage in the host. Positive and negative mechanisms exist in neoplastic melanocytes that control metastasis, exemplifying the dynamic taking place within transformed cells. Factors such as RhoC, an element functioning in the regulation of actin cytoskeletal assembly, is a prometastatic gene that when overexpressed contributes to enhanced mobility of melanoma cells, which is an attribute critical to metastasis. The effects of upregulated RhoC on the metastatic phenotype are counterbalanced by factors such as melastatin, which is a differentiation-associated protein whose expression is detrimental to cell proliferation. Its antiproliferative effects presumably must be circumvented for melanoma cells to begin the process of metastasis.

In general, many, if not most, melanoma genes act within or influence pathways acting on the cell-division cycle. This principal is best illustrated by the cases of CDKN2A, CDK4, and ARF. Emerging information regarding the role of the molecules expressed by these loci offers potential opportunities for developing specific therapeutic strategies that restore a semblance of normal growth control when such control is perturbed by genetic lesions within the susceptibility loci. Proof of this concept can be envisioned for CDKN2A in tumors with inactivating deletions and/or mutations at the locus. Tumor cells with unregulated growth control can be reverted to a semblance of growth regulation on transfection and enforced overexpression of wild type p16 gene product (79). Moreover, small organic molecules that structurally mimic the effects of p16 protein in the cell-division cycle have been synthesized and were shown to have antiproliferative effects in animal models (122). Such preliminary experimental achievements may bode well for future expectations in developing novel therapies that specifically exploit and target pathogenic molecular lesions within melanoma tumors.

REFERENCES

1. Piepkorn MW. Genetic basis of susceptibility to melanoma. J Am Acad Dermatol 1994;31:1022–39.
2. Piepkorn M. Melanoma genetics: an update with focus on the CDKN2A(p16)/ARF tumor suppressors. J Am Acad Dermatol 2000;42:705–22; 723–6.
3. Rocco JW, Sidransky D. p16(MTS-1/CDKN2/INK4a) in cancer progression. Exp Cell Res 2001;264:42–55.
4. Bittner M, Meltzer P, Chen Y, et al. Molecular classification of cutaneous malignant melanoma by gene expression profiling. Nature 2000;406:536–40.
5. Cannon-Albright LA, Goldgar DE, Meyer LJ, et al. Assignment of a locus for familial melanoma, MLM, to chromosome 9p13-p22. Science 1992;258:1148–52. [See Comments.]
6. Bergman W, Gruis NA, Sandkuijl LA, Frants RR. Genetics of seven Dutch familial atypical multiple mole-melanoma syndrome families: a review of linkage results including chromosomes 1 and 9. J Invest Dermatol 1994; 103:122S–5S.
7. Nancarrow DJ, Mann GJ, Holland EA, et al. Confirmation of chromosome 9p linkage in familial melanoma. Am J Hum Genet 1993;53:936–42.
8. Goldstein AM, Dracopoli NC, Engelstein M, et al. Link-

age of cutaneous malignant melanoma/dysplastic nevi to chromosome 9p, and evidence for genetic heterogeneity. Am J Hum Genet 1994;54:489–96.
9. MacGeoch C, Bishop JA, Bataille V, et al. Genetic heterogeneity in familial malignant melanoma. Hum Mol Genet 1994;3:2195–200.
10. Serrano M, Hannon GJ, Beach D. A new regulatory motif in cell-cycle control causing specific inhibition of cyclin D/CDK4. Nature 1993;366:704–7. [See Comments.]
11. Kamb A, Gruis NA, Weaver-Feldhaus J, et al. A cell cycle regulator potentially involved in genesis of many tumor types. Science 1994;264:436–40. [See Comments.]
12. Kumar R, Smeds J, Berggren P, et al. A single nucleotide polymorphism in the 3′ untranslated region of the CDKN2A gene is common in sporadic primary melanomas but mutations in the CDKN2B, CDKN2C, CDK4 and p53 genes are rare. Int J Cancer 2001;95:388–93.
13. Stone S, Jiang P, Dayananth P, et al. Complex structure and regulation of the P16 (MTS1) locus. Cancer Res 1995;55:2988–94.
14. Mao L, Merlo A, Bedi G, et al. A novel p16INK4A transcript. Cancer Res 1995;55:2995–7.
15. Glendening JM, Flores JF, Walker GJ, et al. Homozygous loss of the p15INK4B gene (and not the p16INK4 gene) during tumor progression in a sporadic melanoma patient. Cancer Res 1995;55:5531–5.
16. Liu Q, Neuhausen S, McClure M, et al. CDKN2 (MTS1) tumor suppressor gene mutations in human tumor cell lines. Oncogene 1995;10:1061–7. [See Erratum, 1995;11:2455.]
17. Walker GJ, Flores JF, Glendening JM, et al. Virtually 100% of melanoma cell lines harbor alterations at the DNA level within CDKN2A, CDKN2B, or one of their downstream targets. Genes Chromosomes Cancer 1998;22:157–63.
18. Gonzalgo ML, Bender CM, You EH, et al. Low frequency of p16/CDKN2A methylation in sporadic melanoma: comparative approaches for methylation analysis of primary tumors. Cancer Res 1997;57:5336–47.
19. Straume O, Akslen LA. Alterations and prognostic significance of p16 and p53 protein expression in subgroups of cutaneous melanoma. Int J Cancer 1997;74:535–9.
20. Grover R, Chana JS, Wilson GD, et al. An analysis of p16 protein expression in sporadic malignant melanoma. Melanoma Res 1998;8:267–72.
21. Talve L, Sauroja I, Collan Y, et al. Loss of expression of the p16INK4/CDKN2 gene in cutaneous malignant melanoma correlates with tumor cell proliferation and invasive stage. Int J Cancer 1997;74:255–9.
22. Funk JO, Schiller PI, Barrett MT, et al. p16INK4a expression is frequently decreased and associated with 9p21 loss of heterozygosity in sporadic melanoma. J Cutan Pathol 1998;25:291–6.
23. Keller-Melchior R, Schmidt R, Piepkorn M. Expression of the tumor suppressor gene product p16INK4 in benign and malignant melanocytic lesions. J Invest Dermatol 1998;110:932–8.
24. Polsky D, Young AZ, Busam KJ, Alani RM. The transcriptional repressor of p16/Ink4a, Id1, is up-regulated in early melanomas. Cancer Res 2001;61:6008–11.
25. Reed JA, Loganzo F Jr, Shea CR, et al. Loss of expression of the p16/cyclin-dependent kinase inhibitor 2 tumor suppressor gene in melanocytic lesions correlates with invasive stage of tumor progression. Cancer Res 1995;55:2713–8.
26. Sparrow LE, Eldon MJ, English DR, Heenan PJ. p16 and p21WAF1 protein expression in melanocytic tumors by immunohistochemistry. Am J Dermatopathol 1998;20:255–61.
27. Zhang H, Schneider J, Rosdahl I. Expression of p16, p27, p53, p73 and Nup88 proteins in matched primary and metastatic melanoma cells. Int J Oncol 2002;21:43–8.
28. Flores JF, Pollock PM, Walker GJ, et al. Analysis of the CDKN2A, CDKN2B and CDK4 genes in 48 Australian melanoma kindreds. Oncogene 1997;15:2999–3005.
29. Borg A, Johannsson U, Johannsson O, et al. Novel germline p16 mutation in familial malignant melanoma in southern Sweden. Cancer Res 1996;56:2497–500.
30. Pollock PM, Stark MS, Palmer JM, et al. Mutation analysis of the CDKN2A promoter in Australian melanoma families. Genes Chromosomes Cancer 2001;32:89–94.
31. Monzon J, Liu L, Brill H, et al. CDKN2A mutations in multiple primary melanomas. N Engl J Med 1998;338:879–87. [See Comments.]
32. Auroy S, Avril MF, Chompret A, et al. Sporadic multiple primary melanoma cases: CDKN2A germline mutations with a founder effect. Genes Chromosomes Cancer 2001;32:195–202.
33. Hashemi J, Platz A, Ueno T, et al. CDKN2A germ-line mutations in individuals with multiple cutaneous melanomas. Cancer Res 2000;60:6864–7.
34. Gruis NA, van der Velden PA, Sandkuijl LA, et al. Homozygotes for CDKN2 (p16) germline mutation in Dutch familial melanoma kindreds. Nat Genet 1995;10:351–3.
35. Zhang SY, Klein-Szanto AJ, Sauter ER, et al. Higher frequency of alterations in the p16/CDKN2 gene in squamous cell carcinoma cell lines than in primary tumors of the head and neck. Cancer Res 1994;54:5050–3.
36. Spruck CH III, Gonzalez-Zulueta M, Shibata A, et al. p16 gene in uncultured tumours [Letter]. Nature 1994;370:183–4. [See Comments.]
37. Goldstein AM, Fraser MC, Struewing JP, et al. Increased risk of pancreatic cancer in melanoma-prone kindreds with p16INK4 mutations. N Engl J Med 1995;333:970–4. [See Comments.]
38. Whelan AJ, Bartsch D, Goodfellow PJ. Brief report: a familial syndrome of pancreatic cancer and melanoma with

a mutation in the CDKN2 tumor-suppressor gene. N Engl J Med 1995;333:975–7. [See Comments.]
39. Ciotti P, Strigini P, Bianchi-Scarra G. Familial melanoma and pancreatic cancer. Ligurian Skin Tumor Study Group [Letter]. N Engl J Med 1996;334:469–70. [See Comment; see Discussion, 1996;334:471–2.]
40. Hille ET, van Duijn E, Gruis NA, et al. Excess cancer mortality in six Dutch pedigrees with the familial atypical multiple mole-melanoma syndrome from 1830 to 1994. J Invest Dermatol 1998;110:788–92.
41. Bishop DT, Demenais F, Goldstein AM, et al. Geographical variation in the penetrance of CDKN2A mutations for melanoma. J Natl Cancer Inst 2002;94:894–903.
42. Walker GJ, Hussussian CJ, Flores JF, et al. Mutations of the CDKN2/p16INK4 gene in Australian melanoma kindreds. Hum Mol Genet 1995;4:1845–52.
43. Liu L, Lassam NJ, Slingerland JM, et al. Germline p16INK4A mutation and protein dysfunction in a family with inherited melanoma. Oncogene 1995;11:405–12.
44. Reymond A, Brent R. p16 proteins from melanoma-prone families are deficient in binding to CDK4. Oncogene 1995;11:1173–8.
45. Ranade K, Hussussian CJ, Sikorski RS, et al. Mutations associated with familial melanoma impair p16INK4 function [Letter]. Nat Genet 1995;10:114–6.
46. Serrano M, Lee H, Chin L, et al. Role of the INK4a locus in tumor suppression and cell mortality. Cell 1996;85:27–37.
47. Chin L, Pomerantz J, Polsky D, et al. Cooperative effects of INK4a and ras in melanoma susceptibility in vivo. Genes Dev 1997;11:2822–34.
48. Sharpless NE, Bardeesy N, Lee KH, et al. Loss of p16Ink4a with retention of p19Arf predisposes mice to tumorigenesis. Nature 2001;413:86–91.
49. Krimpenfort P, Quon KC, Mooi WJ, et al. Loss of p16Ink4a confers susceptibility to metastatic melanoma in mice. Nature 2001;413:83–6.
50. Walker GJ, Hayward NK. p16INK4A and p14ARF tumour suppressors in melanoma: lessons from the mouse. Lancet 2002;359:7–8.
51. Clark WH Jr, Elder DE, Guerry D, et al. A study of tumor progression: the precursor lesions of superficial spreading and nodular melanoma. Hum Pathol 1984;15:1147–65.
52. Cowan JM, Halaban R, Francke U. Cytogenetic analysis of melanocytes from premalignant nevi and melanomas. J Natl Cancer Inst 1988;80:1159–64.
53. Parmiter AH, Nowell PC. The cytogenetics of human malignant melanoma and premalignant lesions. Cancer Treat Res 1988;43:47–61.
54. Lee JY, Dong SM, Shin MS, et al. Genetic alterations of p16INK4a and p53 genes in sporadic dysplastic nevus. Biochem Biophys Res Commun 1997;237:667–72.
55. Boni R, Zhuang Z, Albuquerque A, et al. Loss of heterozygosity detected on 1p and 9q in microdissected atypical nevi [Letter]. Arch Dermatol 1998;134:882–3.
56. Park WS, Vortmeyer AO, Pack S, et al. Allelic deletion at chromosome 9p21(p16) and 17p13(p53) in microdissected sporadic dysplastic nevus. Hum Pathol 1998;29:127–30.
57. Wang Y, Becker D. Differential expression of the cyclin-dependent kinase inhibitors p16 and p21 in the human melanocytic system. Oncogene 1996;12:1069–75.
58. Matsumura Y, Nishigori C, Miyachi Y. Analysis of the p16 gene status of non-familial dysplastic nevus syndrome patients. Arch Dermatol Res 2001;293:540–2.
59. Puig S, Ruiz A, Castel T, et al. Inherited susceptibility to several cancers but absence of linkage between dysplastic nevus syndrome and CDKN2A in a melanoma family with a mutation in the CDKN2A (P16INK4A) gene. Hum Genet 1997;101:359–64.
60. Birindelli S, Tragni G, Bartoli C, et al. Detection of microsatellite alterations in the spectrum of melanocytic nevi in patients with or without individual or family history of melanoma. Int J Cancer 2000;86:255–61.
61. Healy E, Sikkink S, Rees JL. Infrequent mutation of p16INK4 in sporadic melanoma. J Invest Dermatol 1996;107:318–21. [See Comments.]
62. Welch J, Millar D, Goldman A, et al. Lack of genetic and epigenetic changes in CDKN2A in melanocytic nevi. J Invest Dermatol 2001;117:383–4.
63. Gruis NA, Sandkuijl LA, van der Velden PA, et al. CDKN2 explains part of the clinical phenotype in Dutch familial atypical multiple-mole melanoma (FAMMM) syndrome families. Melanoma Res 1995;5:169–77.
64. Hashemi J, Linder S, Platz A, Hansson J. Melanoma development in relation to non-functional p16/INK4A protein and dysplastic naevus syndrome in Swedish melanoma kindreds. Melanoma Res 1999;9:21–30.
65. Harland M, Meloni R, Gruis N, et al. Germline mutations of the CDKN2 gene in UK melanoma families. Hum Mol Genet 1997;6:2061–7.
66. Wachsmuth RC, Harland M, Bishop JA. The atypical-mole syndrome and predisposition to melanoma [letter]. N Engl J Med 1998;339:348–9.
67. Nevins JR. E2F: a link between the Rb tumor suppressor protein and viral oncoproteins. Science 1992;258:424–9.
68. Schulze A, Zerfass K, Spitkovsky D, et al. Activation of the E2F transcription factor by cyclin D1 is blocked by p16INK4, the product of the putative tumor suppressor gene MTS1. Oncogene 1994;9:3475–82.
69. Johnson DG. Regulation of E2F-1 gene expression by p130 (Rb2) and D-type cyclin kinase activity. Oncogene 1995;11:1685–92.
70. Soucek T, Pusch O, Hengstschlager-Ottnad E, et al. Expression of the cyclin-dependent kinase inhibitor p16 during the ongoing cell cycle. FEBS Lett 1995;373:164–9.

71. Hall M, Bates S, Peters G. Evidence for different modes of action of cyclin-dependent kinase inhibitors: p15 and p16 bind to kinases, p21 and p27 bind to cyclins. Oncogene 1995;11:1581–8.
72. Ragione FD, Russo GL, Oliva A, et al. Biochemical characterization of p16INK4- and p18-containing complexes in human cell lines. J Biol Chem 1996;271:15942–9.
73. Coleman KG, Wautlet BS, Morrissey D, et al. Identification of CDK4 sequences involved in cyclin D1 and p16 binding. J Biol Chem 1997;272:18869–74.
74. Tam SW, Shay JW, Pagano M. Differential expression and cell cycle regulation of the cyclin-dependent kinase 4 inhibitor p16Ink4. Cancer Res 1994;54:5816–20.
75. Li Y, Nichols MA, Shay JW, Xiong Y. Transcriptional repression of the D-type cyclin-dependent kinase inhibitor p16 by the retinoblastoma susceptibility gene product pRb. Cancer Res 1994;54:6078–82.
76. Hara E, Smith R, Parry D, et al. Regulation of p16CDKN2 expression and its implications for cell immortalization and senescence. Mol Cell Biol 1996;16:859–67.
77. Zhang B, Peng Z. Defective folding of mutant p16(INK4) proteins encoded by tumor-derived alleles. J Biol Chem 1996;271:28734–7.
78. Wick ST, Dubay MM, Imanil I, Brizuela L. Biochemical and mutagenic analysis of the melanoma tumor suppressor gene product/p16. Oncogene 1995;11:2013–9.
79. Piepkorn M. The expression of p16(INK4a), the product of a tumor suppressor gene for melanoma, is upregulated in human melanocytes by UVB irradiation. J Am Acad Dermatol 2000;42:741–5.
80. Quelle DE, Zindy F, Ashmun RA, Sherr CJ. Alternative reading frames of the INK4a tumor suppressor gene encode two unrelated proteins capable of inducing cell cycle arrest. Cell 1995;83:993–1000.
81. Zindy F, Quelle DE, Roussel MF, Sherr CJ. Expression of the p16INK4a tumor suppressor versus other INK4 family members during mouse development and aging. Oncogene 1997;15:203–11.
82. David-Pfeuty T, Nouvian-Dooghe Y. Human p14(Arf): an exquisite sensor of morphological changes and of short-lived perturbations in cell cycle and in nucleolar function. Oncogene 2002;21:6779–90.
83. Palmero I, Pantoja C, Serrano M. p19ARF links the tumour suppressor p53 to Ras [Letter]. Nature 1998;395:125–6.
84. Pomerantz J, Schreiber-Agus N, Liegeois NJ, et al. The Ink4a tumor suppressor gene product, p19Arf, interacts with MDM2 and neutralizes MDM2's inhibition of p53. Cell 1998;92:713–23.
85. Dobrowolski R, Hein R, Buettner R, Bosserhoff AK. Loss of p14ARF expression in melanoma. Arch Dermatol Res 2002;293:545–51.
86. Randerson-Moor JA, Harland M, Williams S, et al. A germline deletion of p14(ARF) but not CDKN2A in a melanoma-neural system tumour syndrome family. Hum Mol Genet 2001;10:55–62.
87. Rizos H, Darmanian AP, Holland EA, et al. Mutations in the INK4a/ARF melanoma susceptibility locus functionally impair p14ARF. J Biol Chem 2001;276:41424–34.
88. Hewitt C, Lee Wu C, et al. Germline mutation of ARF in a melanoma kindred. Hum Mol Genet 2002;11:1273–9.
89. Wolfel T, Hauer M, Schneider J, et al. A p16INK4a-insensitive CDK4 mutant targeted by cytolytic T lymphocytes in a human melanoma. Science 1995;269:1281–4.
90. Sotillo R, Garcia JF, Ortega S, et al. Invasive melanoma in Cdk4-targeted mice. Proc Natl Acad Sci USA 2001;98:13312–7.
91. Goldstein AM, Chidambaram A, Halpern A, et al. Rarity of CDK4 germline mutations in familial melanoma. Melanoma Res 2002;12:51–5.
92. Box NF, Duffy DL, Chen W, et al. MC1R genotype modifies risk of melanoma in families segregating CDKN2A mutations. Am J Hum Genet 2001;69:765–73.
93. Pavey S, Gabrielli B. Alpha-melanocyte stimulating hormone potentiates p16/CDKN2A expression in human skin after ultraviolet irradiation. Cancer Res 2002;62:875–80.
94. Wikberg JE, Muceniece R, Mandrika I, et al. New aspects on the melanocortins and their receptors. Pharmacol Res 2000;42:393–420.
95. Aoki H, Moro O. Involvement of microphthalmia-associated transcription factor (MITF) in expression of human melanocortin-1 receptor (MC1R). Life Sci 2002;71:2171–9.
96. Schaffer JV, Bolognia JL. The melanocortin-1 receptor: red hair and beyond. Arch Dermatol 2001;137:1477–85.
97. Pavey S, Conroy S, Russell T, Gabrielli B. Ultraviolet radiation induces p16CDKN2A expression in human skin. Cancer Res 1999;59:4185–9.
98. Jimenez-Cervantes C, Olivares C, Gonzalez P, et al. The Pro162 variant is a loss-of-function mutation of the human melanocortin 1 receptor gene. J Invest Dermatol 2001;117:156–8.
99. Scott MC, Wakamatsu K, Ito S, et al. Human melanocortin 1 receptor variants, receptor function and melanocyte response to UV radiation. J Cell Sci 2002;115:2349–55.
100. Bastiaens M, ter Huurne J, Gruis N, et al. The melanocortin-1-receptor gene is the major freckle gene. Hum Mol Genet 2001;10 1701–8.
101. Flanagan N, Healy E, Ray A, et al. Pleiotropic effects of the melanocortin 1 receptor (MC1R) gene on human pigmentation. Hum Mol Genet 2000;9:2531–7.
102. Flanagan N, Ray AJ, Todd C, et al. The relation between melanocortin 1 receptor genotype and experimentally assessed ultraviolet radiation sensitivity. J Invest Dermatol 2001;117:1314–7.

103. Palmer JS, Duffy DL, Box NF, et al. Melanocortin-1 receptor polymorphisms and risk of melanoma: is the association explained solely by pigmentation phenotype? Am J Hum Genet 2000;66:176–86.
104. Valverde P, Healy E, Sikkink S, et al. The Asp84Glu variant of the melanocortin 1 receptor (MC1R) is associated with melanoma. Hum Mol Genet 1996;5:1663–6.
105. Kennedy C, ter Huurne J, Berkhout M, et al. Melanocortin 1 receptor (MC1R) gene variants are associated with an increased risk for cutaneous melanoma which is largely independent of skin type and hair color. J Invest Dermatol 2001;117:294–300.
106. Gruis NA, van der Velden PA, Sandkuijl LA, et al. Variants of the melanocyte-stimulating hormone receptor gene modify melanoma risk in familial atypical multiple mole-melanoma (FAMMM) syndrome families. Melanoma Res 1997;7(Suppl 1):S9.
107. van der Velden PA, Sandkuijl LA, Bergman W, et al. Melanocortin-1 receptor variant R151C modifies melanoma risk in Dutch families with melanoma. Am J Hum Genet 2001;69:774–9.
108. Bates S, Phillips AC, Clark PA, et al. p14ARF links the tumour suppressors RB and p53 [Letter]. Nature 1998;395:124–5.
109. Ha T, Rees JL. Melanocortin 1 receptor: what's red got to do with it? J Am Acad Dermatol 2001;45:961–4.
110. Clark EA, Golub TR, Lander ES, Hynes RO. Genomic analysis of metastasis reveals an essential role for RhoC. Nature 2000;406:532–5.
111. Yoshida BA, Sokoloff MM, Welch DR, Rinker-Schaeffer CW. Metastasis-suppressor genes: a review and perspective on an emerging field. J Natl Cancer Inst 2000;92:1717–30.
112. Duncan LM, Deeds J, Hunter J, et al. Down-regulation of the novel gene melastatin correlates with potential for melanoma metastasis. Cancer Res 1998;58:1515–20.
113. Deeds J, Cronin F, Duncan LM. Patterns of melastatin mRNA expression in melanocytic tumors. Hum Pathol 2000;31:1346–56.
114. Duncan LM, Deeds J, Cronin FE, et al. Melastatin expression and prognosis in cutaneous malignant melanoma. J Clin Oncol 2001;19:568–76.
115. Fang D, Setaluri V. Expression and Up-regulation of alternatively spliced transcripts of melastatin, a melanoma metastasis-related gene, in human melanoma cells. Biochem Biophys Res Commun 2000;279:53–61.
116. Wehrli P, Viard I, Bullani R, et al. Death receptors in cutaneous biology and disease. J Invest Dermatol 2000;115:141–8.
117. Shukuwa T, Katayama I, Koji T. Fas-mediated apoptosis of melanoma cells and infiltrating lymphocytes in human malignant melanomas. Mod Pathol 2002;15:387–96.
118. Bullani RR, Wehrli P, Viard-Leveugle I, et al. Frequent downregulation of Fas (CD95) expression and function in melanoma. Melanoma Res 2002;12:263–70.
119. Redondo P, Solano T, Vazquez B, et al. Fas and Fas ligand: expression and soluble circulating levels in cutaneous malignant melanoma. Br J Dermatol 2002;147:80–6.
120. Urquhart JL, Meech SJ, Marr DG, et al. Regulation of Fas-mediated apoptosis by N-ras in melanoma. J Invest Dermatol 2002;119:556–61.
121. Raisova M, Hossini AM, Eberle J, et al. The Bax/Bcl-2 ratio determines the susceptibility of human melanoma cells to CD95/Fas-mediated apoptosis. J Invest Dermatol 2001;117:333–40.
122. Davis ST, Benson BG, Bramson HN, et al. Prevention of chemotherapy-induced alopecia in rats by CDK inhibitors. Science 2001;291:134–7.

CHAPTER 4

Circumscribed Pigmented Lesions Composed of Basilar Melanocytes

Raymond L. Barnhill

FRECKLES (EPHELIDES)

Ephelides are small, well-circumscribed pigmented macules found only on sun-exposed skin (1–5). Ephelides are common in individuals with fair skin color (phototypes 1 and 2) (1), especially in combination with blond or red hair. They are not present at birth but usually appear in the first few years of life. However, the tendency to develop ephelides decreases with advancing age. An autosomal dominant inheritance is possible since freckling can be seen in some families over generations (1). Recently, a significant association has been shown between melanocortin 1 receptor (MC1R) gene variants and the propensity to develop ephelides (6). The carriers of 1 and 2 MC1R gene variants (there are currently some 27 MC1R gene variants) demonstrated a 3- and 11-fold risk for developing freckles, respectively (both $p < .0001$). The latter relationships are independent of skin phenotype and hair color and are comparable in individuals with and without a history of skin cancer (6).

Rhodes et al. (3) suggested that some ephelides may overlap or represent a subtype of solar lentigo (Table 4-1). There is also a relationship of solar lentigines to MC1R gene variants, although not as strong as with freckles. The lesions studied by Rhodes et al. exhibited melanocytic hyperplasia and occasional cytologic atypia, features shared with solar lentigo. Further studies are needed to clarify the significance of the latter findings. Clinically, ephelides become less prominent with age, but even when clinically inapparent in older individuals under ordinary light, they remain visible upon Wood's lamp examination (4).

Clinical Features

Ephelides occur only on sun-exposed areas of the body, mainly on the face, the dorsal aspects of the arms, and the upper part of the chest and the back (Table 4-1). Ephelides are poorly demarcated, round, oval, or irregular macules; they are usually 1–3 mm in diameter, but some may be several millimeters in diameter. Depending on the intensity of sun exposure, they vary in color from light to dark brown, but almost never become as dark as lentigines or junctional nevi; they may increase in number and distribution and show a tendency to confluency.

Histopathological Features

The epidermis exhibits a normal configuration. The keratinocytes show an increase in melanin content, predominantly in the basal cell layer (Fig. 4-1). Occasionally, melanophages are seen in the papillary dermis. The number of melanocytes in ephelides do not differ significantly from normal. However, examination of DOPA-stained sections has been reported to show both significantly fewer melanocytes (5) and an increased number of melanocytes per unit area in ephelides (3). The differences in the latter results are probably related to examination of epidermal sheets en face (5) versus standard vertical histologic sections (3). The melanocytes in ephelides are larger, have more branching of dendrites, and have a higher DOPA-positivity than those in adjacent normal epidermis, apparently indicating greater functional activity.

Differential Diagnosis

Histologically, the freckle cannot be distinguished from café-au-lait macule, melanotic macule of Albright, and melasma. Discrimination of freckle from the latter entities must be based solely on clinical findings. The solar and simple lentigines may also enter into the differential diagnosis of freckle (Table 4-1). The simple lentigo differs from the freckle by showing elongated epidermal rete ridges and melanocytic hyperplasia. The solar lentigo usually has prominently club-shaped rete; melanocytic hyperplasia may or may not be present.

TABLE 4-1 Freckles, solar lentigo, and lentigo simplex.

Characteristic	Freckles (ephelides)	Solar lentigo	Lentigo simplex
Clinical features			
Onset	Early childhood	Often >30 years	Childhood, adolescence, later
Skin phototypes	1 and 2 (Celtic), common		All
Sun exposure	Responsive to sun exposure; tendency to fade	Follows repeated sun exposure; persistent	Some probably related to sun exposure; persistent
Size of macules	1–3 mm	5–15 mm or larger	Usually 1–5 mm
Color	Light to medium brown	Medium to dark brown	Light, medium, dark brown; black
Shape	Round; polycyclic	Round, oval, polycyclic	Homogenous pigment pattern
Borders	Jagged; poorly defined	Regular or slightly irregular	Round, oval; symmetric; regular borders; well circumscribed
Location	On all sun-exposed areas, face, forearms, back	Sun-exposed skin, face, neck, forearms, dorsal hands	Anywhere, including sun-protected skin
Histopathological features			
Epidermis	Normal configuration	Elongated, club-shaped epidermal rete ridges; often anastomosing	Elongated, club-shaped epidermal rete ridges
Basal layer	Hyperpigmentation of epidermis	Hyperpigmentation of epidermis; accentuated on lower poles of rete ridges	Hyperpigmentation; accentuated lower poles of rete
Basilar melanocytes	Reduced, normal, or slightly increased numbers	Normal or increased in frequency	Increased numbers, concentrated on tips of rete ridges
Melanophages	In papillary dermis	In papillary dermis	In papillary dermis
Other		Solar elastosis, common; some degree of cytologic atypia of melanocytes, occasionally; transition to large-cell acanthoma, occasionally; transition to reticulated seborrheic keratosis, occasionally; transition to lichenoid keratosis occasionally,	
Differential diagnosis	Café-au-lait macule; melasma; solar lentigo; simple lentigo	Freckle; pigmented actinic keratosis; lentigo simplex; solar intraepidermal melanocytic proliferation, with atypia; melanoma in situ	Freckle; café-au-lait macule; Becker's nevus (melanosis); solar lentigo; lentiginous junctional nevus, with or without atypia

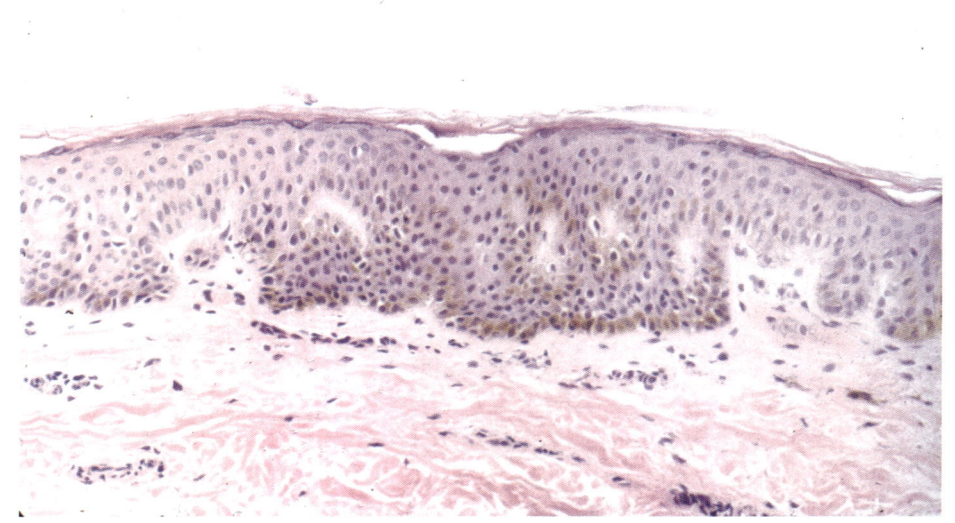

FIGURE 4-1 Freckle. There is basal layer hyperpigmentation in an otherwise unremarkable epidermis. The number of basilar melanocytics do not appear to be significantly increased. (Courtesy of Dr. A.R. Rhodes.)

CAFE-AU-LAIT MACULE

Café-au-lait macules (CALMs) are well-circumscribed, uniformly light to dark brown spots (Table 4-2). CALMs can occur as isolated lesions or as multiple lesions; the latter may be a marker for multisystem disease and can occur in various syndromes (7–18). Single CALMs are found in 10–20% of the normal population, and about 1% of all healthy young adults have up to three CALMs. They may be present at birth but usually develop in early childhood and increase in size with age. CALMs grow proportionately to body growth and remain stable in size after body growth has ceased. They demonstrate no tendency toward malignancy.

Clinical Features

The term *café-au-lait* refers to these lesions' characteristic homogeneous color of coffee with milk, which can be light to dark brown. CALMs are completely flat and often have an oval morphology; the margins are well defined and usually regular. They may be located anywhere on the body, except the mucous membranes. CALMs are usually 2.0–5.0 cm in diameter in adults, but may vary from freckle-like lesions of < 2.0 mm) to macules of > 20 cm in size.

Histopathological Features

The epidermis has a normal configuration with slightly increased melanin content in the basilar keratinocytes (Fig. 4-2). The number of melanocytes is normal or slightly increased. The adnexal epithelium is spared of hyperpigmentation and only rarely does one see melanophages in the upper dermis. In DOPA-stained epidermis from most patients with neurofibromatosis the density of melanocytes is higher in both CALM and normal adjacent skin, in comparison to healthy individuals (10). The melanocytic density in isolated CALM of otherwise normal persons, however, is usually less than in surrounding skin (11). Melanin macroglobules (large pigment particles) which may be found in CALM are not specific for neurofibromatosis as they are occasionally found in isolated CALM without underlying disease and occur in several other conditions such as simple lentigines, Becker's

TABLE 4-2 Café-au-lait macule.

Clinical features
- Onset in childhood
- Single CALM: 10–20% of population
- Associated with neurofibromatosis and other multisystem diseases
- 2–5 cm oval macules
- Well defined
- Usually regular borders
- Homogenous light to dark brown

Histopathological features
- Normal configuration of epidermis
- Increased melanin in basilar keratinocytes
- Normal or slightly increased number of basilar melanocytes

Differential diagnosis
- Freckle
- Melasma

FIGURE 4-2 Café-au-lait macule. The lesion is characterized by a normal configuration of the epidermis and basal layer hyperpigmentation.

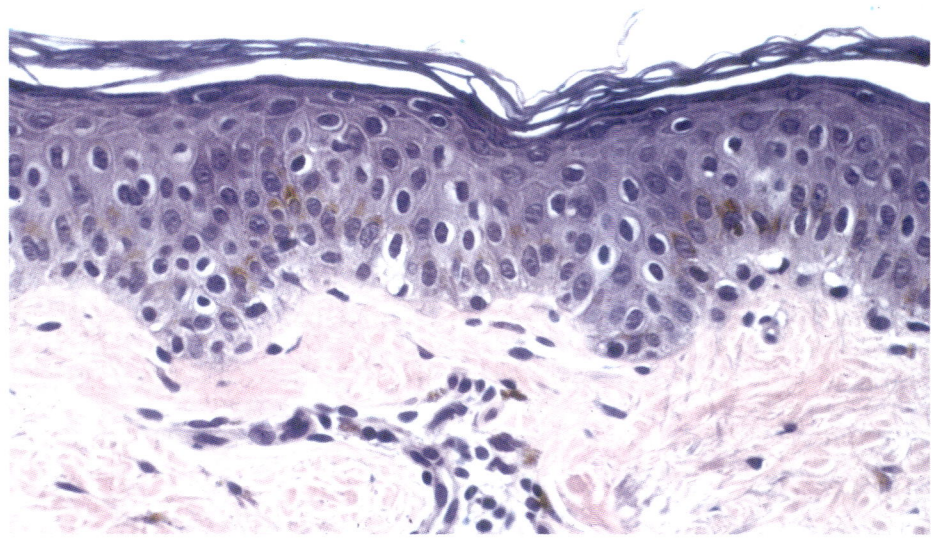

TABLE 4-3 Diseases and syndromes associated with café-au-lait macules.

Disease or syndrome	Pertinent features	Reference
Neurofibromatosis	See text	
Albright's syndrome	See text	
Tuberous sclerosis (epiloa)	Autosomal dominant; epilepsy; mental retardation; adenoma sebaceum; shagreen patch; periungual fibromas; "ash-leaf" (hypopigmented) macules	14
Silver-Russell syndrome	CALM in 45% of patients; short stature; skeletal asymmetry; shortened, incurved fifth fingers; abnormal sexual development	15
Watson syndrome	Pulmonary stenosis; mental retardation; perineal freckling	16
Westerhof syndrome	Mental retardation; growth retardation; hypopigmented macules	17
Bloom syndrome	CALM in >50% of patients; growth retardation; congenital facial telangiectactic erythema; photosensitivity	18

nevus, congenital nevi, dysplastic nevi, and sometimes even in normal skin (11,19–21).

On electron microscopy, the melanosomes are usually dispersed singly in melanocytes and are usually homogenous, electron-dense and ellipsoidal when fully melanized (19).

Associated Diseases and Syndromes

Neurofibromatosis (von Recklinghausen disease) is an autosomal dominant disease of neural crest–derived cells (7,8,12,13) (Table 4-3). Its cutaneous manifestations may occur in conjunction with systemic conditions, which mainly affect the central nervous system. Besides neurofibromata and multiple freckle-like macules in the axillae and other intertriginous areas, multiple CALMs are the leading cutaneous features in neurofibromatosis; they are present in >99% of all such patients. Usually they are present at birth, but they can occur months later. The presence of six or more CALMs > 1.5 cm in diameter in adults or five or more such macules that are ≥ 0.5 cm in diameter in children younger than 5 years has been considered diagnostic, but more reliable are the pigmented hamartomas of the iris, called Tisch nodules (12,13).

Albright syndrome includes polyostotic fibrous dysplasia of the bones, endocrine dysfunction that causes precocious puberty (more often in females than in males), and melanotic macules that are present in nearly two thirds of patients (10,13). The macules may be present at birth but more commonly develop in the first few years of life. They are usually several centimeters in diameter, are few in number, and may be indistinguishable both clinically and histologically from CALM in neurofibromatosis. However, the distribution of the lesions may be somewhat helpful for diagnosis: They favor the forehead, nuchal area, sacrum, and buttocks. They also tend to be unilateral in a linear or segmented arrangement with irregular margins, often involving the same side as the bone lesions and situated directly above them. Axillary freckling does not occur in Albright disease.

Differential Diagnosis

Hyperpigmented macules potentially confused with CALMs histologically include freckle, melasma, postinflammatory hyperpigmentation, and occasionally Becker's melanosis. Clinical findings should allow separation of CALM from the latter entities in most instances. In general, melasma has a distinctive clinical appearance, commonly involving the face in a symmetric pattern, particularly the malar areas but also the forehead and upper lip (22). Women are most commonly affected, and there is a relationship to pregnancy and oral contraceptives, suggesting an endocrine factor. Histologically, one generally observes varying degrees of basal layer hyperpigmentation and numbers of melanophages in the papillary dermis. Basilar melanocytes are normal or slightly increased in number, but the epidermal morphology is otherwise unchanged. Epidermal forms of melasma may be indistinguishable from CALMs. Otherwise, melanoma differs from CALM because of the greater numbers of melanophages. Postinflammatory hyperpigmentation is also distinguished from CALM by prominent pigment incontinence (melanophages) and delicate fibroplasia, often in the papillary dermis.

Becker's melanosis (discussed below), in addition to clinical differences such as hypertrichosis, is usually characterized by variable papillomatosis, elongation of rete ridges, and slight melanocytic hyperplasia.

LENTIGO SIMPLEX (see Chapter 5)
SOLAR LENTIGO (LENTIGO SENILIS, LIVERSPOT, INK-SPOT LENTIGO)

The solar lentigo occurs on sun-exposed skin, generally in somewhat older individuals (6, 23–26) (Table 4-1). Solar lentigines are observed in > 90% of the white population over the age of 60 years (23) (see also Chapter 5). Such lesions and the relatively flat seborrheic keratoses are popularly referred to as "liver spots." Some solar lentigines have resemblance to freckles but are distinguished from common freckles by their persistence despite absence of sun exposure. Solar lentigines are a prominent finding in xeroderma pigmentosum. As previously mentioned, carriers of one or two of the MC1R gene variants have a 1.5- to 2-fold increased risk for the development of numerous solar lentigines (6).

Photochemotherapy (PUVA) induced lentigo has been observed in patients receiving long-term methoxsalen photochemotherapy for psoriasis (27–30).

Clinical Features Solar lentigines are well-circumscribed round, oval, or irregularly bordered macules of yellow, tan, or brown color. More lightly pigmented lesions are usually homogenous, whereas darker ones tend to have a mottled appearance. Solar lentigines usually appear as multiple lesions; they vary in size from 1 to 3 cm in diameter, with a tendency to confluency. Solar lentigines occur on sun-exposed areas, predominantly the dorsal aspects of hands and forearms, the face, and upper chest and back. One variant, termed *sunburn*, hypermelanotic, or *ink-spot* solar lentigo, is characterized by a striking jet black color and a stellate outline (31). PUVA lentigo has a close clinical resemblance to solar lentigo, particularly the hypermelanotic type. The latter macules occur on light-exposed skin and range from 3 to 8 mm in greatest diameter (27–30).

Histopathological Features In general, the solar lentigo is notable for elongated, club-shaped epidermal rete ridges, basal-layer hyperpigmentation most prominent at the tips of the rete, and an increased frequency of basilar melanocytes; however, in some instances, the melanocytes are not increased in number (23,26) (Fig. 4-3). The epidermis between rete ridges is usually atrophic. On occasion, there is slight cytologic atypia of basilar melanocytes (3). There may also be hyperkeratosis and rather prominent elongation and anastomosis of rete. Some varieties of solar lentigo are characterized by an effaced epidermis—for example the epidermal rete ridges are diminished in length or absent. Varying degrees of solar elastosis are almost always present in the dermis. Accumulation of melanin-laden macrophages and slight lymphocytic infiltration are other frequent findings.

The solar lentigo may show transitions to reticulated seborrheic keratosis, large-cell acanthoma, and lichenoid keratosis (32,33). Sometimes there are two or more patterns of these various entities in the same lesion. Reticulated seborrheic keratosis is in reality an exaggerated form of solar lentigo: The epidermal rete are more elongated and exhibit a greater degree of anastomosis than does solar lentigo. The large cell acanthoma is a relatively flat pigmented lesion on sun-exposed skin that histologically contains enlarged monotonous keratinocytes, either in the lower half or thoughout most of the epidermis. The basilar epidermis is often hyperpigmented and thus often overlaps to some degree with solar lentigo. Some solar lentigines develop an associated lichenoid dermatitis and hence are termed *lichenoid* or *lichen planus-like* keratosis. Such lesions usually undergo regression and may show considerable resemblance to or be indistinguishable from a regressing melanocytic nevus.

Similar to solar lentigines, the PUVA lentigo exhibits lentiginous melanocytic hyperplasia, and low-grade cytologic atypia of melanocytes is occasionally noted (28,29).

Differential Diagnosis The most common differential diagnosis for the solar lentigo includes distinction from solar intraepidermal melanocytic proliferations (SIMPs) with varying degrees of atypia (Tables 4-4 and 4-5), solar lentiginous nevi with or without atypia, solar melanoma in situ, and pigmented actinic keratosis. SIMP occupy a continuum between solar lentigo and melanoma in situ (discussed below and in Chapter 10). The term *lentigo maligna* has been used for both melanoma in situ and also probably for virtually any atypical lentiginous melanocytic proliferation developing in chronically sun-exposed skin (see Chapter 10). In general, SIMP and melanoma in situ, particularly when present on the central face, are characterized by an absence or diminution of the epidermal rete pattern in contrast to solar lentigo. In addition, there is usually a greater frequency of basilar melanocytes in SIMP and melanoma in situ than in solar lentigo. Finally, solar melanoma in situ is characterized by a contiguous or near contiguous proliferation of basilar melanocytes, prominent involvement of adnexal epithelium by the lentiginous proliferation of melanocytes, nesting of melanocytes, the beginnings of pagetoid spread, and striking cytologic atypia of basilar melanocytes that should not be seen in solar lentigo and is generally not present in SIMP. Lentiginous nevi, either junctional or compound, developing in sun-damaged skin may also show varying degrees of atypia and may overlap with SIMP and melanoma in situ. Such nevi are differentiated from solar lentigines by well-defined junctional nesing and usually more significant lentiginous proliferation of melanocytes.

Pigmented actinic keratosis is distinguished from solar lentigo by the presence of disorder and cytologic atypia of basilar keratinocytes, "budding" of the atypical epidermis, and overlying parakeratosis in most instances. It should be borne in mind that occasional pigmented actinic keratoses may be difficult to separate from large-cell acanthoma or solar lentigines with features or a component of large cell acanthoma. Actinic keratosis can usually be distinguished by the presence of "crowding," pleo-

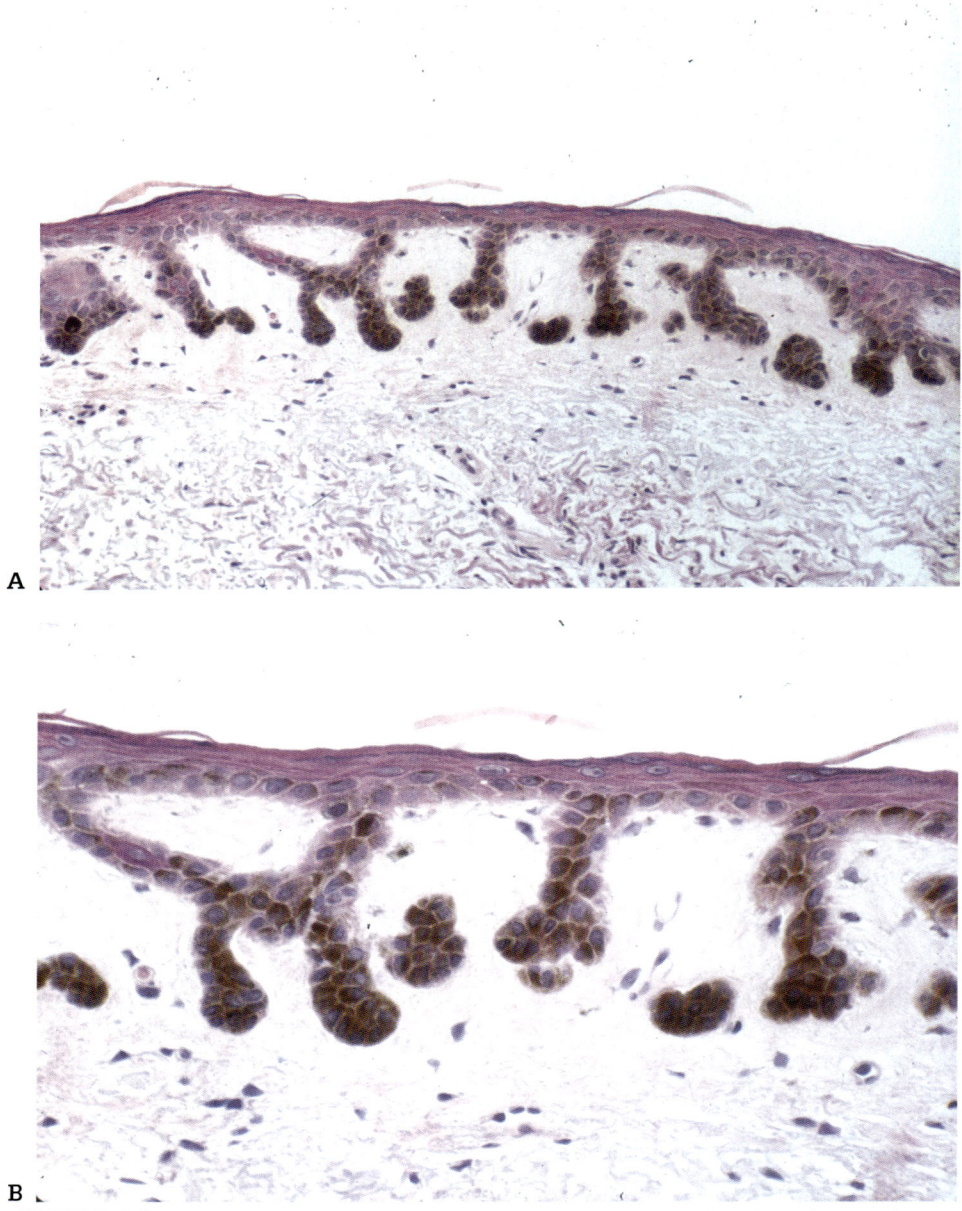

FIGURE 4-3 Solar lentigo. **A,** The lesion exhibits elongated club-shaped epidermal rete with prominent basal layer hyperpigmentation. **B,** There is anastomosis of the elongated rete ridges. The basilar melanocytes are not increased in frequency in this lesion.

morphism, and nuclear atypia of basilar keratinocytes versus the monomorphous enlarged keratinocytes typical of large-cell acanthoma.

Solar Intraepidemal Melanocytic Proliferations with Atypia

Considerable controversy has surrounded the terminology and definitions for and management of atypical melanocytic proliferations developing in chronically sun-exposed skin. These controversies are related to the lack of precise definition of the term *lentigo maligna,* the pronounced heterogeneity of such atypical melanocytic proliferations developing in chronically sun-exposed skin, overlap with atypical lentiginous nevi, and the distinction of true solar neoplastic melanocytic proliferations from melanocytic hyperplasia of chronically sun-exposed skin (solar melanocytic hyperplasia). The term *lentigo maligna* has been used by some authors as equivalent to melanoma

TABLE 4-4 Solar lentigo and solar intraepidermal melanocytic proliferations with atypia.

Characteristic	Solar lentigo	Solar intraepidermal melanocytic proliferation with atypia (historically lentigo maligna)
Clinical features		
Onset	>30–40 years of age	Generally >40–50 years of age
Location	Sun-exposed skin, face, dorsal hands	Sun-exposed skin, cheek is common
Size of macules	5–15 mm or larger	10–40 mm or larger
Color	Medium to dark brown, some variation in color	Tan, brown, dark brown, black, often some variegation
Surface	Slightly rough surface	Varnish-like stain in some cases
Shape	Some asymmetry	Asymmetry often
Borders	Regular or slightly irregular	Irregular
Histopathological features		
Circumscribed	Usually well circumscribed	Usually poorly circumscribed
Shape	Symmetry	Usually some asymmetry
Epidermis	Elongated, club-shaped rete ridges	Often effacement of epidermis
Basal layer	Increased number of basilar melanocytes often	Increased frequency of basilar melanocytes
Rete ridges	Melanocytes more frequent on tips of rete	No particular affinity
Intraepidermal nests of melanocytes	Usually not present	Usually not present
Pagetoid spread	No	Usually no
Basilar melanocytes	Usually do not involve adnexae	Sometimes involve adnexal epithelium
Cytologic atypia of melanocytes	Occasional variable atypia	Greater atypia; melanocytes often pleomorphic, with high nuclear/cytoplasmic ratio; spindle-shaped; atypia graded as slight to severe

in situ of sun-exposed skin, almost irrespective of the histopathologic features present, and by others to encompass not only atypical melanocytic proliferations lacking sufficient criteria for melanoma in situ but also melanoma in situ. As a result, the term has become in many ways a wastebasket for almost any solar atypical melanocytic proliferation. The ensuing confusion surrounding the term can translate into confusion about the

TABLE 4-5 Features of solar intraepidermal melanocytic lesions.

Feature	Solar melanocyte hyperplasia[a]	Solar lentigo	Solar lentiginous nevus	Solar intraepidermal melanocytic proliferation (historically lentigo maligna) with sepia	Solar melanoma in situ (melanoma in situ, lentigo maligna type)
Epidermal rete	Unchanged	Elongated or unchanged	Usually elongated	Variable; elongated or effaced	Often effaced
Lentiginous melanocytic proliferation	Variable; usually slight	Slight or none	Present	Present	Present
Frequency of melanocytes	Slightly increased	Normal or slightly increased	Increased	Increased	Increased; contiguous or near contiguous
Nesting of melanocytes	Usually absent	Absent	Present; usually cohesive	Usually absent	Usually present; often discohesive
Proliferation of melanocytes along adnexae	Usually absent	Usually absent	Usually absent	Usually absent	Usually present and extensive
Pagetoid spread	Absent	Absent	Usually absent	Usually absent	Often present
Cytologic atypia	Often absent or slight pleomorphism	Usually absent	Present or absent	Variable; usually slight to moderate	Often uniform; usually moderate to severe

[a]Chronic photoactivation.

biologic potential of such atypical proliferations and the appropriate clinical management of patients.

We believe that the term *lentigo maligna* should probably be abandoned because of this confusion. However, as discussed in Chapter 10, it is unlikely that this will happen soon because of its historical usage as a clinicopathologic entity. We maintain that the pathologist should try to categorize solar intraepidermal melanocytic lesions into one of the following categories, according to criteria outlined in this text: (a) solar lentigo, (b) lentiginous nevi with or without atypia, (c) solar intraepidermal melanocytic proliferation with varying degrees of atypia, and (d) melanoma in situ. Thus SIMP constitutes a spectrum of lesions generally intermediate between solar lentigo and melanoma in situ. The management of such lesions should include adequate sampling or complete removal with clear margins to exclude melanoma in situ.

Clinical Features

Solar intraepidermal melanocytic proliferations (SIMPs) are macular pigmented lesions generally with features intermediate between solar lentigo and melanoma in situ (Table 4-4). Thus they are likely to be somewhat larger in size (1–4 cm or more in diameter) with tan, brown, or dark brown coloration and borders often less regular than solar lentigo.

Histopathological Features

The spectrum of SIMP includes the following features (Tables 4-4 and 4-5; Fig. 4-4): (a) an increased number of basilar melanocytes, beyond that of a solar lentigo and possibly almost contiguous; (b) solar elastosis; (c) atrophy and effacement of the epidermis; (d) possibly some extension down appendageal structures by the melano-cytic proliferation; (e) a variably atypical population of melanocytes with usually slight to moderate, atypia; (f) absence of appreciable intraepidermal nesting or pagetoid spread.

Differential Diagnosis

As discussed above, the principal differential diagnosis includes solar lentigo and melanoma in situ (Tables 4-4 and 4-5). The criteria for melanoma in situ are as follows: (a) solar elastosis, (b) atrophy and effacement of the epidermis, (c) possibly some extension down appendageal structures by melanocytic proliferation, (d) contiguous or near contiguous lentiginous melanocytic proliferation, (e) nesting of melanocytes, (f) pagetoid spread of individual or nests of melanocytes, and (g) more significant and uniformly appearing cytologic atypia of melanocytes than with SIMP. The latter features including at least one or more of (d), (e), or (f), involving at least a single high-power field ($\times 400$) constitute the minimal essential criteria for a diagnosis of solar melanoma in situ.

BECKER'S MELANOSIS (BECKER'S NEVUS, BECKER'S PIGMENTARY HAMARTOMA, NEVOID MELANOSIS, PIGMENTED HAIRY EPIDERMAL NEVUS)

Becker's melanosis (BM) is a unilateral, hyperpigmented and often hypertrichotic macule or slightly elevated patch (34–42). Although it is usually acquired, some cases are congenital (40). The lesions mostly occur in the second and third decade of life and are six times more common in males than in females. Familial occurrence of both acquired and congenital cases has been reported. The prevalence among 19,302 army recruits aged 17–26 was 0.52% (34).

Becker's melanosis (BM) is believed to be an organoid hamartoma of ectodermally and mesodermally derived tissues, and a segmental increase in androgen receptors and probable heightened sensitivity to androgens has been postulated (39). The latter characteristics would explain its onset during or after puberty, leading to its clinical and histologic manifestations, which include hirsutism, acanthosis, dermal thickening, acne, and hypertrophic sebaceous glands. Androgen stimulation would also explain the accentuated smooth-muscle elements often found in the dermis of BM patients. Hyperpigmentation, similar to that found in "sexual skin," is due to increased melanin content in the epidermal keratinocytes and is often preceded by extensive sun exposure that has resulted in sunburns.

After development, BM enlarges slowly for a year or two but then remains stable in size. The color may fade with time, but hypertrichosis usually persists. BM is a benign lesion, and malignant transformation has not been reported.

In contrast to the hyperplasia of the ectodermal and mesodermal tissues in BM, occasional developmental abnormalities have been found associated with BM (termed the Becker's nevus syndrome) and are generally hypoplastic in nature (41). These abnormalities include hypoplasia of the ipsilateral breast, areola, nipple, and arm; ipsilateral arm shortening; lumbar spina bifida; thoracic scoliosis; pectum carinatum; and enlargement of the ipsilateral foot (38,41). In cases of BM with associated abnormalities, the male/female ratio is reversed (2:5) in comparison to patients with BM without abnormalities. Rarely, BM may be associated with a connective tissue nevus (42).

Clinical Features

The onset of BM is usually noted in the second or third decade of life, often after intense sunbathing (Table 4-6).

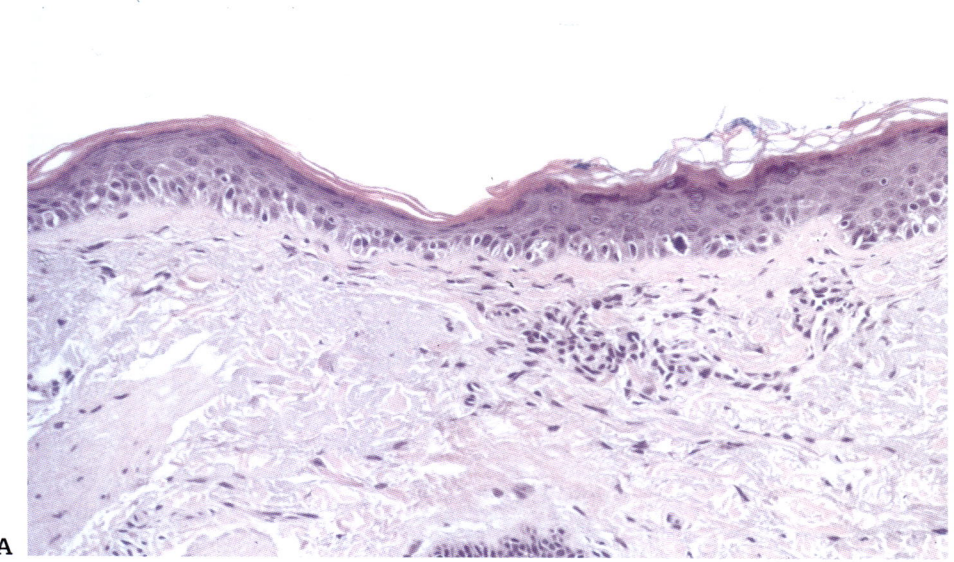

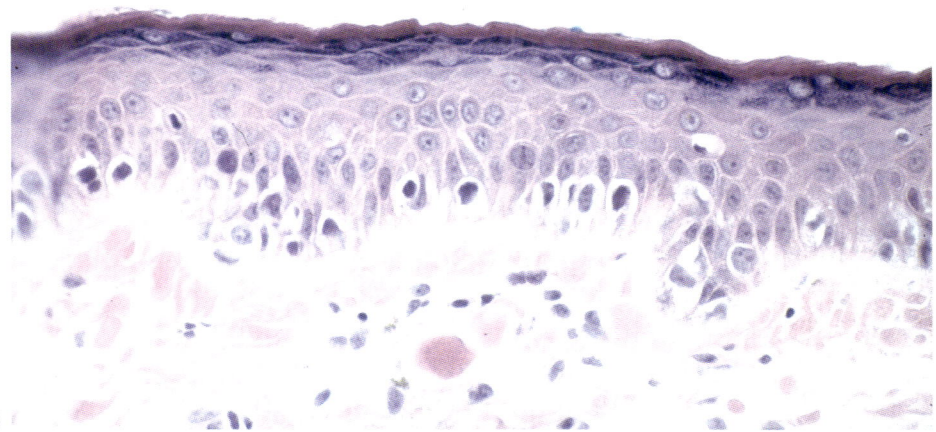

FIGURE 4-4 Solar intraepidermal melanocytic proliferation (SIMP) with atypia. **A,** There is an increased number of basilar melanocytes demonstrating nuclear atypia. The cytologic atypia is graded as slight to moderate, based on nuclear size and other nuclear characteristics relative to the surrounding keratinocytes. The lesion lacks sufficient atypia for melanoma in situ based on the low cellular density of melanocytes, the lack of more pronounced cytologic atypia, the absence of nesting, and the absence of pagetoid spread. Historically, many pathologists would designate this lesion as lentigo maligna, and some melanoma in situ. **B,** Atypical basilar melanocytes at increased frequency (higher magnification). The proliferation demonstrates neither nesting nor pagetoid spread.

The lesions commonly have a unilateral distribution on the shoulders, the submammary area, and the back, but they have also been described on the forehead, cheeks, eyelids, neck, abdomen, hips, lower leg, and buttocks (34). Normally, BM appears as a single lesion, but multiple lesions have been reported. The arrangement may be linear or zosteriform. BM ranges in size from a few centimeters in diameter to palm size or larger. There may

TABLE 4-6 Becker's melanosis.
Clinical features
Onset in childhood, adolescence
Congenital, on occasion
Unilateral location—shoulder, back, inframammary area, other sites
Usually solitary macular or slightly raised lesion
A few centimeters to palm size or larger
Tan to dark brown
Usually has prominent coarse hair
Usually irregular borders
Becker's nevus syndrome
Ipsilateral hypoplasia of breast
Skeletal anomalies—scoliosis, spina bifida, ipsilateral hypoplasia of a limb
Histopathological features
Epidermal configuration varies from almost normal to papillomatous or lentiginous (elongated rete ridges)
Increased melanin in basal layer
Melanocytes normal or slightly increased in frequency
Smooth muscle elements often increased in dermis (smooth muscle hamartoma)
Prominent pilosebaceous units
Associated connective tissue nevus rarely
Differential diagnosis
Café-au-lait macule
Lentigo simplex
Epidermal nevus
Congenital melanocytic nevus

be slow centrifugal extension of pigmentation. Hyperpigmentation varies from uniformly tan to dark brown. The lesions are well demarcated, but the margins are usually irregular. The center of the lesion may show slight thickening and corrugation of the skin. Hairiness usually develops after pigmentation and the hairs become coarser and darker with time. Sometimes hypertrichosis is subtle and can be appreciated only by comparison to the contralateral side. The hypertrichosis and pigmentation may not overlap completely. In some cases, perifollicular papules may be a marker for co-existent proliferation of the muscular arrectores pilorum. Acneiform lesions strictly limited to the area of hyperpigmentation have also been reported (35).

Histopathological Features

The configuration of the epidermis may vary from virtually normal to having variable degrees of papillomatosis, elongation of the epidermal rete ridges, or both (34) (Table 4-6). Thus the epidermal pattern may resemble an epidermal nevus or lentigo simplex (Fig. 4-5). The melanin content of the basilar keratinocytes is increased, whereas the number of melanocytes is normal or only slightly increased. Melanophages may be found in the papillary dermis. There may be prominence or hypertrophy of pilosebaceous units. A concomitant smooth-muscle hamartoma is often but not invariably present in the dermis (36). Rarely, alterations of the dermis such as coarse and thickened collagen bundles consistent with a connective tissue nevus may be present (42).

Differential Diagnosis

The principal entities to be considered in the histologic differential diagnosis include café-au-lait macule, lentigo simplex, epidermal nevus, and congenital melanocytic nevus (Table 4-6). In general, Becker's nevus is distinguished histologically from CALM based on epidermal changes (e.g., papillomatosis and elongated rete ridges) and dermal findings (e.g., prominent pilosebaceous and smooth-muscle components) that are not observed in CALM. Both entities may or may not have slight basilar melanocytic hyperplasia. Clinical findings should also allow rapid discrimination in most instances since BM is often raised and displays hypertrichosis. Histologic overlap may occur between Becker's nevus and lentigo, but gross morphologic features are usually distinctly different. Large (often congenital) varieties of lentigo may be difficult to distinguish from some forms of BM, for example, those that are macular and lack hypertrichosis. BM may potentially be discriminated from such lentigines by irregular borders and the presence of papillomatosis and other hamartomatous features, such as smooth-muscle hamartoma. Lesions showing only features of lentigo are probably best designated as such.

Both Becker's melanosis and epidermal nevus are cutaneous hamartomas and show some degree of clinical and histologic similarity. Epidermal nevus differs from BM by usually having more exaggerated epidermal changes (e.g., acanthosis and papillomatosis), the absence of melanocytic hyperplasia, and usually the absence of dermal hamartomatous features (e.g., smooth muscle hamartoma).

The congenital melanocytic nevus may clinically resemble BM but is immediately discriminated from BM by the presence of nevus cells histologically.

MELANOTIC MACULES AND LENTIGINES OF MUCOCUTANEOUS SITES

Certain pigmented macules may involve mucosal sites such as the conjunctiva, oral mucosa, the vermillion border of the lip (labial lentigo), and genitalia (genital lentigo

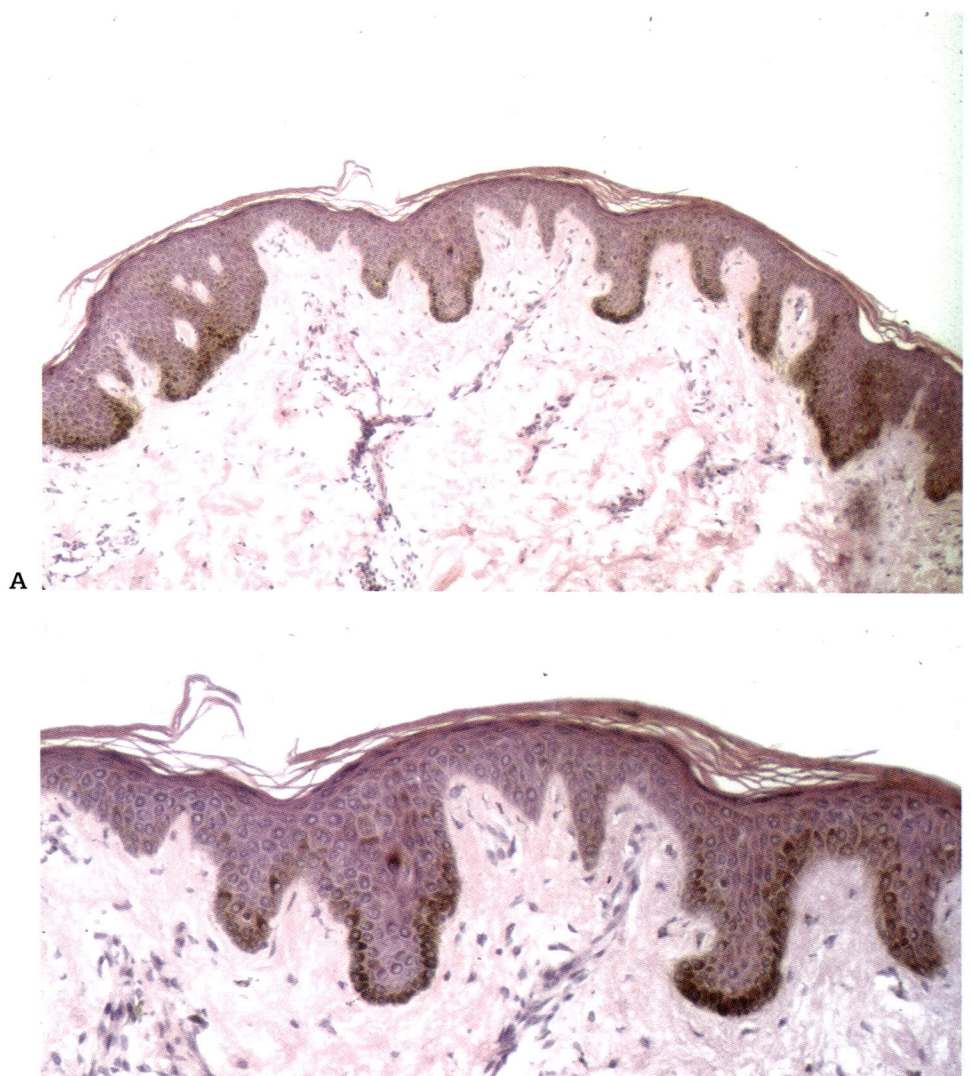

FIGURE 4-5 Becker's melanosis. **A,** The epidermis is characterized by elongated hyperplastic epidermal rete ridges. **B,** There is also significant basal layer hyperpigmentation, most prominently involving the lower-most aspects of the rete ridges. Although the basilar melanocytes are not increased in number, the overall histologic pattern resembles a lentigo.

and lentiginosis) (43–62). Multiple lentigines may involve the oral mucosa and vermillion border as part of the Peutz-Jeghers syndrome (59–61).

Clinical Features

These lesions are usually solitary or multiple macules, measuring 1–5 mm, and are often characterized by uniform light to dark brown or black homogeneous color (43–62) (Table 4-7). The borders are generally regular and well defined. The occurrence of such lesions on the lower lips of young women is commonly observed and is not associated with increased melanoma risk. Occasional lesions on the genitalia in particular are notable for a mottled appearance and large size, measuring up

TABLE 4-7 Melanotic macules, lentigines, and lentiginosis of mucocutaneous sites.

Clinical features
- Onset at almost any age
- Any mucosal site involved, especially lower lip (labial lentigo), vulva, penis
- Solitary, occasionally multiple
- Usually 1–5 mm macule but occasionally up to 40–50 mm
- Light to dark brown, or black
- Sometimes mottled
- Usually regular, well-defined borders
- Round, oval
- Occasionally polycyclic with irregular borders
- Usually symmetric

Histopathological features
- Well circumscribed
- Symmetric
- Variable acanthosis
- Tendency to elongated rete (lip, penis, vulva)
- Basal layer hypermelanosis
- Normal to increased numbers of solitary basilar melanocytes
- Usually no melanocytic atypia
- Melanophages usually present
- Sparse lymphocytic infiltrates

Differential diagnosis
- Melanocytic nevus
- Atypical melanocytic proliferations
- Melanoma

to 50 mm in greatest diameter (49–52,54–57). The latter clinical appearance suggests melanoma, but such lesions generally do not show atypical changes histologically (see below) or eventuate in melanoma on subsequent follow-up (51,52).

Histopathological Features

The histologic spectrum of these lesions may vary from slight acanthosis of epithelium, presence or absence of club-shaped rete, and presence or absence of basilar melanocytic hyperplasia (Fig. 4-6). The lesions without

FIGURE 4-6 Vulvar lentigo. The lesion is notable for elongated rete ridges, basal-layer hyperpigmentation, and slightly increased numbers of basilar melanocytes.

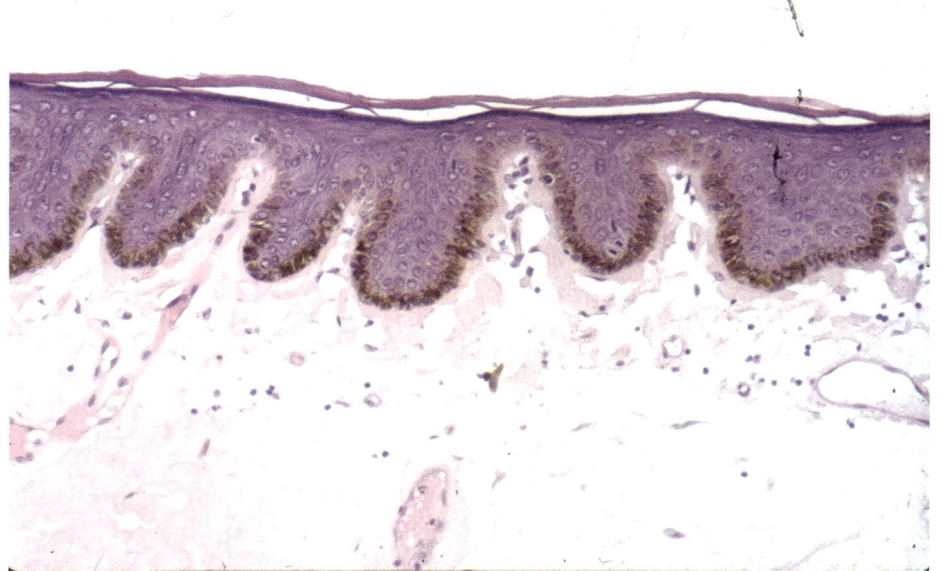

melanocytic hyperplasia may be designated as a melanotic macule or melanosis. The presence of melanocytic hyperplasia is best termed a lentigo. As with other simple lentigines, there is hyperpigmentation of the basilar epithelium. Melanophages and little or no lymphocytic infiltrate are present in the stroma.

Differential Diagnosis

The differential diagnosis includes melanocytic nevi of mucosal sites, atypical melanocytic proliferations, and melanoma. In general, as with melanocytic lesions located on other sites, progressively greater clinical atypicality raises concern about atypical histologic changes and melanoma. For example, asymmetry, size > 5–6 mm, irregular borders, irregularity and complexity of color, blue-black color, and bleeding should raise concern about melanoma.

Histologically atypical melanocytic lesions and melanoma on mucosae are characterized by progressively greater frequency of basilar melanocytes and prominent cytologic atypia. In the case of melanoma, the basilar melanocytes often reach confluence along the basal layer in a lentiginous pattern. The melanocytes exhibit continuous marked cytologic atypia. Pagetoid spread is variable and may be absent, minimal, or prominent.

REFERENCES

1. Fitzpatrick TB. Soleil et peau. J Med Esthet 1975;2(7):33–4.
2. Brues AM. Linkage of body build with sex, eye color and freckling. Am J Hum Genet 1950;2:215–39.
3. Rhodes AR, Albert L, Barnhill RL, Weinstock MA. Sun-induced freckles in children and young adults: a correlation of clinical and histopathologic features. Cancer 1991;67:1990–2001.
4. Gilchrest BA, Fitzpatrick TB, Anderson RR, Parrish JA. Localization of melanin pigmentation in the skin with Wood's lamp. Br J Dermatol 1977;96:245–8.
5. Breathnach AS. Melanocyte distribution in forearm epidermis of freckled human subjects. J Invest Dermatol 1957;29:253–61.
6. Bastiaens M, ter Huurne J, Gruis N, et al. The melanocortin-1-receptor gene is the major freckle gene. Hum Mol Genet 2002;10:1701–08.
7. Crowe FW, Schull WJ. Diagnostic importance of café-au-lait spot in neurofibromatosis. Arch Intern Med 1953;91:758–66.
8. Crowe FW, Schull WJ, Noel JV. A clinical, pathological and genetic study of multiple neurofibromatosis. Springfield, IL: Thomas, 1956.
9. Whitehouse D. Diagnostic value of the café-au-lait spot in children. Arch Dis Child 1966;41:316–9.
10. Benedict PH, Szabó G, Fitzpatrick TB, Sinesi SJ. Melanotic macules in Albright's syndrome and in neurofibromatosis. J Am Med Assoc 1968;205:72–80.
11. Johnson BL, Charneco DR. Café-au-lait spot in neurofibromatosis and in normal individuals. Arch Dermatol 1970;102:442–6.
12. Riccardi VM. Von Recklinghausen neurofibromatosis. N Engl J Med 1981;305:1617–27.
13. Mosher DB, Fitzpatrick TB, Hori Y, Ortonne J-P. Disorders of pigmentation. In: Fitzpatrick TB, Eisen AZ, Wolff K, et al., eds. Dermatology in general medicine. 4th ed. New York: McGraw-Hill, 1993;903–95.
14. Bell SD, MacDonald DM. The prevalence of café-au-lait patches in tuberous sclerosis. Clin Exp Dermatol 1985;10:562–5.
15. Silver HK. Asymmetry, short stature, and variations in sexual development: a syndrome of congenital malformations. Am J Dis Child 1964;107:495–515.
16. Watson GH. Pulmonary stenosis, café-au-lait spots, and dull intelligence. Arch Dis Child 1967;42:303–7.
17. Westerhof W, Beemer FA, Cormane BH, et al. Hereditary congenital hypopigmented and hyperpigmented macules. Arch Dermatol 1978;114:931–6.
18. Bloom D. Congenital telangiectatic erythema resembling lupus erythematosus in dwarfs. Probably a syndrome entity. Am J Dis Child 1954;88:754–8.
19. Jimbow K, Szabó G, Fitzpatrick TB. Ultrastructure of giant pigment granules (macromelanosomes) in the cutaneous pigmented macules of neurofibromatosis. J Invest Dermatol 1973;61:300–9.
20. Silvers DN, Greenwood RS, Helwig EB. Café-au-lait spots without giant pigment granules: occurrence in suspected neurofibromatosis. Arch Dermatol 1974;110:87–8.
21. Nakagawa H, Hori Y, Sato S, et al. The nature and origin of the melanin macroglobule. J Invest Dermatol 1984;83(2):134–9.
22. Sanchez WP, Pathak MA, Sato S. Melasma: a clinical, light microscopic, ultrastructural, and immunofluorescence study. J Am Acad Dermatol 1981;4:698–710.
23. Hodgson C. Senile lentigo. Arch Dermatol 1963;87:197–207.
24. Braun-Falco O, Schoefinius H-H. Lentigo senilis. Übersicht und eigene Untersuchungen. Hautarzt 1971;7:277–83.
25. Bean WB. Senile freckles. J Am Med Assoc 1975;234(10):1059.
26. Montagna W, Hu F, Carlisle K. A reinvestigation of solar lentigines. Arch Dermatol 1980;116:1151–4.
27. Miller RA. Psoralens and UVA-induced stellate hyperpigmented freckling. Arch Dermatol 1982;118:619–20.
28. Rhodes AR, Harrist TJ, Momtaz KT. The PUVA-induced pigmented macule: a lentiginous proliferation of large, sometimes cytologically atypical, melanocytes. J Am Acad Dermatol 1983;9:47–58.

29. Rhodes AR, Stern RS, Melski JW. The PUVA lentigo: an analysis of predisposing factors. J Invest Dermatol 1983;81:459–63.
30. Kanerva L, Niemi K-M, Lauharanta J. A semiquantitative light and electron microscopic analysis of histopathologic changes in photochemotherapy-induced freckles. Arch Dermatol Res 1984;276:2–11.
31. Bolognia JL. Reticulated black solar lentigo ("ink spot" lentigo). Arch Dermatol 1992;128:934–40.
32. Roewert HJ, Ackerman AB. Large-cell acanthoma is a solar lentigo. Am J Dermatopathol 1992;14:122–32.
33. Mehregan AH. Lentigo senilis and its evolutions. J Invest Dermatol 1975;65:429–33.
34. Copeman PM, Wilson Jones E. Pigmented hairy epidermal nevus (Becker). Arch Dermatol 1965;92:249–51.
35. Burgreen BL, Ackerman AB. Acneiform lesions in Becker's nevus. Cutis 1978;21:617–19.
36. Urbanek RW, Johnson WC. Smooth muscle hamartoma associated with Becker's nevus. Arch Dermatol 1978;114:104–6.
37. Tymen R, Forrestier JF, Bontet B, Colomb B. Nevus tardif de Becker. Ann Dermatol Venereol 1981;108:41–6.
38. Glinick, SE, Alper JC, Bogaars H, Brown JA. Becker's melanosis: associated abnormalities. J Am Acad Dermatol 1983;9:509–15.
39. Person JR, Longcope C. Becker's nevus: an androgen-mediated hyperplasia with increased androgen receptors. J Am Acad Dermatol 1984;10:235–8.
40. Book SE, Glass AT, Laude TA. Congenital Becker's nevus with a familial association. Pediatric Dermatol 1997;14:373–5.
41. Happle R, Koopman RJJ. Becker nevus syndrome. Am J Med Genet 1997;68:357–61.
42. Dai-Ho K, Chung-Won K, Tae-Yoon K. Becker's naevus associated with connective tissue naevus. Acta Derm Venerol 1999;79:393–4.
43. Shapiro L, Zegarelli DJ. The solitary labial lentigo: a clinicopathologic study of 20 cases. Oral Surg Oral Med Oral Pathol 1971;31:87–92.
44. Weathers DR, Corio RL, Crawford BE, et al. The labial melanotic macule. Oral Surg Oral Med Oral Pathol 1976;42:196–205.
45. Page LR, Corio RL, Crawford BE, et al. The oral melanotic macule. Oral Surg Oral Med Oral Pathol 1977;44:219–26.
46. Powell JP, Cummings CW. Melanoma and the differential diagnosis of oral pigmented lesions. Laryngoscope 1978;88:1252–67.
47. Buchner A, Hansen LS. Melanotic macule of the oral mucosa: a clinicopathologic study of 105 cases. Oral Surg 1979;48:244–9.
48. Spann CR, Owen CG, Hodge SJ. The labial melanotic macule. Arch Dermatol 1987;123:1029–31.
49. Tsukada Y. Benign melanosis of the vagina and cervix. Am J Obstet Gynecol 1976;124:211–2.
50. Jackson R. Melanosis of the vulva. J Dermatol Surg Oncol 1984;10:119–21.
51. Sison-Torre EQ, Ackerman AB. Melanosis of the vulva: a clinical simulator of malignant melanoma. Am J Dermatopathol 1985;7(Suppl):51–60.
52. Barnhill RL, Albert LS, Shama SK, et al. Genital lentiginosis: a clinical and histopathologic study. J Am Acad Dermatol 1990;22:453–60.
53. Cullen SI. Incidence of nevi: Report of survey of the palms, soles, and genitalia of 10,000 young men. Arch Dermatol 1962;86:41–3.
54. Landthaler M, Stolz W, Braun-Falco O. Lentigo der glans penis. Hautarzt 1989;40:221–5.
55. Kopf AW, Bart RS. Tumor conference 43. Penile lentigo. J Dermatol Surg Oncol 1982;8:637–9.
56. Bhawan J, Cahn TM. Atypical penile lentigo. J Dermatol Surg Oncol 1984;10:99–100.
57. Revuz J, Clerici T. Penile melanosis. J Am Acad Dermatol 1989;20:567–70.
58. Folberg R, McLean IW. Primary acquired melanosis and melanoma of the conjunctiva: terminology, classification and biologic behavior. Hum Pathol 1985;16:129–35.
59. Jeghers H, McKusick BA, Katz KH. Generalized intestinal polyposis and melanin spots of the oral mucosa, lips and digits. N Engl J Med 1949;241:993–1005, 1031–6.
60. Utsunomiya J, Gocho H, Miyanaga T, et al. Peutz-Jeghers syndrome: its natural course and management. Johns Hopkins Med J 1975;136:71–82.
61. Blank AA, Schneider BV, Panizzon R. Pigmentfleckenpolypose (Peutz-Jeghers-syndrome). Hautarzt 1981;32:296–300.
62. Rahman SB, Bhawan J. Lentigo. Int J Dermatol 1996;35:229–39.

CHAPTER 5

Common Acquired and Atypical (Dysplastic) Melanocytic Nevi

Michael Piepkorn and Raymond L. Barnhill

Arising embryologically from the neural crest, the cutaneous melanocyte takes residence in the epidermis and provides the histogenetic source of such melanocytic proliferations as lentigines and melanocytic nevi. Common acquired and atypical melanocytic nevi of the skin are described in this chapter.

HISTOGENESIS OF MELANOCYTIC NEVI

Beyond establishing the embryonic origin of melanocytic nevi from neural crest–derived cells, the histogenesis of these melanocytic proliferations has not been adequately elucidated (1–3). The conventional viewpoint is that nevi arise from proliferation of intraepidermal melanocytes within growth centers, termed junctional nests or theques. According to this model, nevus cells are considered a morphologic variant of melanocytes that have assumed a more epithelioid and less dendritic configuration. From evolution of the lesions, researchers hold that cells "drop off"—"*Abtropfung*" of Unna (4)—into the dermis (5,6). The *Abtropfung* hypothesis derives from cross-sectional observations correlating histologic findings in nevi with chronologic aging (7–15).

Alternative hypotheses regarding the genesis of nevi include the proposal that nevus cells arise from cutaneous nerves, from a pluripotential cell of nerve sheath origin (16) and by contributions from both neural and non-neural dermal sources (17–19). Proof for these theories has been constrained by the possibility that neural crest cells may phenotypically display both melanocytic and neural differentiation to varying degrees (7,20,21).

Whether melanocytic nevi are hamartomas or neoplasms has been subject to long-standing debate (7,17,22).

The common finding of other tissue elements in excess within nevi, such as epidermal hyperplasia, hypertrophy of adnexal structures, and connective tissue alterations, has been interpreted by some authorities as supporting the proposition that nevi are indeed developmental malformations; thus the term *nevus* is often used synonymously with *malformation* or *hamartoma*.

Contrarily, accumulating data support the hypothesis that the melanocytic nevus is a neoplasm and, putatively, the first stage in tumor progression of the melanocytic system (3,23–27). Stages in the putative progression model may not be obligate precursors to the subsequent stages, but rather could represent end stages at any point in the process. In support of this model are the gross morphologic and cytologic differences between melanocytes and nevus cells, the expression on nevus cells of markers of tumor progression that are not present on intraepidermal basilar melanocytes by immunophenotyping (27), and the growth advantages of nevus cells over epidermal melanocytes in cell culture (25–27). In attempts to resolve the issue of whether nevi are clonal and thus neoplastic in nature, researchers have performed clonality studies on nevus cells assessing the expression of X-linked genes and loss of heterozygosity analyses at relevant genomic loci, but the data are conflicting. Both polyclonality, which would support a hamartomatous origin for nevi (28), and clonality have been asserted (29–31).

Genetic and environmental factors clearly influence the development of melanocytic nevi (32–38). Increased numbers of nevi aggregate in some families, and the phenotype of multiple nevi and/or enlarged nevi is linked to melanoma-prone kindreds and, in fact, is the strongest epidemiologic risk factor for melanoma (32,33,36). These familial associations indicate a genetic basis for the growth and development of nevi. Correlations of nevus counts and nevus densities (nevus counts normalized to the skin surface area) are much higher between monozygous twins than between dizygous twins, with concordance values of 0.94 and 0.61, respectively (39). The twin data indicate that the emergence of nevi during adolescence is under strong genetic control. Quantification of total nevus number and total nevus density in melanoma kindreds has also shown familial (hereditary) correlations, but the nevus phenotype does not readily model genetically as a simple Mendelian trait resulting from the transmission of a dominant locus (33,40). With respect to environmental factors, sun exposure, especially during early childhood, promotes the initiation and development of nevi in susceptible individuals (34). This effect is reflected in the observation that nevi have a predilection for sun-exposed sites, especially sites that receive intermittent, but occasionally intense, ultraviolet (UV) exposure. Moreover, nevus counts are higher at tropical than at temperate latitudes (39). From these empirical observations, we may view nevi as clonal proliferations of initiated cells with a growth advantage over their progenitors, the intraepidermal melanocytes (7).

Lentigines and melanocytic nevi most likely represent sequential developmental stages of melanocyte proliferation and migration within the skin (7,9,12). Proliferation of an initiated basal epidermal melanocyte or, alternatively, an embryonic stem cell (melanoblast) within the epidermis constitutes the basis for the first morphologically recognizable lesion within this developmental pathway—namely the lentigo. With further development, according to the model, melanocytes phenotypically transition to a more epithelioid configuration and begin to aggregate as nests along the basal epidermal zone, thereby defining the junctional nevus (5–7). At this stage of development, the component cells within the nests are generally designated *nevus* (or *nevic*) *cells*. The morphologic transition during this process suggests that the cells have been functionally altered as either a reflection of or secondary to the aggregative pattern of growth (8). The cells lose the dendritic processes that are characteristic of solitary basilar melanocytes and have more abundant cytoplasms, larger nuclei, and somewhat more prominent nucleoli. In common with basal melanocytes, nevus cells contain single melanosomes at all stages of development. From this and other lines of evidence, some authorities consider nevus cells to be simply melanocytes and summarily dismiss the need for alternative nomenclature.

A reasonable hypothesis regarding the natural history of melanocytic nevi is that they arise as a lentiginous (i.e., lentigo-like) proliferation of single cell units along the basal zone of elongated and hyperpigmented rete ridges.

TABLE 5-1 Events in the involution of melanocytic nevi.

Declining proliferative activity of intraepidermal melanocytes
Loss of proliferative activity with descent of nevus cells into the dermis
Decline of cell density
Terminal differentiation and neurotization with dermal descent
Replacement of nevus cells by connective tissue

At some point thereafter, the melanocytes undergo a morphologic transition into the epithelioid nevus cells with their propensity to aggregate as junctional nests. Following this stage of development as a *junctional nevus*, further cellular development and proliferation results in the migration or dropping off of nevus cells and their organization into nests within the papillary dermis (4,5). According to this generally accepted model, eventually all intraepidermal proliferation of melanocytes ceases, and the nevus becomes entirely intradermal (5,6).

Nevus cells residing within the dermis have reduced proliferative and metabolic activity, except for the formation of melanosomes (5,6,41) (Table 5-1). With the decline of replication, the nevus cell population is gradually replaced by mesenchymal elements, including fibrous matrix, glycosaminoglycans, and adipose tissue (6). Most dermal nevi are believed to undergo progressive involution, some eventuating as acrochordons and others shedding (10). This developmental sequence may, presumably, be arrested at any stage, so that a lentigo, junctional nevus, or compound nevus may persist indefinitely. Because the model has been developed from largely cross-sectional data, alternative theories of development have been proposed, including a model invoking a reverse order of development (16,19).

CLASSIFICATION OF MELANOCYTIC NEVI

Melanocytic nevi may be classified according to a number of clinical and histologic attributes (Tables 5-2 and 5-3). Although a discussion of clinical features of nevi is beyond the scope of this chapter, it warrants emphasis that clinical characteristics are important in arriving at a pathologic diagnosis. An example of this is that the presence of a nevus at birth enables conclusive identification of a congenital nevus. Similarly, a bluish color of a nevus argues for a diagnosis of blue nevus, unless the histologic features are unusual, as in a tattoo or regressed melanocytic lesion.

TABLE 5-2 Clinical criteria used for the classification of melanocytic nevi.

Age of onset
   Congenital or acquired
Size
   Small congenital nevus: < 1.5 cm
   Medium-sized congenital nevus: > 1.5–≤ 20 cm
   Large congenital nevus: > 20 cm
   Garment or bathing trunk nevus
   Segmental nevus
Anatomic location
   Glabrous skin
   Acral
   Mucosal
   Genital
Appearance
   Border characteristics: symmetry, circumscription
   Surface topography: macular, papular, papillomatous, verrucoid
   Pattern of coloration: variegated, homogeneous
   Colors present: flesh, tan, brown, black, blue, gray, white, pink, red
   Speckled, targetoid, agminated, zosteriform

TABLE 5-3 Histologic criteria for the classification of melanocytic nevi.

Location of melanocytes in the skin (depth)
   Superficial
      Intraepidermal
      Papillary dermis
      Upper half of reticular dermis
   Deep
      Lower half of reticular dermis
      Subcutaneous
      Fascial
Disposition of melanocytes
   Intraepidermal
      Basilar melanocytes, single cell unit pattern
         Normal numbers
         Increased density
            With elongated rete (lentiginous)
            Without elongated rete
      Pagetoid pattern
      Nested pattern
         With lentiginous pattern
         Without lentiginous pattern
   Dermal
      Diffuse, interstitial
      Inverted wedge[a]
      Patchy or plexiform pattern[b]
      Bulbous aggregates, nodules[c]
      Alveolar pattern
      Maturation/differentiation
Stroma (e.g., desmoplasia, sclerosis, mucinosis)
Cell type
   Small, round, or oval
   Fusiform or spindle
   Epithelioid cell (enlarged, with abundant cytoplasm)
   Dendritic cell (lengthy, delicate cellular processes)
   Intermediate or indeterminate
   Degree of melaninization

[a]Deep apex of nests or fascicles of melanocytes extend into reticular dermis or subcutis.
[b]Discrete nests or fascicles associated with neurovascular or adnexal structures of reticular dermis with intervening normal dermis.
[c]Cellular nests or fascicles with rounded contours, usually extending into reticular dermis or subcutis.

HISTOLOGIC CRITERIA FOR MELANOCYTIC LESIONS

Location of Melanocytes in the Skin

The prevailing criterion for histologic classification of nevi has long been the location of melanocytes within the skin or contiguous epithelia (20) (Table 5-3). This criterion refers specifically to the spatial disposition of the cells relative to the anatomic levels of the skin. A superficial category within this classification, for example, comprises lesions represented by a proliferation of single-cell melanocytic units within the basilar zone, such as lentigines, atypical nevi, acral nevi, and pigmented patches on mucous membranes. Another superficial category includes proliferations represented by the dispersion of single cells and nests of cells above the basal zone, referred to variously as *pagetoid scatter* or *pagetoid melanocytosis,* because of its resemblance to Paget disease of the breast. In addition to its importance as a criterion for melanoma, pagetoid scatter can be found in various other settings, such as acral nevi, childhood nevi, atypical nevi, persistent/recurrent nevi, and Spitz and pigmented spindle cell nevi. Moreover, trauma such as UV irradiation can transiently induce pagetoid alterations in otherwise banal nevi (42).

Nested aggregates of cells are the most characteristic feature of melanocytic nevi. Further diagnostic characterization derives from the depth of the lesion, architectural features, stroma, and cytologic characteristics. Some nevi contain particular arrangements of nevus cells. For example, interstitial disposition of melanocytes between reticular dermal collagen fibers, perivascular arrays of melanocytes, plexiform arrangements of melanocytes in relation to microvessels and nerves, and nests of melanocytes within sebaceous glands are features characteristic of congenital nevi (Chapter 6).

Stroma

Alterations within the stroma of melanocytic nevi are not well understood from a mechanistic standpoint but may reflect the diverse cellular–stromal interactions of cells derived from the neural crest. At one extreme, certain nevi exhibit sclerosis of their dermal elements with some regularity (6). These include desmoplastic Spitz nevi, blue nevi, and their variants.

Cell Type
Cytologic characteristics of the melanocytes are considered in the classification of nevi. Although there is often both maturation/differentiation and some degree of heterogeneity in melanocytic lesions, most nevi are composed of essentially one nevus cell type. In the case of most acquired and congenital nevi, this cell type is a small, round to oval "nevus" or "nevic" cell.

LENTIGO SIMPLEX (SIMPLE LENTIGO, NEVOID LENTIGO)

In at least some instances, a lentigo simplex is the first recognizable stage in the histogenetic development of a melanocytic nevus. In other instances, it represents a fully developed lesion in and of itself. Clinically, lentigo simplex is a sharply demarcated macule of either uniform or variegated hyperpigmentation located anywhere on the body, without predilection for sun-exposed skin (7,43). These lesions are common in children and adults, occur in all races, are equally distributed between the genders. They may be present at birth (44). In darkly pigmented skin, lentigo simplex is the most common pattern of pigmented lesion on acral skin (45). Lentigines simplex can increase in number during childhood or puberty and may occur in an eruptive form as lentiginosis, with or without obvious precipitating factors (46,47). Lesions with the histologic pattern of lentigo simplex can also be found in the nail matrix epithelium, producing pigmented bands that are common in black but rare in white individuals (48–50).

Clinical Features
Lentigines are regular, well-circumscribed macules, usually ranging from 1 to 5 mm in diameter, that have a uniform light to dark brown color (43). The simple lentigo may occur in a localized or a widespread pattern as in lentiginosis profusa or as a component of certain syndromes, including LEOPARD, LAMB (Carney complex), and Peutz-Jeghers (51–56) (Table 5-4).

Histopathological Features
Architecturally, lentigo simplex is often a circumscribed process. These lesions can be defined by three histologic features: increased density of melanocytes along the basilar epidermis; elongated, club-shaped epidermal rete; and hyperpigmentation of the basilar epidermis, which has a predilection for the tips of the rete but can extend to the upper epidermis, including the stratum corneum (7,9,12) (Fig. 5-1). The melanocytic proliferation also has a predilection for the tips of the rete, so that the density of cells diminishes along the sides of the rete and overlying the dermal papillae. This spatial predilection corresponds to the zones of greatest pigmentation. Within the subjacent stroma, melanophages and sparse perivascular lymphocytic infiltrates are present, and fibrosis envelops the accentuated rete.

Differential Diagnosis
The principal entities to be discriminated from lentigo simplex are freckles (ephilids) and solar lentigo. The simple lentigo differs from a freckle by the presence of elongated rete ridges and increased density of melanocytic cells along the basilar epidermis. Solar lentigines occur in association with actinic elastosis and tend to have longer and more complexly anastomosing rete ridges and somewhat less melanocytic hyperplasia compared to simple lentigines.

TABLE 5-4 Syndromes associated with multiple lentigines.

Syndrome	Onset	Distribution	Associations	Inheritance
Lentiginosis profusa	Birth to childhood	Widespread; mucosa spared	None	None
Multiple lentigines (LEOPARD syndrome)	Infancy	Widespread; mucosa spared	Cardiac conduction defects; ocular hypertelorism; pulmonary stenosis; hypogonadism; growth retardation; neural deafness	Autosomal dominant
Carney complex (LAMB syndrome)	Childhood	Widespread skin and mucosal sites	Atrial myxoma; cutaneous myxomas; blue nevi; schwannomas	Autosomal dominant
Peutz-Jeghers syndrome	Childhood	Perioral; vermillion border; oral mucosa; dorsal fingers	Multiple gastrointestinal polyps; adenocarcinoma	Autosomal dominant

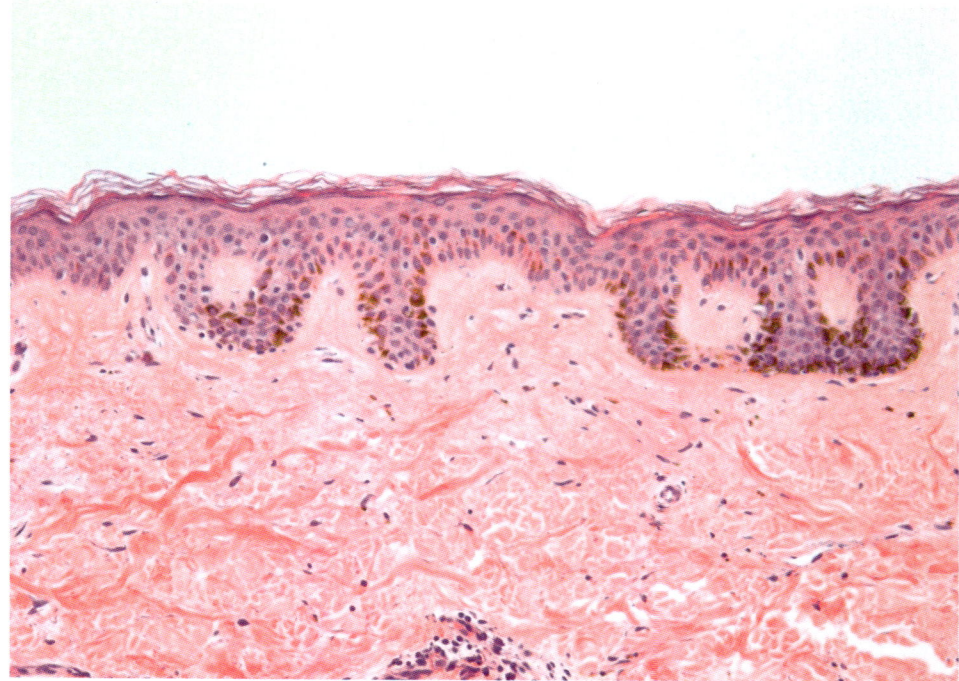

FIGURE 5-1 Lentigo simplex. Note the elongated epidermal rete and basilar hyperpigmentation, most prominent at the tips of the retia.

The histologic pattern of simple lentigo overlaps that of common acquired and atypical (dysplastic) nevi, perhaps suggesting a common histogenesis. The melanocytic nevus may have all of the described features of a lentigo simplex, but the added feature of nests of nevoid cells situated at the junctional zone defines the first recognizable stage of a junctional nevus (12). Historically, the designations *jentigo* and *nevus incipiens* have been applied to those lesions presenting an overlapping histologic phenotype. To reflect common histogenetic mechanisms between junctional nevi and simple lentigines, however, the designation *junctional lentiginous nevus* is preferable for lesions with an overlapping phenotype. These lesions are rather common in histopathologic practice. Atypical nevi are distinguished by increased density of basilar melanocytes resulting in a multilayered, coalescent growth pattern and by cytologic atypia of the intraepidermal melanocytic cells, as discussed later in this chapter.

COMMON ACQUIRED MELANOCYTIC NEVI (NEVOCELLULAR NEVUS; MOLE)

Exhibiting a wide variety of phenotypic patterns, acquired nevi may range from small, well-circumscribed, pigmented macules to larger, less well circumscribed lesions to raised, flesh-colored nevi. Each stage is principally defined by anatomic location of nevus cell aggregates within the skin. Junctional nevi have intraepidermal collections of nevus cells; dermal (or intradermal) nevi have nevus cells in the dermis, and in compound nevi, the cells are situated at both locations (5,6).

The natural history of acquired nevi, as mentioned previously, is not well understood, but inferences have been made as to their developmental sequence across cross-sectional, descriptive analyses (5,6). The prevalence of nevi is related to age and race, as well as to genetic and environmental factors (32–34,36,37). Few nevi are present in early childhood, but they increase in number thereafter, reaching a peak in the third decade of life and gradually declining with increasing age (9,10,12–14). Puberty represents a period of active growth of nevi, and nevus density reaches a peak among individuals aged 20–29 years (15). During the first decade of life, average nevus number has been reported to be 2–3, increasing to 22–33 during the third decade (15). There is no substantial gender difference in numbers of nevi (14,15). Among the races, whites have the highest number of nevi, and a direct correlation exists between lightness of skin color and number of nevi (57,58). Contrarily, melanocytic nevi of volar skin, nail beds, and conjunctiva are more prevalent in blacks than in whites (45,59).

Genetic factors appear to play a substantive permissive role in the development of nevi, controlling the numbers of nevi that may develop as a result of exogenous stimuli, especially early childhood sun exposure (34). The role of heredity is reflected in the clustering of large numbers of nevi in some families, particularly those kindreds at increased risk for melanoma (33). The pattern of inheritance for susceptibility to large numbers and sizes of nevi is complex and does not fit a simple pattern of Mendelian inheritance (33). However, the genetic control of nevi is reflected in the significant concordance in the nevus phenotype between identical twins (32). The role of solar exposure is shown in epidemiologic studies that have directly correlated increased numbers of nevi with residence in sunny climates (34).

Clinical Features

Melanocytic nevi are well to somewhat poorly circumscribed, round or ovoid lesions that typically range from 2 to 6 mm in maximal dimension (60,61) (Table 5-5). Most have overall architectural symmetry and regular margins. As noted above, the consensus opinion is that nevi follow an orderly process of natural progression from junctional nevus to compound nevus, then to intradermal nevus and gradual involution (5,6,10). Many nevi may originate as a lesion morphologically indistinguishable from a lentigo simplex. However, reliable, long-term natural history data to confirm this model of development and involution are lacking. Moreover, any given lesion may arrest its development at any of the observable stages.

Junctional nevi are macular and exhibit slight accentuation of the skin markings by side lighting. They are often uniformly medium to dark brown, but minor degrees of color variegation are not uncommon, especially with lentiginous junctional nevi. Compound nevi are elevated to varying degrees and are usually lighter shades of brown than junctional lesions. Dermal nevi are more elevated and have lost much or all of their pigmentation, evolving to flesh-colored papules. It warrants emphasis that there is considerable clinical overlap among the three recognized categories of nevi (11). Dermal and compound nevi can be papillomatous or verrucoid, resembling seborrheic keratoses or warts. Some nevi, most often of the elevated types, contain dark, coarse hairs.

TABLE 5-5 Common acquired melanocytic nevi.

Characteristic	Junctional nevus	Compound nevus	Dermal nevus
Clinical features			
Onset	Childhood, adolescence	Childhood, adolescence, third decade	First, second, third decade or later
Size	2–5 mm, macule	3–6 mm, papule	3–6 mm, papule; often dome shaped or papillomatous
Shape	Round, oval	Round, oval	Round, oval
Symmetry	Symmetrical	Symmetrical	Symmetrical
Borders	Well-defined, regular borders	Well-defined, regular borders	Well-defined, regular borders
Color	Homogeneous brown, dark brown	Homogeneous tan to dark brown	Light brown to flesh tones
Histopathological features			
Symmetry	Symmetry	Symmetry	Symmetry
Circumscription	Well circumscribed	Well circumscribed	Well circumscribed
Nesting	Regular junctional nesting	Regular junctional nesting	Dome shaped or papillomatous
Arrangement	Uniform size, shape, and placement of nests	Uniform size, shape, and placement of nests	Orderly arrangement of nevus cells in dermis
Location	Nests often at tips of retia	Nests often at tips of retia	Transition from epithelioid to lymphocytoid to spindled cells with dermal descent
Cohesiveness	Cohesive nests, usually	Cohesive nests, usually	
Pagetoid scatter	No or little scatter	no or little scatter	
Other	Lentiginous proliferation, common	Nevus cells often confined to papillary or superficial reticular dermis	Nevus cells often confined to papillary or superficial reticular dermis
		Transition from epithelioid to lymphocytoid to spindled cells with dermal descent	Transition from epithelioid to lymphocytoid to spindled cells with dermal descent
		Mitotic figures rare in dermis	Mitotic figures rare in dermis
		Minimal nuclear pleomorphism	Minimal pleomorphism

On volar skin, nevi are usually macular and have regular borders, although varying degrees of asymmetry are not uncommon. Most often, they are uniformly brown or dark brown. Nevi of the nail bed usually present as uniformly pigmented, brown or dark brown longitudinal bands with regular and distinct margins, termed *melanonychia striata* (48–50,62).

Histopathological Features

Nests of nevus cells arrayed along the basal epidermal zone define the junctional nevus (4–6). A junctional nest (occasionally referred to as a *theque* in the older literature) has been arbitrarily defined as being made up of five or more cells in close apposition, situated at or above the basement membrane (11,12) (Fig. 5-2). In prototypic lesions, which are not especially common in histopathologic practice, the characteristics of these nests, such as size, shape, location, and spacing within the epidermis, tend to be regular and homogeneous within a given nevus. Exceptions to this rule, however, are common, particularly within junctional lentiginous nevi (see below). The cells are usually cohesive, giving the nests a syncytial appearance (17) (Fig. 5-3). Junctional nests have a spatial predilection for the tips of rete, rather than the sides or overlying the dermal papillae.

Constituting a common pigmented lesion in histopathologic practice, the lentiginous nevus by definition incorporates histologic features of both lentigo simplex and junctional nevus. Lentiginous nevi are of junctional or compound type. The lesions appear common in practice because clinically their appearance overlaps that of the atypical nevus, accounting for their frequent removal for biopsy examination. Variably sized and shaped nests of nevus cells are situated in a somewhat heterogeneous distribution at the junctional zone and occasionally suprabasally. The nests are often poorly formed and are separated from one another by a *lentiginous* pattern of melanocytic proliferation, to wit: a proliferation of melanocytes as single-cell units spaced at more or less regular distances within elongated rete of the basal epidermal zone (Fig. 5-4). The hyperplastic cells have a predilection for the tips of the rete, essentially recapitulating the histologic pattern of a lentigo simplex. Rete affected by the melanocytic proliferation are usually enveloped by new collagenous connective tissue, in a pattern termed *concentric fibroplasia*. The peripheral extension of lentiginous nevi in histologic section is often poorly delimited. Histologically, lentiginous nevi overlap the histologic phenotype of atypical (dysplastic) nevi, and the threshold for discriminating the two lesions is probably rather subjective. This matter is discussed in more depth later in the chapter.

The compound nevus contains nevus cells within the dermis as well as at the junctional zone, whereas the dermal nevus, by definition, has evolved past the stage with junctional nevoid cells (5) (Figs. 5-4 to 5-8; Table 5-5).

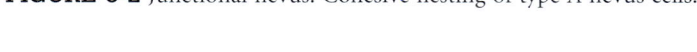

FIGURE 5-2 Junctional nevus. Cohesive nesting of type A nevus cells.

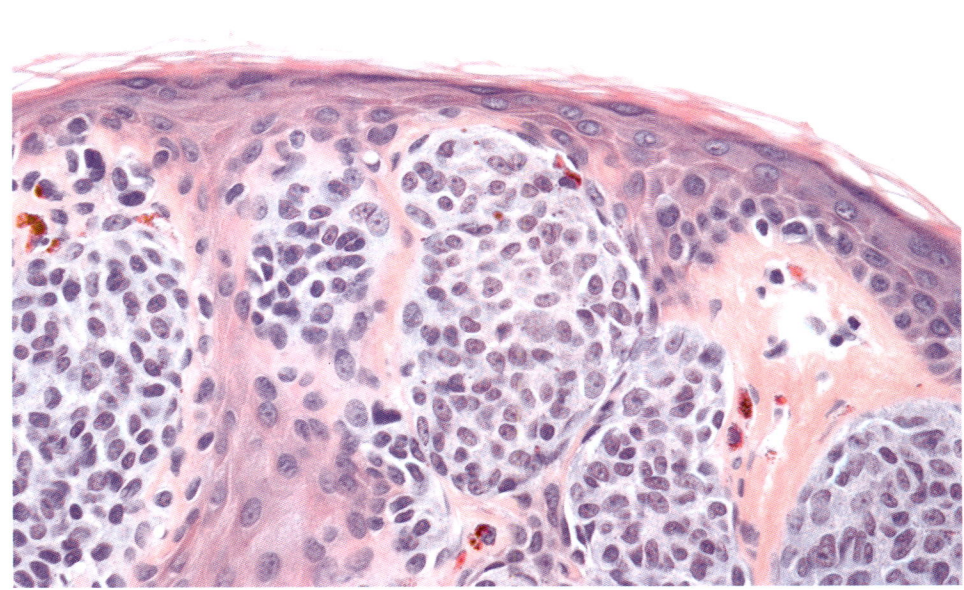

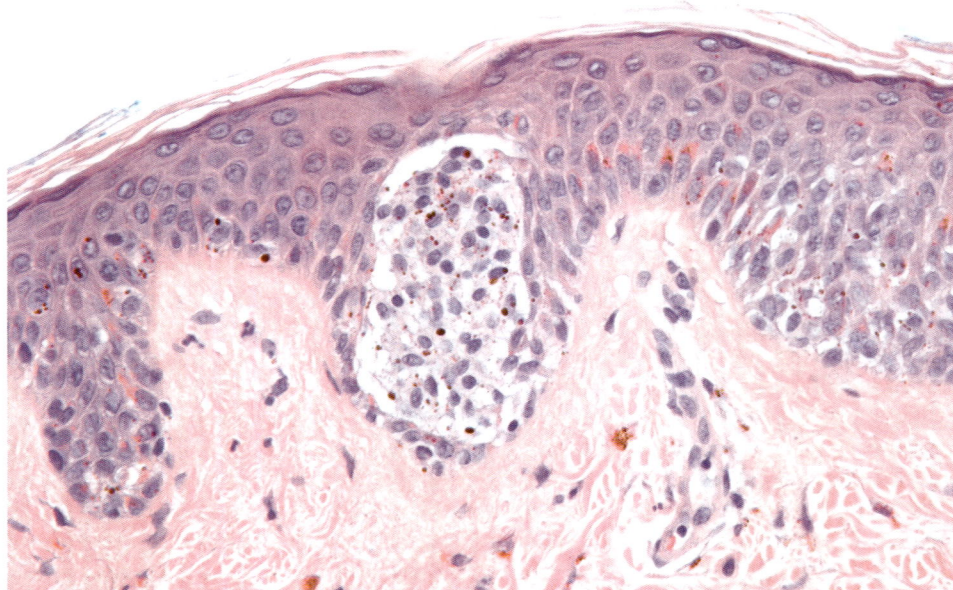

FIGURE 5-3 Junctional nevus containing syncytial aggregate of type A nevus cells. Note the round, oval, and slightly elongate nuclei with evenly dispersed, ground-glass chromatin. Occasional small nucleoli are present in some nuclei.

FIGURE 5-4 Lentiginous compound nevus. Within the epidermis is a mixed lentiginous and nested pattern of melanocyte hyperplasia.

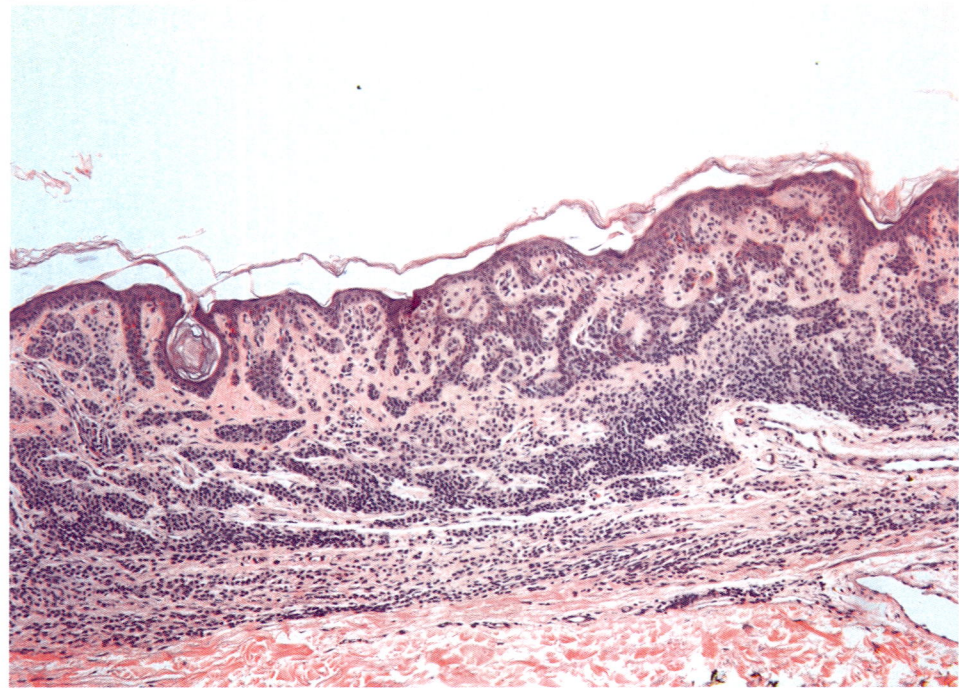

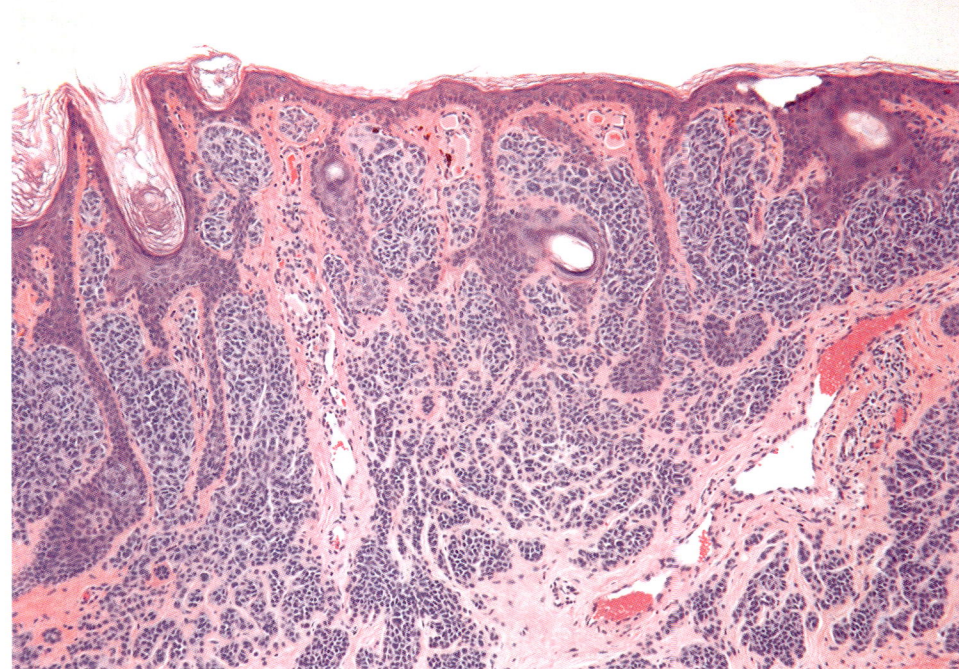

FIGURE 5-5 Compound nevus. Most of the nevus cells are disposed as cords with the papillary dermis.

FIGURE 5-6 Compound nevus of acral skin. Nests of epithelial nevus cells are situated within the epidermis and dermis. There has occurred focally an upward migration of cells into the stratum spinosum, which is a finding common to nevi of the acra.

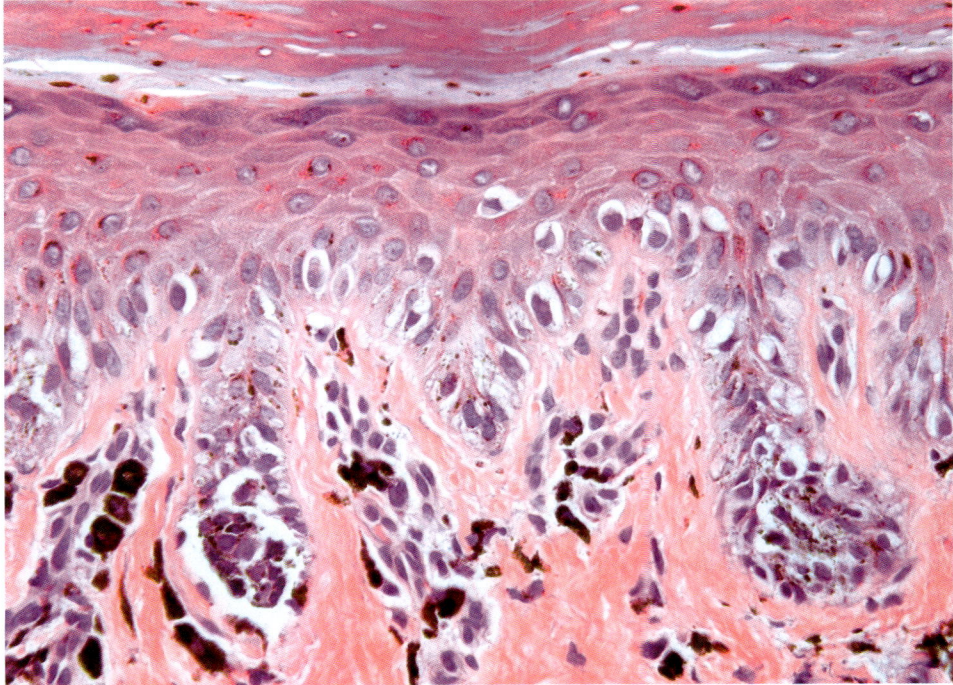

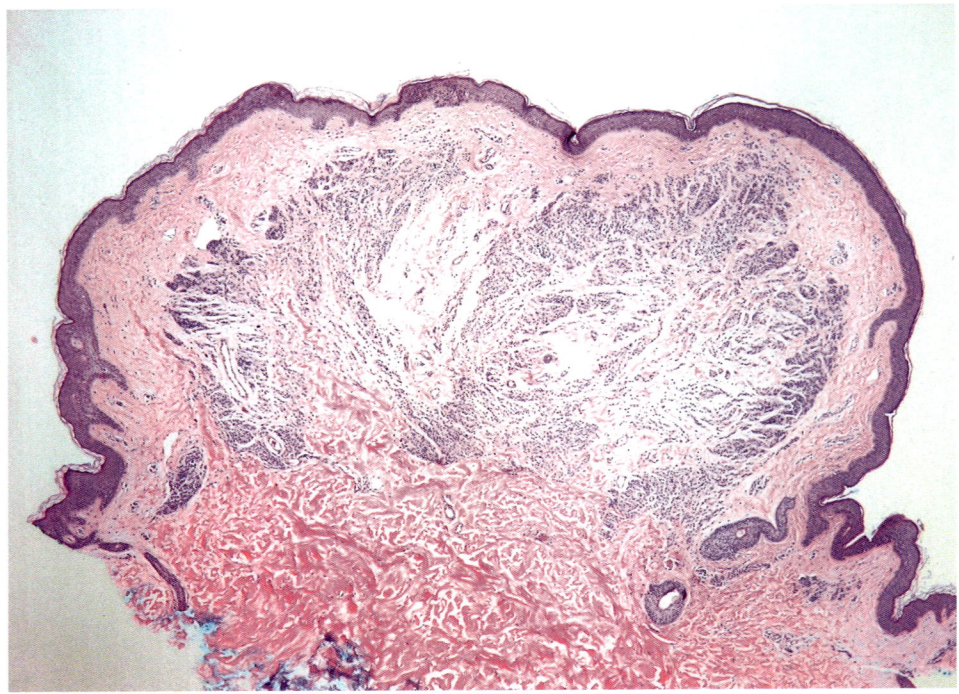

A

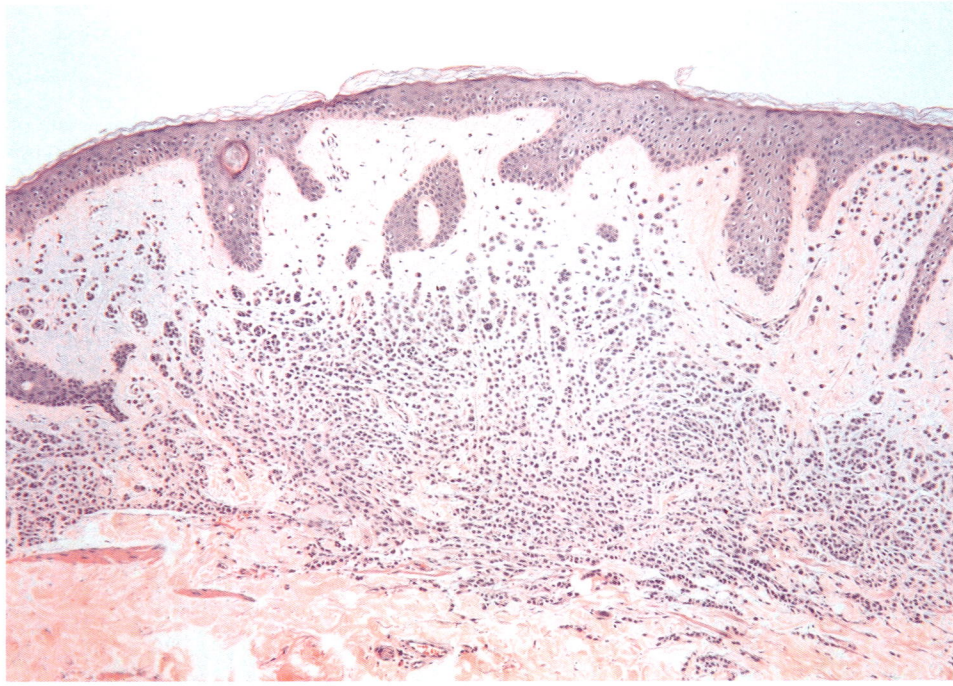

B

FIGURE 5-7 Dermal nevus. **A,** A dome-shaped lesion that evokes a symmetrical silhouette. **B,** The disposition of nevus cells within the papillary dermis is orderly.

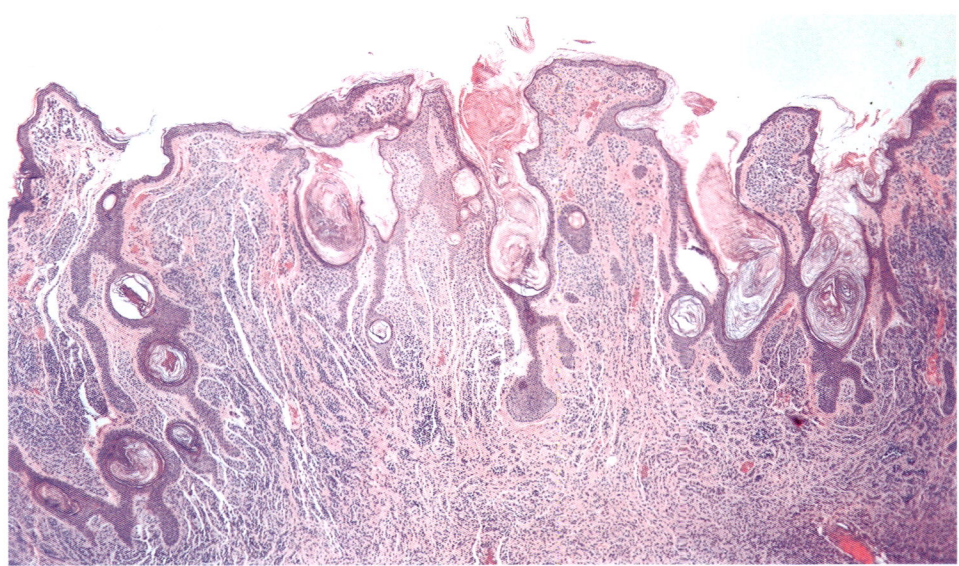

FIGURE 5-8 Papillomatous (or papillary) dermal nevus. The epidermal surface is papillated.

The compound nevus is more common by histologic criteria than the dermal nevus (11). In most acquired nevi, dermal involvement by nevus cells is largely restricted to the adventitial dermis—that is, the finely textured collagenous stroma of the papillary dermis and surrounding adnexae and the vasculature (Fig. 5-5). Dermal nevus cells mainly proliferate within and expand the papillary dermis, resulting in progressive elevation of nevus contours commensurate with the volume of nevus cells (Figs. 5-7 and 5-8).

Cytology

Nevus cells within the intraepidermal component or superficial dermis are characterized by a pattern of cohesive, rounded nesting of cells, a tendency to synthesis of melanin, and cytologic resemblance to epithelial cells (5,6,17,20,41) (Fig. 5-3). The epithelial quality refers to the moderate amount of eosinophilic cytoplasm within the cells and to their rounded or polygonal silhouette. This cell type is sometimes referred to as *type A* nevus cell (17). The nuclei, which often are slightly larger than those of basilar melanocytes, contain uniformly dispersed chromatin with a ground-glass basophilic quality and are bordered by delicate nuclear membranes (5,8,17,41). Nucleoli, where observable, are small and regular in configuration. When situated within the subjacent papillary dermis, type A nevus cells focally begin to metamorphose to small cells with little cytoplasm that resemble lymphocytes, which are referred to as the *type B* or *lymphocytoid* cells (Fig. 5-9A,B) (17,41). They tend to organize into compact cords and nests of cells (Fig. 5-9B) and have lost the capacity to synthesize melanin (5,6,17,41). The final, histologically recognizable stage of cellular transition is to that of an elongate or spindle-shaped cells separated from one another by delicate fibrous tissue (5,6,17,41) (Fig. 5-9C,D). At this final stage of transition or maturation, the nevoid melanocytes resemble Schwannian cells and are designated *type C* cells.

Nevus cells not uncommonly display some degree of pleomorphism (i.e., anisokaryosis or variation in nuclear size and shape) and variation in chromasia, or staining of chromatin (20). When present, the cellular changes should be interpreted in the overall context of the lesion. For example, lower grades of cellular pleomorphism and variation in chromasia are permissible if other histologic characteristics, such as architectural abnormalities and host inflammatory response, are absent. This caveat pertains especially to nevi of infants and young children, the cells of which can on occasion be pleomorphic.

Nevus giant cells are a common component in melanocytic nevi but also can be found in atypical nevi and melanoma (5). Intradermal giant cells with tightly packed, molded nuclei and scant cytoplasm have been designated mulberry-type giant cells (Fig. 5-9E) and can give the mistaken impression of a bizarre, atypical nevus cell. Another pattern is that of a wreath-like arrangement of nuclei at the periphery of the cells, creating a central zone of eosinophilic to slight basophilic cytoplasm. These cells, which may be situated at the basilar epidermis as well as within the papillary dermis, resemble the Touton giant cells of such histiocytic proliferations as juvenile xanthogranuloma.

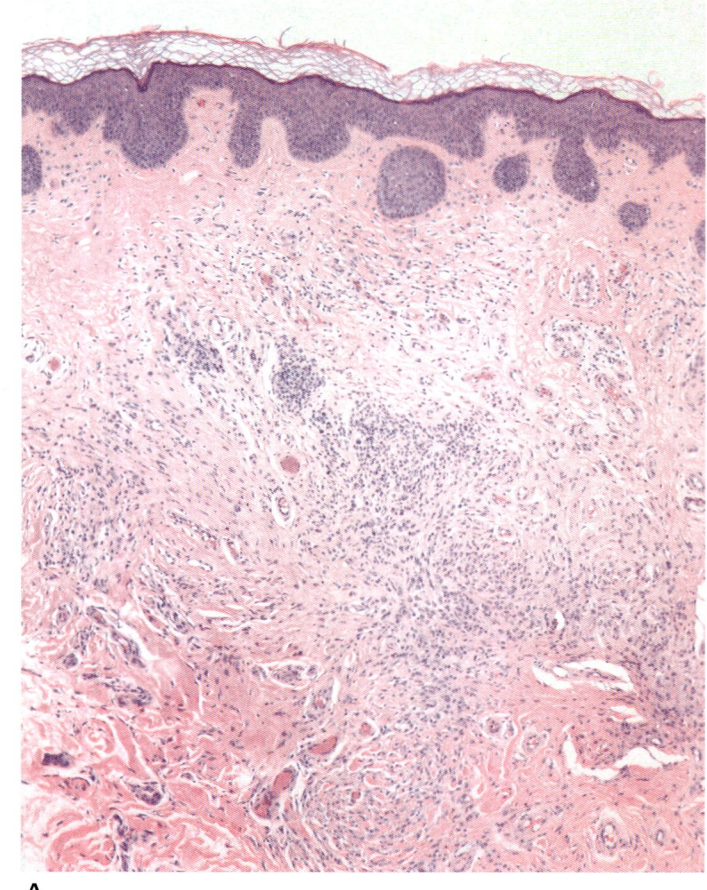

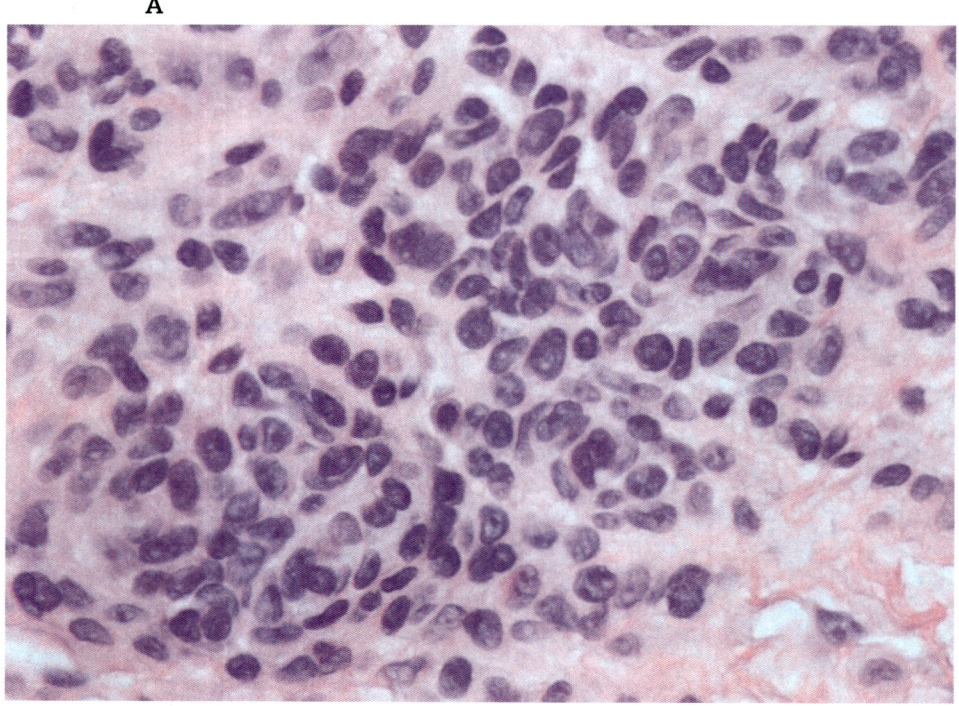

FIGURE 5-9 Dermal nevus. **A,** Maturation of type B nevus cells of the upper dermis to type C cells with dermal descent. **B,** Type B (lymphocytoid) nevus cells in dermis. The cells have minimal cytoplasm and contain uniform, round to oval nuclei.

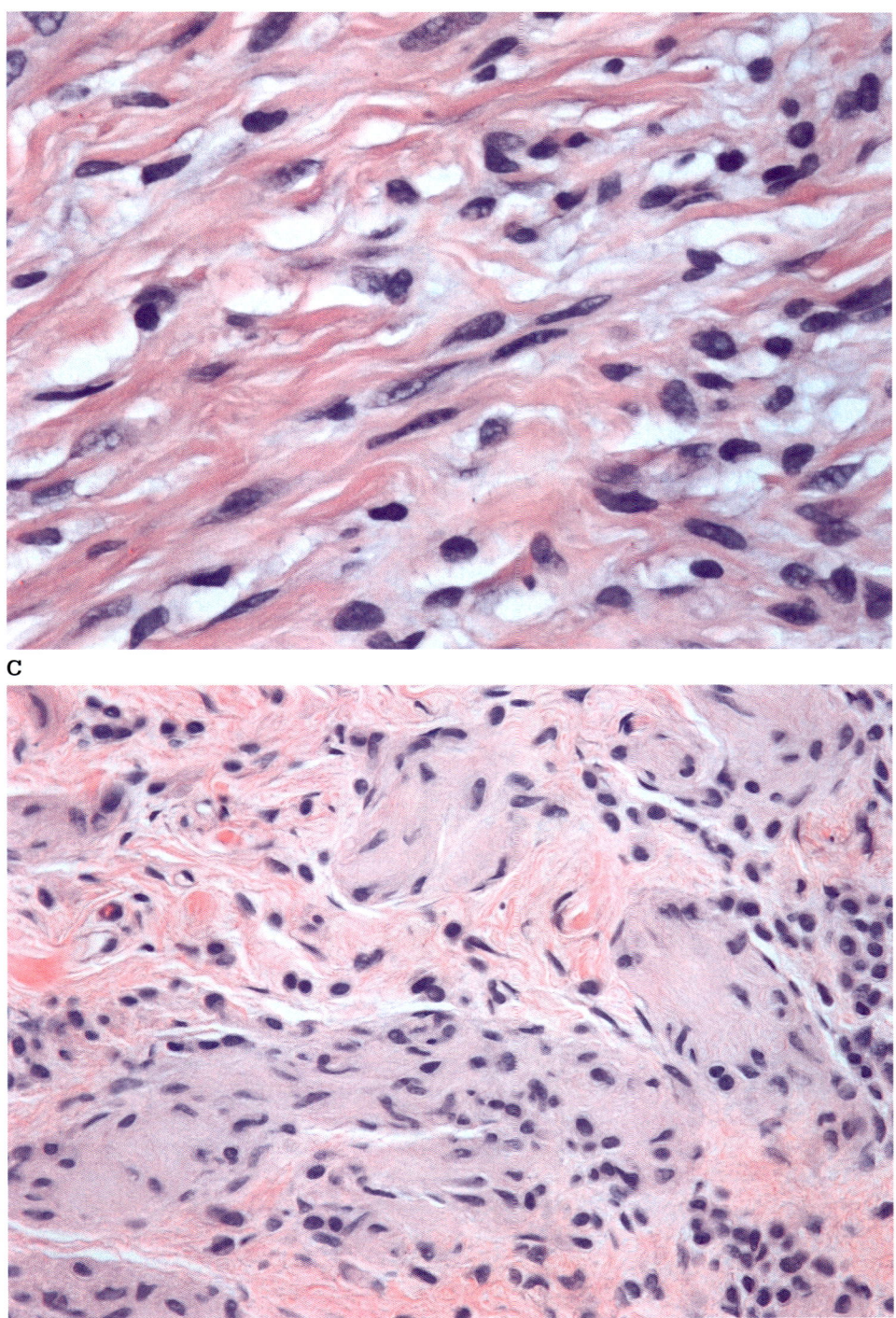

FIGURE 5-9 *Continued.* **C,** Type C (Schwannian) nevus cells. The cells are less nested and are enveloped by delicate connective tissue. **D,** Neurotization in a dermal nevus. These structures resemble Wagner-Meissner corpuscles.

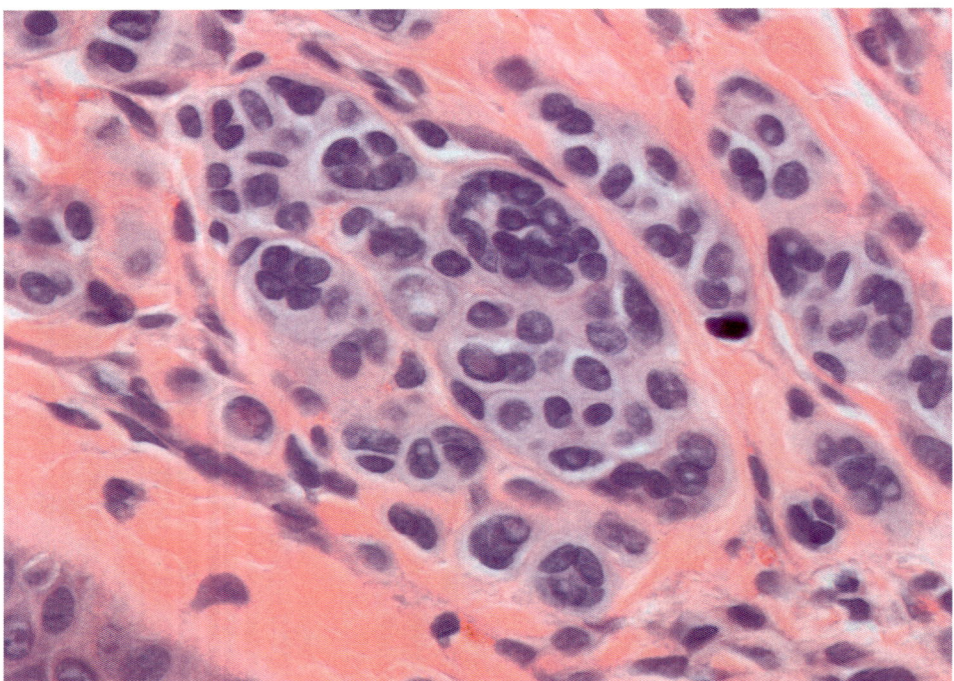

E
FIGURE 5-9 Continued. **E,** Multinucleate (mulberry-type) nevus giant cells within a nest of type A cells.

Inclusion-like structures can be found in the nuclei of nevus cells (63) (Fig. 5-9B). The appearance is created by an invagination of cytoplasm into the nuclear membrane, which when viewed on cross section seems to lie within the nucleus. The histologic staining properties of the interior of these pseudoinclusions therefore resemble that of the nevus cell cytoplasm.

HISTOLOGIC VARIATIONS WITHIN COMMON ACQUIRED NEVI

General Architecture

Melanocytic nevi are generally symmetrical and have a well-circumscribed configuration (Fig. 5-7A). The principal exceptions are lentiginous nevi, which, in contrast to other common acquired nevi (7), may extend beyond the dermal component, if present. The surface topography of the common acquired nevus may vary from flat to dome shaped, polypoid, or papillomatous (61). The cross-sectional silhouette correlates with the stage in nevus development—junctional nevi are relatively macular; compound nevi are slightly raised; and dermal nevi are dome shaped, polypoid, or papillomatous. The anatomic site often influences the surface configuration of nevi. Those situated at the acra are flat or only slightly raised, as a rule (5,6,11–13) (Fig. 5-6).

In contrast, many nevi of the head and neck are dome-shaped to polypoid, compound or dermal nevi (Fig. 5-8), influenced of course by the natural history of the lesions and by the age of the individual.

Epidermal Changes

Variations in the epidermis within a nevus may include little or no acanthosis, elongation of the rete ridges in a lentiginous pattern, papillomatous hyperplasia mimicking seborrheic keratoses, and effacement of the retia as in some intradermal nevi (64). Those lesions with papillated epidermal hyperplasia have been known by various designations, including papillary nevus and keratotic nevus. Those lesions, which in silhouette resemble seborrheic keratoses by virtue of the epidermal hyperplasia, hyperkeratosis, papillomatosis, and horn pseudocyst formation, represent about 6% of all common nevi and have a predilection for the torso (65). Papillomatous changes in nevi can be a response to estrogenic hormones (66).

Occasionally are seen predominantly intradermal nevi that display increased numbers of melanocytes arrayed at uneven intervals as single cell units along the basilar epidermal layer. The cells may have abundant pale to clear cytoplasms, increased nuclear:cytoplasmic ratios, and prominent nucleoli. They are distinguished from melanoma by absence of several features, including lateral spread beyond the dermal component, pagetoid scatter, advanced nuclear atypia, finely granular cytoplasms, mitotic activity, and host inflammatory response (67).

Dermal Variations

The proportion of cells that are type A, B, and C varies between nevi and may be related to the age of the nevus and to other poorly understood factors (5–7,17,41) (Fig. 5-9). The failure within some nevi of the dermal component to mature beyond type A cells is believed to be a maturational disturbance and is discussed in more detail later in this chapter under atypical nevi. In any given nevus, the dermal constituents may be largely type A, type B, or type C cells (5–7,17,41).

An uncommon variation that may simulate melanoma on occasion is the *ancient melanocytic nevus* (68). These lesions, most of which occur on the face of older individuals, contain a mixed dermal population, one of which consists of cells resembling the epithelioid cell of a Spitz nevus. The nuclei are pleomorphic, and mitotic figures, although not common, can be found in some sections. Thus the lesion may present a difficult differential diagnosis of melanoma arising within a nevus (68).

Balloon cell alterations within nevi are considered to be a degenerative or senescent change. Balloon cells are found in approximately 2% of nevi (69–71). These cells are substantially enlarged and contain abundant vacuolated cytoplasms and centrally situated nuclei. Electron microscopic examination indicated that the alteration is due to vacuolar degeneration of melanosomes (72,73).

Variations that in the past were considered to indicate congenital nevi are now recognized as not entirely specific (74). These include distribution of nevus cells within the upper reticular dermis and dispersal of cellular strands between collagen fibers, around blood vessels in an angiocentric pattern, and within the adventitia of the appendages. Other findings that may indicate a congenital lesion are large junctional nests and a diffuse, cohesive pattern of growth that fills the papillary dermis.

Desmoplasia, or sclerosis, is defined as increased density of fibrous tissue within the stroma of nevi (6) (Fig. 5-10). Nests of nevus cells can be distributed within this matrix. The desmoplastic (sclerotic) nevus combines a population of predominantly spindled melanocytes situated within a fibrotic stroma (75). In these lesions, the epidermis is frequently hyperplastic, the stroma may contain keloidal collagen, and increased numbers of factor XIIIa-positive dendritic cells are present interstitially (75). Although discontinuously distributed, cytologically atypical cells can be found. The absence of mitotic activity and low expression of the proliferation marker Ki-67 help distinguish these nevi from desmoplastic melanoma (75).

FIGURE 5-10 Desmoplasia (sclerosis) in a dermal nevus.

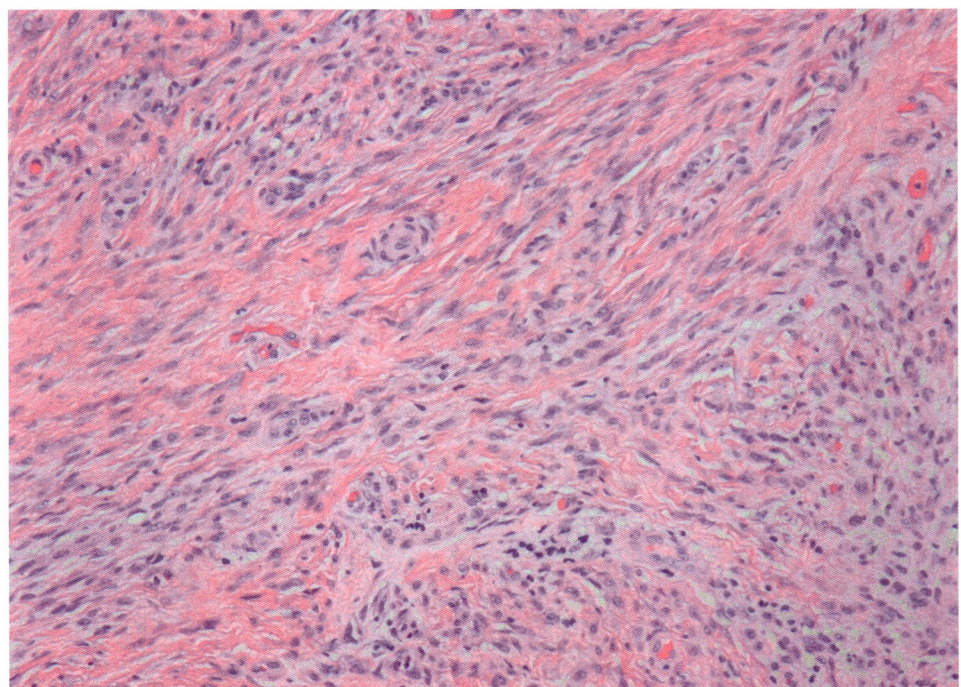

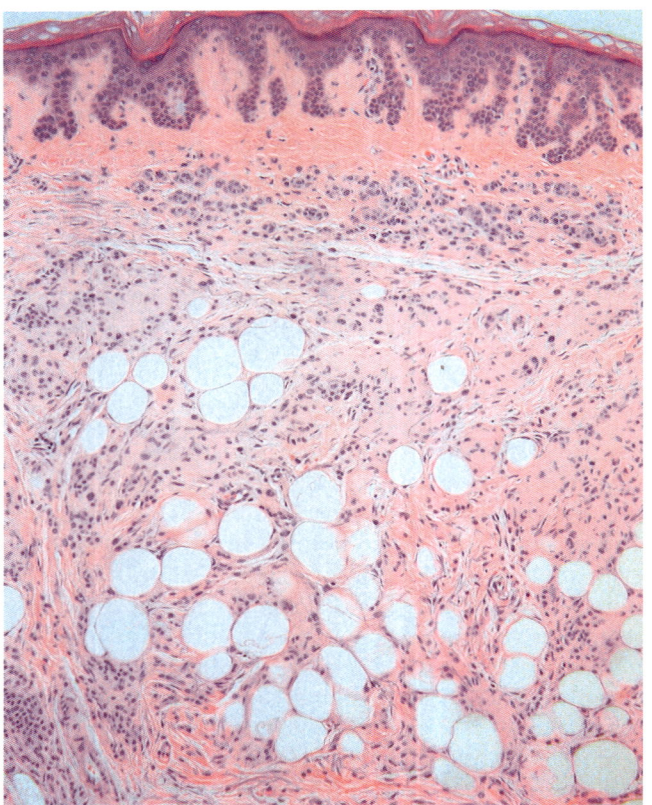

FIGURE 5-11 Lipomatous metaplasia in a dermal nevus.

Current understanding of nevus evolution postulates that many, if not most, nevi will ultimately undergo gradual involution mediated by progressive replacement of the dermal nevus cells by delicate fibrous tissue or by adipocytes (5,6,10). The final stage in the lifespan of a nevus may therefore resemble an acrochordon or an angiofibroma (6,10,76).

The progressive accumulation of adipocytes that occurs within some nevi correlates with age of the individual (6) (Fig. 5-11). In most cases, the change probably represents one component in the process of involution of a nevus. This histologic finding should not be taken by itself as evidence for a diagnosis of nevus lipomatosis superficialis.

Interstitial accumulation of mucin is a common finding within nevi (6). The deposition of this ground substance occurs most commonly in dermal nevi and, in unusual cases, may give rise to confluent pools of the basophilic material.

Within the dermis of compound or intradermal nevi, the cells may array about anastomosing clear spaces, conveying the appearance of vascular structures (Fig. 5-12).

Neurotization refers to the histologic pattern of neural differentiation, with prominence of type C cells in the dermal component of a nevus (5–7,13,17,18,41) (Fig. 5-9C). The predominant cell type is spindled, and the cells may organize into neuroidal structures resembling Wagner-Meissner corpuscles (Fig. 5-9D). Both Schwannian and perineurial differentiation may occur. Encasing the cells is a delicate fibrous stroma, which when mucinous can resemble the stroma of a neurofibroma (17,77). Table 5-6 lists other uncommon changes that can be found histologically within nevi.

ATYPICAL (DYSPLASTIC) NEVI

Atypical nervi are also referred to as dysplastic nevi, Clark nevi, B-K mole, and (lentiginous) nevi with architectural disorder and cytologic atypia.

TABLE 5-6 Uncommon findings in, or presentation of, melanocytic nevi.

Variant	Comment(s)	Reference(s)
Agminated (speckled) lentiginosis or melanocytic nevus	Circumscribed grouping of hyperpigmented macules and/or papules similar to nevus spilus but with no background macule; hyperpigmented foci are lentigines or junctional or compound nevi	78
Amyloid deposition	Degenerative nevus cells	79
Angiomatous, pseudovascular pattern	Nevus cell pattern resembling vascular or lymphatic spaces, possibly an artifact from tissue processing (Fig. 5-12)	80, 81
Cockarde (Cockade) nevus	Peripheral pigmented halo with intervening, nonpigmented annulus about central nevus	82–85
Keratinous cyst rupture, folliculitis, abscess formation	Clinical enlargement or color change, simulating melanoma	86–89
Meyerson nevus	Subacute eczematous epidermal changes associated with nevus, often forming eczematous halos	90–93
Nevus (osteonevus) of Nanta	Bone formation in a nevus (osseous metaplasia)	94, 95
Perinevoid alopecia	Hair loss associated with scalp nevi; inflammatory reaction resembling halo nevus but associated with hair follicles	96
Psammoma bodies	Degenerative change within a nevus	97

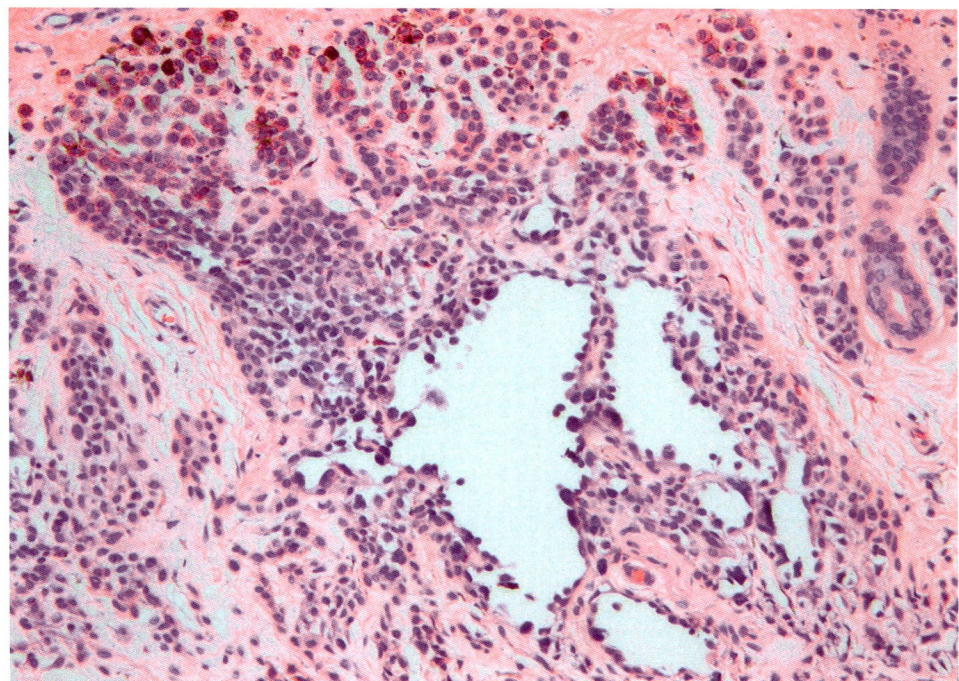

FIGURE 5-12 Pseudovascular structures within an acquired nevus. Dermal nevus cells line clear spaces that mimic vascular lumina.

The search for lesions that are precursors to melanoma has intrigued investigators for many years, since a substantial proportion of melanomas (20–80%, depending on the study) arise in association with a preexisting nevus by clinical history, and about a third to half of melanomas in histologic section contain remnants of a nevus (98–101). Moreover, many melanoma patients have increased numbers and/or unusual nevi (102–107).

As a result of the search for melanoma precursor lesions, attention came to be focused on melanocytic proliferations with disordered architectural arrangements and cytologic atypia, commonly referred to as the dysplastic nevus but designated herein as the *atypical nevus*. This focus of attention has generated substantial controversy. Considered broadly, the category of atypical nevus is essentially situated within a continuum of morphologic abnormality extending from "typical" acquired nevi at one extreme to melanoma at the other (Fig. 5-13). The salient issues subject to ongoing debate regarding these lesions are whether they are markers of increased melanoma risk (Table 5-7) and whether they are precursors to melanoma. The more practical concern in the present context is their histologic distinction from melanoma.

The original descriptions (105–107) of what later came to be most commonly referred to as the dysplastic nevus stimulated rather intense focus on the curious association between nevi and melanoma, providing new information and insights into putative mechanisms of tumor progression. This maelstrom of unbridled controversy unleashed by the focus on atypical nevi, however, generated many unanswered questions about the pathophysiologic relationship of nevi in general to melanoma.

FIGURE 5-13 Continuum of melanoma risk associated with clinical phenotypes.

Low	Melanoma Risk	High
No nevi	⟶ Increasing number of nevi ⟶	Numerous nevi
No atypical nevi	⟶ Increasing number of atypical nevi ⟶	Atypical nevi
No family history of melanoma or dysplastic nevi	⟶ Increasing genetic component ⟶	Hereditary melanoma

TABLE 5-7 Summary of prevalence, melanoma risk, and genetics associated with clinically atypical nevi.

Prevalence of atypical nevi (by clinical criteria)
    Hereditary melanoma, 54%
    Sporadic melanoma, 33%
    General population, 7–10%
Melanoma risk, relative
    Hereditary melanoma kindreds
        Patient with previous melanoma and atypical nevi, 500
        Patient with atypical nevi, 150
        Individual with no atypical nevi, 2–12
    No family history
        Patient with previous melanoma and no atypical nevi, 9
        Individual with sporadic atypical nevi, 7–20
Genetics
    Partly genetic, partly environmental (e.g., solar radiation)
    Mode of inheritance uncertain, probably polygenic
    Not proved to be linked to the CDKN2A/p16 melanoma tumor-suppressor locus

The atypical nevus is not a new entity. The presence of multiple nevi on individuals with hereditary melanoma was noted as early as 1820 (102,103) (Table 5-8). Much later, nevi with atypical histologic features that we now associate with this entity were described as "active," "activated," or "atypical" junctional nevi (104,108,109). In fact, Lund and Kraus (109) outlined a sequence of progression of the atypical junctional nevus to melanoma very similar to what has been proposed in more recent decades (7). The significance of atypical nevi, however, did not become the focus of more general interest until the widely promoted descriptions of individuals bearing those peculiar nevi in hereditary melanoma kindreds by Frichot et al. (105), Lynch et al. (106), and Clark et al. (107) (Table 5-8).

A large body of clinical, histologic, and experimental data acquired since the 1980s tends to support in broad terms the legitimacy of atypical nevi as intermediate stage(s) in the clinicopathologic continuum from nevi to melanoma (Fig. 5-13; Table 5-9). Because of the apparent histologic, as well as clinical, spectrum from ordinary nevi to melanoma, however, it has proved difficult to define the upper and lower limits that distinguish the atypical nevus on the one hand and melanoma on the other (110). This one factor has largely contributed to the considerable controversy as to the criteria for, and the prevalence of, the atypical nevus. Now after more than two decades of intensive study, there is still no consensus as to the minimum essential criteria for the atypical nevus; consequently, there is considerable latitude in the diagnostic criteria for these lesions.

One aspect to the ongoing controversy has been the appropriate nomenclature for the lesion and the clinical syndrome (111,112). To some, the terms *dysplasia* and *dysplastic* when applied to nevi or a nevus phenotype are ambiguous because the terms have been used to denote both developmental anomaly and architectural and cytologic atypia of tissue. Because of the controversy, a consensus conference convened by the National Institutes of Health (NIH) recommended that the designation *dysplastic nevus* be abandoned in favor of *nevus with architectural disorder and cytologic atypia* (113). The term *dysplasia* as applied to melanocytic proliferations, however, has probably encompassed both usages mentioned above (110). In one sense, the term has been used to indicate

TABLE 5-8 Chronology of descriptions of atypical nevi.

Year	Researcher(s)	Description
1820	Norris	First description of hereditary melanoma and observation that family members have numerous moles
1952	Cauley	Multiple atypical nevi in families prone to melanoma
1977	Frichot et al.	Cutaneous phenotype of atypical nevi in family members of hereditary melanoma kindreds
1978	Clark et al.	B-K mole syndrome; individuals in familial melanoma kindreds have atypical moles
1978	Lynch et al.	Familial atypical multiple mole-melanoma syndrome (FAMMM) introduced
1980	Greene et al.	Dysplastic nevus syndrome introduced
1980	Elder et al.	Sporadic dysplastic nevus syndrome introduced
1992	NIH Consensus Conference	Nevus with architectural disorder and/or cytologic atypia introduced to replace dysplastic nevus

TABLE 5-9 Empirical support for the atypical nevus as a precursor to melanoma.

Clinical behavior	Occasionally progression to melanoma
Clinical features	Intermediate in size, asymmetry, and color variegation
Histologic features	Intermediate in architectural disorder and cytologic atypia
Melanocyte-associated antigens	Intermediate in expression of antigens such as HLA-DR, epidermal growth factor (EGF) receptor, nerve growth factor (NGF) receptor, gangliosides
DNA content	Intermediate
Cytogenetics	Intermediate in chromosomal aberrations
Melanosomal alterations	Intermediate in frequency of abnormal melanosomes

abnormal development of nevi, represented by persistent lentiginous proliferation with reduced tendency to undergo the usual maturational sequence or regression of nevi (7). On the other hand, the most common usage has been to denote a stage of tumor progression intermediate between the common nevus and melanoma (7). Because the matter has not been settled, varying terminologies will undoubtedly persist into the foreseeable future. Although the designation *dysplastic nevus* continues to have wide currency in dermatologic practice, *atypical nevus* and *atypical nevus* syndrome will be used herein for either the clinical or the histologic presentation.

The arguments for and against the case of the atypical nevus as a significant risk indicator and precursor lesion to melanoma are summarized in the following section. Regardless of the controversial aspects of the dysplastic nevus, a large majority of dermatologists accept its legitimacy as an entity that conveys an increased risk of melanoma (114). Because the literature on the subject is voluminous, no attempt is made here to provide an exhaustive review. Representative literature, however, is presented on both sides of the controversial aspects of the atypical nevus, with the intent of avoiding an untenable, polarized position on the subject.

The Significance of the Atypical Nevus

Markers of Increased Risk of Melanoma In hereditary melanoma kindreds, the presence of *clinically* atypical nevi confers a significantly increased risk for the development of melanoma (105–107,115–117) (Tables 5-7 and 5-10). Within this familial setting, the presence of atypical nevi is associated with nearly a 50% cumulative risk for melanoma by age 50 years (117). During prospective follow up of melanoma kindreds, only those family members with atypical nevi develop melanoma at a rate of 14.3/1000 patient-years in one dataset (115) and 1710/100,000 patient-years in a subsequent analysis (118).

Atypical nevi are also found sporadically within the general population and serve as risk markers for melanoma, although at not nearly as great a level as observed in the familial setting (119–126). Sporadic, clinically atypical nevi are associated with a relative risk for melanoma ranging from ~2 to > 20, depending on numbers of atypical nevi and on criteria for diagnosis of an atypical nevus (Tables 5-11 and 5-12). The prevalence of atypical nevi in the general population has been difficult to gauge, partly because of the lack of uniformity in its definition and partly because of incomplete ascertainment of subjects within study populations. A commonly

TABLE 5-10 Stratification of risk factors for cutaneous melanoma.

Factor	Estimated relative risk[a]
Changing pigmented lesion	Very high
Xeroderma pigmentosa	500
Melanoma-atypical nevus kindred	
Prior melanoma	500
No prior melanoma	150
Numerous common nevi	5–65
Atypical nevi	2–>20
Giant congenital nevus	5–15
Previous melanoma	9
Lentigo maligna	5–10
Immunosuppression	4–7
Red or blond hair	2–7
Tendency to freckle	2–4
Sun sensitivity	2–3
Excessive sun exposure	2–4
Melanoma in first-degree relative	2–12
Few or no common nevi	0.3
Asian, Hispanic, or African American pigmentation	0.08–0.15
Age < 15 years	0.01

Source: Adapted from Williams and Sagebiel (1994).
[a]Average risk = 1; estimates derived from references.

TABLE 5-11 Melanoma risk associated with clinically atypical nevi: comparison of melanoma patients and controls.

Study	Country	Definition	One or more atypical nevi		
			Patients (%)	Controls (%)	Relative risk
Roush (1986), Nordlund (1985)	Australia	5 mm, irregular border and pigmentation	34	7	7.7
MacKie (1985)	Scotland	> 5 mm, either irregular border or pigmentation, or inflammation	38	20	2.1–4.5[a]
Holly (1987)	USA	> 5 mm, irregular border or pigmentation, erythema	55	17	3.8–6.3[b]
Grob (1990)	France	≥ 5 mm, irregular border, irregular pigment	18	5	2.77[c]
Halpern (1991)	USA	> 4 mm, macular component irregular color and border	39	7	8.8
Garbe (1989)	Germany	> 5 mm, irregular border, color variation, macular and papular components	45	5	7
Augustsson (1990)	Sweden	≥ 5 mm, ill-defined border, speckled pigmentation, erythema or pebbled surface	28	9	2.5–5.6[d]
Rieger (1995)	Germany	≥ 5 mm, ill-defined border, irregular outline, non-uniform color, partly macular	41	18	4.0[e]
Carli (1995)	Italy	> 6 mm, ill-defined border variegated pigment, background erythema	16	3	8.4[f]
Grulich (1996)	Australia	≥ 5 mm, ill-defined border, irregular pigmentation	13	2	9.0[g]
Bataille (1996)	Britain	≥ 5 mm, irregular border, irregular pigmentation	10	1	14.3[h]
Tucker (1997)	USA	> 5 mm, flatness, color variation, irregular borders	59	24	2–12[i]
Rodenas (1997)	Spain	≥ 5 mm, irregular border, irregular pigmentation, background erythema	20	8	3.6[j]
Bataille (1998)	Britain	≥ 5 mm, irregular border, irregular pigmentation	16	1	4.6[k]
	Australia		24	5	51.7[k]

Source: Adapted and updated from Williams and Sagebiel (1994).
[a]For 1–2 atypical nevi, 2.1; for ≥ 3 atypical nevi, 4.5.
[b]For 1–5 atypical nevi, 3.8; for ≥ 6 atypical nevi, 6.3.
[c]For > 1 atypical nevus.
[d]For 1–2 atypical nevi, 2.5; for ≥ 3 atypical nevi, 5.6.
[e]For ≥ 1 or more atypical nevi on the trunk of men.
[f]For ≥ 1 or more atypical nevi.
[g]For ≥ 5 or more atypical nevi.
[h]For ≥ 4 or more atypical nevi.
[i]For 1 atypical nevus, 2; for ≥ 10, 12.
[j]For ≥ 1 atypical nevi on the back.
[k]For ≥ 3 atypical nevi.

cited range for the general population prevalence of atypical nevi by clinical criteria is 7–20% (120–122,127–131).

One constraint that is relevant to this determination is that interobserver concordance by κ statistics among expert observers in judging clinical atypia of nevi is in the range of 50–62%, which is considered only slight to fair reliability (118,132). This is not surprising because, with the exception of lesional diameter, the criteria for the individual clinical features constituting the atypical nevus are intrinsically subjective. In fact, the interobserver cor-

TABLE 5-12 Relative risk of melanoma in relation to numbers of nevi.

Study	Country	Nevus definition	Number of nevi	Relative risk
Holly (1987)	USA	≥ 2 mm, "nondysplastic"	11–25	1.6
			26–50	4.4
			51–100	5.4
			> 100	9.8
Swerdlow and Green (1987)	Scotland	≥ 2 mm, whole body	10–24	4.4
			25–49	8.7
			≥ 50	64
Green (1985)	Australia	≥ 2 mm, left arm	2–4	16
			5–10	15
			> 10	20
Grob (1990)	France	> 1 mm, whole body	0–10	1.0
			11–20	1.17
			21–40	3.84
			41–80	3.46
			81–120	4.14
			> 120	16.06
Augustsson (1990)	Sweden	≥ 2 mm, whole body	75–149	1.2
			≥ 150	2.6
Weiss (1991)	Germany	"Benign" nevi	10–50	4.3
			> 50	15
Kruger (1992)	Germany	≥ 2 mm, trunk, males	5–10	2.9
			11–20	5.5
			> 20	33
			> 40	133
Rieger (1995)	Germany	≥ 2 mm, trunk, males	≥ 40	20.6
		≥ 2 mm, legs, women	≥ 20	11.7
Carli (1995)	Italy	> 2 mm, whole body	> 30	22.3
Grulich (1996)	Australia	≥ 2 mm, whole body	> 100	7.4
Bataille (1996)	Britain	≥ 2 mm, whole body	> 100	7.7
Rodenas (1997)	Spain	> 2 mm, whole body	> 50	6.9
Tucker (1997)	USA	≥ 2 mm, whole body	> 100	3.4
Bataille (1998)	Britain	≥ 2 mm, whole body	> 100	16.5
	Australia	≥ 2 mm, whole body	> 100	12.7

Source: Adapted and updated from Williams and Sagebiel (1994).

relation coefficients range from ~0.1 to 0.64, depending on the criterion, with especially low rates of interobserver agreements for assessing coloration (133).

Estimates for the prevalence of the atypical nevus syndrome (dysplastic nevus syndrome) have been even more intractable because there is no minimum criterion for numbers of nevi and sizes of nevi, although the arbitrary standard of 50–100 or more nevi has been offered (100,110) (Table 5-13). Risk stratification protocols have been formulated to facilitate the assessment of melanoma risk and the management of patients (Tables 5-7 and 5-10). Regardless of these efforts to categorize risk, it should be emphasized that the nevus phenotype is best described as a continuous trait, and the derivative relative risk values probably represent points on a continuous scale (Fig. 5-13). The factors that enter into any formulation of risk include family history of melanoma, total number of nevi, total number of clinically atypical nevi, and personal history of melanoma.

Another aspect fueling the controversy concerns the fact that the increased relative risk for melanoma associated in epidemiologic studies with the lesion derives largely from *clinical* and not *histologic* criteria. For example, the relative risk values for melanoma that range from 1.6 to > 60 in case-control studies reflects the dose-response effects of increasing total numbers of nevi and increasing size (i.e., > 6 mm) of nevi, with or without clinical atypia (100,121,122,124,134–144) (Tables 5-11 and 5-12). Only one case-control study to date has addressed the relative risk for melanoma conferred by a histologic diagnosis of atypical nevus. That analysis reported a frequency of histologically atypical nevus in 40% of cases and 8% of controls, giving an adjusted relative risk of 4.6 (130). It has been estimated that the phenotype of increased numbers of nevi may be the major risk factor for as many as 29–79% of all melanomas (124). Irrespective of the presence or absence of histologic atypia, the finding of clinically atypical nevi—defined as increased size,

TABLE 5-13 Nevus phenotypes.

Parameter	Normal nevus pattern	Abnormal nevus phenotype
Number	None to few (< 25) nevi	Many (> 50) nevi
Size	< 5 mm	Variable: small to large, often several > 5 mm
Color and borders	Uniform or homogeneous color, well circumscribed	Some to many nevi with irregular or haphazard color, erythema, irregular or ill-defined borders

irregular borders, and variegated color—is also clearly associated with increased melanoma risk (15,100,121,122, 124–126,131,138,139,141–143,145) (Table 5-12). The effects of increasing nevus number and increased nevus size and atypia are overlapping because the phenotypes are related, or *covariate,* traits. In other words, those people with increased numbers of nevi tend to have, on average, more large and irregular nevi than those without increased numbers (146). There is, in fact, a highly significant correlation between number of benign nevi and the presence of at least one clinically atypical nevus—for example, it was reported that women with 100 more banal nevi had a 26-fold increased likelihood of having an atypical nevus (147). Suffice it to say that both the nevus phenotype and the relationship between nevi and melanoma are complex.

It is important to point out that, although correlations exist, the concordance between clinical atypia and histologic atypia is rather poor (110,132,133,148,149). Moreover, the predictive value of the clinical examination for histologic atypia will vary substantially in different patient populations, being rather low in the general population (150). Clinically atypical nevi may lack histologic atypia, and vice versa. In a multiobserver analysis, clinically typical nevi exhibited histologic atypia in 4–46% of cases, depending on observer (151). Thus, a not insignificant proportion of nevi with histologic atypia are clinically rather unremarkable (148,151–153). This indicates a low sensitivity of the clinical examination in predicting histologic atypia, estimated at 0.29 in one study in which 71% of histologically atypical nevi were judged clinically not atypical (148). Furthermore, another systematic study found that 69.7% of clinically nonatypical nevi judged were histologically atypical (149). The overall sensitivity of the clinical examination in predicting histologic atypia in the latter study was 58.4%, with a specificity of 66.6% and a κ value of 0.17. Thus the clinical criteria appeared to be poorly sensitive and scarcely specific for histologic atypia, prompting the authors to conclude that the atypical nevus cannot be considered a distinct entity (149). The practical effect of the low sensitivity of the clinical examination in predicting histologic atypia is that the true population prevalence of histologic atypia is probably much higher than generally recognized, certainly higher than the oft-cited prevalence of 7–10%, based on the clinical criteria of increased size and border and color irregularity of nevi.

Atypical Nevi as Precursors to Melanoma Although atypical nevi are much more prevalent than melanoma and are in most instances stable lesions, they are thought to occasionally progress to melanoma (7,154) (Fig. 5-14). The basis for this belief follows from the serial photography of individual nevi and from the spatial co-existence within pigmented lesions of both melanoma and atypical nevus (7,155). Remnants of atypical nevi within histologic sections of melanoma have been reported at a frequency of < 20–50% (7,98–101,156–159). Any estimate of the frequency with which nevi are associated with melanomas is constrained by potential difficulties in discriminating melanomas in situ from atypical nevi and by the rather high rate at which melanomas are associated with remnants of common, banal nevi in histologic sections. For example, in a study of a series of thin melanomas, histologic remnants of a nevus were found in 51% of cases, and of these, 56% were atypical nevi and 41% were banal nevi (101). In another systematic analysis yielding substantially contradictory conclusions, nevus remnants were found in 21% of melanomas, of which only one (~4%) was an atypical nevus (160). Suffice it to say that firm conclusions regarding the actual proportion of melanomas attributable to atypical nevi as precursor lesions remain intractable.

The hypothesis that atypical nevi serve as potential precursors to melanoma predicts that those nevi sustain genetic alterations at loci that are critical in the development of melanoma. In some molecular analyses of DNA content, the nuclei of atypical nevi more often contained > 2N DNA content (i.e., hyperdiploidy) than did common nevi (161,162), but they did not display the aneuploidy of melanoma (162). Other independent analyses failed to confirm significant rates of hyperdiploidy in atypical nevi (163,164), which could be explained in part by differences either in histological criteria or in composition of the respective samples. In one systematic analysis, the tumor antigen profile expressed by atypical nevus

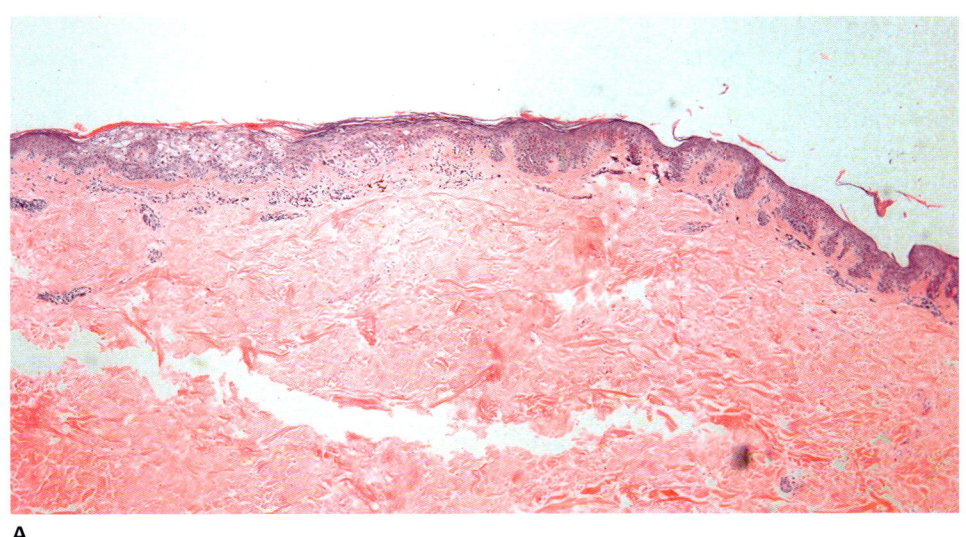

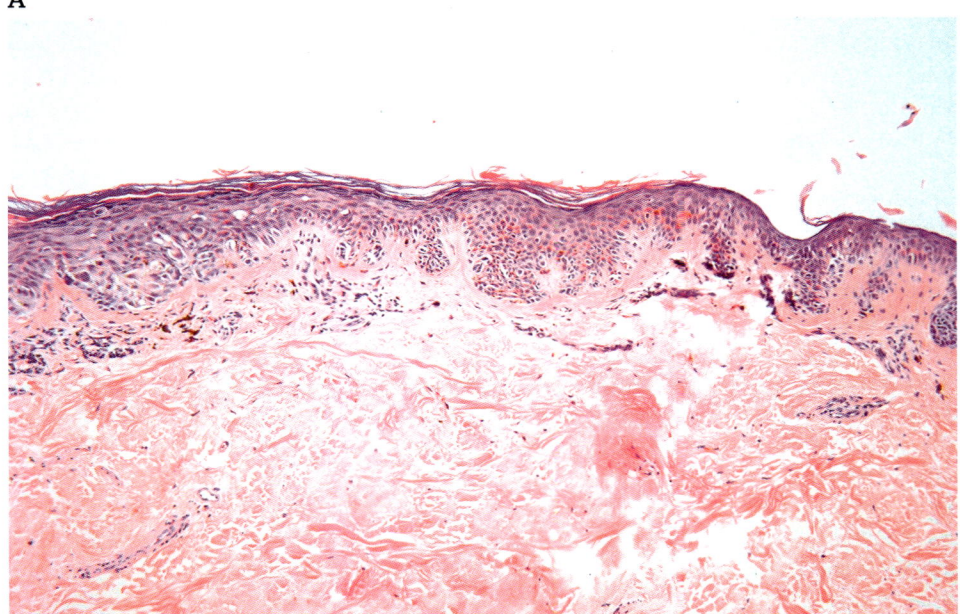

FIGURE 5-14 Malignant melanoma arising in association with an atypical nevus. **A,** On scanning magnification, an atypical nevus is present on the right side of the field and a superficially invasive melanoma on the left. **B,** The transition from atypical nevus to melanoma is shown at higher magnification.

cells was intermediate between that expressed by common nevus cells and that expressed by melanoma (165). In that study, expression levels of such tumor-related antigens as epidermal growth factor (EGF) receptor and nerve growth factor (NGF) receptor increased progressively in the following sequence: melanocytes, banal nevus cells, atypical nevus cells, radial growth phase melanoma, vertical growth phase melanoma, and metastatic melanoma (165).

The major melanoma gene thus far identified is CDKN2A, also known as p16, which accounts for up to 40% of all cases of familial melanoma; inactivation in the germ cell line at that tumor-suppressor locus on chromosome 9p21 by point mutations or deletions is putatively an initiating event in melanoma development (166). There is as of yet no consensus as to whether atypical nevi sustain genetic lesions in the p16 gene, because the p16 protein and mRNA are expressed at normal levels in atypical as well as in banal nevi, but at reduced levels in many melanomas (167–169); moreover, the atypical nevus phenotype does not readily link genetically by the use of polymorphic markers to the CDKN2A locus (170). Several reports have suggested, however, that in atypical nevi, as in melanoma, there may be point mutations or allelic deletions in the vicinity of that critical locus on chromosome 9p (171–173). On the other hand, chromosomal loss, sequence mutations in the p16 exonic sequence, and promoter methylation were not found in a detailed genetic analysis of 45 typical nevi, the data being consistent with the hypothesis that variants in the coding and noncoding regions of the p16 gene are not the major genetic determinants of the nevus phenotype (174). Atypical nevi, as well as melanoma, express DNA mismatch repair genes at a lower level (175), and have a higher rate of microsatellite instability at markers near the CDKN2A (p16) locus (176), than do common nevi. Atypical, as well as common, nevi from CDKN2A mutation carriers and noncarriers have a low proliferation index (<1–2% of cells), compared to indices > 7% in melanomas in situ and higher levels yet in invasive and metastatic melanomas (177).

Correlation of Histologic Melanocytic Atypia with Increased Melanoma Risk The link between atypical nevi and melanoma risk is almost entirely based on quantitative and qualitative clinical criteria. Histologic melanocytic atypia in isolation has not been sufficiently studied at this time to conclude that it is a definite risk factor for melanoma. It also warrants emphasis that the histologic features of atypical nevi (discussed below) cover a continuum from common nevi to melanoma (110). The sensitivity and specificity of the diagnostic criteria as both a melanoma risk indicator and a potential precursor lesion will therefore vary according to the placement of the threshold for diagnosis. If the threshold for recognition of atypical alterations is low, then the criteria will lose specificity. Contrarily, a high threshold for diagnosis will result in reduced sensitivity. Presently, the issue of the appropriate diagnostic threshold is unresolved. This is an important problem because the architectural alterations attributed to atypical nevi were found in 53% of nevi sampled from the general population of Utah by one observer (153) and in 7–32% of nevi employing a multiobserver study design of the Utah database (151). Histologic atypia was commonly observed in clinically normal nevi in a separate study (152). There is some correlation, however, between histologic atypia and total number of nevi (153). It nevertheless does appear likely that a certain threshold of atypia, and in particular cytologic atypia, must be achieved to have significance in terms of melanoma risk.

Limited attempts to correlate increased atypia within nevi of patients with melanoma, compared to controls without melanoma, have provided preliminary evidence that atypia may be somewhat greater in the nevi of melanoma patients (161,178). Other studies have not clearly supported this observation (151,179). Variation in histologic criteria for atypical nevi could account for differences in conclusions among the studies. Clearly, it is not the case at present that histologic analysis by itself is able to identify with substantial reliability a type of nevus that constitutes a marker of significant melanoma risk irrespective of the clinical phenotype. Thus the important matter of sensitive and specific histologic criteria for diagnosis of the atypical nevus merits further study.

Clinical Features

On any given individual, the numbers of clinically atypical nevi may vary from only one or two to several hundred or more (105–107,115,155,158,180). The minimum number of nevi and degree of clinical atypia required for diagnosis of the atypical nevus syndrome, however, have not been formulated as of yet (Table 5-13). Because the phenotype is most probably a continuous trait, any assignment of a minimum number would be arbitrary in the absence of persuasive empirical data that link the clinical parameters with biologic phenomena, such as disease outcome. One important hallmark of the atypical nevus phenotype is the tendency for considerable variation in size, shape, and coloration from nevus to nevus. The distribution of atypical nevi on affected individuals has a predilection for the trunk, but there is a curious propensity in some patients for the scalp, female breasts, buttocks, and feet (Table 5-14). A sizable fraction (42%) of nevi from the scalp in the pediatric population is atypical clinically and histologically (181). Nevi situated at sun-protected sites in patients with an atypical nevus phenotype may not be enlarged or atypical (182).

Individual atypical nevi exhibit clinical features that are often intermediate between those of common, acquired nevi and melanoma (105–107,110,115,158,183). With occasional exceptions, the lesions are larger than ba-

TABLE 5-14 Clinical features of atypical nevi.
Global phenotype
Increased numbers of typical and atypical nevi
Variations in gross morphologic features among nevi
Increased numbers of nevi on scalp, female breasts, buttocks
Nevus characteristics
Increased size (4–12 mm), but with exceptions
Asymmetry
Macular component
Irregular and ill-defined border
Altered topography, pebbled or cobblestone surface
Haphazard, variegated, or complexity of coloration

nal nevi and range from 4 to 12 mm in greatest diameter. Asymmetry is common, borders are often irregular and ill defined, and at least some portion of each lesion is macular. The surface may be pebbled. Some degree of color variegation is usual, and there may be more than two colors distributed within a lesion in a haphazard pattern (e.g., tan, brown, dark brown). Despite the subjective nature of the clinical criteria, the average rate of interobserver agreement in clinically identifying atypical nevi has been reported to be 77% (184).

Histopathological Features

The histological criteria for atypical nevi include parameters of architectural disorder, cytologic atypia, and host immune response (7,98,107,110,113,119,150,153,155,158, 159,161,178,179,185–194) (Figs. 5-15 to 5-22, Table 5-15). Controversy continues as to which of these criteria are most important for diagnosis and which are merely secondary features (183). Much of the debate has been focused on the criterion of cytologic atypia (111–113,153). As the controversy has matured since the 1980s, it has become more generally accepted that cytologic (or more precisely, nuclear) atypia is a fundamental component of the diagnosis. Without a requirement for nuclear atypia, it appears that the findings of architectural disorder and host response are quite common in nevi from the general white population and thus lack specificity as a reasonable risk marker for melanoma (153). Nuclear atypia in general does not occur without the architectural disorder (195–197). If one accepts the requirement for nuclear atypia, the matter resolves itself into recognizing gradations of nuclear alterations along a continuum from minimum to severe. Unfortunately, objective criteria for evaluating nuclear atypia have not been standardized, and defining the threshold at which point nuclear atypia first appears is difficult and possibly not easily reproducible. In one systematic study, interobserver concordance between expert observers from different institutions in the histologic diagnosis of atypia averaged 56%, with a κ value of 0.34 indicating "fair" reproducibility; intraobserver concordance ranged from 78 to 85%, with κ values (0.63–0.71) indicating substantial agreement (151). Another analysis found that the rates of interobserver agreement for diagnosis of atypical nevus ranged from 32 to 71% (198). Somewhat better interobserver concordance was reported in yet another analysis (199), and among expert observers working at the same institution, an overall concordance rate of 77% (κ = 0.55–0.84) was achieved in diagnosing atypical nevi (200). It is clear that the histologic diagnosis of the atypical nevus remains subjective. The documentation of a spectrum of DNA aneuploidy and abnormal nuclear area by image analysis that parallels grade of nuclear atypia in these lesions provides some objective validation of the subjective histologic rating of nuclear atypia (201,202). It seems reasonable to conclude at this time that, although rating of atypia within nevi is subjective, nuclear atypia does exist within nevi outside the context of fully evolved melanoma.

In efforts to resolve the issue of the relative importance of the various histologic features in atypical nevi, architectural and host-response parameters were correlated with nuclear atypia in a series of atypical and banal nevi (193). By multivariate analysis, both lentiginous melanocytic proliferation and variation in size, shape, and placement of junctional nests showed a statistically significant correlation with nuclear atypia after adjustment for co-variate factors. Other features generally assigned to atypical nevi, such as lateral extension of the intraepidermal component, lymphocytic infiltrates, and papillary dermal fibrosis, did not correlate significantly with nuclear atypia. Additional studies examining histologic criteria, although differing in experimental design, reached somewhat similar conclusions (189,190). It bears emphasis, in any event, that none of the individual histologic criteria for the atypical nevus is, by itself, unique to atypical nevi because it is shared in varying degrees by common nevi and melanoma (153,195,196,203–205).

To summarize, the most important histologic features for diagnosis of the atypical nevus are essentially (a) disordered intraepidermal melanocytic proliferation and (b) nuclear atypia of intraepidermal melanocytes (Table 5-15). The other attributes that have been assigned to the atypical nevus are most probably derivative or secondary to those criteria.

Diagnostic Criteria

Architecture More than three quarters of atypical nevi are of compound type; the remainder are junctional (192). Most are relatively macular, with only slight expansion of the papillary dermis by a limited dermal component. With a few exceptions, atypical nevi manifest a lentiginous pattern of melanocytic proliferation, in which melanocytes as variable nests and single-cell units are arrayed along the basilar aspect of elongated, club-shaped, and hyperpigmented rete (110,193) (Figs. 5-15 to 5-17). The lentiginous proliferation of compound atypical nevi extends laterally in a poorly circumscribed fashion beyond the dermal melanocytic cell population. This *shoulder phenomenon* gradually diminishes in cellularity toward the periphery and correlates with the macular annulus observed clinically with many atypical nevi. Although shoulder phenomena, by definition, are absent in junctional atypical nevi, such nevi also tend to be poorly circumscribed at their peripheries.

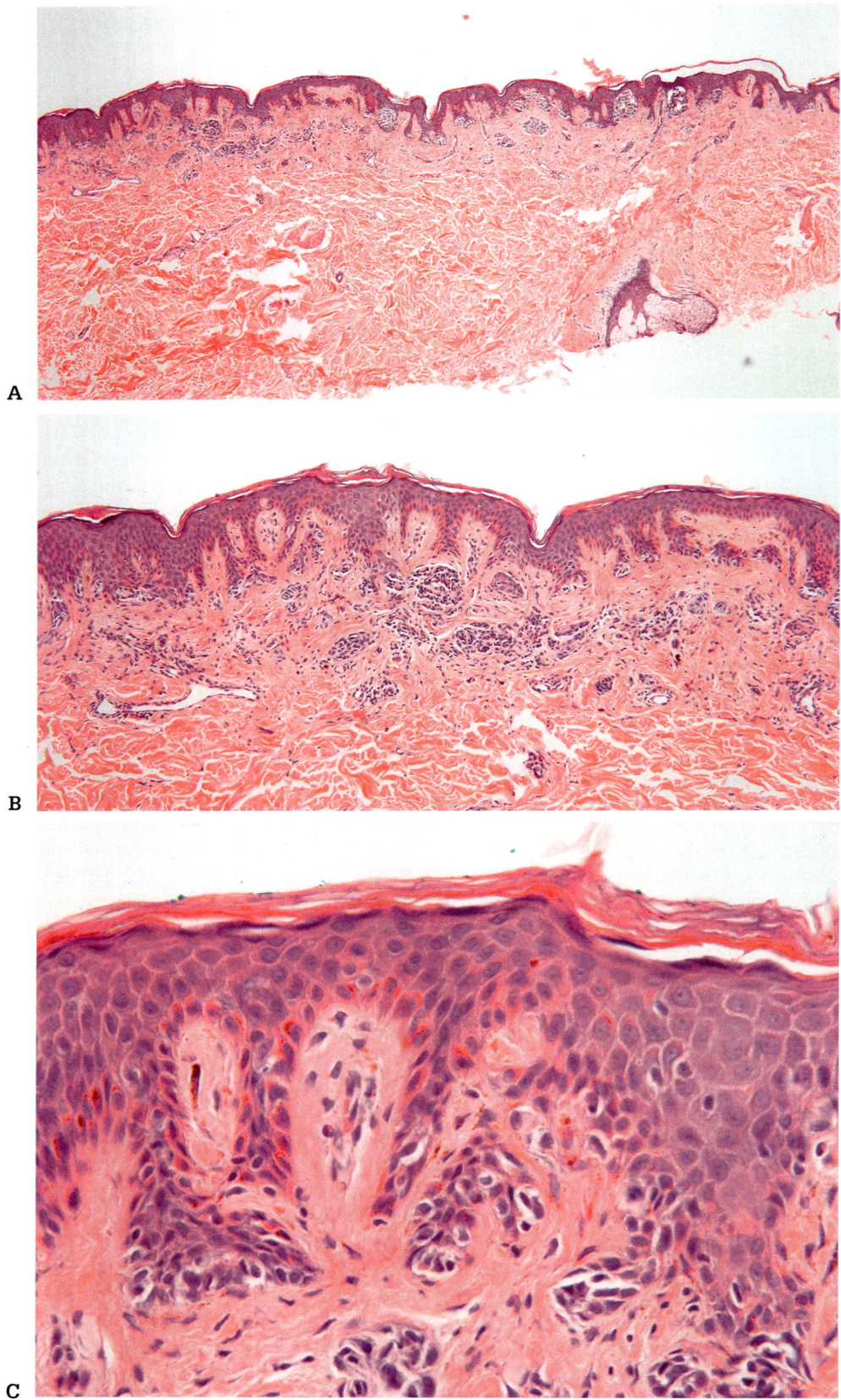

FIGURE 5-15 Compound atypical nevus. **A,** Low-power magnification showing the flat topography of an atypical nevus. The lesion is poorly circumscribed. **B,** The lentiginous architecture is shown in this field. The rete are elongated, enveloped by concentric fibroplasia, and associated with perivascular lymphoid infiltrates within the adjacent stroma. **C,** Variation in the nesting pattern and prominent lentiginous proliferation are seen at higher magnification.

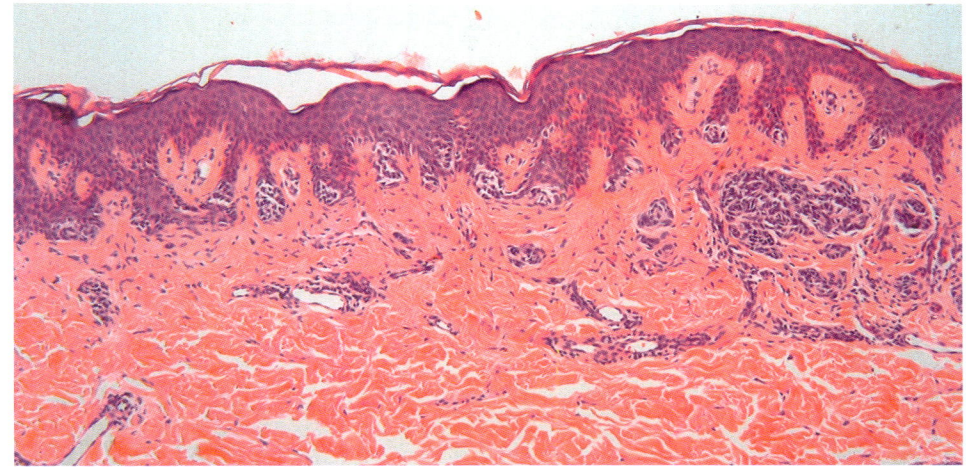

FIGURE 5-16 Compound atypical nevus. The intraepidermal component extends beyond the dermal nevus component.

FIGURE 5-17 Junctional atypical nevus. **A,** The lentiginous pattern at the junction is prominent. The basilar melanocytes are confluent along the elongated rete. **B,** There is variation in the size, shape, and nuclear chromasia of the basilar melanocytes. Some melanocytes contain nuclei that are larger than those of the spinous keratinocytes.

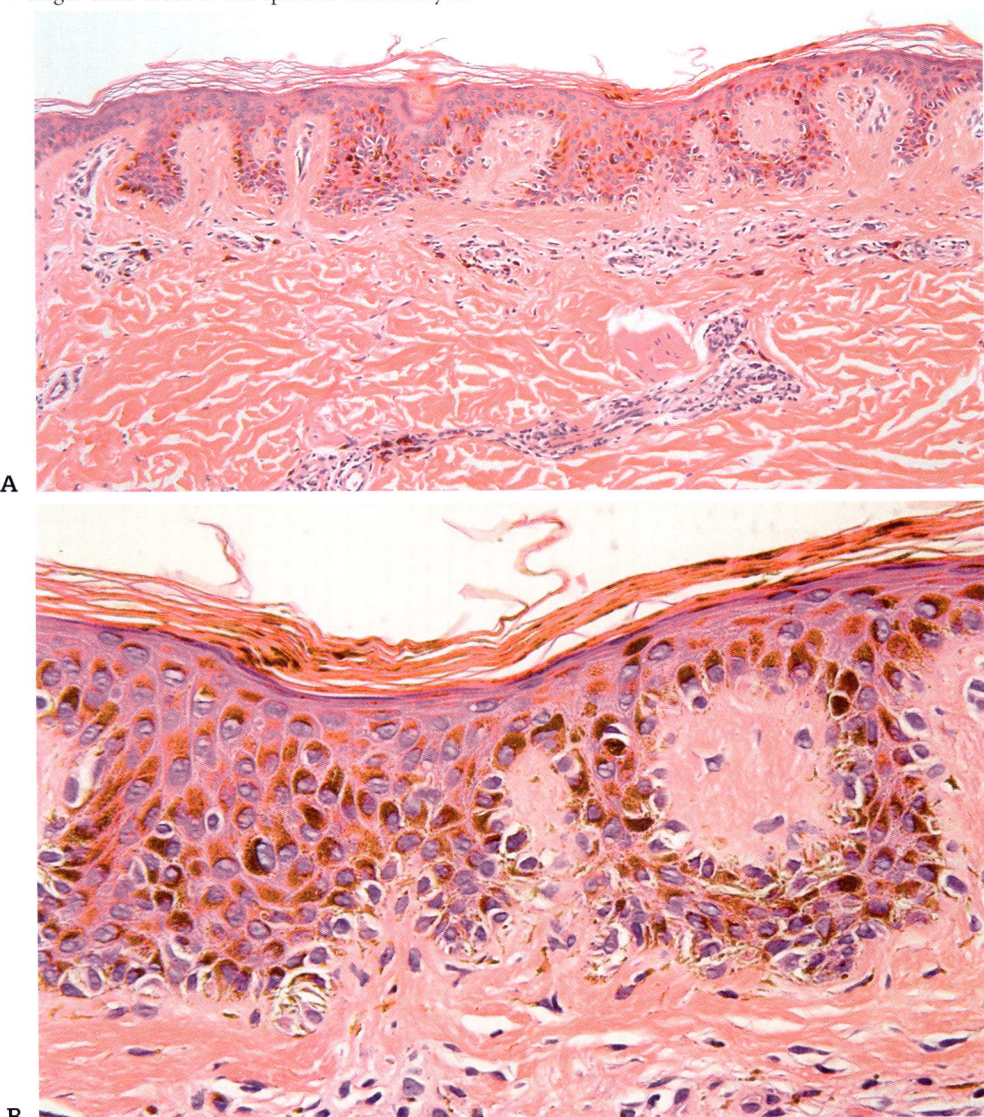

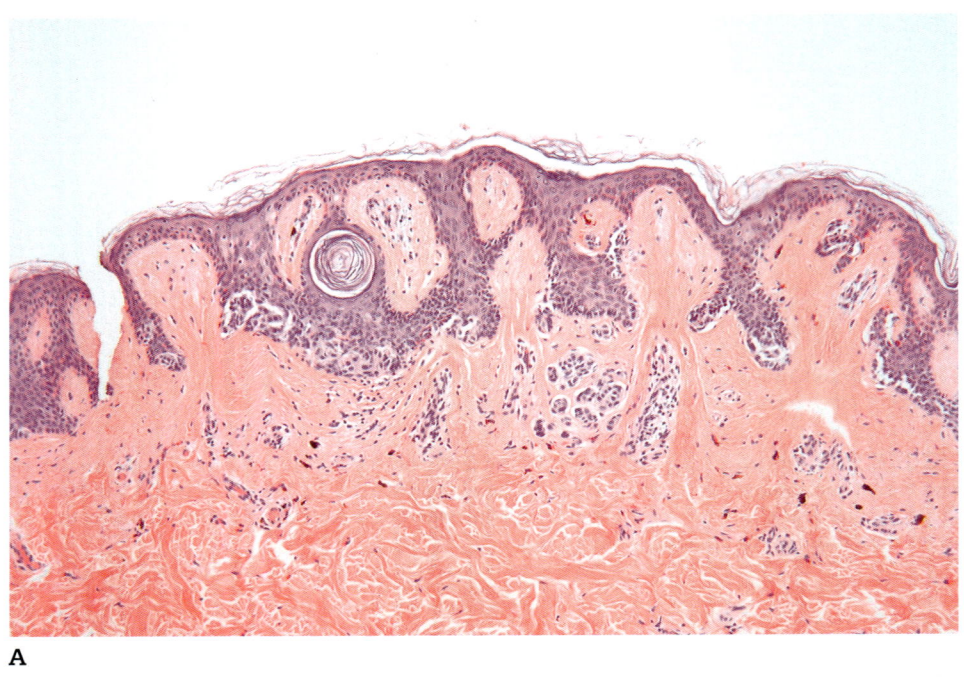

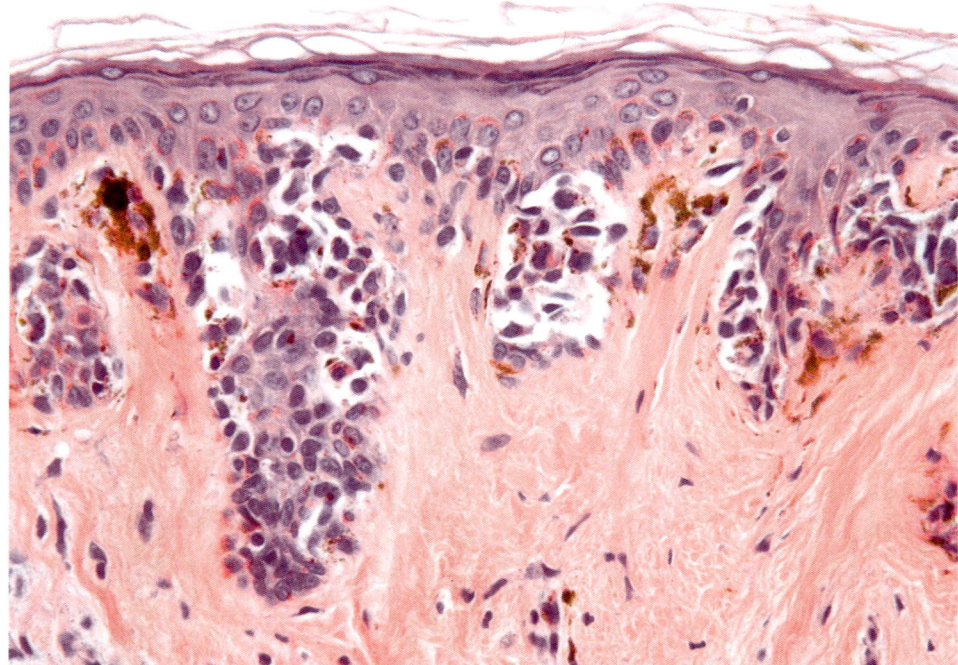

FIGURE 5-18 Compound atypical nevus. **A,** Although the pattern is nested, there is variation in the size, shape, and placement of the junctional nests. **B,** On higher magnification the variation in nesting and the nuclear characteristics of the melanocytes are seen.

The principal architectural feature of atypical nevi is disordered intraepidermal melanocytic proliferation (110,193). This criterion encompasses both single-cell melanocytic arrays along the basilar zone and disordered or irregular junctional nesting. Both alterations are generally present within a given lesion. Because the lentiginous proliferation is fundamentally the pattern of a lentigo simplex, this criterion requires increased numbers of basilar melanocytes, both along the sides and tips of the retia and above the dermal papillae. The increased density of the cells often reaches the state of confluency, displacing basal keratinocytes. In more advanced lesions, the proliferation may result in coalescent, multiple layers along the dermoepidermal junction, bridging adjacent rete. Retraction spaces, when present about the lesional melanocytes, impart a vacuolated appearance to the basal

FIGURE 5-19 Variation in nesting patterns of an atypical nevus. **A,** Irregular nests have coalesced along the junctional zone of this compound lesion. The basilar melanocytes vary appreciably in size, shape, and staining qualities. **B,** A nest of melanocytes is situated between the rete. Nuclear atypia is focally advanced.

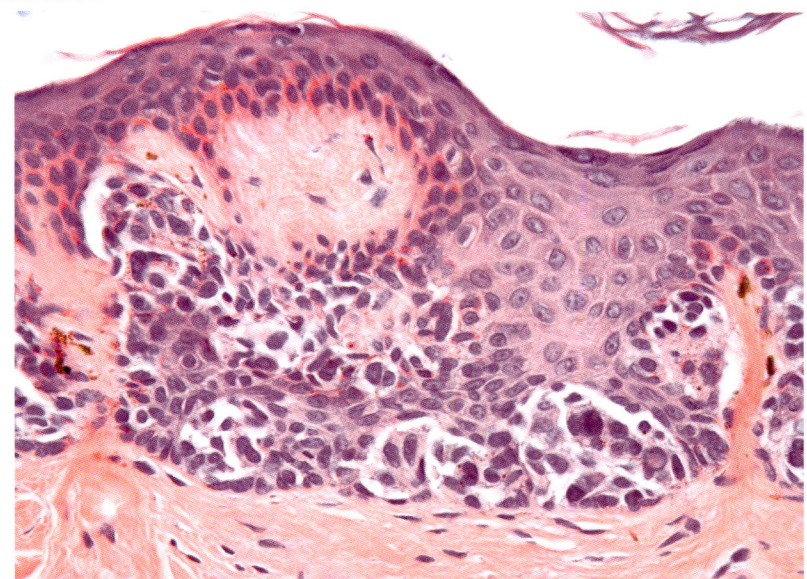

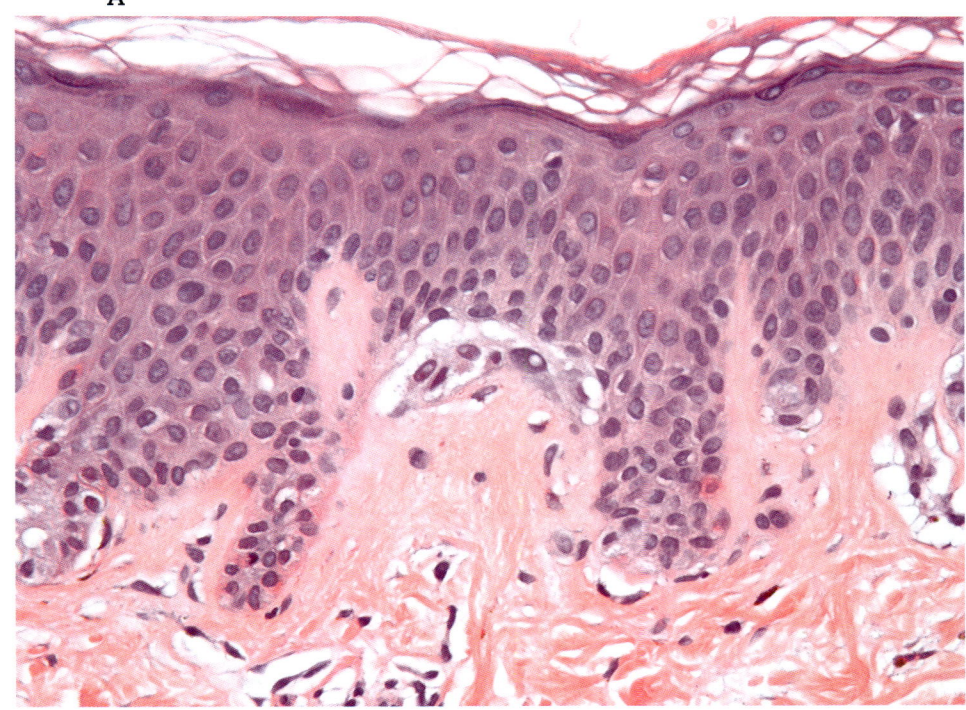

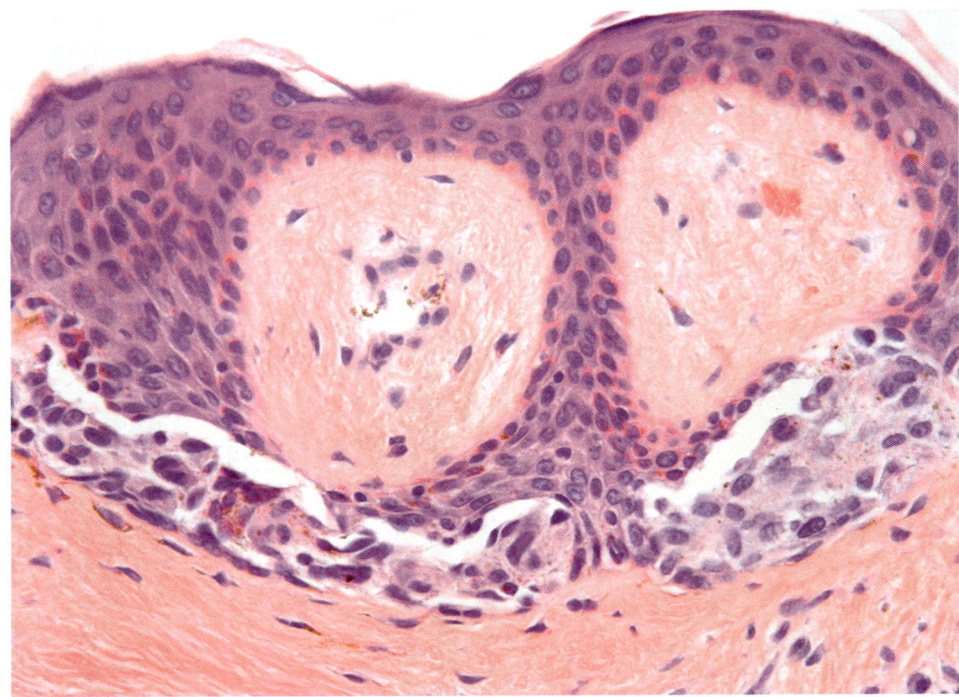

FIGURE 5-19 *Continued.* **C,** Confluence and bridging of nested cells are well developed in this lesion. The component cells are atypical. Lamellar fibroplasia is present below the confluent nests.

FIGURE 5-20 High-grade cytologic atypia within a nevus. **A,** Nuclear enlargement and pleomorphism of basilar melanocytes are advanced.

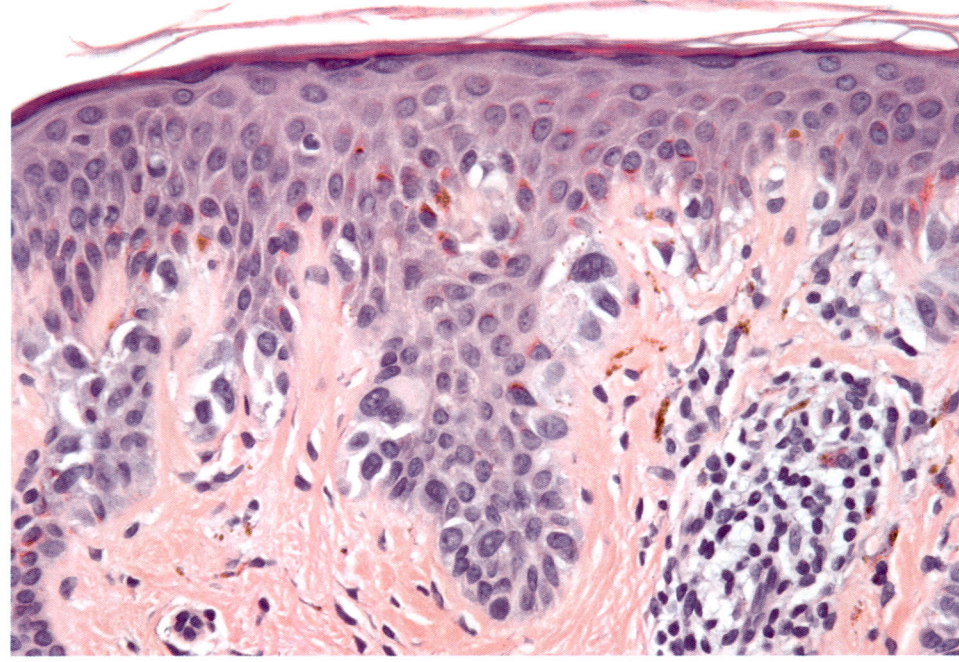

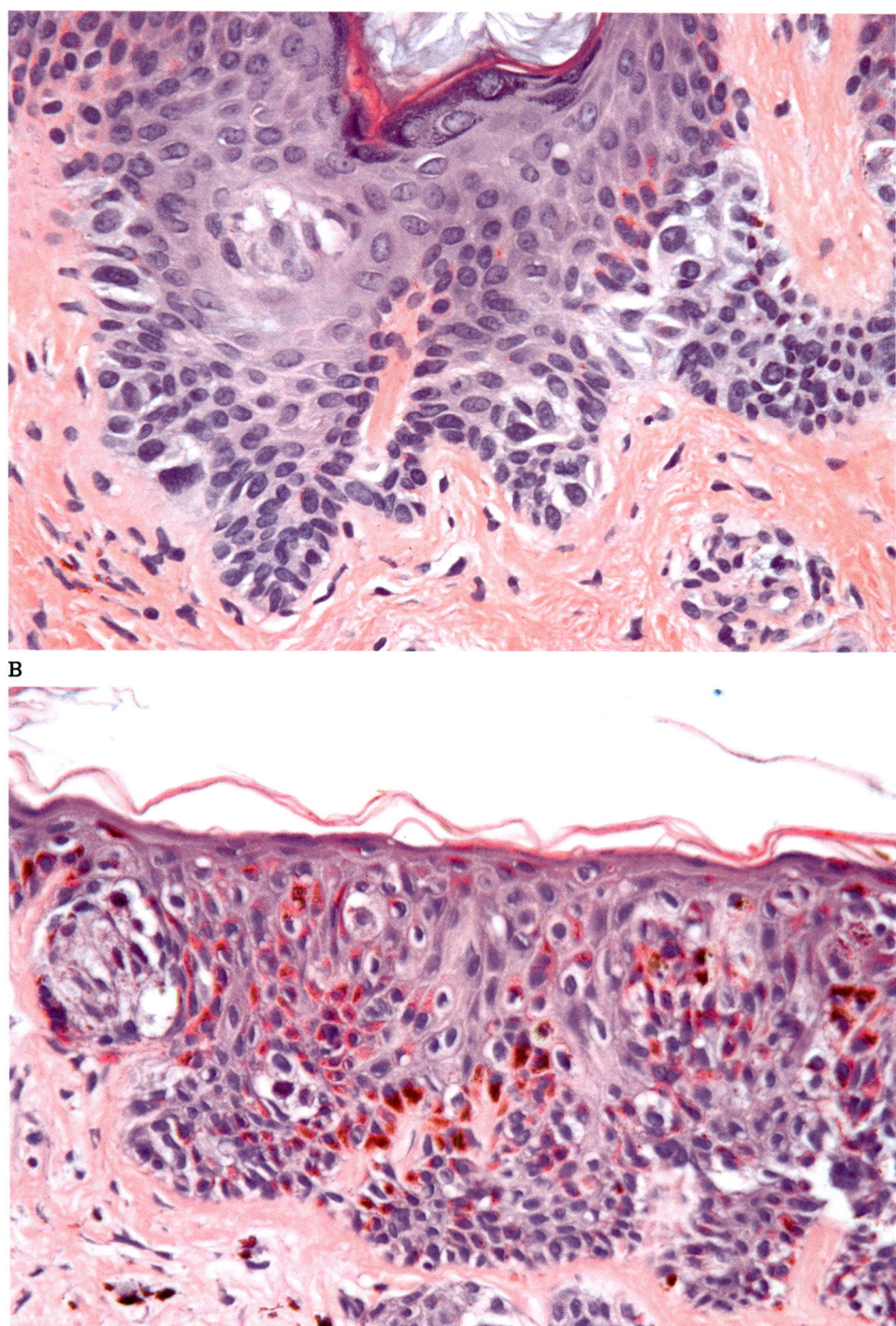

FIGURE 5-20 *Continued*. **B,** In this lesion, severe nuclear atypia is present but in a discontinuous pattern. In contrast, most melanomas contain cells with monotonous or continuous atypia. **C,** Melanoma in situ has elvoved within an atypical nevus. Note the large melanocytes with abundant cytoplasms that contain pleomorphic nuclei and variably prominent nucleoli.

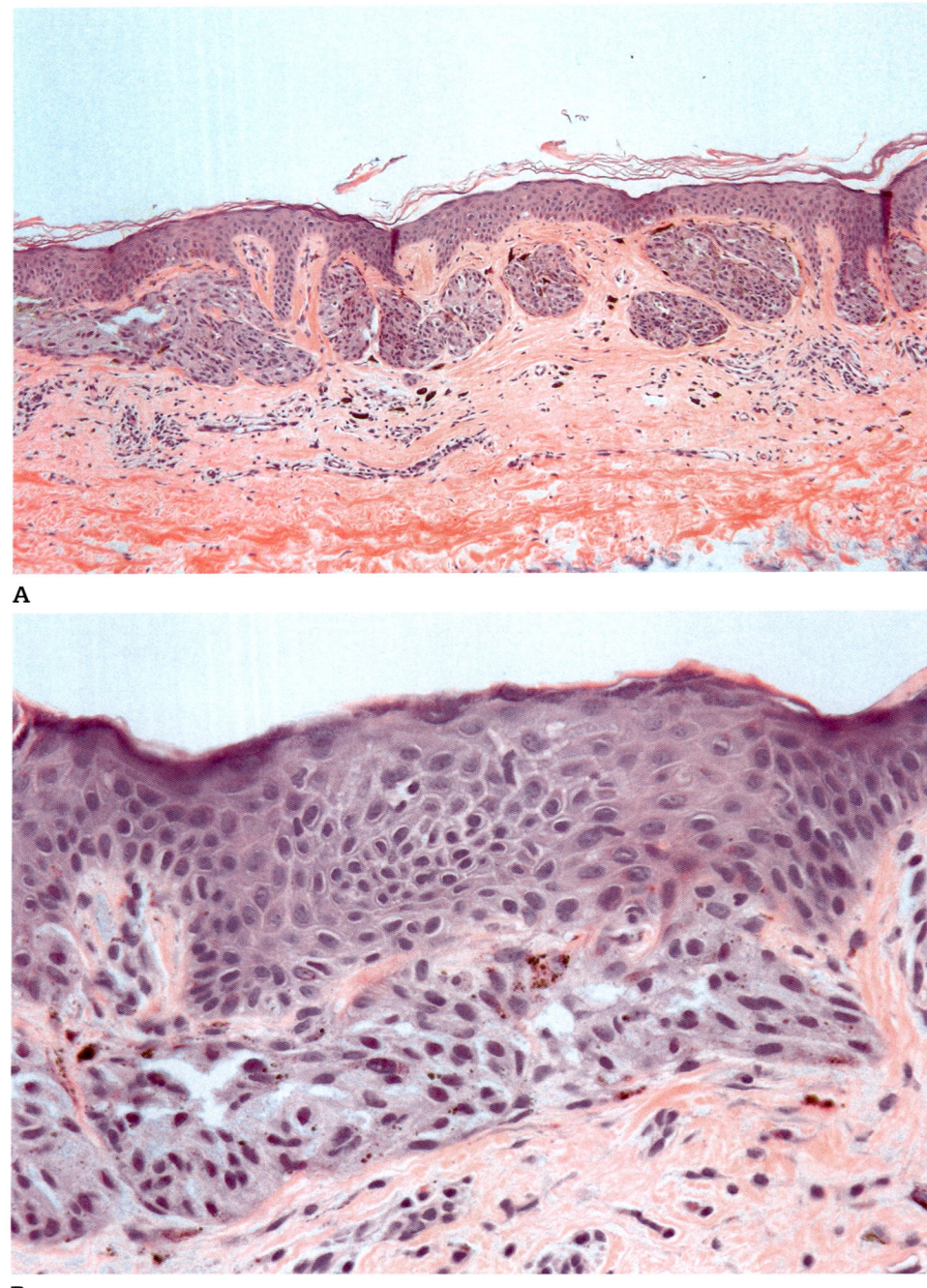

FIGURE 5-21 Compound atypical nevus, epithelioid cell variant. **A,** The junctional nests vary in size and configuration. **B,** Abundant, "dusty" cytoplasms are present within the junctional epithelioid cells. The junctional nests have coalesced.

layer. Pleomorphic nuclei with angulated contours are commonly present within the vacuolated cells (110,193) (Fig. 5-17).

Variations in intraepidermal nesting of melanocytes are reflected in general asymmetry and a chaotic pattern of cellular aggregation. Individual nests vary appreciably in size, shape, and spacing, such that the nests are not arrayed at equidistant intervals. In contrast to the preferential distribution of nests at the tips of the rete in banal nevi, the nests in atypical nevi are irregularly distributed

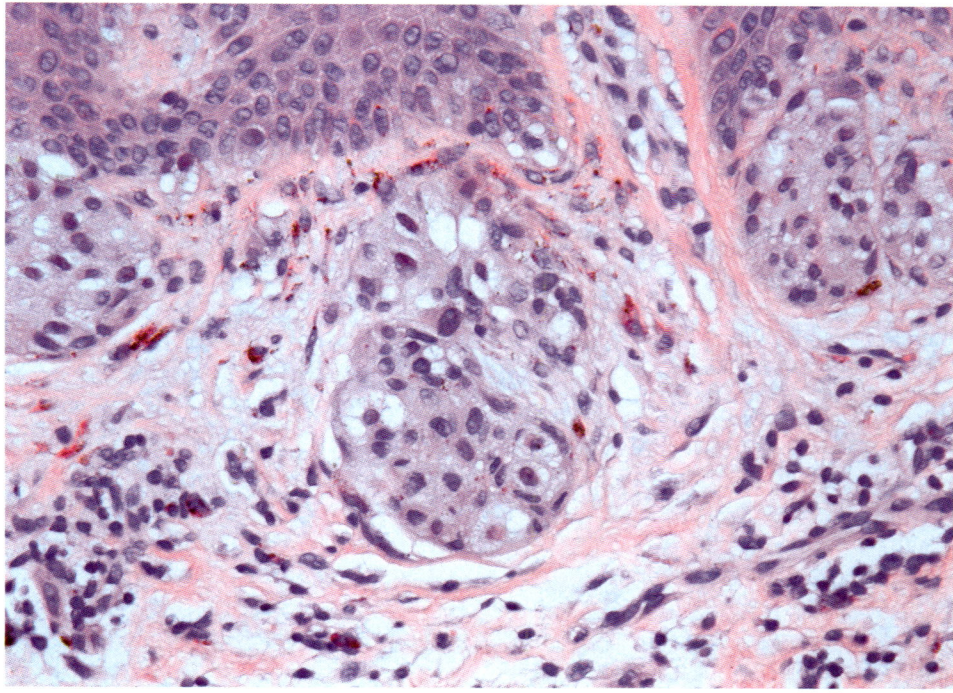

FIGURE 5-21 *Continued.* **C,** On higher magnification, the melanocytic nuclei vary substantially in size, shape, and chromasia.

along the sides of the rete and over the dermal papillae. Bridging of adjacent rete by aggregated melanocytes is another feature of the abnormal nesting pattern, and in advanced cases, confluence of the nesting may encompass three or four adjacent rete ridges (Fig. 5-19). Within the nests, loss of cellular cohesion may occur; the individual cells appear literally to fall apart. Although pagetoid scatter of cells into the spinous layer is not a common feature of atypical nevi, focal or limited suprabasal extension of the melanocytes can occur on occasion. Table 5-16 summarizes the spectrum of architectural alterations found within atypical nevi.

Cytologic Features The cell types that make up atypical nevi include variations of basilar melanocytes with retracted cytoplasms, small rounded nevus cells, spindled cells with variable pigmentation, and epithelioid cells (7,110,186,193) (Fig. 5-21). In the atypical nevi with a predominantly lentiginous architectural pattern, basilar melanocytes with retraction of cytoplasm are commonly observed; the epithelioid cell type may be present in the much less prevalent, predominantly nested form of the atypical nevus. Across cell types, however, the presence of variable (discontinuous) cytologic atypia of intraepidermal melanocytes is currently considered the most fundamental criterion for diagnosis of the atypical nevus (110,186,192,193). Discontinuous atypia means that the cells are not uniformly atypical but rather the degree of nuclear atypia varies from cell to cell, such that some, and indeed most, cells may not be atypical at all. Indeed, the original descriptions of the atypical nevus held that the proportion of atypical cells is on the order of 5% or less (7,98,107,119,186).

Nuclear atypia occurs along a continuum characterized by gradual nuclear enlargement, pleomorphism, variation in nuclear chromatin pattern, and the eventual development of prominent nucleoli. At the low-grade end of the spectrum, nuclear atypia may be nearly imperceptible and thus not reproducible between observers. In low-grade lesions, cytoplasms commonly retract about the cells, giving a vacuolated appearance. The size of the nuclei is increased and approximates that of or is slightly larger than the nuclei of spinous keratinocytes (191) (Figs. 5-17B and 5-18B). The nuclei range from oval to rhomboidal or angulated in configuration (Fig. 5-17A). Chromatin is evenly dispersed, and nucleoli inconspicuous.

In lesions with more advanced nuclear atypia, many cells are clearly larger than the spinous keratinocytes, the melanocytic cytoplasms may become more abundant (Figs. 5-19C and 5-21C), and the nuclei are more pleomorphic. Nucleoli gain in prominence. With severe or high-grade atypia, the melanocytes may contain abundant

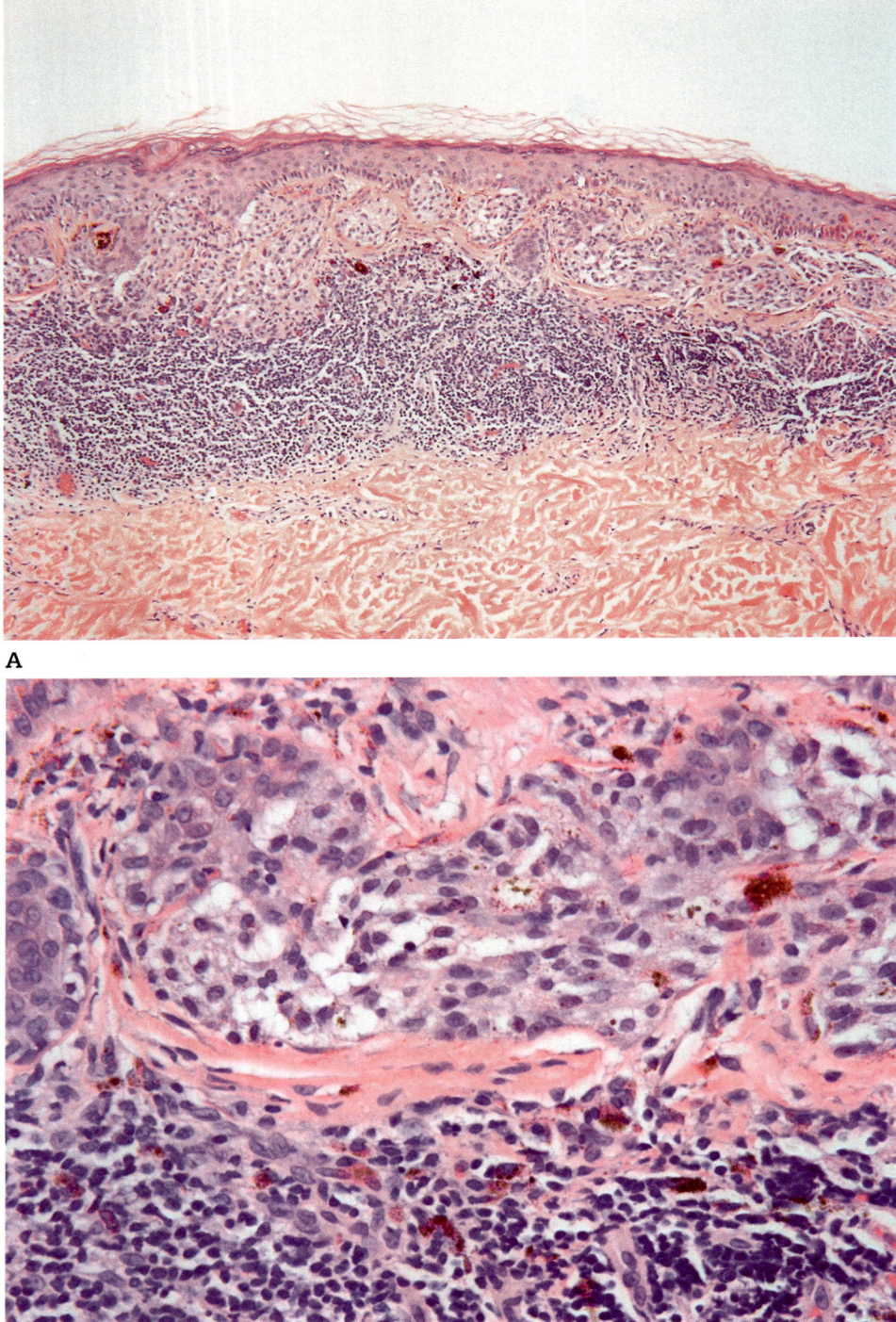

FIGURE 5-22 Compound atypical nevus with halo phenomenon. **A,** A dense lymphocytic infiltrate fills the papillary dermis. **B,** There is confluence of variably atypical basilar melanocytes in addition to the prominent mononuclear infiltrate of the papillary dermis.

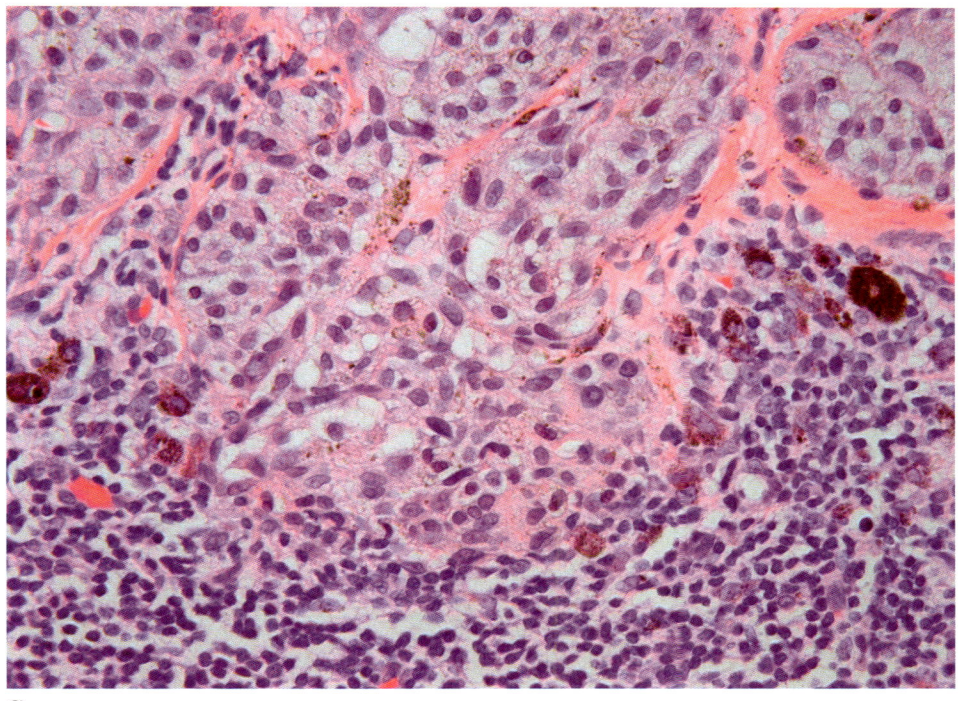

FIGURE 5-22 *Continued.* **C,** On higher magnification of the nevus shown in panel B, the discontinuous nature of the nuclear hyperchromasia and pleomorphism of the nevus are seen.

TABLE 5-15 Histologic features of atypical nevi.
Architectural features
Lentiginous melanocytic proliferation[a]
Variation in size, shape, location of junctional nests with bridging or confluence[a]
Lack of cellular cohesion within nests
Lateral extension (shoulder phenomenon) of junctional component
Asymmetry, commonly
Poor circumscription of intraepidermal component
Cytologic features
Spindle cell pattern
Epithelioid cell pattern
Discontinuous nuclear atypia (not all nuclei atypical)[a]
Nuclear enlargement
Nuclear pleomorphism
Nuclear hyperchromasia
Prominent nucleoli
Prominent pale or dusty cytoplasms
Large melanin granules
Stroma response
Lymphocytic infiltrates
Fibroplasia
Concentric eosinophilic pattern
Lamellar pattern
Prominent vascularity

[a]Feature essential for diagnosis.

cytoplasms that are granular or filled with finely divided (dusty) melanin (191) (Fig. 5-20). Nuclei may be twice or more the size of those within the spinous keratinocytes (Fig. 5-20B). The enlarged nucleoli may be eosinophilic (Fig. 5-20C). The ultimate end point is a continuously atypical population of cells, which marks the advent of melanoma.

Host Response Mononuclear cell infiltrates, fibroplasia, and prominent vascularity constitute the host response in atypical nevi. Of these, the first two have received the most attention as components of the diagnostic criteria (7,110,155,186–188,193). Lymphocytic infiltrates are ubiquitous within the lesions but vary from a sparse perivascular arrangement of cells (Fig. 5-18A) to dense, band like arrays filling the papillary dermis and mimicking that found in halo nevi (Fig. 5-22). Monocytes and melanophages are present to varying degrees within the infiltrates of most lesions.

Dermal fibroplasia as observed in atypical nevi is of two types. The most common is designated *concentric fibroplasia* and is characterized by hyalinized collagen that is compactly disposed about the epidermal rete ridges (Fig. 5-17). This alteration is fairly nonspecific, being

TABLE 5-16 Guidelines for grading architectural disorder and cytologic atypia in melanocytic proliferations.

	Spectrum of changes[a]		
	Low grade	⟶	High grade
Architectural features		Asymmetry, lateral extension[b]	
	Lentiginous melanocytic proliferation[b]		Confluence of cells at basal layer
	Little or no pagetoid scatter[b]	Upward migration	Prominent pagetoid scatter
	Little variation in nesting[b]	Variation in nesting with bridging	Confluence of nests; marked variation in size, shape, spacing
	Cohesion of cells in nests		Diminished cohesion
	Elongated rete		Effacement of rete
Cytologic features	Dermal maturation of cells[b]	Partial loss of maturation	Expansile nests without maturation
	Discontinuous atypia[b]		Continuous atypia (most cells atypical)
		Cellular enlargement[b]	
		Nuclear enlargement[b]	
		Nuclear pleomorphism[b]	
		Prominent nucleoli[b]	
		Hyperchromatism[b]	
	Uniform, nongranular cytoplasm	Abundant cytoplasm	Abundant granular or dusty cytoplasm

[a]Each parameter is a continuous variable from low grade to high grade. For example, the variable *asymmetry* represents a spectrum from little or no asymmetry (low grade) to prominent asymmetry (high grade). Thus either the extremes for each parameter are indicated or the parameter is simply stated without qualification of the extremes.

[b]Principal features for grading architectural and cytologic atypia.

found rather ubiquitously in common lentigines and lentiginous nevi. The other, *lamellar fibroplasia,* is less commonly observed and is represented by delicate stacking of horizontally disposed collagen subjacent to the epidermal rete (Fig. 5-19). Mesenchymal, spindle cells line the filamentous strands of collagen.

With respect to alterations in the papillary dermal vascular plexus, atypical nevi do not differ from ordinary nevi with respect to the numbers of microvessels in the papillary dermis (206). The appearance of prominent vascularity in these lesions is probably secondary to vascular dilatation and hypertrophy rather than actual angiogenesis, which is an attribute of melanoma.

Histologic Variants of Atypical Nevi

Epithelioid Cell Atypical Nevus One relatively uncommon lesion contains cells that resemble the epithelioid cells observed in superficial spreading melanoma, albeit with somewhat less cytologic atypia (7,186) (Figure 5-21). These enlarged cells are oval or polygonal, contain abundant eosinophilic or dusty cytoplasms, and are almost exclusively nested in their distribution. Paradoxically, the nuclei are often small and round, lacking nuclear alterations of high grade atypia.

Halo Nevus Variant There are variants of atypical nevi that contain dense mononuclear infiltrates filling the papillary dermis and obscuring the dermal nevus cells (Fig. 5-22). The aberrant architectural and cytologic features of the underlying atypical nevus distinguish these lesions from halo nevi (207).

Differential Diagnosis

The atypical nevus requires discrimination from lentiginous nevi, in situ and invasive melanoma, atypical lentiginous melanocytic proliferations arising in sun-damaged skin, pigmented spindle cell nevus, Spitz tumor, halo nevus, congenital nevus, and recurrent nevus. By far the most common situation is the differential diagnosis of lentiginous nevus. Here, the main problem, of course, is one of threshold. In other words, for a particular lesion is there sufficiently disordered architecture and cytologic atypia for the diagnosis of the atypical nevus? In the broad context, a complex histologic spectrum exists across the parameters of architectural and cytologic atypia, and attempts at categorical assignment of individual lesions to either the common lentiginous or atypical nevus categories belie the histologic complexity of melanocytic proliferations (205). Factors to be considered in this distinction include circumscription, symmetry, degree of cell density along the basal zone, irregularity of nesting, and—most important—cytologic atypia of intraepidermal melanocytes. Lesions having equivocal changes may be diagnosed as either lentiginous nevi, nevi with architectural disorder, or nevi without unequivocal melanocytic atypia.

TABLE 5-17 The differential diagnosis of severely atypical nevus and melanoma.[a]

Severely atypical severely atypical nevus	In situ or microinvasive melanoma
Some asymmetry	Prominent asymmetry
Poorly circumscribed	Poorly circumscribed
Some maintenance of nesting pattern	Loss of orderly nesting pattern
Some diminished cohesion of nests	Diminished cohesion of nests may be prominent
Lentiginous proliferation concentrated on rete ridges	Loss of rete-oriented melanocytic proliferation
Pagetoid scatter absent or minimal	Pagetoid spread prominent
Discontinuous cytologic atypia	Continuous cytologic atypia
Some maturation of dermal elements	Often no dermal maturation
Usually no dermal mitoses	Dermal mitoses may be present
Usually perivascular but occasionally band-like lymphocytic infiltrates	Tendency to band-like lymphocytic infiltrates

[a]These guidelines represent the most common presentations; however, there is considerable variation among lesions.

One of the most difficult, if not the most common, problems is the discrimination of severely atypical nevi from in situ or microinvasive melanoma. The most salient points are summarized in Table 5-17. In one sense, the distinction can be disturbingly arbitrary and subjective, because no consensus exists regarding separating the two entities. The presence of well-developed pagetoid melanocytosis and continuous, high-grade nuclear atypia, however, are useful criteria for assigning a diagnosis of melanoma. Immunostaining of specimens with monoclonal antibodies to proliferation markers, such as Ki-67, has been used as an ancillary test in the discrimination of atypical nevi from melanoma. In these studies, proliferation markers label < 2% of dermal melanocytes in atypical and common nevi but > 10% of cells in melanoma (208–210).

On occasion, atypical nevi and lentigo maligna (i.e., actinic melanocytosis and melanoma in situ) show histologic similarities and may be difficult to discriminate. In most instances, lentigo maligna is an abnormal melanocytic proliferation secondary to cumulative sun exposure that develops on actinically damaged skin of patients over 60 years of age (Table 5-18). The most common sites are the cheek and nose, which are unusual locations for atypical nevi. In lentigo maligna, there is a basilar proliferation of variably atypical melanocytes represented by single-cell units and occasional small or elongate nests containing discohesive, pigmented, and spindle cells. The cells have a striking propensity to spread down along pilar and occasionally eccrine and epithelium, which is a finding unusual to atypical nevi. The rete ridge pattern is generally effaced, and solar elastosis is prominent within the papillary dermis. In contrast, atypical nevi are characterized in most instances by elongated rete ridges with a concentration of basilar melanocytes and junctional nests along the exaggerated rete. Solar elastosis, if present at all, is minimal. Finally, lentigo maligna is a de novo melanocytic proliferation, whereas 80% or so of atypical

TABLE 5-18 The differential diagnosis of atypical nevus and lentigo maligna.

Feature	Atypical Nevus	Lentigo Maligna
Clinical		
Age	≥ 10 years	≥ 60 years
Site	Intermittently sun-exposed or covered skin—trunk > buttock, scalp, extremities > face (unusual)	Markedly sun-exposed skin—face (cheek, nose) most common
Histopathology		
Circumscription	Poorly circumscribed	Poorly circumscribed
Rete ridges	Elongated	Effaced
Nesting	Usually lentiginous and junctional nesting	Mainly lentiginous, but occasional nesting
Adnexae	Little or no involvement	Striking involvement
Spindle cells	On occasion	Pigmented cells, common
Solar elastosis	Inconspicuous	Prominent

nevi contain dermal nevic cell elements (99). There are cases, however, in which the discrimination of atypical nevus from lentigo maligna is not possible, especially in instances of lentigo maligna associated with a preserved or accentuated rete ridge pattern. The discriminating features favoring lentigo maligna in those cases may include a mainly lentiginous pattern of melanocytic proliferation, prominent involvement of appendages, presence of pigmented spindle cells, and solar elastosis. If resolution of the differential cannot be achieved with reasonable confidence, a reasonable approach is a descriptive diagnosis.

Various types of melanocytic nevi such as pigmented spindle cell nevus, Spitz tumor/nevus, and congenital nevus may on occasion demonstrate disordered architectural patterns and cytologic atypia but, at the same time, retain many of the histologic features that make them distinctive—for example, fascicles of slender pigmented spindle cells in pigmented spindle cell nevus, large epithelioid cells in Spitz nevus, and extensive involvement of the reticular dermis in congenital nevus. The problem is particularly germane with atypical variants of pigmented spindle cell nevi (211) and Spitz nevi (212). These lesions may be characterized by peripheral extension of the intraepidermal component, poor circumscription, prominent lentiginous melanocytic hyperplasia, irregular junctional nesting, horizontal confluence of nests, and cytologic atypia. Whether spindle cell nevi with the preceding attributes are termed *dysplastic nevi, atypical spindle cell nevi,* or *spindle cell nevi with architectural disorder and cytologic atypia* is subjective, because atypical alterations within spindle cell and the other various types of nevi have not been the subject of sufficient empirical investigation; thus their significance has not been determined. It is nevertheless reasonable to acknowledge the atypical changes when present and communicate them in the pathology reported, under the hypothesis that such nevi, especially those with high-grade or severe atypia, have increased risk for progression to melanoma and should be treated accordingly.

Recurrent melanocytic nevi may enter into the differential diagnosis and may in fact represent recurrent atypical nevi. Recurrence usually occurs from 6 weeks to 6 months after incomplete saucerization of a banal nevus. Such nevi may contain a variable intraepidermal component localized to the area of the scar and not beyond. Effacement of the epidermis is commonly present, and a dermal nevus remnant often lies beneath the scar. Irregular nesting, single-cell hyperplasia, and occasion pagetoid scatter of cells can occur. The melanocytes often take on an epithelioid appearance, but nuclear atypia is usually minimal or absent. A review of the initial biopsy material is important in the process of determining whether significant atypicality was present in the original lesion. In any event, extension of the recurrent intraepidermal component beyond the scar is a sufficiently abnormal feature that should prompt scrutiny to rule out melanoma.

Grading and Histopathological Reporting

Any attempt at grading atypia within melanocytic nevi should have relevance to the management of patients. Fundamentally, the objective is to segregate the lesions that may have significant risk of progression to melanoma from lesions with lesser degrees of risk. A grading scheme should guide clinicians in the practical management of individual lesions, to wit: which lesions should be excised with particular margins or simply left alone. Moreover, grading schemes should be reproducible among pathologists. The grading scheme outlined in Table 5-19 has been subjected to interobserver agreement studies, which indicated fair to good agreement among observers working at the same institution, with an overall concordance rate of 77% ($\kappa = 0.55$–0.84) in diagnosing atypical nevi and 35–58% ($\kappa = 0.38$–0.47) in grading nevi (200). Such data, if corroborated independently by other research groups, would suggest that grading of atypical nevi is feasible and reproducible.

In the absence of a standardized or formal scheme for grading, the following guidelines are suggested: (a) It is important that severely atypical and high-grade nevi are recognized because of their overlap with melanoma in situ. This recognition is of particular significance because

TABLE 5-19 Histopathological reporting of atypical nevi.

Grade of lesion	Reexcision if margins involved
Low-grade lesions	
Junctional or compound nevus with architectural disorder and no cytologic atypia	No
Junction or compound nevus with mild atypia	No
High-grade lesions	
Junctional or compound nevus with moderate atypia	Yes
Junctional or compound nevus with severe atypia	Yes, 5-mm margins

melanoma in situ may potentially undergo rapid progression to invasive melanoma. For these reasons, severely atypical nevi are best managed by complete excision with 5-mm margins. (b) Because DNA aneuploidy has been demonstrated in moderately atypical nevi (202), there may possibly be grater potential for progression to melanoma than less atypical lesions, and their excision with histologically clear margins is a reasonable management objective. (c) There is at present no compelling empirical evidence that atypical nevi with slight or mild atypia require complete removal. These lesions appear to be quite common in the general population, there is no reason to believe that they are more likely to constitute melanoma precursor lesions than are banal acquired nevi, and their reproducible distinction from lentiginous nevi may not be generally achievable in histopathologic practice.

To summarize, the most important aspect in the reporting of melanocytic lesions is that the pathologist communicates clearly to the clinician the nature of the lesion and its significance, regardless of the terminology used. The immediate concern is to ensure proper management of the individual lesion based on its degree of atypia (Table 5-19). More generally, the results of the histologic analysis should be correlated with the clinical nevus phenotype and the family history with respect to occurrence of melanoma. In the context of an atypical clinical nevus phenotype (i.e., increased numbers of nevi with or without enlarged, clinically atypical nevi) and/or a personal or family history of melanoma, management of the individual patient can be formulated by the clinician with supporting guidance by the pathologist. This cooperative approach works in the best interest of patients and ensures the best available risk stratification.

OTHER VARIANTS OF MELANOCYTIC NEVI

Acral Nevus

Regardless of the age of the individual, most nevi situated at acral sites have a junctional component, with or without a dermal component. These lesions not uncommonly pose diagnostic problems because both the clinical and the histologic presentation can appear atypical. Notwithstanding the atypical features, the natural history of these lesions conforms to that of benign acquired melanocytic nevi.

Clinical Features Acral nevi are usually macular but occasionally can be slightly elevated (Table 5-20). They are generally < 5 mm in diameter but may be larger. Pigmentation is uniformly brown to dark brown. When of lighter shade, they resemble simple lentigines.

TABLE 5-20 Melanocytic nevus of acral skin.

Clinical features
  All ages
  Size usually 3–6 mm
  Macular or only slightly raised
  Uniform brown of dark brown pigmentation
  Symmetry
  Regular and well-defined borders
Histologic features
  Symmetrical, well-demarcated silhouette
  Regular, evenly spaced nesting at the junctional zone
  Lentiginous melanocytic proliferation along the basal layer of elongated rete
  Pagetoid scatter of cells common but orderly
  Little or no inflammatory reaction within the stroma
  When of compound type, the dermal nests are well formed and cells mature with dermal descent
Differential diagnosis
  Atypical nevi
  Acral lentiginous melanoma

Histologic Features Nevi at the acra share the histologic features of common acquired nevi (Table 5-5), although they may exhibit atypical features, as noted above. The overall architecture is usually symmetrical, and the lateral margin is circumscribed, although the plane of sectioning with respect to dermatoglyphic lines apparently influences the architectural silhouette (213) (Table 5-20). Nests of cells at the junctional zone, although occasionally enlarged, are well formed, round to oval in shape, and uniform in size and spacing (Fig. 5-6). Acral nevi, however, have a propensity for a lentiginous pattern of single-cell melanocytic proliferation along the basilar epidermis and for upward scatter of cells in a pattern resembling pagetoid melanocytosis. Pagetoid scatter to some degree is found in > 60% of nevi of the palms and soles (213,214). A similarly high rate of pagetoid melanocytosis (68%) was reported in a series of acral nevi in children, and the junctional nesting in that population may be irregular or confluent, posing a difficult differential diagnosis with melanoma (215). Lesions with elongation of rete ridges, continuous proliferation of melanocytes along the basilar epidermis, pagetoid scatter of cells suprabasally, and poor lateral circumscription have been referred to as acral-lentiginous nevi (216). Caution is necessary lest these features result in overinterpretation as evolving melanoma. When present, the dermal pattern in acral nevi is characteristic of common acquired nevi in general.

Differential Diagnosis The principal differential diagnostic considerations in the case of nevi situated at the acra are atypical nevus and melanoma and, occasionally, Spitz nevus/tumor. Although atypical nevi and melanoma have greater architectural abnormalities than acral nevi, the principal criterion for resolving the differential is the cytologic detail. The atypical melanocytes of atypical nevi and melanoma are, to varying degrees, enlarged, pleomorphic, and hyperchromatic. Moreover, the density of the cells at the basilar zone and suprabasally is appreciably increased over that found in acral nevi; at higher densities, the cells may be confluently arrayed along the basal layer. Other criteria that favor the interpretation of atypical nevus or melanoma include irregular nesting pattern within the epidermis, poor cohesion of the cells within the nests, advanced pagetoid scatter of cells suprabasally, poor lateral circumscription, and a brisk inflammatory response within the subjacent papillary dermis. Acral-lentiginous nevi pose more difficulties due to the greater architectural alterations, but the absence of cytologic atypia and pagetoid scatter at the periphery are useful criteria in their diagnosis (216). Further discussion regarding atypical acquired nevi can be found elsewhere in this chapter. Its characteristic cell population of enlarged, spindle, and epithelioid melanocytes, which usually possess abundant cytoplasms that stain homogeneously eosinophilic, distinguishes the Spitz nevus/tumor from acral nevi.

Balloon Cell Nevus

Acquired nevi in which more than half of the cells are composed of balloon cells are uncommon, and those composed entirely of balloon cells are exceedingly rare (69–73). Their principal importance is that they can create difficulties in histologic differential diagnosis, especially in regard to melanoma.

Clinical Features Balloon cell lesions do not have any distinguishing features clinically (Table 5-21), although one was reported to have a faint yellow halo surrounding an otherwise ordinary brown nevus (70). Most are < 5 mm in diameter and have predilection for skin of the head and neck (71). Men and women are affected equally, and most cases have been reported in people < 30 years of age (69,71).

Histologic Features The usual pattern is that of balloon cells admixed with ordinary nevus cells. Transitional forms can also be found (69–71) (Fig. 5-23A). The balloon cells are large and contain clear, foamy, or vacuolated cytoplasms (69) (Fig. 5-23B). When vacuolated, the cells resemble sebocytes. The nuclei are not usually enlarged and are centrally situated within the cells. The chromatin is uniformly basophilic. Multinucleate giant cells of balloon type are not uncommon. As with ordinary intradermal nevus cells, the balloon cells mature with dermal descent. Melanin pigmentation is variable and ranges from finely or coarsely granular to clumped (71). By election microscopy, the cytoplasmic vacuolization results from progressive enlargement and lysis of melanosomes, which has been postulated to represent a degenerative phenomenon (72,73).

Differential Diagnosis The primary differential diagnosis is that of balloon cell melanoma, which occurs most often in older individuals (71). In common with the nevus, a balloon cell melanoma may be composed of any proportion of balloon cells. As with other melanomas, it is characterized histologically by mitotic activity and by prominent atypia, with nuclear enlargement, pleomorphism, and hyperchromasia. For those lesions with an inconspicuous nevus cell component, the differential diagnosis may include xanthoma, granular cell tumor, and sebaceous neoplasms (69,71).

Halo Nevus (Leukoderma Acquisitum Centrifugum, Sutton Nevus, Perinevoid Vitiligo, Perinevoid Leukoderma)

By clinical definition, the halo nevus is a nevus that is surrounded by a white (hypopigmented or depigmented) annulus or halo. Histologically, it is characterized by a dense mononuclear inflammatory infiltrate that fills the papillary dermis (217–220). The underlying lesion is usually a common acquired nevus, but on occasion other nevi such as atypical nevi, congenital nevi, and blue nevi may develop halos (217–221).

Halo nevi generally occur in people younger than age 20, and the mean age is approximately 15 years (219,220), with a range in one study of 3 to 42 years (219). The frequency of halo nevi among all nevi in individuals younger than age 20 is < 1% (222). There is an equal gender distribution (219). Some 20% of those with halo nevi also have vitiligo, and halo nevi have been associated with atypical nevi and melanoma (223).

TABLE 5-21 Balloon cell nevus.

Clinical features
  None distinctive
  Size usually < 5 mm
Histologic features
  Balloon cells admixed with common nevus cells
  More than half of nevus composed of nevus cells (by definition)
  Clear, foamy, or vacuolated cytoplasms
Differential diagnosis
  Balloon cell melanoma
  Xanthoma
  Sebaceous tumors

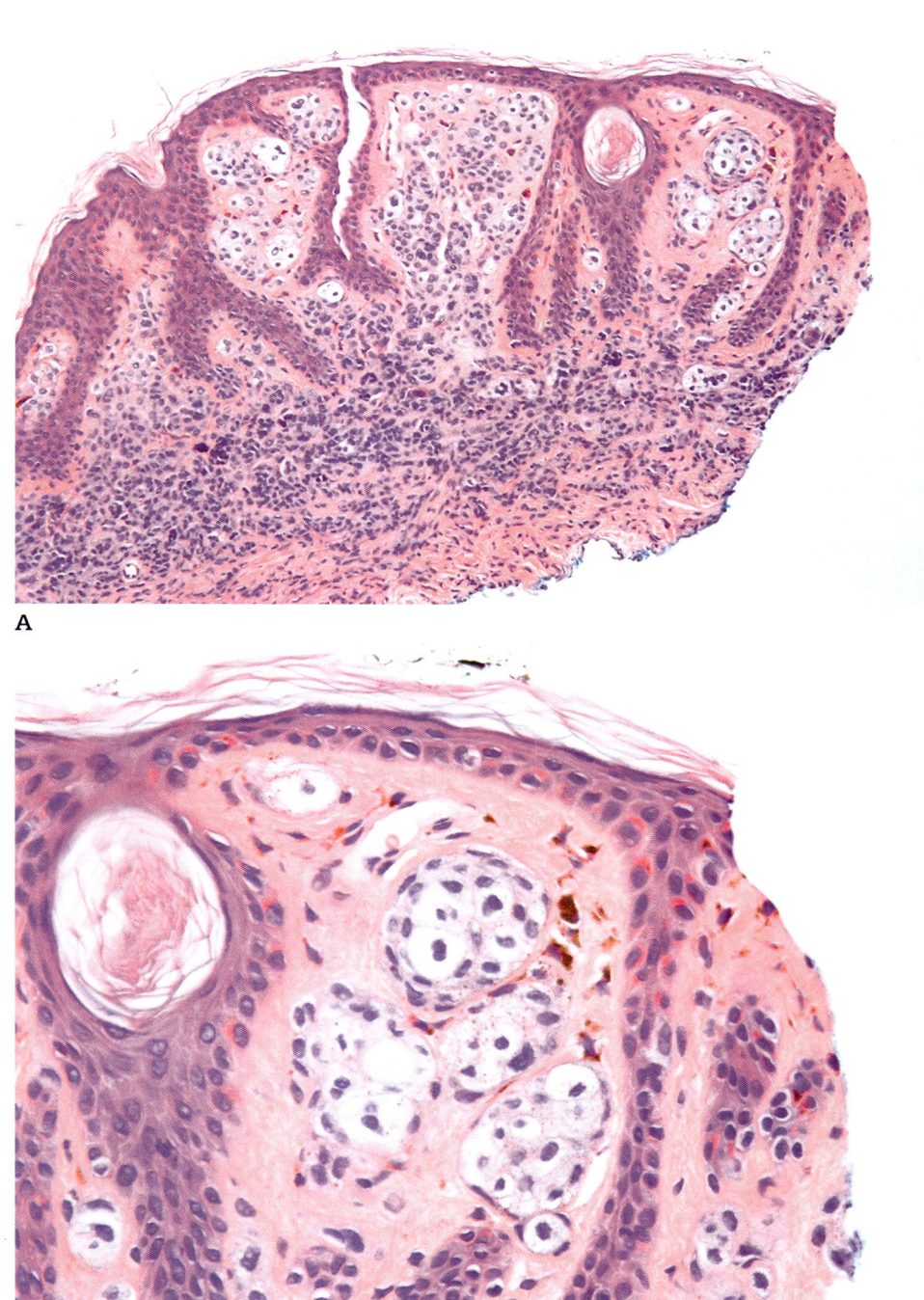

FIGURE 5-23 Balloon cell nevus. **A,** Enlarged, vacuolated cells are situated within the dermis. **B,** Balloon nevus cells contain small, centrally placed nuclei surrounded by clear vacuolated space.

Etiology It has been hypothesized that the halo of depigmentation results from either an immune response against nevus cells expressing neoantigens associated with tumor progression (20,224,225) or cell-mediated and/or humoral (antibody-mediated) reaction targeting nevoid melanocytes altered nonspecifically by physical or chemical means, by autoimmune mechanisms, or by cross-reaction from antigen response at distant sites (224–226). According to the first hypothesis, all halo nevi are atypical because the immune response is associated with tumorigenesis.

Although poorly understood, nevus cell destruction in halo nevi is probably mediated by a combination of humoral and cell-mediated mechanisms (223–225,227, 228). The abundance of antigen-presenting cells and T lymphocytes, including $CD8^+$ cells, within the infiltrate of halo nevi are observations supporting cell-mediated immunity (229). Lymphocytes isolated from patients with halo nevi are cytotoxic to melanoma cells in culture (228), and circulating lymphocytes express HLA-DR and other activation markers at higher levels than control subjects (230). With respect to humoral immunity, the antibodies targeted to the cytoplasm of nevoid cells within halo nevi cross react with melanoma cells (228). It is not clear whether these immune responses are essential in the pathogenesis of halo nevi or are merely an epiphenomenon. The mechanisms responsible for the clinical white annulus, which histologically usually lacks an inflammatory infiltrate, are not well understood but may involve humoral mechanisms or diffusion of a toxic cytokine (219,220).

Clinical Features The central nevus may be macular or raised and varies in color from pink to dark brown (218–220) (Table 5-22). It usually ranges from 3 to 6 mm in diameter, the borders are regular and well defined, and the color is homogeneous. The surface is usually unremarkable but may be scaly or crusted. About the central nevus is a well-demarcated, often symmetrical zone of hypopigmented or depigmented skin that is of uniform width, varying from a few millimeters to several centimeters on rare occasions (218–220). The lesions are most commonly situated on the upper back, but may be found at any location. Between 20 and 50% of affected patients have two or more halo nevi, and on rare occasions multiple lesions can develop rapidly (218–220).

The onset of the clinical ring of pigmentation is thought to occur over a period of weeks to months (218–220). Its subsequent development is variable. The central nevus may persist indefinitely or undergo gradual involution over months to years, with the area of hypopigmentation or depigmentation often persisting (218–220). About half of all lesions undergo complete regression (218).

Histologic Features Although usually of compound type, halo nevi may be junctional or dermal. When fully evolved, the nevus is associated with a dense, well-circumscribed infiltrate of lymphocytes and histiocytes that fills the papillary dermis in a band-like fashion and percolates between the nevus cell nests, obscuring the lower portions of the nevus (Fig. 5-24, Table 5-22). The density of the infiltration is so prominent that is difficult to distinguish nevus cells from the infiltrating inflammatory cells. Degenerating or apoptotic nevus cells with pyknotic nuclei and hypereosinophilic cytoplasms may be identifiable within the infiltrate, especially near the junctional zone. Although most halo nevi do not contain atypical nevus cells, on occasion some nevi may display some cytologic atypia of low grade (20) and rarely they may be associated with moderate to severe atypia. Centrally, there may be thinning and effacement of the epidermis in some cases. The melanocytes may coalesce along the dermal–epidermal junction, sometimes accompanied by discohesive nesting and separation along the junctional zone. The melanocytes often have epithelioid cell features and exhibit nuclear atypia. There is usually maturation with depth; however, uncommon mitoses may be noted in the dermal nevus component. With partial regression, nests of melanocytes may be isolated by dermal fibroplasia. Within the depigmented zone at the perimeter of the lesion, basilar melanocytes and melanin are diminished or absent (220). The papillary dermis in this zone may display reparative changes, but usually no infiltrate is found (220). It warrants mention that, on occasion, nevi with clinical halos may lack inflammatory infiltrates histologically (221,231).

When the lesion regresses clinically, all nevus cells by histologic examination are destroyed. The central zone previously occupied by the nevus is replaced by fibrous tissue with vascular ectasia, mucin deposits on occasion, variable residual mononuclear cell infiltrates, and melanophages (Fig. 5-25). There may be complete depigmentation of the epidermis in this central zone.

By immunophenotype analysis, most of the infiltrating cells are either T lymphocytes or macrophages (223). Helper/inducer ($CD4^+$) and cytotoxic/suppressor ($CD8^+$) T cells are represented in approximately equal numbers. The nevus cells within the infiltrate expression class I HLA antigens to a greater degree than class II antigens. This pattern is similar to that observed in atypical nevi and melanoma (223), suggesting a specific cell-mediated immune response in halo nevi.

Differential Diagnosis The halo nevus must be distinguished primarily from atypical nevi and malignant melanoma. The distinction should focus on the overall architecture of the lesion, the presence or absence of mat-

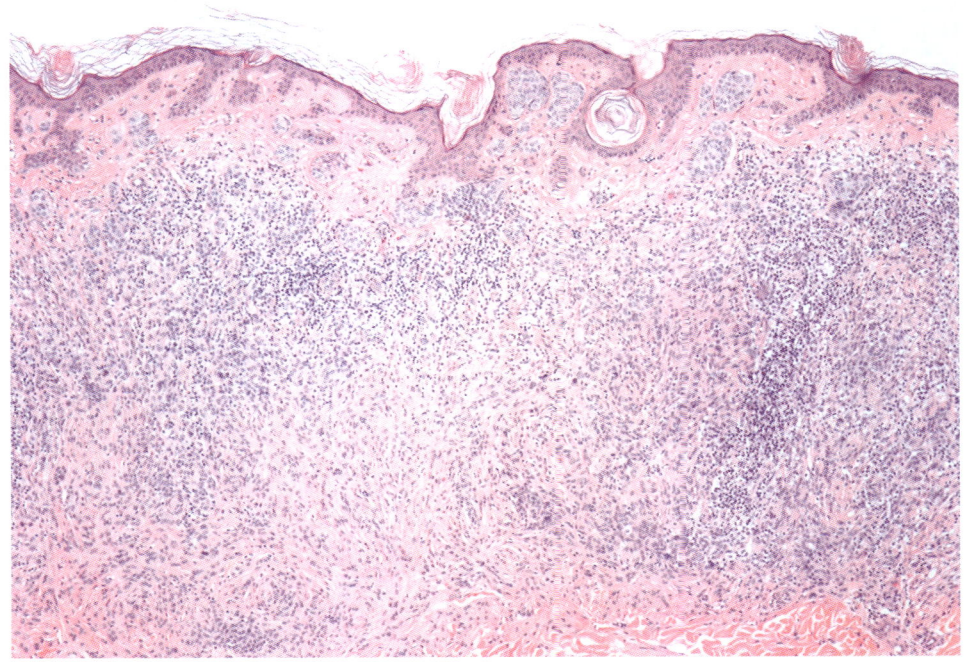

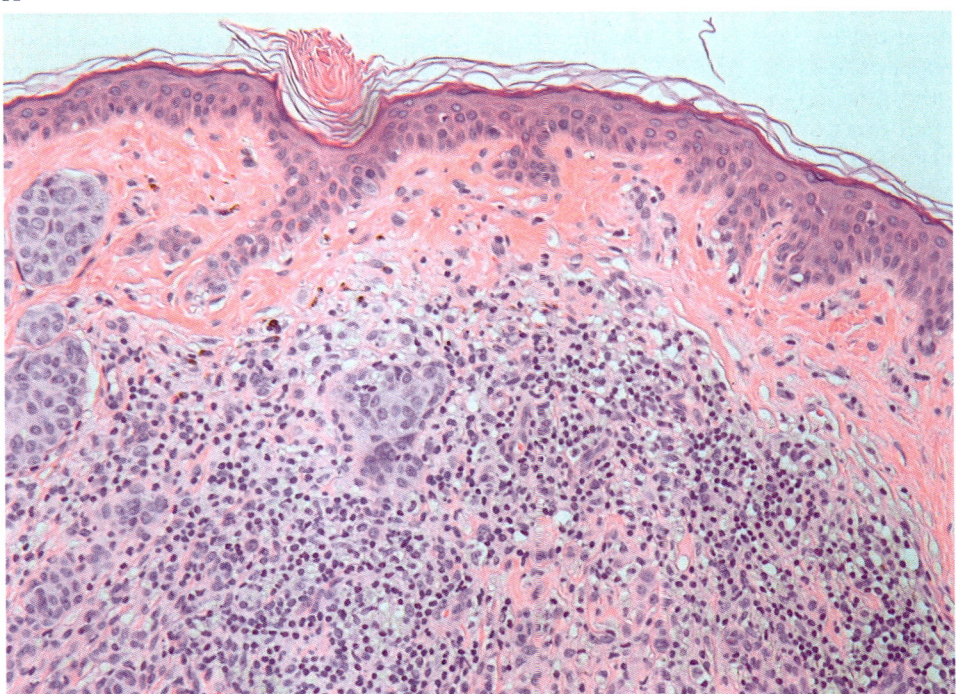

FIGURE 5-24 Halo nevus. **A,** At low magnification, the lesion appears predominantly inflammatory. **B,** A dense, mononuclear infiltrate obscures dermal nests of nevus cells.

TABLE 5-22 Differential diagnosis of halo nevus and malignant melanoma.		
Feature	Halo nevus	Malignant melanoma
Clinical features		
Size	Central nevus, 3–6 mm in diameter	Usually > 6 mm at diagnosis
Symmetry	Symmetry of central nevus and halo	Asymmetry
Borders	Well-circumscribed	Irregular
Color	Central nevus uniformly pigmented	Pigment variegation
Histologic features		
Symmetry	Symmetry	Asymmetry
Circumscription	Usually circumscribed	Poorly circumscribed
Infiltrate pattern	Lymphoid infiltrate orderly, with well-defined lower margin	Variation in pattern of infiltrate
Cell maturity	Nevus cells mature with dermal descent	No maturation
Apoptosis of nevus cell	Common	May occur
Rete ridges	Preserved	May be effaced
Cytologic atypia	Little or none	Prominent
Dermal mitoses	Few or none; no atypical mitoses	Frequent; atypical mitoses may occur

uration, and the cytologic characteristics of the melanocytic population (207). For halo nevi with little or no cytologic atypia, which are in the majority, the distinction from atypical nevi and melanoma with halo phenomenon does not usually pose difficulties (Table 5-22). Such nevi are usually small, symmetrical, and orderly in overall architecture. The lateral borders and base of the infiltrate are sharply marginated, and nevus cells do not as a rule extend lateral to the terminus of the infiltrate. From the superficial to the lower dermal extension of the lesion, the nevus cells with most halo nevi undergo maturation. Atypical nevi with histologic halo phenomenon are recognized by the findings of discontinuous melanocytic atypia of varying degrees and architectural alterations (212). Rarely, markedly atypical halo nevi may suggest "nevoid" melanoma. Consequently, one must weigh the clinical and histologic features collectively when interpreting such lesions. Some lesions may fall into a biologically indeterminate category and should be managed cautiously. More than a few nevus cell mitoses, mitoses toward the base, and atypical mitotic figures should pose concern for the possibility of melanoma.

Neural Nevus (Neurotized Nevus)

Neural nevi include those dermal nevi with a prominent content of Schwannian or type C nevus cells, usually situated toward the base of the lesions (5,6,17,41) (Fig. 5-9C). With advanced neurotization, it may be difficult to distinguish the nevus from a neurofibroma. The presence of nested nevus cells within the upper dermal component, however, serves to discriminate the two entities.

Nevus Spilus (Speckled Lentiginous Nevus)

The nevus spilus is a slightly pigmented macular lesion that contains more pigmented foci or speckles that may be either flat or raised (232–239). Although sometimes present at birth, the lesion more commonly develops in childhood (232). The frequency among white adults has been estimated to be 2.3% (238). There is no gender predilection. The trunk and extremities are most commonly affected.

The lesion generally persists indefinitely, although over time increased degrees of speckling can occur, and the specks may become more prominent after solar exposure (100,107). Melanoma has been documented to occur in these lesions (240–242).

Clinical Features The tan macular component varies from < 1 to > 20 cm in greatest dimension (232–239) (Table 5-23). The skin surface markings are not distorted within this area. The more pigmented speckles may be macular or papular and generally range from 1 to 6 mm in diameter. Large nevi spili may be unilateral, segmental, or zosteriform and involve in extreme cases an entire extremity or half of the trunk (235–237).

Histologic Features The tan macular component of the lesion resembles a lentigo simplex. Increased numbers of singly arranged melanocytes are situated along the basilar zone of elongated rete (Fig. 5-26; Table 5-23). The more pigmented macules may show features of either lentigo simplex or junctional nevus, whereas the papular foci contain junctional or compound nevus elements. Rarely, the histologic changes of Spitz, atypical, or congenital nevi are found within the papules.

Differential Diagnosis Large or congenital lentigo, congenital nevus, and atypical nevus are considered in the differential diagnosis. Biopsy sampling of the tan macular component will display changes indistinguishable from lentigo simplex, and clinical criteria will be required

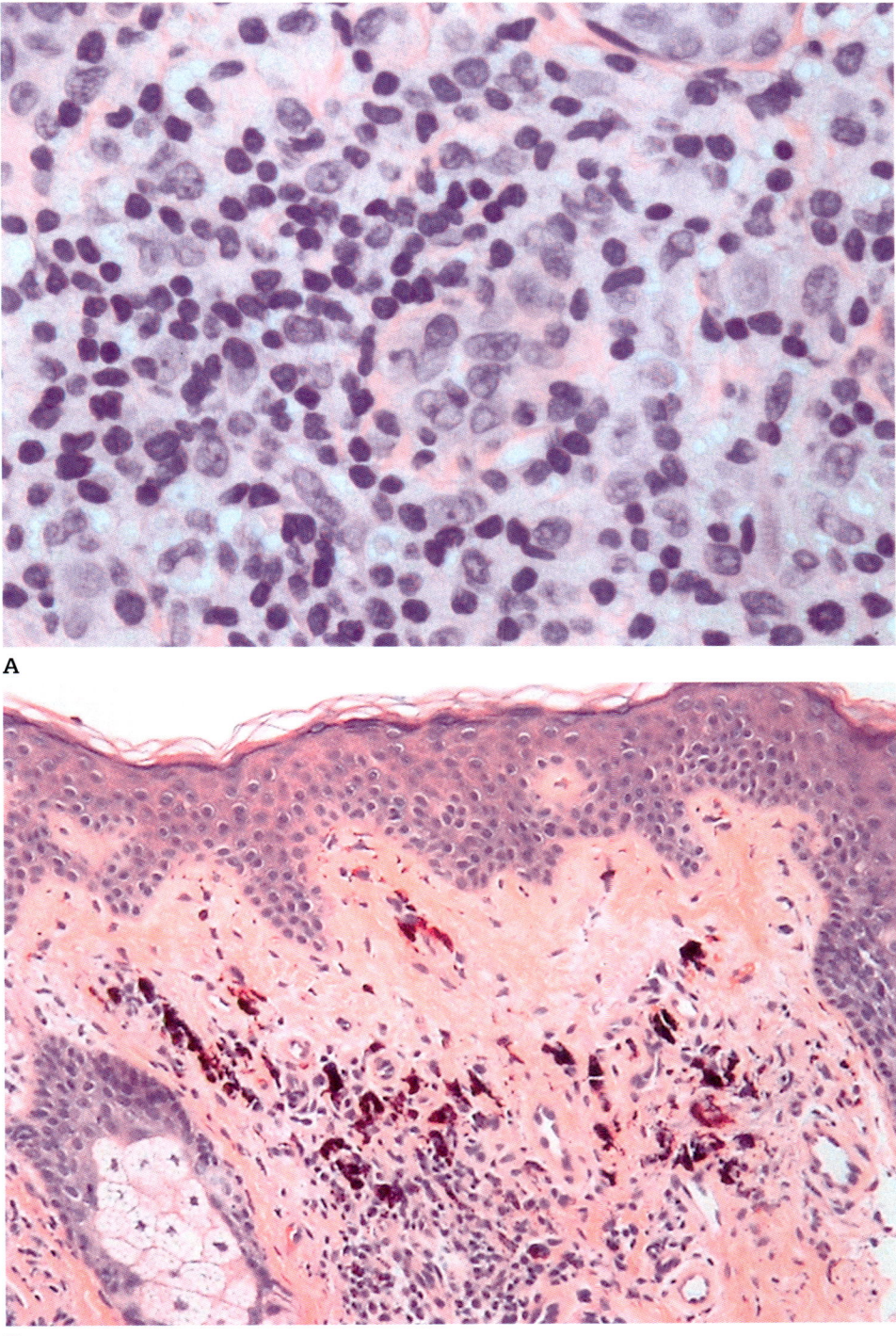

FIGURE 5-25 Halo nevus. **A,** Lymphocytes form rosette arrangements around nevus cells. Apoptotic and degenerating cells represent the effects of active immune-mediated regression. **B,** The stage of complete regression of a halo nevus.

TABLE 5-23 Nevus spilus.
Clinical features
Tan café-au-lait macule, 1–20 cm or larger
Hyperpigmented, macular, or papular speckles on tan macule
Speckles 1–6 mm in diameter
Uncommon segmental or zosteriform variants
Histologic features
Tan macule; resembles lentigo simplex
Speckles; lentiginous nevus to compound nevus
Occasionally, features of Spitz nevus, atypical nevus, or congenital nevus
Differential diagnosis
Large or congenital lentigo
Congenital nevus
Atypical nevus

to resolve the diagnosis. Some nevi spili are congenital and thus simply a curious subtype of congenital nevus. Lesions with histologic changes of atypical nevi have been termed *atypical* (dysplastic) *nevus spilus,* and the same guidelines for evaluating an atypical nevus (discussed elsewhere in this chapter) should be applied to those variants.

Recurrent Melanocytic Nevus (Recurrent/Persistent Melanocytic Nevus)

As defined by clinical criteria, a recurrent melanocytic nevus is a lesion that recurs at the site of previous surgical removal (243–246). With this phenomenon, the primary concern is the possibility of malignant melanoma. Although its prevalence has not been clearly established, it is a relatively common event among individuals with incompletely removed nevi. Most recurrent nevi have been reported in relatively young females, perhaps reflecting a trend to removal of more nevi in women (243–246). The trunk is the most commonly affected area, followed by the head and neck (246). Most follow removal of the antecedent nevus by incomplete saucerization. Recurrence is more likely following incomplete removal of the perimeter of the initial lesion than following transection of the base. Recurrences can also represent proliferation of residual melanocytes from the epidermal appendages (246). Trophic factors associated with the reparative response following initial biopsy may stimulate nevus cell migration or proliferation, giving rise to the clinical recurrence. Half of all cases recur within 6 months of the initial surgery, but delayed recurrences are possible (243,246). Most recurrent nevi are stable after development and persist indefinitely. No increased risk of melanoma has been reported with recurrent nevi.

Clinical Features With these lesions, circumscribed hyperpigmentation develops within a scar from the previous surgical removal of a nevus (243–246) (Table 5-24). The lesion is usually macular. The borders are irregular, and the pigment pattern may be variegated. Stippling, mottling, and loss of pigment may be observed (245,246). Most lesions measure 4–6 mm in greatest dimension.

Histologic Features Intraepidermal melanocytic proliferation is usually, but not always, confined to the area above the dermal scar (243–246) (Fig. 5-27A; Table 5-24). The rete ridge pattern is effaced, and the basal zone contains a variable lentiginous or nested intraepidermal proliferation of melanocytes (Fig. 5-27B). The melanocytes, which contain relatively uniform nuclei, are often heavily pigmented. Pagetoid scatter of melanocytes has been found in 60% of recurrent nevi in one series (214). Occasionally, low-grade nuclear atypia and prominent nucleoli may be present, and the nesting and architectural patterns may be irregular; however, the area with the cytologic and architectural irregularities is confined to the epidermis and dermis immediately above the scar (247). Well-formed nests of residual dermal nevus cells are commonly situated beneath the superficial dermal scar.

Differential Diagnosis

Recurrent nevus presents a differential diagnosis of atypical nevus, lentiginous melanocytic proliferations developing in melanoma scars, and recurrent melanoma. Most often, recurrent nevi remain confined histologically to the area of the dermal scar, appear within 6 months after surgery, and have well-defined margins and banal histologic features. Recurrent atypical nevi have greater architectural and cytologic atypia. Clinical features suggesting melanoma include irregular pigmentation, recurrence beyond the confines of the surgical scar, and a longer interval until recurrence (> 6 months).

When the histologic examination suggests the possibility of recurrent nevus, it is important to establish that a previous surgical procedure occurred at the site and, if so, to review the histologic sections of the original nevus. In this manner, the possibility of progression to melanoma is best evaluated.

Unusual Melanocytic Nevi of Genital Skin

Some nevi occurring on the vulvar skin have distinctive histologic features compared to most nevi from that site as well as to nevi situated on nongenital skin (248–250). Similarly, distinctive nevi may occur in other "special" locations, such as the scrotum or umbilicus and at other flexural sites (251). The significance of unusual nevi arising in the special sites in regard to the risk of progression to melanoma is uncertain and requires further study.

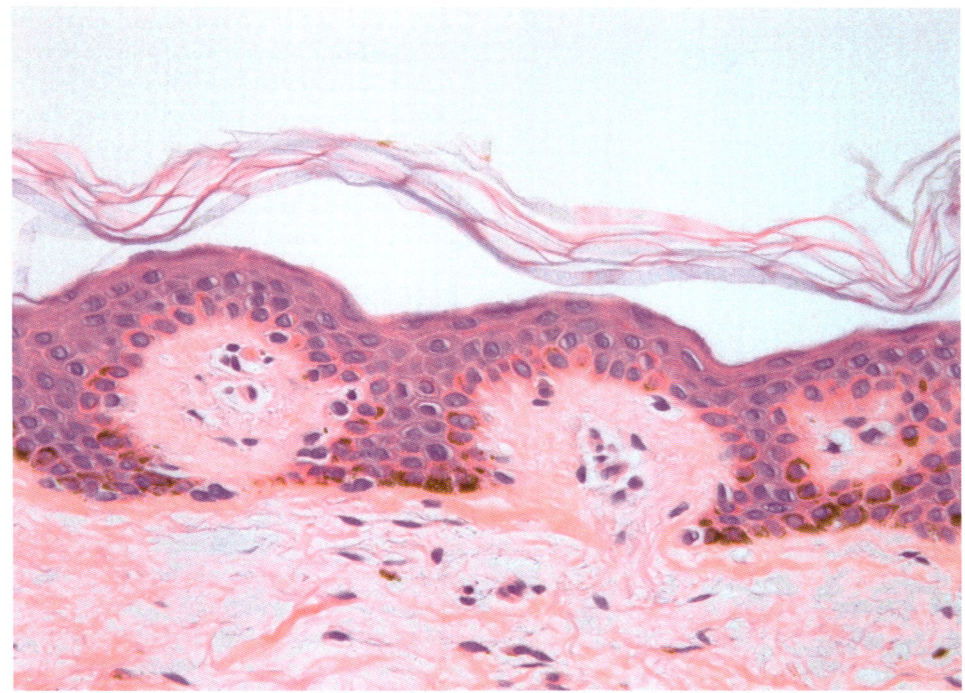

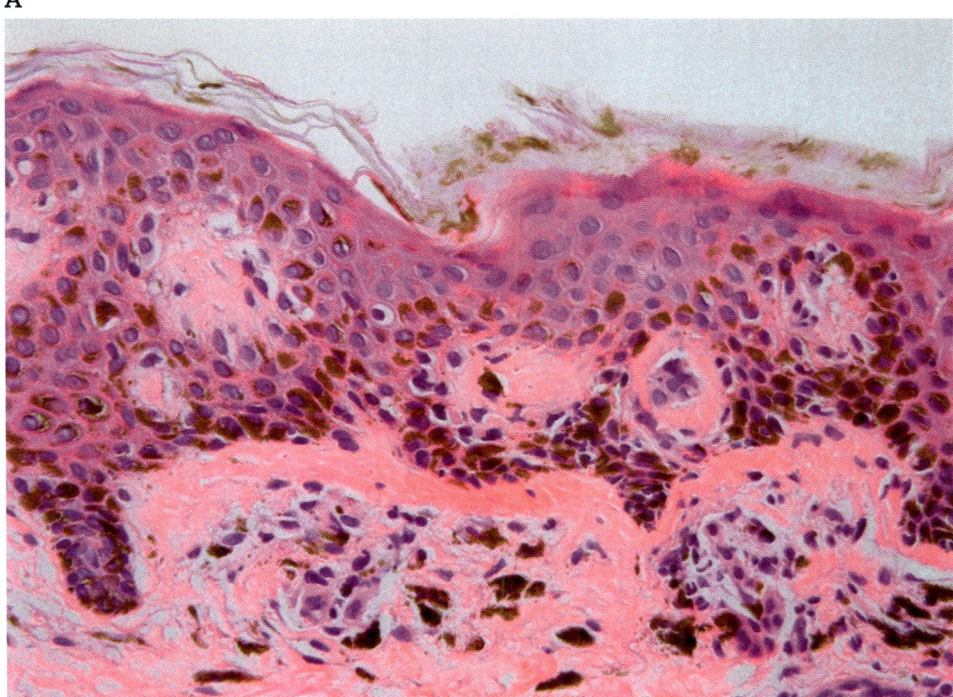

FIGURE 5-26 Nevus spilus. **A,** Within a tan macule, the features are those of a lentigo simplex. **B,** The pattern of a lentiginous nevus is present within a hyperpigmented papule.

TABLE 5-24 Recurrent melanocytic nevus.
Clinical features
Onset ∼ 6 weeks to 6 months after surgery
Macular pigmentation limited to site of scar
Often 4–6 mm in greatest dimension
Border irregularity common
Histologic features
Effacement of epidermal rete
Dermal scar
Intraepidermal melanocytic proliferation confined to area above scar
Melanocytic proliferation nested or lentiginous
Occasional nuclear atypia, but low grade
Differential diagnosis
Atypical nevus
Melanoma

Some of the unusual nevi exhibit features intermediate between those of common nevi and melanoma and may thus be related to atypical nevi.

Clinical Features Of the limited number of cases reported thus far, the majority has occurred in premenopausal women (248,249) (ages 14–40) (Table 5-25).

They appear to be uncommon among all vulvar nevi, perhaps accounting for < 10% of nevi removed (248). Detailed documentation of their clinical features are lacking; however, it is our experience that the nevi are larger (up to 12 mm) than usual for acquired nevi, are often relatively macular, may have irregular margins, and often present with color variegation (e.g., a mixture of tan, brown, and red).

Histologic Features The architectural pattern may be relatively orderly, with overall symmetry, absence of lateral extension beyond the dermal component (if present), and circumscribed borders (248,249). The unusual features are those shared by atypical (dysplastic) nevi—namely, prominent lentiginous melanocytic proliferation, enlarged junctional nests, variation in configuration of the junctional nests, coalescence of nests, and nuclear atypia of the cells, generally of low grade (248,249). The horizontal confluence and dyscohesion of cells within the nests may be pronounced (Fig. 5-28). The atypical basilar proliferation may extend down along appendageal epithelium (Fig. 5-29A). Pagetoid scatter of cells is usually not found. Cytologically, the junctional melanocytes are enlarged and contain abundant cytoplasms, thereby re-

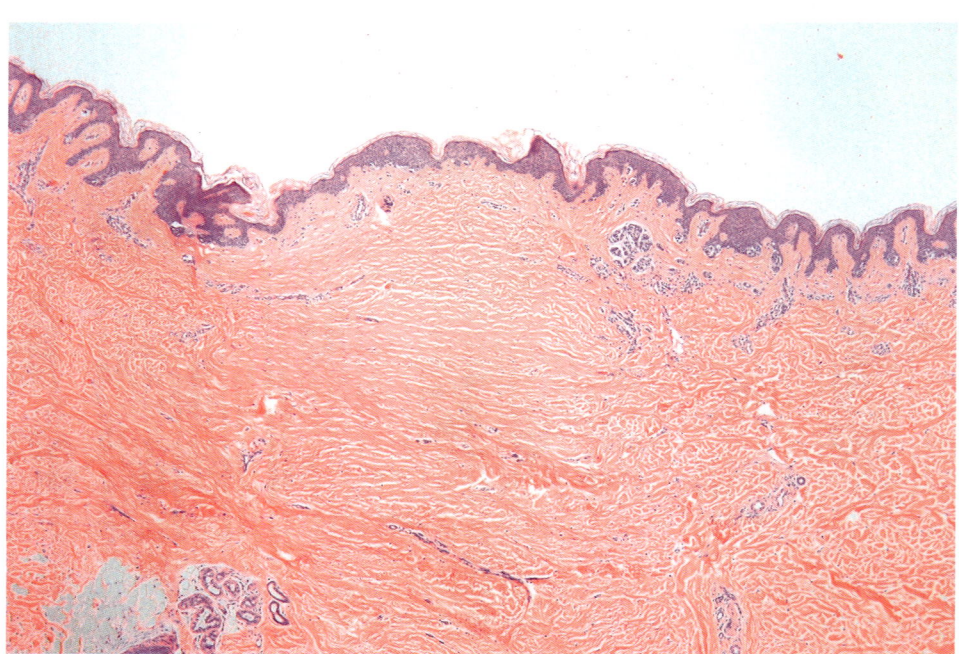

FIGURE 5-27 Recurrent melanocytic nevus. **A,** A dermal scar is associated with remnants of nevus cells.

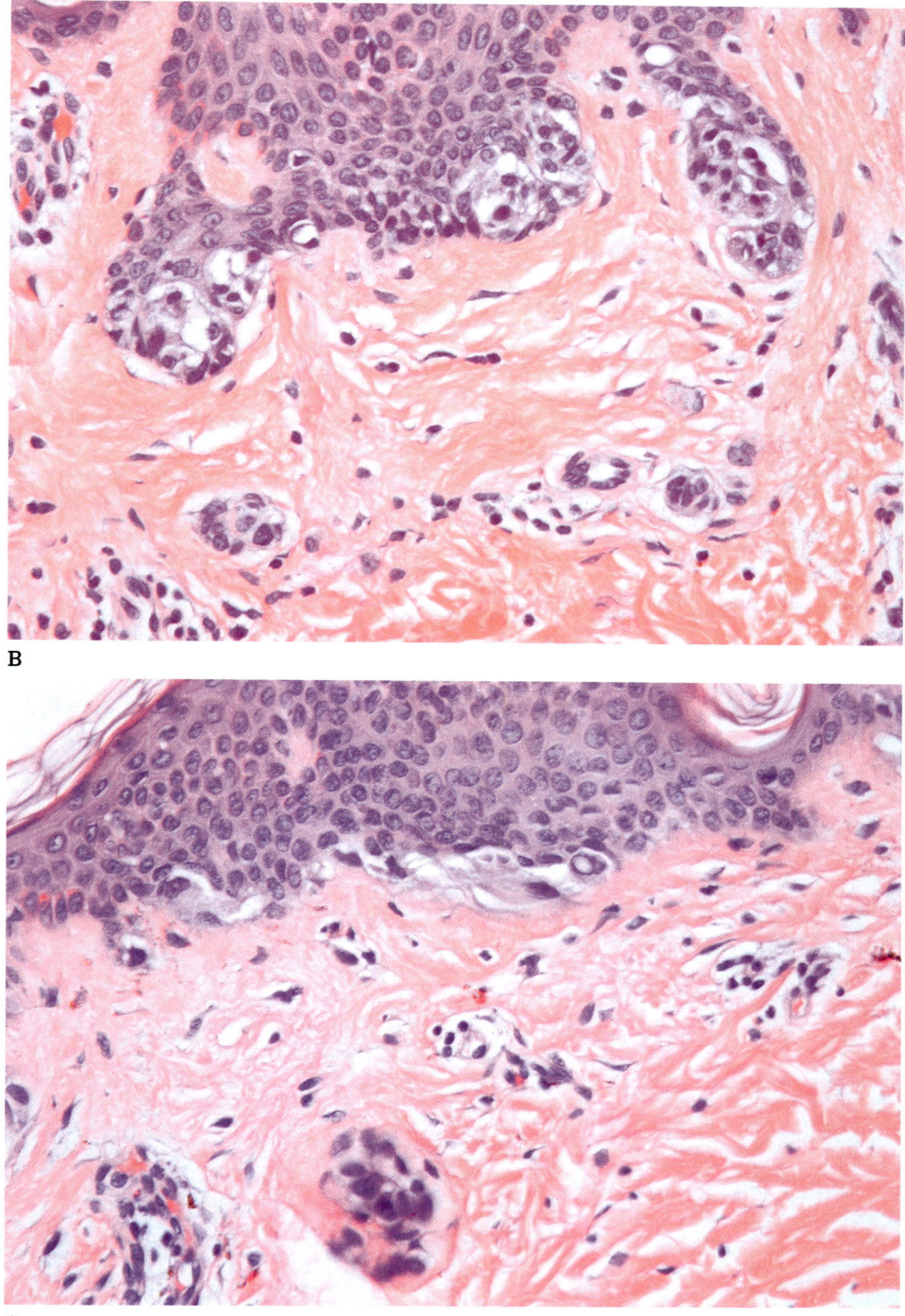

FIGURE 5-27 B, A mixed nested and lentiginous pattern of melanocytic proliferation is present along the basal epidermal zone in association with prominent hyperpigmentation. **C,** This recurrent atypical nevus is associated with irregular junctional and dermal nests and with nuclear atypia.

TABLE 5-25 Unusual vulvar melanocytic nevus.
Clinical features
Occurrence in premenopausal women
Often enlarged, up to 12 mm in diameter
Histologic features
Symmetry and circumscription, usually
Enlarged junctional nests with diminished cohesion
Lentiginous melanocytic proliferation
Confluence of cells and nests along basal epidermis
Variation in size, shape, position of junctional nests
Extension of melanocytes along appendageal epithelium
Generally no pagetoid scatter
Variable lateral extension
Common fibroplasia, often lamellar
Lymphocytic infiltrates
Slight to moderate nuclear atypia
Enlarged epidermal melanocytes with abundant cytoplasms
Multinucleate nevus giant cells
Maturation of dermal cells common
Differential diagnosis
Vulvar melanoma
Spitz nevus
Atypical nevus

sembling to some degree the epithelioid cells of Spitz nevi (Fig. 5-29B).

The stromal fibrotic reaction in vulvar nevi is said to be distinctive (250). Prominent lamellar fibrosis may replace the papillary dermis; and nests of dermal nevus cells, when present, are entrapped in the dense fibrous stroma (248,249). This finding may evoke the possibility of invasive melanoma, but the dermal cells are banal cytologically and mature with dermal descent. Perivascular lymphocytic infiltrates are usually evident within the fibrotic stroma.

Differential Diagnosis The diagnostic considerations are atypical nevus, Spitz tumor/nevus, and melanoma. The architectural and cytologic alterations within these nevi, however, are not as advanced as those found in melanoma, which display greater density of melanocytic proliferation with the basal zone, prominent pagetoid scatter, poorly defined lateral margins, greater cytologic atypia, and more advanced inflammatory response. Vulvar melanomas, moreover, tend to occur in older women (average age approximately 65 years) (Table 5-25). Spitz nevi are distinguished by the presence of a dimorphic population of spindled and epithelioid cells that are moderately enlarged. The pathogenic relationship of unusual vulvar nevi to atypical nevi is debated, and one reasonable hypothesis is that there is a common pathophysiology. In sum, the biologic significance of unusual vulvar nevi has not been adequately elucidated and requires further study.

Nevus with Focal Epithelioid Cell Component (Clonal Nevus, Combined Nevus, Combined Spitz Nevus, Inverted Type A Nevus)

Uncommon variants of otherwise ordinary nevocellular nevi incorporate a seemingly separate "clone" of cells situated within the dermal component of the nevus. These lesions can present a very difficult differential diagnosis with melanoma arising within the dermis. These lesions have undergone a variety of designations over recent decades, and their classification has thus not been standardized.

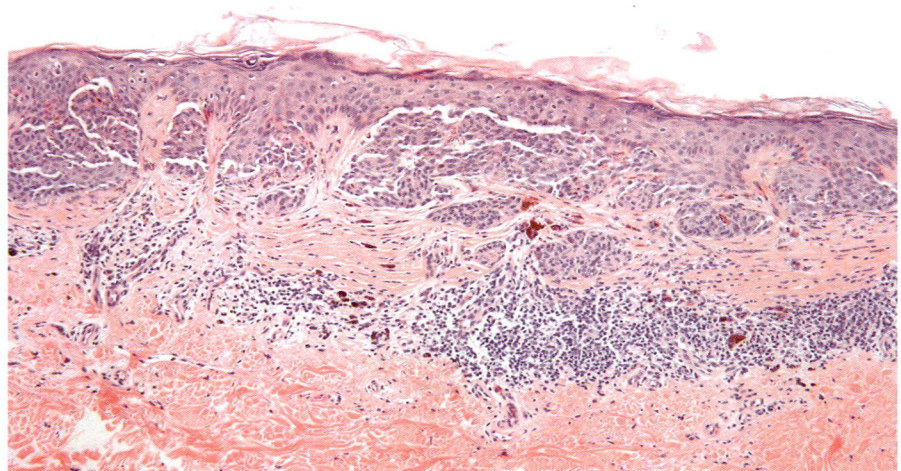

FIGURE 5-28 Vulvar nevus. Nests of nevus cells have coalesced along the dermoepidermal junction.

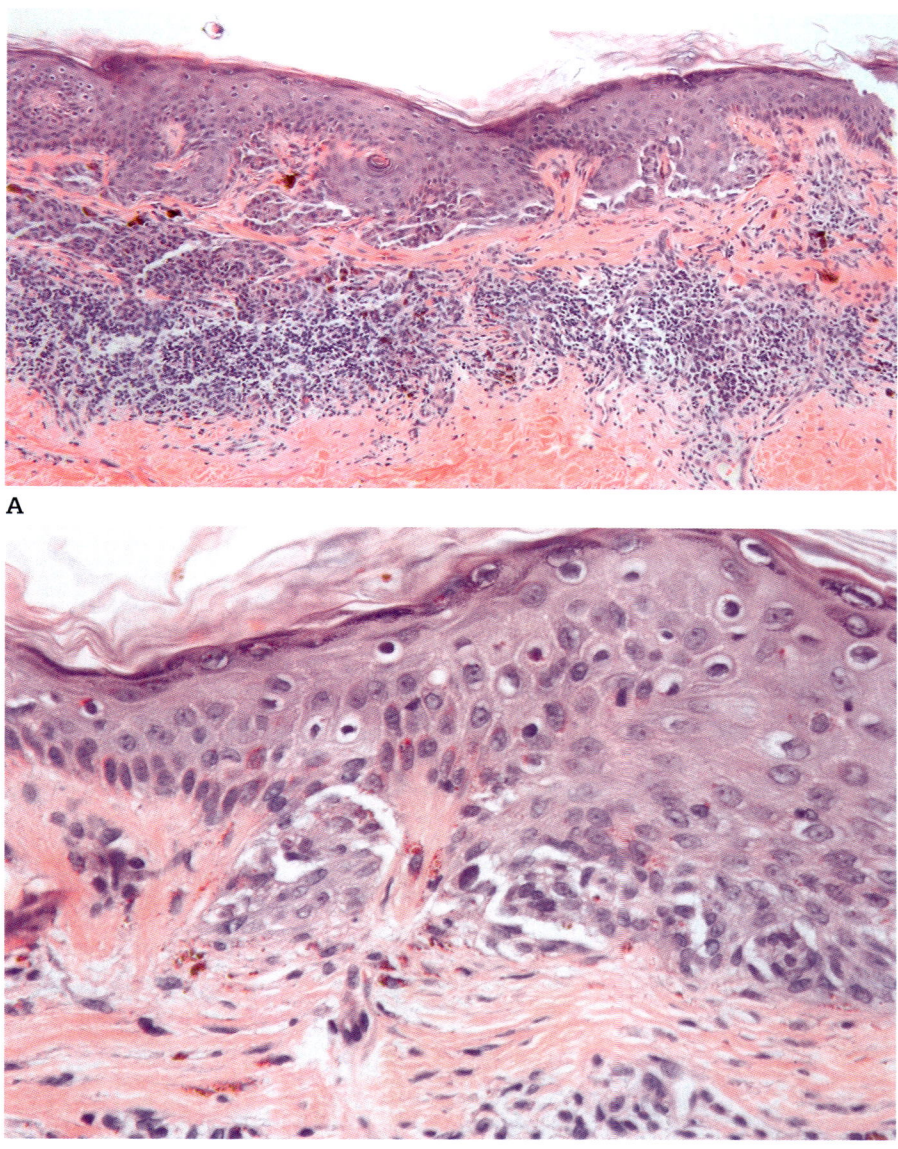

FIGURE 5-29 Scrotal nevus. **A,** Irregular, confluent, and bridging nests are arrayed at the junctional epidermis. **B,** The nevus cells have abundant cytoplasms. Multinucleate nevus giant cells are present.

Clinical Features Most of those variants affect young adults (252), with a mean age of 31 years (253). There is no strict anatomic site predilection, but many have been truncal or situated on the head and neck (253). The lesions most often come to medical attention because of their dark pigmentation or because a dark papule has developed within an existing nevus (253). Mean diameter was 6.2 mm in one series (253). There may be a history of recent growth, which in conjunction with the dark pigmentation prompts clinical concern for melanoma.

Histologic Features The substrate lesions within which these melanocytic tumors arise include banal compound or dermal nevi and, in a proportion of cases, nevi with a congenital pattern, which except for the "clonal" component are otherwise unremarkable. The clonal cells form a separate, spatially distinct, population of enlarged epithelioid cells, which most often are situated near the horizontal center of the nevus, within the upper half of the dermis (253) (Fig. 5-30A). The focus is either well or moderately circumscribed. The lesional cells do not in-

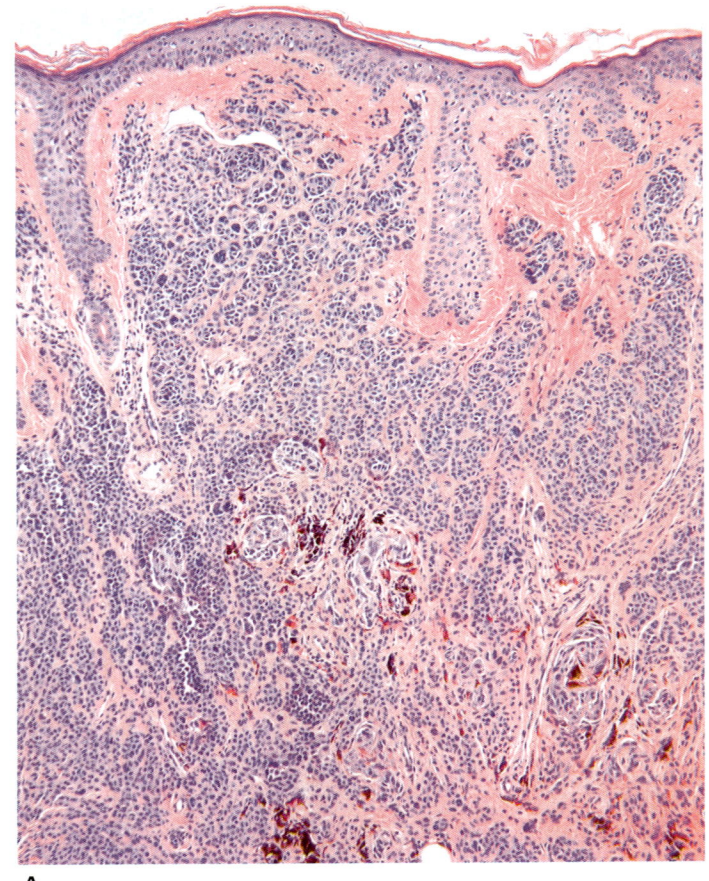

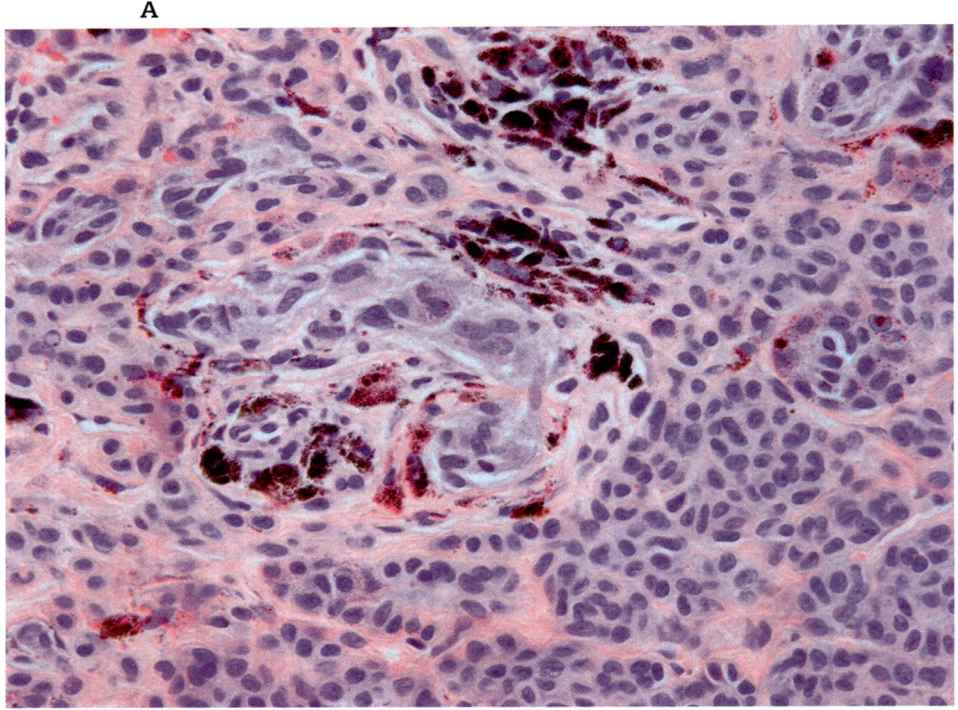

FIGURE 5-30 Clonal nevus. **A,** A distinct population of epithelioid cells is aggregated as nested arrays within the center of this nevocellular nevus. **B,** At higher magnification, the cells have abundant cytoplasms that are melaninized in a granular fashion. Reactive changes are present within the associated stroma, but nuclear atypia of significant degree is not in evidence.

volve the epidermis. The cells are organized into fascicles or small nests. Characteristically, their abundant cytoplasms are heavily melaninized, often in a granular pattern, and melanophages are represented within the contiguous, fibrotic stroma. The nuclei are generally small or slightly enlarged, and they may vary mildly in size and chromasia; however, moderate or advanced nuclear atypia is not present, and mitotic activity is rare or absent (Fig. 5-30B). Typically, there is no maturation with dermal descent. Patchy lymphoid infiltrates are not uncommonly situated in or near the epithelioid cell nests.

Differential Diagnosis The differential diagnosis of clonal nevus versus combined pigmented Spitz nevus of epithelioid type is largely a matter of semantics. The principal differential is with melanoma arising in the dermis of a precursor nevus. Lesions of the latter type and clonal nevi are often fairly well circumscribed and symmetrical, such that the architectural silhouette is not reliable in the diagnostic discrimination, nor is the absence of intraepidermal, pagetoid scatter of cells a practicable negative finding (254). However, a large expansile dermal mass of cells, if present, supports the diagnosis of melanoma, as do the findings of coarse nuclear chromatin, frequent mitoses, or satellitosis (253). Because the growth patterns cannot be relied on in most instances, however, the issue may resolve itself to one of assessing the degree of nuclear abnormality. Enlargement of nuclei, advanced nuclear hyperchromasia and pleomorphism, or indications of mitotic activity should prompt serious consideration of a dermal variant of melanoma.

REFERENCES

1. Weston JA. The migration and differentiation of neural crest cells. Adv Morphol 1971;8:41–114.
2. LeDouarin N. Migration and differentiation of neural crest cells. Curr Top Dev Biol 1980;16:31–85.
3. Quevedo WC Jr, Fleischmann RD. Developmental biology of mammalian melanocytes. J Invest Dermatol 1980;75:116–20.
4. Unna PG. Naevi and naevo-carcinoma. Berl Klin Wochenschr 1893;30:14.
5. Lund HZ, Stobbe GD. The natural history of the pigmented nevus: factors of age and anatomic location. Am J Pathol 1949;25:1117–55.
6. Maize JC, Foster G. Age-related changes in melanocytic naevi. Clin Exp Dermatol 1979;4:49–58.
7. Clark WH Jr, Elder DE, Guerry D, et al. A study of tumor progression: the precursor lesions of superficial spreading and nodular melanoma. Hum Pathol 1984;15:1147–65.
8. Hu F. Melanocyte cytology in normal skin, melanocytic nevi, and malignant melanomas. In Acherman AB, ed. Pathology of Malignant Melanoma. New York: Masson, 1981:1–21.
9. Stegmaier G, Montgomery H. Histopathologic studies of pigmented nevi in children. J Invest Dermatol 1953;20:51–62.
10. Stegmaier OC. Natural regression of the melanocytic nevus. J Invest Dermatol 1959;32:413–9.
11. Kopf AW, Andrade R. A histologic study of the dermaoepidermal junction in clinically "intraepidermal" nevi, employing serial sections: I. junctional theques. Ann NY Acad Sci 1960;100:200–22.
12. Stegmaier O, Becker SJ. Incidence of melanocytic nevi in young adults. J Invest Dermatol 1960;34:125–9.
13. Winkelmann RK, Rocha G. The dermal nevus and statistics: An evaluation of 1200 pigmented lesions. Arch Dermatol 1962;86:310–5.
14. Nicholls EM. Development and elimination of pigmented moles, and the anatomical distribution of primary malignant melanoma. Cancer 1973;32:191–5.
15. MacKie RM, English J, Aitchison TC, et al. The number and distribution of benign pigmented moles (melanocytic naevi) in a healthy British population. Br J Dermatol 1985;113:167–74.
16. Cramer SF. The histogenesis of acquired melanocytic nevi. Based on a new concept of melanocytic differentiation. Am J Dermatopathol 1984;6(Suppl):289–98.
17. Masson P. My conception of cellular nevi. Cancer 1951;4:9–38.
18. Masson P. Melanogenic system: nevi and melanomas. Pathol Annu 1967;2:351–97.
19. Worret WI, Burgdorf WH. Which direction do nevus cells move? Abtropfung reexamined. Am J Dermatopathol 1998;20:135–9.
20. Reed RJ, Ichinose H, Clark WH Jr, Mihm MC Jr. Common and uncommon melanocytic nevi and borderline melanomas. Semin Oncol 1975;2:119–47.
21. Aso M, Hashimoto K, Eto H, et al. Expression of Schwann cell characteristics in pigmented nevus. Immunohistochemical study using monoclonal antibody to Schwann cell associated antigen. Cancer 1988;62:938–43.
22. Whimster IW. What are moles? Am J Dermatopathol 7 1985;Suppl:A8–A15.
23. Herlyn M, Herlyn D, Elder DE, et al. Phenotypic characteristics of cells derived from precursors of human melanoma. Cancer Res 1983;43:5502–8.
24. Balaban G, Herlyn M, Guerry D, et al. Cytogenetics of human malignant melanoma and premalignant lesions. Cancer Genet Cytogenet 1984;11:429–39.
25. Herlyn M, Thurin J, Balaban G, et al. Characteristics of cultured human melanocytes isolated from different stages of tumor progression. Cancer Res 1985;45:5670–6.
26. Herlyn M, Clark WH, Rodeck U, et al. Biology of tumor progression in human melanocytes. Lab Invest 1987;56:461–74.

27. Mancianti ML, Herlyn M, Weil D, et al. Growth and phenotypic characteristics of human nevus cells in culture. J Invest Dermatol 1988;90:134–41.
28. Harada M, Suzuki M, Ikeda T, et al. Clonality in nevocellular nevus and melanoma: an expression-based clonality analysis at the X-linked genes by polymerase chain reaction. J Invest Dermatol 1997;109:656–60.
29. Robinson WA, Lemon M, Elefanty A, et al. Human acquired naevi are clonal. Melanoma Res 1998;8:499–503.
30. Hui P, Perkins A, Glusac E. Assessment of clonality in melanocytic nevi. J Cutan Pathol 2001;28:140–4.
31. Maitra A, Gazdar AF, Moore TO, Moore AY. Loss of heterozygosity analysis of cutaneous melanoma and benign melanocytic nevi: laser capture microdissection demonstrates clonal genetic changes in acquired nevocellular nevi. Hum Pathol 2002;33:191–7.
32. Easton DF, Cox GM, Macdonald AM, Ponder BA. Genetic susceptibility to naevi—a twin study. Br J Cancer 1991;64:1164–7.
33. Goldgar DE, Cannon-Albright LA, Meyer LJ, et al. Inheritance of nevus number and size in melanoma and dysplastic nevus syndrome kindreds. J Natl Cancer Inst 1991;83:1726–33.
34. Armstrong BK, de Klerk NH, Holman CD. Etiology of common acquired melanocytic nevi: constitutional variables, sun exposure, and diet. J Natl Cancer Inst 1986;77:329–35.
35. Green A, Bain C, MacLennan R. Risk factors for cutaneous melanama in Queensland. In: Gallagher R, ed. Recent Results in Cancer Research: Epidimilogy of Malignant Melanoma. Berlin: Springer-Verlag, 1986;102:76–97.
36. Armstrong BK, English DR. The epidemiology of acquired melanocytic naevi and their relationship to malignant melanoma. In: Elwood JM, ed. Melanoma and Naevi. Basel: Karger, 1988:27–47.
37. Hughes BR, Cunliffe WJ, Bailey CC. Excess benign melanocytic naevi after chemotherapy for malignancy in childhood. Br Med J 1989;299:88–91.
38. de Wit PEJ, de Vaan GAM, de Boo TM. Prevalence of nevocytic nevi after chemotherapy for childhood cancer. Med Pediatr Oncol 1990;18:336–8.
39. Wachsmuth RC, Gaut RM, Barrett JH, et al. Heritability and gene-environment interactions for melanocytic nevus density examined in a U.K. adolescent twin study. J Invest Dermatol 2001;117:348–52.
40. Goldgar DE, Cannon-Albright LA, Meyer LJ, et al. Inheritance of nevus number and size in melanoma/DNS kindreds. Cytogenet Cell Genet 1992;59:200–2.
41. Mishima Y. Macromolecular changed in pimentary disorders. Arch Dermatol 1965;91:519–57.
42. Tronnier M, Smolle J, Wolff HH. Ultraviolet irradiation induces acute changes in melanocytic nevi. J Invest Dermatol 1995;104:475–8.
43. Lucky PA, Nordlund JJ. The biology of the pigmentary system and its disorders. Dermatol Clin 1985;3:197–216.
44. Alper JC, Holmes LB. The incidence and significance of birthmarks in a cohort of 4,641 newborns. Pediatr Dermatol 1983;1:58–68.
45. Coleman WP III, Gately LE III, Krementz AB, et al. Nevi, lentigines, and melanomas in blacks. Arch Dermatol 1980;116:548–51.
46. Coskey RJ. Eruptive nevi (Letter). Arch Dermatol 1975;111:1658.
47. Eady RA, Gilkes JJ, Jones EW. Eruptive naevi: report of two cases, with enzyme histochemical, light and electron microscopical findings. Br J Dermatol 1977;97:267–78.
48. Leyden JJ, Spott DA, Goldschmidt H. Diffuse and banded melanin pigmentation in nails. Arch Dermatol 1972;105:548–50.
49. Kawamura T, Nishihara K, Kawasakiya S. Pigmentatio longitudinalis striata unguium and the pigmentation of nail plate in Addison's disease [Abstract]. Jpn J Dermatol 1958;68:10.
50. Kopf AW, Waldo E. Melanonychia striata. Australas J Dermatol 1980;21:59–70.
51. Voron DA, Hatfield HH, Kalkhoff RK. Multiple lentigines syndrome. Case report and review of the literature. Am J Med 1976;60:447–56.
52. Rhodes AR, Silverman RA, Harrist TJ, Perez-Atayde AR. Mucocutaneous lentigines, cardiomucocutaneous myxomas, and multiple blue nevi: the "LAMB" syndrome. J Am Acad Dermatol 1984;10:72–82.
53. Carney JA, Gordon H, Carpenter PC. The complex of myxomas, spotty pigmentation, and endocrine overactivity. Medicine 1985;64:270–83.
54. Jeghers H, McKusick VA, Katz KH. Genernalized intestinal polyposis and melanin spots of the oral mucosa, lips, and digits: a syndrome of diagnostic significance. N Engl J Med 1949;241:993–1005.
55. Utsunomiya J, Gocho H, Miyanaga T, et al. Peutz-Jeghers syndrome: its natural course and management. Johns Hopkins Med J 1975;136:71–82.
56. Carney JA. Carney complex: the complex of myxomas, spotty pigmentation, endocrine overactivity, and schwannomas. Semin Dermatol 1995;14:90–8.
57. Rampen FH, de Wit PE. Racial differences in mole proneness. Acta Derm Venereol 1989;69:234–6.
58. Sigg C, Pelloni F. Frequency of acquired melanonevocytic nevi and their relationship to skin complexion in 939 schoolchildren. Dermatologica 1989;179:123–8.
59. Pack G, Davis J. The relation of race and complexion to the incidence of moles and melanomas. Ann NY Acad Sci 1963;100:719–42.
60. Shaffer B. Pigmented nevi: a clinical appraisal in the light of present-day histopathologic concepts. Arch Dermatol 1955;72:120–32.

61. Pack GT, Davis J. The pigmented mole. Postgrad Med 1960;27:370–82.
62. Tosti A, Baran R, Piraccini BM, et al. Nail matrix nevi: a clinical and histopathologic study of twenty-two patients. J Am Acad Dermatol 1996;34:765–71.
63. Barr RJ, King DF. The significance of pseudoinclusions within the nuclei of melanocytes of certain neoplasms. In: Ackerman AB, ed. Pathology of Malignant Melanoma. New York: Masson, 1981:269–72.
64. Bentley-Phillips CB, Marks R. The epidermal component of melanocytic naevi. J Cutan Pathol 1976;3:190–4.
65. Horenstein MG, Prieto VG, Burchette JL Jr, Shea CR. Keratotic melanocytic nevus: a clinicopathologic and immunohistochemical study. J Cutan Pathol 2000;27:344–50.
66. Morgan MB, Raley BA, Vannarath RL, et al. Papillomatous melanocytic nevi: an estrogen related phenomenon. J Cutan Pathol 1995;22:446–9.
67. Okamura JM, Barr RJ, Cantos KA. Benign atypical junctional melanocytic hyperplasia associated with intradermal nevi: a common finding that may be confused with melanoma in situ. Mod Pathol 2000;13:857–60.
68. Kerl H, Soyer HP, Cerroni L, et al. Ancient melanocytic nevus. Semin Diagn Pathol 1998;15:210–5.
69. Schrader WA, Helwig EB. Balloon cell nevi. Cancer 1967;20:1502–14.
70. Lewis BL. Clinical appearance of a balloon cell nevus. Arch Dermatol 1969;100:312–3.
71. Goette DK, Doty RD. Balloon cell nevus. Summary of the clinical and histologic characteristics. Arch Dermatol 1978;114:109–11.
72. Hashimoto K, Bale GF. An electron microscopic study of balloon cell nevus. Cancer 1972;30:530–40.
73. Okun MR, Donnellan B, Edelstein L. An ultrastructural study of balloon cell nevus. Relationship of mast cells to nevus cells. Cancer 1974;34:615–25.
74. Rhodes AR, Silverman RA, Harrist TJ, Melski JW. A histologic comparison of congenital and acquired nevomelanocytic nevi. Arch Dermatol 1985;121:1266–73.
75. Harris GR, Shea CR, Horenstein MG, et al. Desmoplastic (sclerotic) nevus: an underrecognized entity that resembles dermatofibroma and desmoplastic melanoma. Am J Surg Pathol 1999;23:786–94.
76. McGibbon DH, Jones EW. Fibrous papule of the face (nose). Fibrosing nevocytic nevus. Am J Dermatopathol 1979;1:345–8.
77. Weedon D. Unusual features of nevocellular nevi. J Cutan Pathol 1982;9:284–92.
78. Thompson GW, Diehl AK. Partial unilateral lentiginosis. Arch Dermatol 1980;116:356.
79. MacDonald DM, Black MM. Secondary localized cutaneous amyloidosis in melanocytic naevi. Br J Dermatol 1980;103:553–6.
80. Soderstrom KO. Angiomatous type of intradermal nevi. Am J Dermatopathol 1987;9:549–51.
81. Collina G, Eusebi V. Naevocytic naevi with vascular-like spaces. Br J Dermatol 1991;124:591–5.
82. Mehregan AH, King JR. Multiple target-like pigmented nevi. Arch Dermatol 1972;105:129–30.
83. Happle R. Kokardennaevus. Hautarzt 1974;25:594–96.
84. Warin AP. Cockarde naevus. Clin Exp Dermatol 1976;1:221–4.
85. James MP, Wells RS. Cockade naevus: an unusual variant of the benign cellular naevus. Acta Derm Venereol 1980;60:360–3.
86. Saunders TS. Abscess formation in pigmented nevi: report of three cases. Arch Dermatol 1957;76:189–92.
87. Freeman RG, Knox JM. Epidermal cysts associated with pigmented nevi. Arch Dermatol 1962;85:590–4.
88. Haber H. Some observations on common moles. Br J Dermatol 1962;74:224–8.
89. Canizares O. Subnevic folliculitis resembling melanoma. Arch Dermatol 1968;97:363.
90. Meyerson LB. A peculiar papulosquamous eruption involving pigmented nevi. Arch Dermatol 1971;103:510–2.
91. Krivanek JF, Cains GD, Paver K. Halo eczema and junctional naevi: a case report. Australas J Dermatol 1977;18:81–3.
92. Weedon D, Farnsworth J. Spongiotic changes in melanocytic nevi. Am J Dermatopathol 1984;6(Suppl):257–9.
93. Elenitsas R, Halpern AC. Eczematous halo reaction in atypical nevi. J Am Acad Dermatol 1996;34:357–61.
94. Burgdorf W, Nasemann T. Cutaneous osteomas: a clinical and histopathologic review. Arch Dermatol Res 1977;260:121–35.
95. Delacretaz J, Frenk E. Zur pathogenese des osteo-naevus nanta. Hautarzt 1964;15:487–9.
96. Yesudian P, Thambiah AS. Perinevoid alopecia. An unusual variety of alopecia areata. Arch Dermatol 1976;112:1432–4.
97. Weitzner S. Intradermal nevus with psammoma body formation. Arch Dermatol 1968;98:287–9.
98. Elder DE, Greene MH, Bondi EE, Clark WHJ. Acquired melanocytic nevi and melanoma: the dysplastic nevus syndrome. In: Ackerman AB, ed. Pathology of Malignant Melanoma. New York: Masson, 1981:185–215.
99. Gruber SB, Barnhill RL, Stenn KS, Roush GC. Nevomelanocytic proliferations in association with cutaneous malignant melanoma: a multivariate analysis. J Am Acad Dermatol 1989;21:773–80.
100. Williams ML, Sagebiel RW. Melanoma risk factors and atypical moles. West J Med 1994;160:343–50.
101. Skender-Kalnenas TM, English DR, Heenan PJ. Benign melanocytic lesions: risk markers or precursors of cutaneous melanoma? J Am Acad Dermatol 1995;33:1000–7.
102. Norris W. A case of fungoid disease. Edinb Med Surg J 1820;16:562–5.
103. Cawley EP. Genetic aspects of malignant melanoma. AMA Arch Dermatol 1952;65:440–50.

104. Munro DD. Multiple active junctional naevi with family history of malignant melanoma. Proc R Soc Med 1974;67: 594–5.
105. Frichot BC III, Lynch HT, Guirgis HA, et al. New cutaneous phenotype in familial malignant melanoma. Lancet 1977;1:864–5.
106. Lynch HT, Frichot BC III, Lynch JF. Familial atypical multiple mole-melanoma syndrome. J Med Genet 1978;15: 352–6.
107. Clark WH Jr, Reimer RR, Greene M, et al. Origin of familial malignant melanomas from heritable melanocytic lesions. "The B-K mole syndrome." Arch Dermatol 1978; 114:732–8.
108. Allen AC, Spitz S. Malignant melanoma: a clinicopathological analysis of the criteria for diagnosis and prognosis. Cancer 1953;6:1–45.
109. Lund HZ, Kraus JM. Melanotic tumors of the skin. In Atlas of Tumor Pathology. Washington, DC: Armed Forces Institue of Pathology 1962;sect 1(fasc 3):86–9.
110. Barnhill RL. Current status of the dysplastic melanocytic nevus. J Cutan Pathol 1991;18:147–59.
111. Ackerman AB, Mihara I. Dysplasia, dysplastic melanocytes, dysplastic nevi, the dysplastic nevus syndrome, and the relation between dysplastic nevi and malignant melanomas. Hum Pathol 1985;16:87–91.
112. Ackerman AB. What naevus is dysplastic, a syndrome and the commonest precursor of malignant melanoma? A riddle and an answer. Histopathology 1988;13:241–56.
113. Conference NC. Precursors to malignant melanoma. J Am Med Assoc 1984;251:1864–6.
114. Tripp JM, Kopf AW, Marghoob AA, Bart RS. Management of dysplastic nevi: a survey of fellows of the American Academy of Dermatology. J Am Acad Dermatol 2002;46: 674–82.
115. Greene MH, Clark WH Jr, Tucker MA, et al. High risk of malignant melanoma in melanoma-prone families with dysplastic nevi. Ann Intern Med 1985;102:458–65.
116. MacKie RM, McHenry P, Hole D. Accelerated detection with prospective surveillance for cutaneous malignant melanoma in high-risk groups. Lancet 1993;341:1618–20.
117. Tucker MA, Fraser MC, Goldstein AM, et al. Risk of melanoma and other cancers in melanoma-prone families. J Invest Dermatol 1993;100:350S–5S.
118. Carey WP Jr, Thompson CJ, Synnestvedt M, et al. Dysplastic nevi as a melanoma risk factor in patients with familial melanoma. Cancer 1994;74:3118–25.
119. Elder DE, Goldman LI, Goldman SC, et al. Dysplastic nevus syndrome: a phenotypic association of sporadic cutaneous melanoma. Cancer 1980;46:1787–94.
120. Nordlund JJ, Kirkwood J, Forget BM, et al. Demographic study of clinically atypical (dysplastic) nevi in patients with melanoma and comparison subjects. Cancer Res 1985;45: 1855–61.
121. Swerdlow AJ, English J, Mackie RM. Benign melanocytic naevi as a risk factor for malignant melanoma. Br Med J Clin Res Ed 1986;292:1555–9.
122. Holly EA, Kelly JW, Shpall SN, Chiu SH. Number of melanocytic nevi as a major risk factor for malignant melanoma. J Am Acad Dermatol 1987;17:459–68.
123. Rigel DS, Rivers JK, Friedman RJ, Kopf AW. Risk gradient for malignant melanoma in individuals with dysplastic naevi. Lancet 1988;1:352–3.
124. Roush GC. Abnormal nevi, excess total nevi, and melanoma: an epidemiologic perspective. Cancer Treat Rev 1988;43:85–100.
125. Roush GC, Nordlund JJ, Forget B, et al. Independence of dysplastic nevi from total nevi in determining risk for nonfamilial melanoma. Prev Med 1988;17:273–9.
126. MacKie RM, Freudenberger T, Aitchison TC. Personal risk-factor chart for cutaneous melanoma. Lancet 1989;2: 487–90.
127. Crutcher WA, Sagebiel RW. Prevalence of dysplastic naevi in a community practice. Lancet 1984;1:729.
128. Cooke KR, Spears GF, Elder DE, Greene MH. Dysplastic naevi in a population-based survey. Cancer 1989;63:1240–4.
129. Garbe C, Kruger S, Stadler R, et al. Markers and relative risk in a German population for developing malignant melanoma. Int J Dermatol 1989;28:517–23.
130. Augustsson A, Stierner U, Suurkula M, Rosdahl I. Prevalence of common and dysplastic naevi in a Swedish population. Br J Dermatol 1991;124:152–6.
131. Halpern AC, Guerry D, Elder DE, et al. Dysplastic nevi as risk markers of sporadic (nonfamilial) melanoma. A case-control study. Arch Dermatol 1991;127:995–9.
132. Meyer LJ, Piepkorn M, Goldgar DE, et al. Interobserver concordance in discriminating clinical atypia of melanocytic nevi, and correlations with histologic atypia. J Am Acad Dermatol 1996;34:618–25.
133. Barnhill RL, Roush GC, Ernstoff MS, Kirkwood JM. Interclinician agreement on the recognition of selected gross morphologic features of pigmented lesions. Studies of melanocytic nevi V. J Am Acad Dermatol 1992;26:185–90.
134. Holman CDJ, Armstrong BK. Pigmentary traits, ethnic origin, benign nevi, and family history as risk factors for cutaneous malignant melanoma. J Am Med Assoc 1984; 251:1864–6.
135. Green A, MacLennan R, Siskind V. Common acquired naevi and the risk of malignant melanoma. Int J Cancer 1985;35:297–300.
136. Weiss J, Bertz J, Jung EG. Malignant melanoma in southern Germany: different predictive value of risk factors for melanoma subtypes. Dermatologica 1991;183:109–13.
137. Kruger S, Garbe C, Buttner P, et al. Epidemiologic evidence for the role of melanocytic nevi as risk markers and direct precursors of cutaneous malignant melanoma. Results of a case control study in melanoma patients and

nonmelanoma control subjects. J Am Acad Dermatol 1992;26:920–6.
138. Carli P, Biggeri A, Giannotti B. Malignant melanoma in Italy: risks associated with common and clinically atypical melanocytic nevi. J Am Acad Dermatol 1995;32:734–9.
139. Rieger E, Soyer HP, Garbe C, et al. Overall and site-specific risk of malignant melanoma associated with nevus counts at different body sites: a multicenter case-control study of the German Central Malignant-Melanoma Registry. Int J Cancer 1995;62:393–7.
140. Bataille V, Bishop JA, Sasieni P, et al. Risk of cutaneous melanoma in relation to the numbers, types and sites of naevi: a case-control study. Br J Cancer 1996;73:1605–11.
141. Grulich AE, Bataille V, Swerdlow AJ, et al. Naevi and pigmentary characteristics as risk factors for melanoma in a high-risk population: a case-control study in New South Wales, Australia. Int J Cancer 1996;67:485–91.
142. Rodenas JM, Delgado-Rodriguez M, Farinas-Alvarez C, et al. Melanocytic nevi and risk of cutaneous malignant melanoma in southern Spain. Am J Epidemiol 1997;145:1020–9.
143. Tucker MA, Halpern A, Holly EA, et al. Clinically recognized dysplastic nevi. A central risk factor for cutaneous melanoma. J Am Med Assoc 1997;277:1439–44.
144. Bataille V, Grulich A, Sasieni P, et al. The association between naevi and melanoma in populations with different levels of sun exposure: a joint case-control study of melanoma in the UK and Australia. Br J Cancer 1998;77:505–10.
145. Swerdlow AJ, Green A. Melanocytic naevi and melanoma: an epidemiological perspective. Br J Dermatol 1987;117:137–46.
146. Carli P, Biggeri A, Nardini P, et al. Epidemiology of atypical melanocytic naevi: an analytical study in a Mediterranean population. Eur J Cancer Prev 1997;6:506–11.
147. Titus-Ernstoff L, Mansson-Brahme E, Thorn M, et al. Factors associated with atypical nevi: a population-based study. Cancer Epidemiol Biomarkers Prev 1998;7:207–10.
148. Grob JJ, Andrac L, Romano MH, et al. Dysplastic naevus in non-familial melanoma. A clinicopathological study of 101 cases. Br J Dermatol 1988;118:745–52.
149. Annessi G, Cattaruzza MS, Abeni D, et al. Correlation between clinical atypia and histologic dysplasia in acquired melanocytic nevi. J Am Acad Dermatol 2001;45:77–85.
150. Roush GC, Barnhill RL, Duray PH, et al. Diagnosis of the dysplastic nevus in different populations. J Am Acad Dermatol 1986;14:419–25.
151. Piepkorn MW, Barnhill RL, Cannon-Albright LA, et al. A multiobserver, population-based analysis of histologic dysplasia in melanocytic nevi. J Am Acad Dermatol 1994;30:707–14.
152. Klein LJ, Barr RJ. Histologic atypia in clinically benign nevi. A prospective study. J Am Acad Dermatol 1990;22:275–82.
153. Piepkorn M, Meyer LJ, Goldgar D, et al. The dysplastic melanocytic nevus: a prevalent lesion that correlates poorly with clinical phenotype. J Am Acad Dermatol 1989;20:407–15.
154. Seykora J, Elder D. Dysplastic nevi and other risk markers for melanoma. Semin Oncol 1996;23:682–7.
155. Greene MH, Clark WH Jr, Tucker MA, et al. Acquired precursors of cutaneous malignant melanoma. The familial dysplastic nevus syndrome. N Engl J Med 1985;312:91–7.
156. Rhodes AR, Harrist TJ, Day CL, et al. Dysplastic melanocytic nevi in histologic association with 234 primary cutaneous melanomas. J Am Acad Dermatol 1983;9:563–74.
157. Duray PH, Ernstoff MS. Dysplastic nevus in histologic contiguity with acquired nonfamilial melanoma. Clinicopathologic experience in a 100-bed hospital. Arch Dermatol 1987;123:80–4.
158. Barnhill RL, Hurwitz S, Duray PH, Arons MS. The dysplastic nevus: recognition and management. Plast Reconstr Surg 1988;81:280–9.
159. Black WC. Residual dysplastic and other nevi in superficial spreading melanoma. Clinical correlations and association with sun damage. Cancer 1988;62:163–73.
160. Massi D, Carli P, Franchi A, Santucci M. Naevus-associated melanomas: cause or chance? Melanoma Res 1999;9:85–91.
161. Bergman W, Ruiter DJ, Scheffer E, van Vloten WA. Melanocytic atypia in dysplastic nevi. Immunohistochemical and cytophotometrical analysis. Cancer 1988;61:1660–6.
162. Fleming MG, Wied GL, Dytch HE. Image analysis cytometry of dysplastic nevi. J Invest Dermatol 1990;95:287–91.
163. Sangueza OP, Hyder DM, Bakke AC, White CR Jr. DNA determination in dysplastic nevi. A comparative study between flow cytometry and image analysis. Am J Dermatopathol 1993;15:99–105.
164. Bjornhagen V, Bonfoco E, Brahme EM, et al. Morphometric, DNA, and proliferating cell nuclear antigen measurements in benign melanocytic lesions and cutaneous malignant melanoma. Am J Dermatopathol 1994;16:615–23.
165. Elder DE, Rodeck U, Thurin J, et al. Antigenic profile of tumor progression stages in human melanocytic nevi and melanomas. Cancer Res 1989;49:5091–6.
166. Piepkorn M. Melanoma genetics: an update with focus on the CDKN2A(p16)/ARF tumor suppressors. J Am Acad Dermatol 2000;42:705–22; 723–6.
167. Keller-Melchior R, Schmidt R, Piepkorn M. Expression of the tumor suppressor gene product p16INK4 in benign and malignant melanocytic lesions. J Invest Dermatol 1998;110:932–8.

168. Grover R, Chana JS, Wilson GD, et al. An analysis of p16 protein expression in sporadic malignant melanoma. Melanoma Res 1998;8:267–72.
169. Sparrow LE, Eldon MJ, English DR, Heenan PJ. p16 and p21WAF1 protein expression in melanocytic tumors by immunohistochemistry. Am J Dermatopathol 1998;20:255–61.
170. Puig S, Ruiz A, Castel T, et al. Inherited susceptibility to several cancers but absence of linkage between dysplastic nevus syndrome and CDKN2A in a melanoma family with a mutation in the CDKN2A (P16INK4A) gene. Hum Genet 1997;101:359–64.
171. Boni R, Zhuang Z, Albuquerque A, et al. Loss of heterozygosity detected on 1p and 9q in microdissected atypical nevi. Arch Dermatol 1998;134:882–3.
172. Park WS, Vortmeyer AO, Pack S, et al. Allelic deletion at chromosome 9p21(p16) and 17p13(p53) in microdissected sporadic dysplastic nevus. Hum Pathol 1998;29:127–30.
173. Birindelli S, Tragni G, Bartoli C, et al. Detection of microsatellite alterations in the spectrum of melanocytic nevi in patients with or without individual or family history of melanoma. Int J Cancer 2000;86:255–61.
174. Welch J, Millar D, Goldman A, et al. Lack of genetic and epigenetic changes in CDKN2A in melanocytic nevi. J Invest Dermatol 2001;117:383–4.
175. Korabiowska M, Brinck U, Ruschenburg I, et al. Expression of DNA mismatch repair genes in naevi. In Vivo 1999;13:251–4.
176. Hussein MR, Sun M, Tuthill RJ, et al. Comprehensive analysis of 112 melanocytic skin lesions demonstrates microsatellite instability in melanomas and dysplastic nevi, but not in benign nevi. J Cutan Pathol 2001;28:343–50.
177. Florell SR, Boucher KM, Holden JA, et al. Failure to detect differences in proliferation status of nevi from CDKN2A mutation carriers and non-carriers. J Invest Dermatol 2002;118:386–7.
178. Black WC, Hunt WC. Histologic correlations with the clinical diagnosis of dysplastic nevus. Am J Surg Pathol 1990;14:44–52.
179. Ahmed I, Piepkorn MW, Rabkin MS, et al. Histopathologic characteristics of dysplastic nevi. Limited association of conventional histologic criteria with melanoma risk group. J Am Acad Dermatol 1990;22:727–33.
180. Kelly JW, Crutcher WA, Sagebiel RW. Clinical diagnosis of dysplastic melanocytic nevi. A clinicopathologic correlation. J Am Acad Dermatol 1986;14:1044–52.
181. Fernandez M, Raimer SS, Sanchez RL. Dysplastic nevi of the scalp and forehead in children. Pediatr Dermatol 2001;18:5–8.
182. Abadir MC, Marghoob AA, Slade J, et al. Case-control study of melanocytic nevi on the buttocks in atypical mole syndrome: role of solar radiation in the pathogenesis of atypical moles. J Am Acad Dermatol 1995;33:31–6.
183. Barnhill RL, Roush GC. Correlation of clinical and histopathologic features in clinically atypical melanocytic nevi. Cancer 1991;67:3157–64.
184. Hartge P, Holly EA, Halpern A, et al. Recognition and classification of clinically dysplastic nevi from photographs: a study of interobserver variation. Cancer Epidemiol Biomarkers Prev 1995;4:37–40.
185. Sagebiel RW. Histopathology of borderline and early malignant melanomas. Am J Surg Pathol 1979;3:543–52.
186. Elder DE. The dysplastic nevus. Pathology 1985;17:291–7.
187. Sagebiel RW. Histopathology of precursor melanocytic lesions. Am J Surg Pathol 1985;9:41–52.
188. Sagebiel RW. Diagnosis and management of premalignant melanocytic proliferations. Pathology 1985;17:285–90.
189. Balkau D, Gartmann H, Wischer W, et al. Architectural features in melanocytic lesions with cellular atypia. Dermatologica 1988;177:129–37.
190. Steijlen PM, Bergman W, Hermans J, et al. The efficacy of histopathological criteria required for diagnosing dysplastic naevi. Histopathology 1988;12:289–300.
191. Rhodes AR, Mihm MC Jr, Weinstock MA. Dysplastic melanocytic nevi: a reproducible histologic definition emphasizing cellular morphology. Mod Pathol 1989;2:306–19.
192. Barnhill RL, Roush GC. Histopathologic spectrum of clinically atypical melanocytic nevi. II. Studies of nonfamilial melanoma. Arch Dermatol 1990;126:1315–8.
193. Barnhill RL, Roush GC, Duray PH. Correlation of histologic and cytoplasmic features with nuclear atypia in atypical (dysplastic) nevomelanocytic nevi. Hum Pathol 1990;21:51–8.
194. Clemente C, Cochran AJ, Elder DE, et al. Histopathologic diagnosis of dysplastic nevi: concordance among pathologists convened by the World Health Organization Melanoma Programme. Hum Pathol 1991;22:313–9.
195. Piepkorn M. A hypothesis incorporating the histologic characteristics of dysplastic nevi into the normal biological development of melanocytic nevi. Arch Dermatol 1990;126:514–8.
196. Piepkorn MW. An appraisal of the dysplastic nevus syndrome concept. Adv Dermatol 1991;6:35–55; 56.
197. Seywright MM, Doherty VR, MacKie RM. Proposed alternative terminology and subclassification of so called "dysplastic naevi." J Clin Pathol 1986;39:189–94.
198. Duray PH, DerSimonian R, Barnhill R, et al. An analysis of interobserver recognition of the histopathologic features of dysplastic nevi from a mixed group of nevomelanocytic lesions. J Am Acad Dermatol 1992;27:741–9.
199. Weinstock MA, Barnhill RL, Rhodes AR, et al. Reliability of the histopathologic diagnosis of melanocytic dysplasia. Arch Dermatol 1997;133:953–8.

200. Duncan LM, Berwick M, Bruijn JA, et al. Histopathologic recognition and grading of dysplastic melanocytic nevi: an interobserver agreement study. J Invest Dermatol 1993; 100:318S–21S.
201. Bruijn JA, Berwick M, Mihm MC Jr, Barnhill RL. Common acquired melanocytic nevi, dysplastic melanocytic nevi and malignant melanomas: an image analysis cytometric study. J Cutan Pathol 1993;20:121–5.
202. Schmidt B, Weinberg DS, Hollister K, Barnhill RL. Analysis of melanocytic lesions by DNA image cytometry. Cancer 1994;73:2971–7.
203. Cook MG, Fallowfield ME. Dysplastic naevi—an alternative view. Histopathology 1990;16:29–35.
204. Piepkorn M. Whither the atypical (dysplastic) nevus? Am J Clin Pathol 2001;115:177–9.
205. Urso C. Atypical histologic features in melanocytic nevi. Am J Dermatopathol 2000;22:391–6.
206. Barnhill RL, Fandrey K, Levy MA, et al. Angiogenesis and tumor progression of melanoma. Quantification of vascularity in melanocytic nevi and cutaneous malignant melanoma. Lab Invest 1992;67:331–7.
207. Mooney MA, Barr RJ, Buxton MG. Halo nevus or halo phenomenon? A study of 142 cases. J Cutan Pathol 1995; 22:342–8.
208. Rudolph P, Schubert C, Schubert B, Parwaresch R. Proliferation marker Ki-S5 as a diagnostic tool in melanocytic lesions. J Am Acad Dermatol 1997;37:169–78.
209. Kanter L, Blegen H, Wejde J, et al. Utility of a proliferation marker in distinguishing between benign naevocellular naevi and naevocellular naevus-like lesions with malignant properties. Melanoma Res 1995;5:345–50.
210. Rudolph P, Lappe T, Schubert C, et al. Diagnostic assessment of two novel proliferation-specific antigens in benign and malignant melanocytic lesions. Am J Pathol 1995;147:1615–25.
211. Barnhill RL, Barnhill MA, Berwick M, Mihm MC Jr. The histologic spectrum of pigmented spindle cell nevus: a review of 120 cases with emphasis on atypical variants. Hum Pathol 1991;22:52–8.
212. Toussaint S, Kamino H. Dysplastic changes in different types of melanocytic nevi. A unifying concept. J Cutan Pathol 1999;26:84–90.
213. Signoretti S, Annessi G, Puddu P, Faraggiana T. Melanocytic nevi of palms and soles: a histological study according to the plane of section. Am J Surg Pathol 1999; 23:283–7.
214. Haupt HM, Stern JB. Pagetoid melanocytosis. Histologic features in benign and malignant lesions. Am J Surg Pathol 1995;19:792–7.
215. Evans MJ, Gray ES, Blessing K. Histopathological features of acral melanocytic nevi in children: study of 21 cases. Pediatr Dev Pathol 1998;1:388–92.
216. Clemente C, Zurrida S, Bartoli C, et al. Acral-lentiginous naevus of plantar skin. Histopathology 1995;27:549–55.
217. Sutton RL. An unusual variety of vitiligo (leucoderma acquisitum centrifugum). J Cutan Dis 1916;34:797–800.
218. Frank SB, Cohen HJ. The halo nevus. Arch Dermatol 1964;89:367–73.
219. Kopf A, Morrill SIS. Broad spectrum of leukoderma acquisitum centrifugum. Arch Dermatol 1965;92:14–35.
220. Wayte DM, Helwig EB. Halo nevi. Cancer 1968;22:69–90.
221. Brownstein MH, Kazam BB, Hashimoto K. Halo congenital nevus. Arch Dermatol 1977;113:1572–5.
222. Larsson PA, Liden S. Prevalence of skin diseases among adolescents 12–16 years of age. Acta Derm Venereol 1980; 60:415–23.
223. Bergman W, Willemze R, de Graaff-Reitsma C, Ruiter DJ. Analysis of major histocompatibility antigens and the mononuclear cell infiltrate in halo nevi. J Invest Dermatol 1985;85:25–9.
224. Copeman PW, Lewis MG, Phillips TM, Elliott PG. Immunological associations of the halo naevus with cutaneous malignant melanoma. Br J Dermatol 1973;88:127–37.
225. Bennett C, Copeman PW. Melanocyte mutation in halo naevus and malignant melanoma? Br J Dermatol 1979; 100:423–6.
226. Whimster IW. The halo naevus and cutaneous malignant melanoma [Letter]. Br J Dermatol 1974;90:111–3.
227. Roenigk HH, Deodhar SD, Krebs JA, Barna B. Microcytotoxicity and serum blocking factors in malignant melanoma and halo nevus. Arch Dermatol 1975;111:720–5.
228. Mitchell MS, Nordlund JJ, Lerner AB. Comparison of cell-mediated immunity to melanoma cells in patients with vitiligo, halo nevi or melanoma. J Invest Dermatol 1980;75:144–7.
229. Zeff RA, Freitag A, Grin CM, Grant-Kels JM. The immune response in halo nevi. J Am Acad Dermatol 1997;37:620–4.
230. Baranda L, Torres-Alvarez B, Moncada B, et al. Presence of activated lymphocytes in the peripheral blood of patients with halo nevi. J Am Acad Dermatol 1999;41: 567–72.
231. Gauthier Y, Surleve-Bazeille JE, Texier L. Halo nevi without dermal infiltrate. Arch Dermatol 1978;114:1718.
232. Cohen HJ, Minkin W, Frank SB. Nevus spilus. Arch Dermatol 1970;102:433–7.
233. Matsudo H, Reed WB, Homme D, et al. Zosteriform lentiginous nevus. Arch Dermatol 1973;107:902–5.
234. Stewart DM, Altman J, Mehregan AH. Speckled lentiginous nevus. Arch Dermatol 1978;114:895–6.
235. Port M, Courniotes J, Podwal M. Zosteriform lentiginous naevus with ipsilateral rigid cavus foot. Br J Dermatol 1978;98:693–8.
236. Pritchett RM, Pritchett PS. Zosteriform speckled lentiginous nevus with giant melanosomes. Cutis 1982;30:329–34.

237. Nguyen KQ, Pierson DL, Rodman OG. Mosaic speckled lentiginous nevi. Cutis 1982;30:65–8.
238. Kopf AW, Levine LJ, Rigel DS, et al. Prevalence of congenital-nevus-like nevi, nevi spili, and cafe au lait spots. Arch Dermatol 1985;121:766–9.
239. Falo LD Jr, Sober AJ, Barnhill RL. Evolution of a naevus spilus. Dermatology 1994;189:382–3.
240. Rhodes AR, Mihm MC Jr. Origin of cutaneous melanoma in a congenital dysplastic nevus spilus. Arch Dermatol 1990;126:500–5.
241. Stern JB, Haupt HM, Aaronson CM. Malignant melanoma in a speckled zosteriform lentiginous nevus. Int J Dermatol 1990;29:583–4.
242. Kurban RS, Preffer FI, Sober AJ, et al. Occurrence of melanoma in "dysplastic" nevus spilus: report of case and analysis by flow cytometry. J Cutan Pathol 1992;19:423–8.
243. Schoenfeld RJ, Pinkus H. The recurrence of nevi after incomplete removal. Arch Dermatol 1958;78:30–35.
244. Cox AJ, Walton RA. The induction of junctional changes in pigmented nevi. Arch Pathol 1965;79:428–34.
245. Kornberg R, Ackerman AB. Pseudomelanoma: recurrent melanocytic nevus following partial surgical removal. Arch Dermatol 1975;111:1588–90.
246. Park HK, Leonard DD, Arrington JH III, Lund HZ. Recurrent melanocytic nevi: clinical and histologic review of 175 cases. J Am Acad Dermatol 1987;17:285–92.
247. Hoang MP, Prieto VG, Burchette JL, Shea CR. Recurrent melanocytic nevus: a histologic and immunohistochemical evaluation. J Cutan Pathol 2001;28:400–6.
248. Christensen WN, Friedman KJ, Woodruff JD, Hood AF. Histologic characteristics of vulvar nevocellular nevi. J Cutan Pathol 1987;14:87–91.
249. Friedman RJ, Ackerman AB. Difficulties in the hisologic diagnosis of melanocytic nevi on the vulvae of premenopausal women. In: Ackerman AB, ed. Pathology of Malignant Melanoma. New York: Masson, 1981:119–127.
250. Clark WH Jr, Hood AF, Tucker MA, Jampel RM. Atypical melanocytic nevi of the genital type with a discussion of reciprocal parenchymal-stromal interactions in the biology of neoplasia. Hum Pathol 1998;29:S1–24.
251. Rongioletti F, Ball RA, Marcus R, Barnhill RL. Histopathological features of flexural melanocytic nevi: a study of 40 cases. J Cutan Pathol 2000;27:215–7.
252. Rogers GS, Advani H, Ackerman AB. A combined variant of Spitz's nevi. How to differentiate them from malignant melanomas. Am J Dermatopathol 1985;7(Suppl):61–78.
253. Ball NJ, Golitz LE. Melanocytic nevi with focal atypical epithelioid cell components: a review of seventy-three cases. J Am Acad Dermatol 1994;30:724–9.
254. Wong TY, Duncan LM, Mihm MC Jr. Melanoma mimicking dermal and Spitz's nevus ("nevoid" melanoma). Semin Surg Oncol 1993;9:188–93.

CHAPTER 6

Congenital Melanocytic Nevi and Associated Neoplasms, Congenital and Childhood Melanoma

Raymond L. Barnhill

CONGENITAL MELANOCYTIC NEVI

By definition, the term *congenital nevus* denotes presence at birth (1,2) (Table 6-1). However, congenital melanocytic nevi (CMN) are also defined by striking differences from common acquired nevi. In general, these differences include (a) overall size, (b) depth of involvement by nevus cells, (c) adnexal or vascular involvement, and (d) diversity of neurocristic differentiation (3). Most melanocytic nevi > 1.5 cm in diameter are probably congenital (1), if not acquired atypical (dysplastic) nevi or melanoma. However, smaller CMN may be indistinguishable from acquired nevi (2,4–6). Thus documentation at birth by reliable means such as physicians, parents, photography, or medical records is necessary to confirm a congenital onset for nevi > 1.5 cm. The larger CMN are distinctive because of their size (1,6–8). A small subset of nevi are remarkable for clinical and histologic features that are indistinguishable from typical CMN but are associated with an onset at several months to 2 years after birth. Such nevi have been termed congenital nevi tardive (9).

A variety of methods have been used to classify CMN according to size: surface area, the relationship to other anatomic structures such as the palm, longest diameter of the nevus, and difficulty of surgical removal (9–16). All are arbitrary, and none is entirely satisfactory. Kopf et al. (15) classified all nevi < 1.5 cm as small, nevi 1.5–19.9 cm as medium, and nevi > 20 cm as large or giant (Tables 6-2 to 6-4) (15). The terms *giant, gigantic, bathing trunk,* and *garment type* of nevus refer to CMN that occupy a major anatomic region or significant portion of the cutaneous surface (7). Some authors have classified CMN based on their ease of surgical removal (13). Small CMN are those that may be removed by simple surgical excision and primary closure. Intermediate or medium CMN often require a skin graft or flap. Giant CMN may prove difficult to remove altogether or require staged excision. It should be pointed out that CMN tend to enlarge proportionately to growth of the individual, and thus the category of the CMN may change (3,9).

Neurocutaneous melanosis (NCM) is a rare congenital syndrome characterized by the presence of either large (> 20 cm) CMN or multiple (more than three) usually smaller CMN, or both. It is associated with meningeal melanosis or melanoma; absence of cutaneous melanoma, except in patients with histologically benign meningeal lesions; and absence of meningeal melanoma, except in patients with histologically benign cutaneous lesions (17–20).

Incidence and Melanoma Risk

Estimates of the incidence of congenital nevi are rather imprecise since distinctions between relatively "small" CMN and acquired nevi are not well defined and histologic patterns vary considerably among CMN (21–29). When histologic confirmation is a criterion, incidence may range as low as 0.64%; another series based on clinical criteria found an incidence of 2.7%. Giant hairy nevi are rare, with an estimated incidence of 0.005% from one study (30). Patients with giant nevi often have multiple smaller (satellite) nevi as well. Familial aggregation of congenital nevi also has been reported. Among 289 patients with large CMN 11.4% presented with clinically obvious NCM (20). The prevalence of the latter condition is thus higher in large CMN.

The significance of CMN, particularly the larger varieties, relates to their risk for progression to melanoma and cosmetic disfigurement (7,12–16,21–32). There has been and continues to be considerable controversy surrounding the melanoma risk and management of CMN of all sizes. Accurate estimates of melanoma risk associated with CMN are difficult to obtain (2,30,33). However, one particular problem associated with estimating melanoma risk

TABLE 6-1 Congenital melanocytic nevi and congenital and childhood melanoma.

Congenital melanocytic nevi
  Prevalence
    All congenital nevi, 1.1%
    Giant congenital nevi, 0.005%
  Classification
    Small, < 1.5 cm
    Medium, > 1.5–19.9 cm
    Large/giant, ≥ 20 cm
    Congenital nevus "tardive," onset between 1 and 24 months of age
  Familial aggregation
    Of small CMN (prevalence rate 11 times the population-based prevalence)
    Of large and medium CMN
    Autosomal dominant inheritance with incomplete penetrance or polygenic inheritance possible
    Association of large CMN of head and neck or posterior midline and underlying leptomeningeal melanocytosis of cranium, spine, or both
  Lifetime melanoma risk
    Relatively small CMN, 5% or less (estimate)
    Very large CMN, 6.3%
Congenital melanoma
  Incidence exceedingly rare
  Subtypes
    Transplacental spread of maternal metastatic melanoma
    De novo primary melanoma
    Primary melanoma arising in association with congenital melanocytic nevi
Childhood melanoma
  Incidence
    Prepubertal, 0.4% (of total melanomas)
    Under age 20 years, 2%
  Rick factors
    Family history of melanoma
    Xeroderma pigmentosum
    Immunosuppression
    Sun exposure
  Subtypes
    Conventional (adult-like) types, epithelioid-cell type (pagetoid, "nodular")
    Small cell type
    Melanomas simulating Spitz nevus/tumor
  Prognosis, 84–87% with 5-year survival

TABLE 6-2 Small congenital nevus.

Clinical features
  Symmetry
  < 1.5 cm
  Round, oval
  Tan, brown, dark brown
  Slightly raised, dome-shaped, papillomatous
  Pebbled surface topography, common
Histopathology
  Lentiginous melanocytic hyperplasia, common
  Junctional, compound, or dermal nevus
  Plaque of nevus cells in papillary dermis, common
  Involvement of upper half of reticular dermis, common
    Interstitial pattern
    Perivascular, periadnexal pattern
Differential diagnosis
  Common acquired nevus
  Atypical (dysplastic) nevus

in small CMN nevi is the lack of specificity of histologic features for CMN of this size (5).

Although all sizes of CMN are susceptible to malignant transformation, historical estimates of melanoma risk have been exaggerated because of referral bias and misdiagnosis of atypical melanocytic proliferations developing in CMN as melanoma. The potential risk is probably related to size of the CMN—that is, the larger the nevus, the greater the risk. At present it is thought that the melanoma risk associated with small CMN is low and probably not much more than that associated with acquired nevi. A recent prospective study of 230 medium CMN in 227 patients followed on average for 6.7 years failed to document the development of a single case of melanoma (29). Similarly, in a cohort study following up 265 patients with medium CMN ranging from 1 to 19 cm, none developed melanoma (26). Thus, in general, the latter studies suggest that medium (and small) CMN are not associated with significant risk for melanoma.

Very high estimates of melanoma risk associated with large/giant CMN have been at least partially explained by

TABLE 6-3 Medium congenital nevus.

Clinical features
  May occur anywhere, but head and neck, common
  Symmetry
  1.5–20 cm
  Round, oval, elongate
  Tan, brown, dark brown, often mahogany; may be black
  Slightly raised plaque
  Pebbled or rugose surface
  Coarse hairs, often
Histopathology
  Lentiginous melanocytic hyperplasia, often
  Junctional, compound, or dermal
  Involvement of reticular dermis, particularly lower half
  Diffuse dermal involvement by nevus cells
  Interstitial pattern
  "Inflammatory" pattern
  Nevus cells within appendages, blood vessels, nerves
Differential diagnosis
  Becker nevus
  Atypical (dysplastic) nevus
  Epidermal nevus
  Congenital lentigo
  Melanoma

TABLE 6-4 Large or giant congenital nevi.

Clinical features
- Symmetry
- > 20 cm
- Involvement of major anatomic area, segmental
- Dorsal involvement, often
- Congenital deformities, occasional
- Well-defined borders
- Brown, dark brown, black
- "Animal pelt" feature, rugose, doughy
- Soft tissue hypertrophy
- Hypertrichosis
- Scattered satellite nevi distant from giant nevus
- Involvement of meninges, common for head and neck nevi

Histopathological features
- Lentiginous melanocytic hyperplasia, common
- Compound or dermal, usually
- Reticular dermal involvement, superficial and deep, usually
  - Diffuse
  - Interstitial
  - Perivascular, periadnexal
- Subcutaneous involvement, septal > lobular
- Maturation
- Neural differentiation, neuroid or neurofibroma-like pattern, on occasion
- Wagner-Meissner-like corpuscles
- Fascial or muscle involvement
- Cellular nodules in reticular dermis, occasional
- Blue nevus component, occasional
- Spindle and epithelioid cell nevus component, occasional
- Hamartomatous elements
  - Cartilaginous differentiation
  - Adipose differentiation

Differential diagnosis
- Becker nevus
- Neurofibromatosis
- Melanoma
- Peripheral nerve sheath tumors

referral bias. Perhaps the most accurate figures of melanoma risk have been associated with studies from the Danish Birth Registry (11). A lifetime risk of approximately 6.3% has been estimated from the latter database (11,22). On the other hand, recent studies have confirmed substantial melanoma risk linked to large or giant (> 20 cm) CMN. In the same cohort study referred earlier, Swerdlow et al. (26) estimated that patients with CMN > 20 cm had a standardized morbidity ratio (SMR) of 1224 for the development of melanoma. In a prospective study of 92 patients with large/giant CMN, 3 patients developed melanoma in extracutaneous sites (brain, central nervous system, retroperitoneum) during follow-up averaging 5.4 years. Marghoob et al. (31) calculated the cumulative 5-year life-table risk for melanoma to be 4.5%. The SMR, calculated to be 239, was highly significant.

An analysis of 289 patients with large CMN culled from the world literature revealed that 34 patients (12%) developed primary cutaneous melanoma within their nevi (32). An additional 2 patients had cutaneous melanomas arise outside the confines of their nevi. All of the latter patients developing melanoma had CMN in an axial location—that is, the head, neck, and trunk. No melanomas were associated with an extremity or satellite CMN. The median age at diagnosis of melanoma was 4.6 years (range: birth to 52 years; average age: 13.2 years). A total of 21 patients developed primary melanomas in the CNS; all of the latter patients had NCM and large CMN in a posterior axial location. The median age at diagnosis was 3 years (range: 1 month to 50 years; average age: 11.6 years) for the latter group. An additional 10 patients presented with metastatic melanoma with unknown primary. All of the latter patients had axial CMN.

Histogenesis

Acquired nevi and CMN demonstrate many of the same histopathologic features: lentiginous melanocytic proliferation, junctional nesting, and maturation in the dermis (1–8). However, there are substantial differences in size, depth, adnexal/vascular infiltration, and neurocristic differentiation (3,8). As already mentioned, little is known about the histogenesis of nevi in general, but this is especially true for CMN. Thus there is no information available on the developmental biology of nevi that might account for the striking differences between acquired nevi and CMN. Cramer (3) suggested that all nevi may originate from nerve sheath precursor cells that migrate to the skin associated with peripheral nerves. These pluripotential cells may then differentiate and migrate to the dermis and epidermis, giving rise to nevi. If this differentiation to nevus cells occurs in larger more proximal nerves, the migration of nevus cells to the area of innervation of such a nerve might account for the large surface area of many CMN. Presumably, acquired nevi would develop from differentiation and migration of precursor cells associated with small distal cutaneous nerves. Such an hypothesis has merit but has not been verified (3).

By definition, all CMN develop in utero, but the time of their appearance or full development may vary. For example, as mentioned, nevi with the gross morphologic features of CMN ("tardive" nevi) may be CMN with migratory cells that reach the superficial skin and achieve full development after birth (9). The congenital divided nevus of the eyelid provides some information on the development of CMN. Because such nevi appear (intact) at a time when the eyelids are fused and before the eyelids reopen, one can estimate that these nevi probably develop between 8 and 24 weeks gestational age (34). However, it is unlikely that this scenario applies to all CMN.

It is presumed that both genetic and environmental factors may be operative in the histogenesis of CMN;

however, there is only limited information currently available on this subject.

Familial Aggregation

Small CMN have been reported to aggregate in families (35), and there is evidence for a similar phenomenon for larger varieties of CMN (9). A clear-cut mode of inheritance, however, has not been established.

Associations

Congenital melanocytic nevi, especially larger or giant forms, have been associated with a number of developmental deformities, such as elephantiasis of the extremities, anatomic asymmetry, hypertrophy of cranial bones, scoliosis, spina bifida, and club foot (7,9,36,37). An association with neurofibromatosis has been suggested because of phenotypic similarity (9), but the relationship has not been proved (27).

Clinical Features

The clinical characteristics of CMN are related to size and age (1,2,4–9,21,36). Small congenital nevi < 1.5 cm in greatest diameter may be indistinguishable from common acquired nevi and documentation at birth may be the only means of confirming a congenital origin (5). In general, CMN in the range of 1.5–20 cm in diameter are well circumscribed, elongate or oval lesions that are usually only slightly elevated (1). Many CMN may be relatively flat and tan or light brown in an infant and may resemble a café-au-lait macule. However, most CMN of this size exhibit a relatively uniform brown or dark brown color with increasing age of the child (1). Some CMN also exhibit a mottled but relatively homogenous coloration with shades of red-brown that has an almost mahogany appearance. Dark brown speckling may also be found in some nevi. Coarse, terminal hair follicles are found on a regular basis.

Intermediate or medium CMN measuring 10–20 cm in the longest diameter frequently have a well-defined, round, oval, or elongate morphology and an orderly distribution of pigment (1). Most of these nevi are brown but can range in color from tan to dark brown to black. A speckled or mottled appearance is also common.

Giant CMN occupy a large area of the cutaneous surface and hence the term *garment* or *bathing trunk nevus* accurately depicts this appearance (1,7,9). Such CMN often involve a large portion of the dorsal surface of the individual. The surface topography of giant nevi shows considerable variation. These nevi are most often raised and exhibit a variably papular, lumpy, rugose, or even verrucous surface. The skin surface may be shiny or contain numerous terminal hairs. Soft tissue hypertrophy may mimic changes found in neurofibromatosis. The color is most often a dark brown or black, but considerable variegation of pigment is often noted. (7,36). Giant CMN are notable for varying numbers of so-called satellite CMN on the skin beyond the giant nevus. In one study, at least 78% of patients with large CMN had satellite CMN. Such lesions typically have characteristics of small congenital CMN. Although CMN change in size with the growth of the individual, they do not spread to cover proportionately larger areas than those defined at their congenital (or tardive) origin. Any extension into previously unaffected normal skin must be viewed with concern.

Congenital nevi, as indicated above, do not increase out of proportion to the anatomic area they occupy. An enlarging lesion may be evidence of a focus of atypical melanocytic proliferation or melanoma supervening in the nevus. CMN can become raised, exhibit changing surface characteristics, or develop halos of hypopigmentation; in rare instances, CMN may regress completely. Giant nevi that darken in childhood may display lightening of coloration over decades.

In fact, all sizes of CMN may develop hypopigmented or depigmented halos, loss of pigmentation either within the nevus or on normal skin, or undergo variable degrees of regression (38).

Important in the biologic behavior of CMN is their potential for malignant degeneration, particularly their relationship to malignant melanoma. Melanocytic atypia in congenital nevi ranges from slight atypicality to fully evolved malignancy. When a malignant melanoma develops in a relatively small CMN, it appears most commonly at the dermoepidermal junction in a fashion similar to that of other conventional melanomas. However, up to two thirds of cutaneous melanomas arising in larger CMN develop in the dermis, subcutaneous fat, or deeper as a distinct nodule. More rarely, a variety of other malignant tumors may occur in these lesions (22).

Neurocutaneous Melanosis

Congenital melanocytic nevi, not necessarily large or giant, involving the scalp, neck, or posterior midline may be associated with melanocytic proliferations localized to the cranial and/or spinal leptomeninges (7–9,17–20) (Table 6-5). Histologically, aggregates of melanotic cells are present in the basal subarachnoid cisterns. Such affected individuals often manifest signs and symptoms of increased intracranial pressure or a mass effect in the first 2 years of life. One may observe seizures, mental retardation, and other neurologic manifestations. In many cases, the syndrome proves fatal at birth or by 12 months of age. It has been established that NCM is a precursor for the development of meningeal melanoma; in a review published in 1991, 62% of reported cases of NCM culminated in leptomeningeal melanoma. Among 33 pa-

TABLE 6-5 Leptomeningeal melanocytosis associated with neurocutaneous melanosis.

Cranial or spinal leptomeningeal involvement
Scalp, neck, or posterior midline CMN
Hydrocephalus, communicating or noncommunicating type
Seizures
Neurologic signs
Mental retardation
Meningeal melanoma

tients having NCM associated with large CMN (> 20 cm) all nevi had a posterior axial location (involving the head, neck, back, or buttocks or any combination); 31 had satellite nevi. MRI is indicated for neonates with large posterior axial CMN and with multiple satellite nevi to screen for NCM (20).

Histopathological Features

The histologic characteristics observed in CMN are related to the size of the nevus primarily and to a lesser degree the age of the individual (2,5,6,22,25,39). Although it has been suggested that the histologic pattern of a CMN changes with age (2,13,40), there is now evidence that the depth of nevus cell involvement throughout the dermis and subcutis is established early and remains for the most part unchanged (41–43). However, the superficial (intraepidermal and superficial dermal) components of a CMN may mature in some instances. It is believed that immature disordered patterns—such as pagetoid spread, large irregular nests, and cytologic atypia—do diminish (or mature) with time (39,40). However, the latter conclusion must be made with some circumspection because of the rather prominent morphologic heterogeneity throughout many CMN (39).

Congenital Nevi in the 1st Year of Life A study of 110 unselected CMN of all sizes from infants < 1 year of age was recently conducted at Children's Hospital in Boston (39). As shown in Table 6-6, 90% of CMN involved the deeper half of the dermis and 47% involved the subcutaneous fat (Fig. 6-1). There was also a striking correlation between nevus size and nevus depth (χ^2; $p < .0001$). Approximately 62% of small CMN, 97% of medium CMN, and 100% of large CMN extended into the lower half of the reticular dermis or subcutis. The only junctional nevi were small CMN (8% of small CMN). A total of 9 CMN (7 were small CMN) involved the superficial reticular dermis only. These findings indicate that the depth of nevus involvement characteristic of CMN is established very early in life and correlates with the size of CMN.

The pattern of dermal involvement also tended to correlate with overall nevus size. The predominant dermal pattern was a diffuse, interstitial infiltration of the reticular dermis by nevus cells in 61% of CMN (Fig. 6-1B). The latter pattern correlated with larger CMN. Smaller CMN tended to exhibit a patchy periadnexal/perivascular pattern (Fig. 6-2). There was a rather striking affinity of nevus cells for eccrine ducts, particularly just after birth (Fig. 6-3A).

Cytologic atypia has been reported to be somewhat more common and prominent in the CMN of neonates and infants (40); even though its biologic significance has been questioned (40). In the above study, 29% of CMN showed cytologic atypia of the intraepidermal component (Table 6-7) but this was only minimal or slight in almost all the cases (39). The presence of cytologic atypia did not correlate with CMN size, anatomic site, or other gross morphologic features. Melanoma was not observed in any CMN. These findings indicate that cytologic atypia is probably not as common as was believed and that melanoma is exceedingly rare if it occurs at all in this age group (see below).

Relatively Small CMN Recent evidence indicates that small CMN display considerable heterogeneity of their histologic features (2,4,5). Some may be entirely junctional and indistinguishable from acquired nevi (2,39,44) (Fig. 6-4). Many small nevi, particularly those measuring < 1.5 cm in diameter, also demonstrate what has been

TABLE 6-6 Frequency distribution of nevus depth versus size of CMN in infants <1 year of age.[a]

Location	Small[b]	Medium[b]	Large[b]	Total[b]
Junctional	2 (1.8)	0 (0.0)	0 (0.0)	2 (1.8)
Superficial	7 (6.4)	2 (1.8)	0 (0.0)	9 (8.2)
Deep dermal	13 (11.8)	29 (26.4)	6 (5.4)	48 (43.6)
Subcutaneous	2 (1.8)	35 (31.8)	14 (12.7)	51 (46.4)
Total	24 (21.8)	66 (60.0)	20 (18.2)	110 (100.0)

[a]χ^2 analysis suggests a significant association between nevus cell depth and the size of the lesion ($p < .0001$).
[b]Percent is given in parentheses.

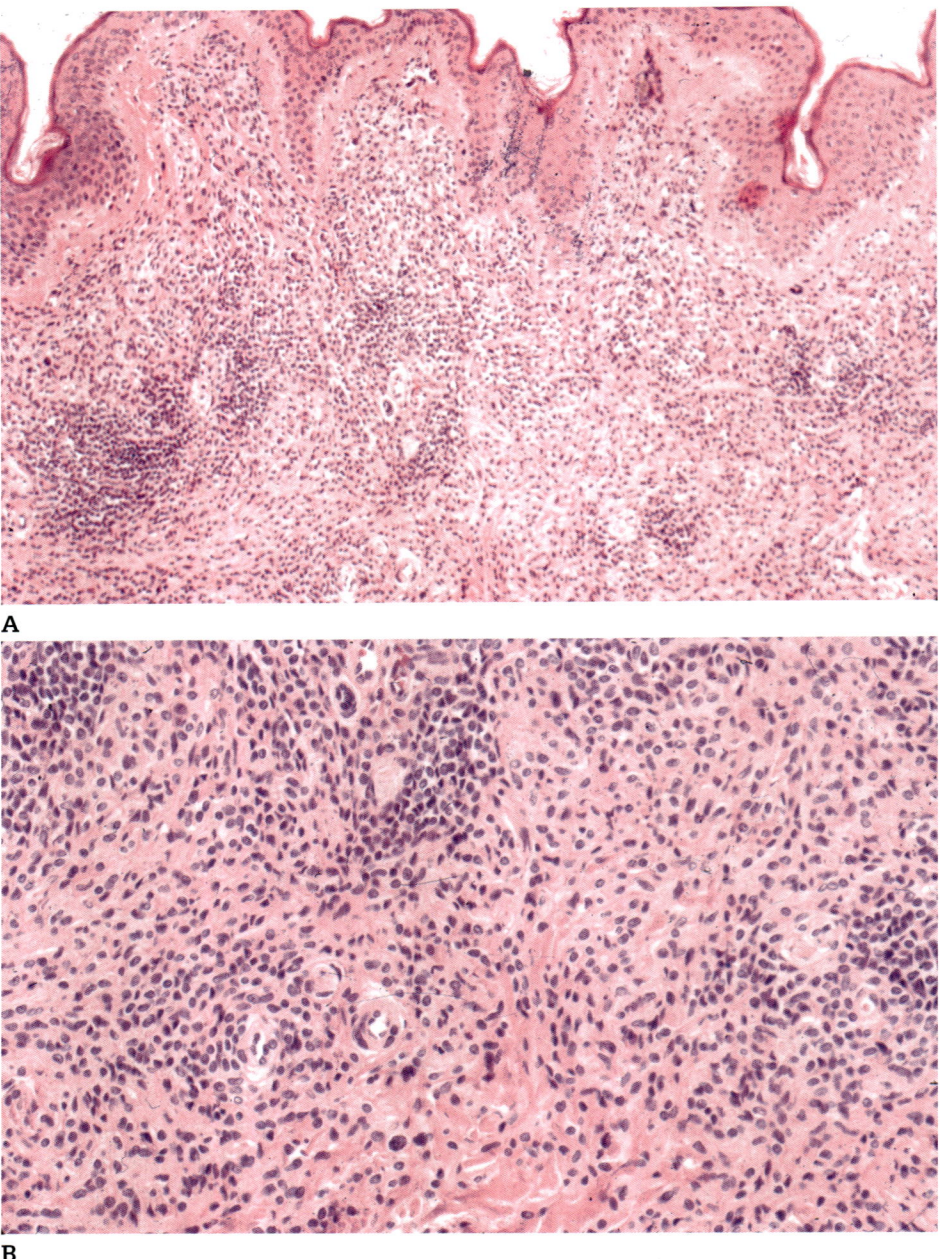

FIGURE 6-1 Large congenital nevus. **A,** Nevus cells diffusely infiltrate the upper dermis. **B,** Maturation with the descent of nevus cells in the reticular dermis. Cellularity decreases from top to bottom as nevus cells are dispersed among collagen bundles at the bottom of the field.

termed a superficial pattern (6,39) (Fig. 6-2A,C). The latter characterization refers to junctional nests of nevus cells alone or as a compound or an entirely dermal pattern with aggregates of nevus cells extending to no greater depth than the upper half of the reticular dermis. Such a pattern may be seen in a significant percentage of acquired nevi. Up to 28% of acquired nevi may also exhibit nevus cells extending into the lower two thirds of the reticular dermis (5).

Thus there is also been increasing evidence that many relatively small CMN do not exhibit the classic histologic features of CMN as originally outlined by Mark et al.

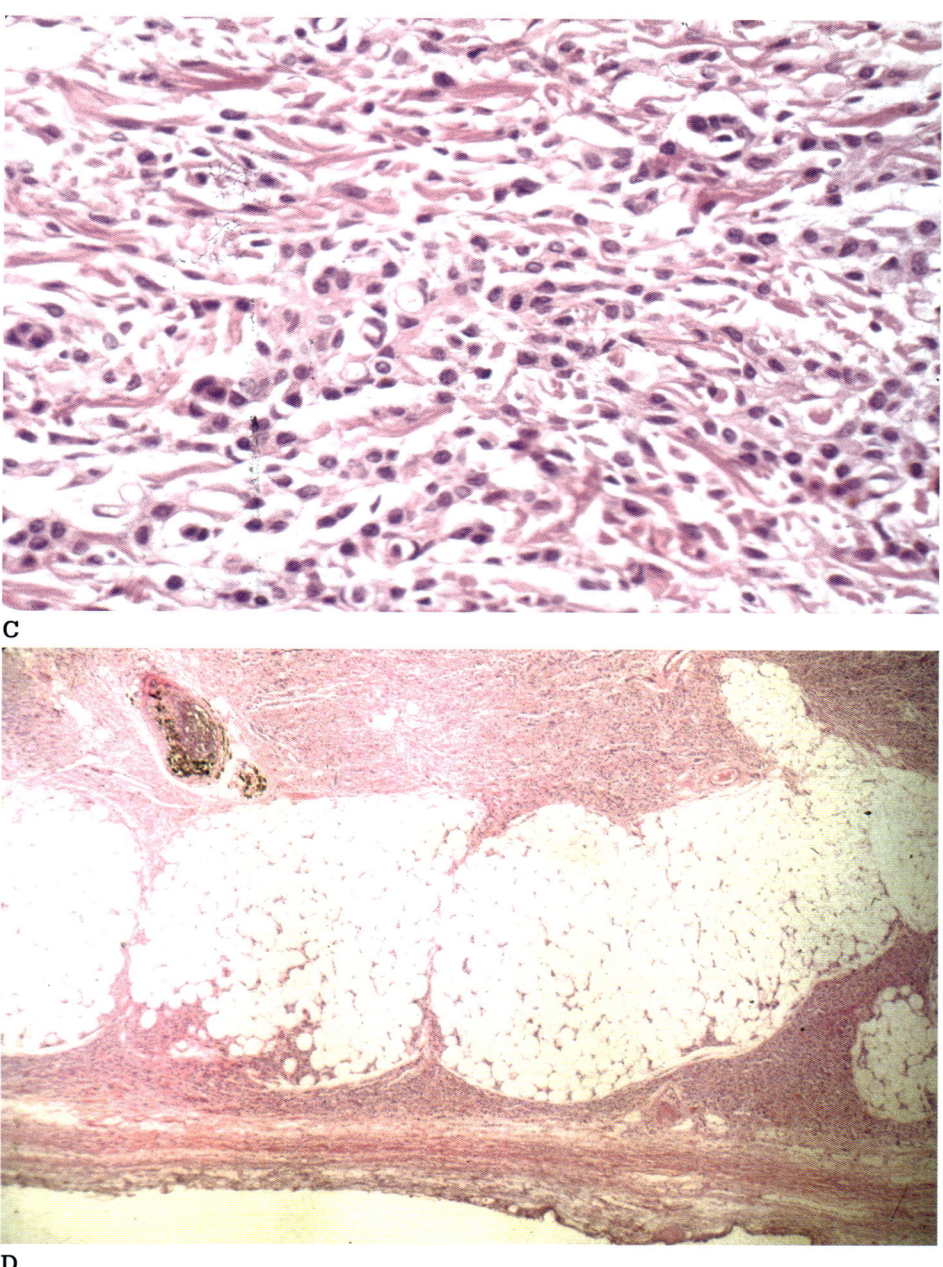

FIGURE 6-1 *Continued.* **C,** Diffuse permeation of the collagen of the reticular dermis by nevus cells. **D,** Nevus cells involve the fibrous trabeculae of subcutaneous fat.

(1,5,6). These features include involvement of the lower third of the reticular dermis by nevus cells, close association of nevus cells with or within appendageal, and neurovascular structures at the middle reticular dermal level or deeper (1). The patterns of reticular dermal involvement by nevus cells are characterized by single cells separated by collagen, single files of nevus cells in an interstitial distribution, nests, cords, and sheets of nevus cells (Figs. 6-1C and 6-2F). According to Mark et al. (1), the latter features were considered to be characteristic of a congenital onset regardless of size. In contradistinction to acquired nevi, CMN are notable for nevus cells being disposed, "fanning out," or splaying collagen bundles of the reticular dermis as single cells, files, and cords of cells (two

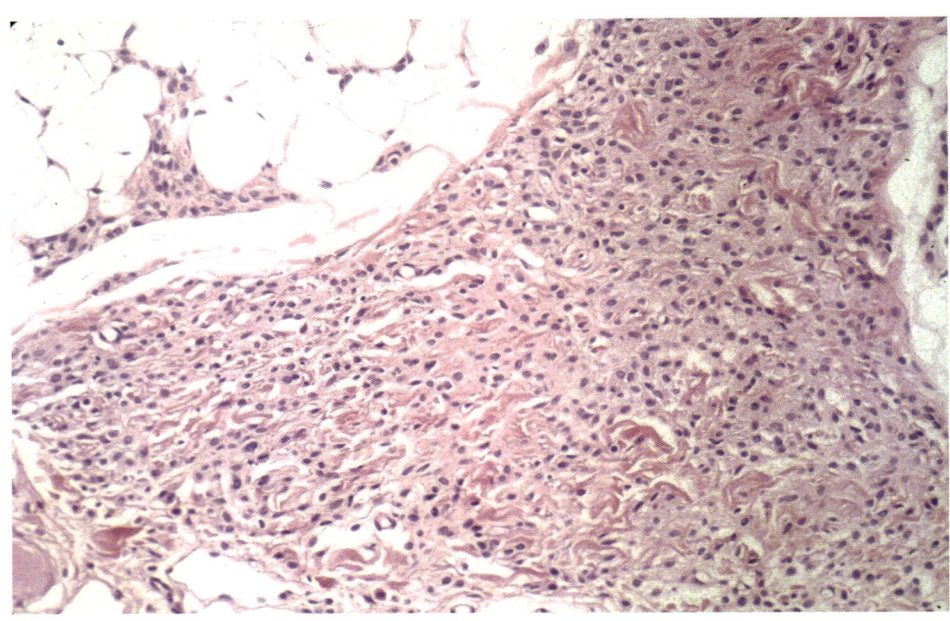

FIGURE 6-1 *Continued.* **E,** Higher magnification of panel D showing diffuse infiltration of the fibrous trabeculae.

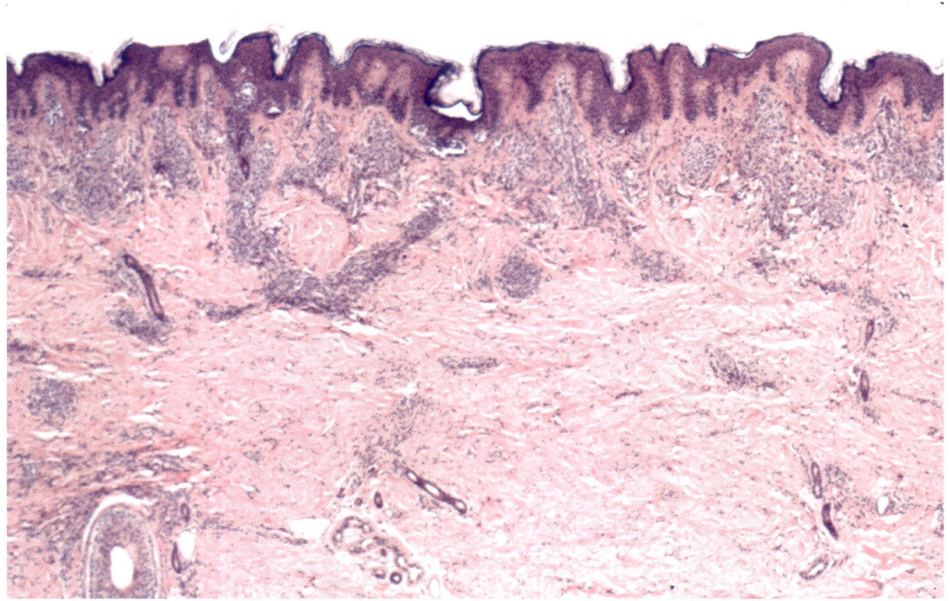

FIGURE 6-2 Small congenital nevus. **A,** There are aggregates of nevus cells in the papillary dermis that are distributed throughout reticular dermis in association with blood vessels and adnexal structures.

cells in tandem) (Fig. 6-2F). CMN also show a typical pattern of maturation of nevus cells from superficial to deep dermis. Near the epidermal surface, nevus cells tend to be aggregated in nests and may exhibit epithelioid cell features (1,39) (Fig. 6-4B). With increasing depth, the nevus cells often demonstrate greater separation (i.e., splaying) and slightly diminished cellular and nuclear sizes (Fig. 6-1B). Extension of nevus cells into the subcutaneous fat is also a common feature, particularly in larger varieties of congenital nevi (1,39) (Fig. 6-1D).

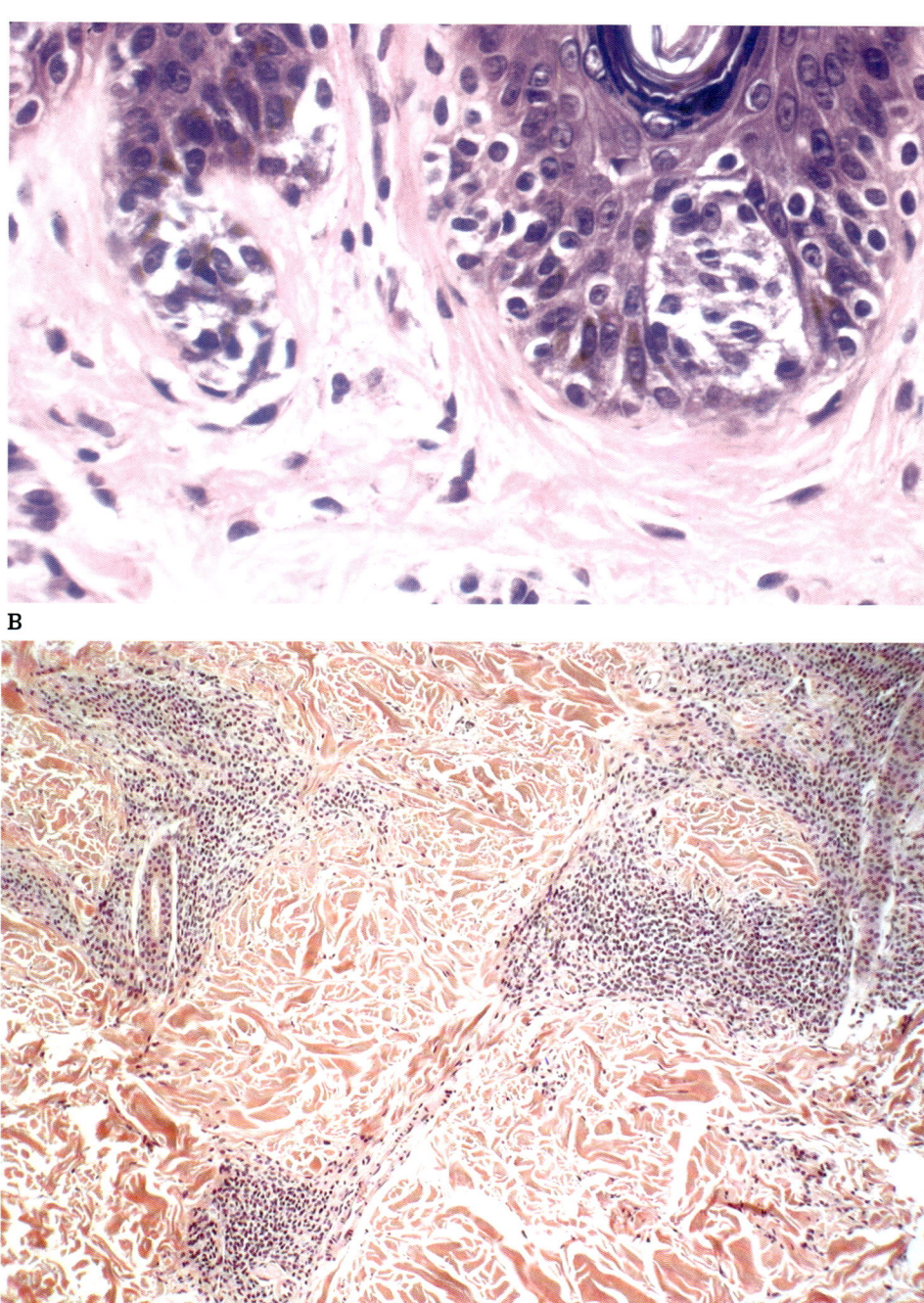

FIGURE 6-2 *Continued.* **B,** Junctional nests are indistinguishable from those in an acquired nevus. **C,** Discrete nests of nevus cells in the reticular dermis simulate inflammatory infiltrates, as in a gyrate erythema.

With increasing sizes of CMN, there is greater tendency for deep dermal, appendageal, and neurovascular involvement (5,6,25,39) (Tables 6-8 and 6-9). However, even some congenital nevi < 1.5 cm in diameter tend to exhibit involvement of eccrine and follicular units at the middle reticular dermal level or deeper, much more commonly than acquired nevi (42).

Larger CMN Giant CMN, most medium CMN, and a small percentage of nevi < 10 cm in diameter tend to ex-

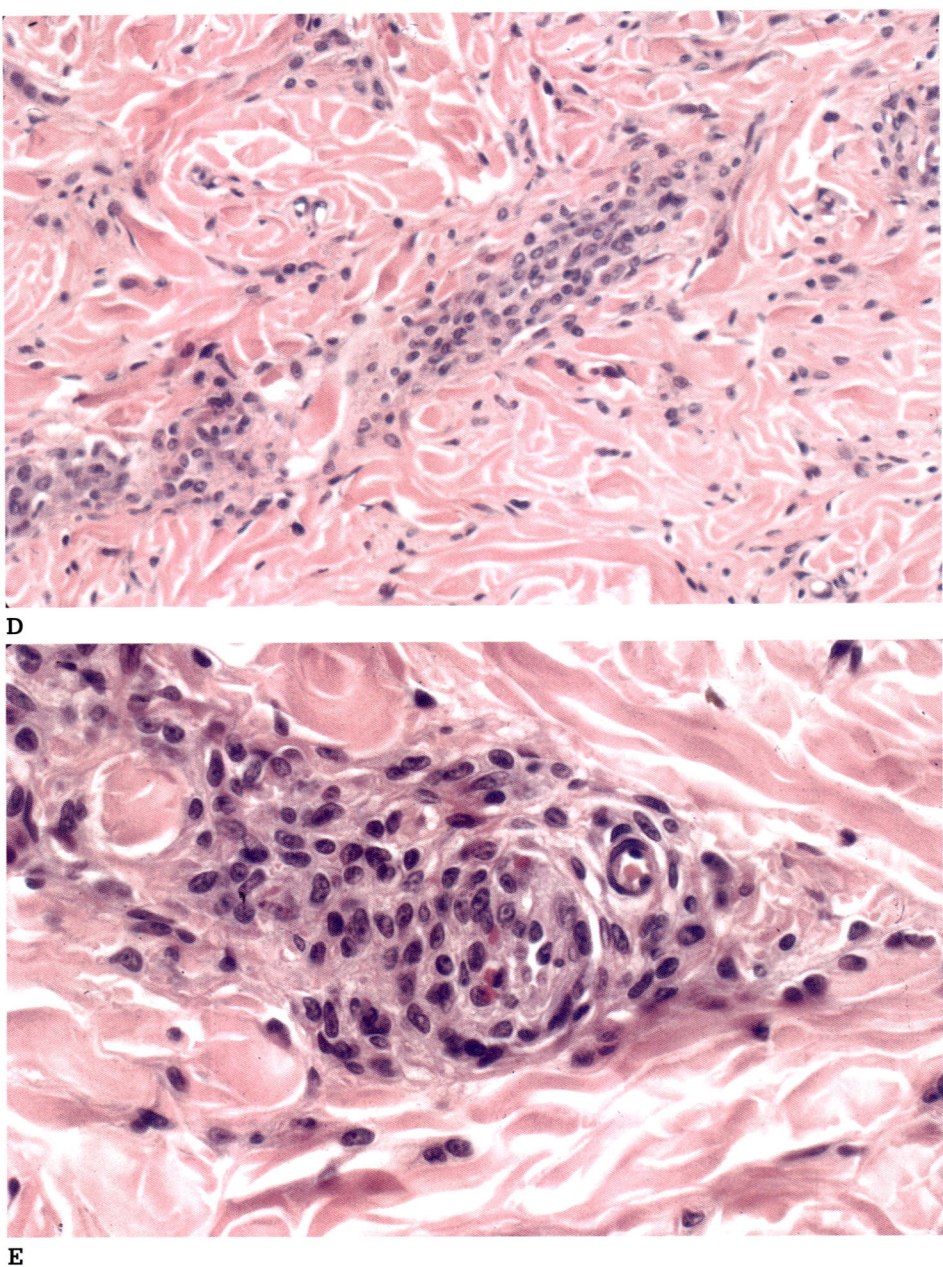

FIGURE 6-2 *Continued.* **D,** Perivascular and interstitial disposition of nevus cells in the reticular dermis. **E,** Nevus cells show perivascular cuffing typical of congenital nevi.

hibit distinctive features (5,6,7,8,25,39) (Tables 6-3, 6-4, 6-8, and 6-9). Probably the most characteristic feature shared by these larger varieties of congenital nevi is the pattern of diffuse proliferation of nevus cells throughout the reticular dermis with frequent extension into the subcutaneous fat (1,6,7,25,39). There is usually a grenz zone separating the epidermis from the dermal infiltration of nevus cells (25,45) (Fig. 6-1A). The nevus cells tend to infiltrate collagen in an orderly and uniform pattern. The nevus cells also often extend along the fibrous trabeculae of the subcutaneous fat (Fig. 6-1E). In some instances, there is infiltration of fat lobules (1,39). Aggregates of nevus cells also tend to cuff or be present within follicular epithelium, sebaceous glands, eccrine ducts and glands,

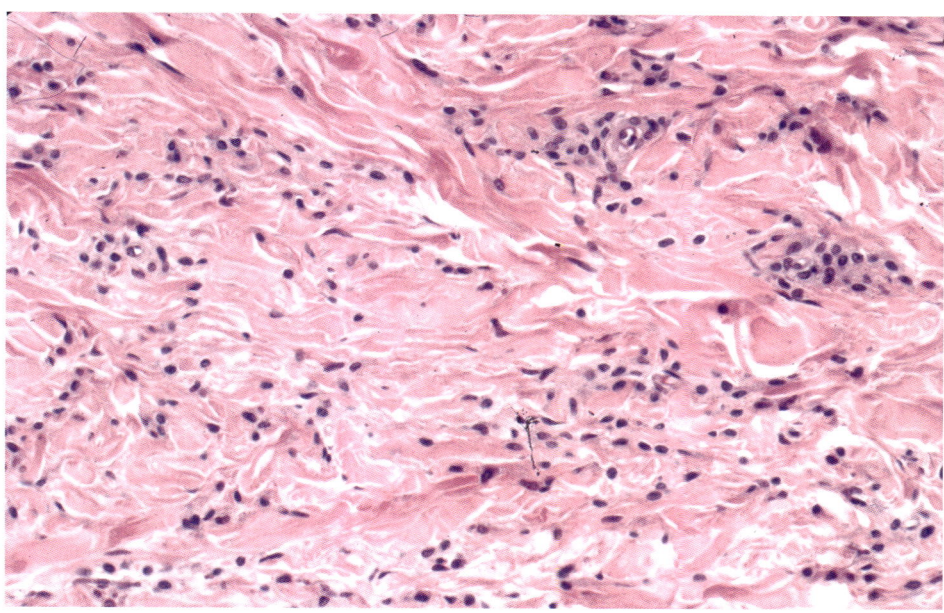

FIGURE 6-2 *Continued.* **F,** Splaying of nevus cells among the collagen bundles as single cells and files of cells.

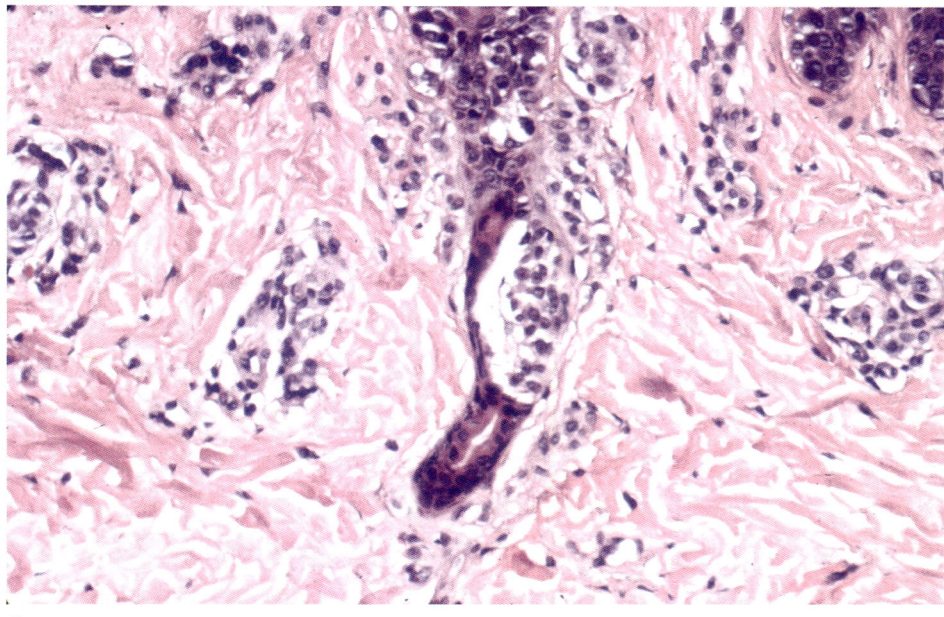

FIGURE 6-3 Congenital nevus. **A,** Nest of nevus cells within an eccrine sweat duct.

the perineurium of nerve twigs, and the walls of vascular structures (1,4,5,39) (Figs. 6-2C,D,E and 6-3). The rather striking perivascular and periadnexal cuffing of nevus cells in some congenital nevi may closely resemble an inflammatory process, such as a gyrate erythema (Fig. 6-2C). Such a presentation may be designated as an "inflammatory pattern" of congenital nevi. The nevus cells usually exhibit small uniform nuclei comparable to those

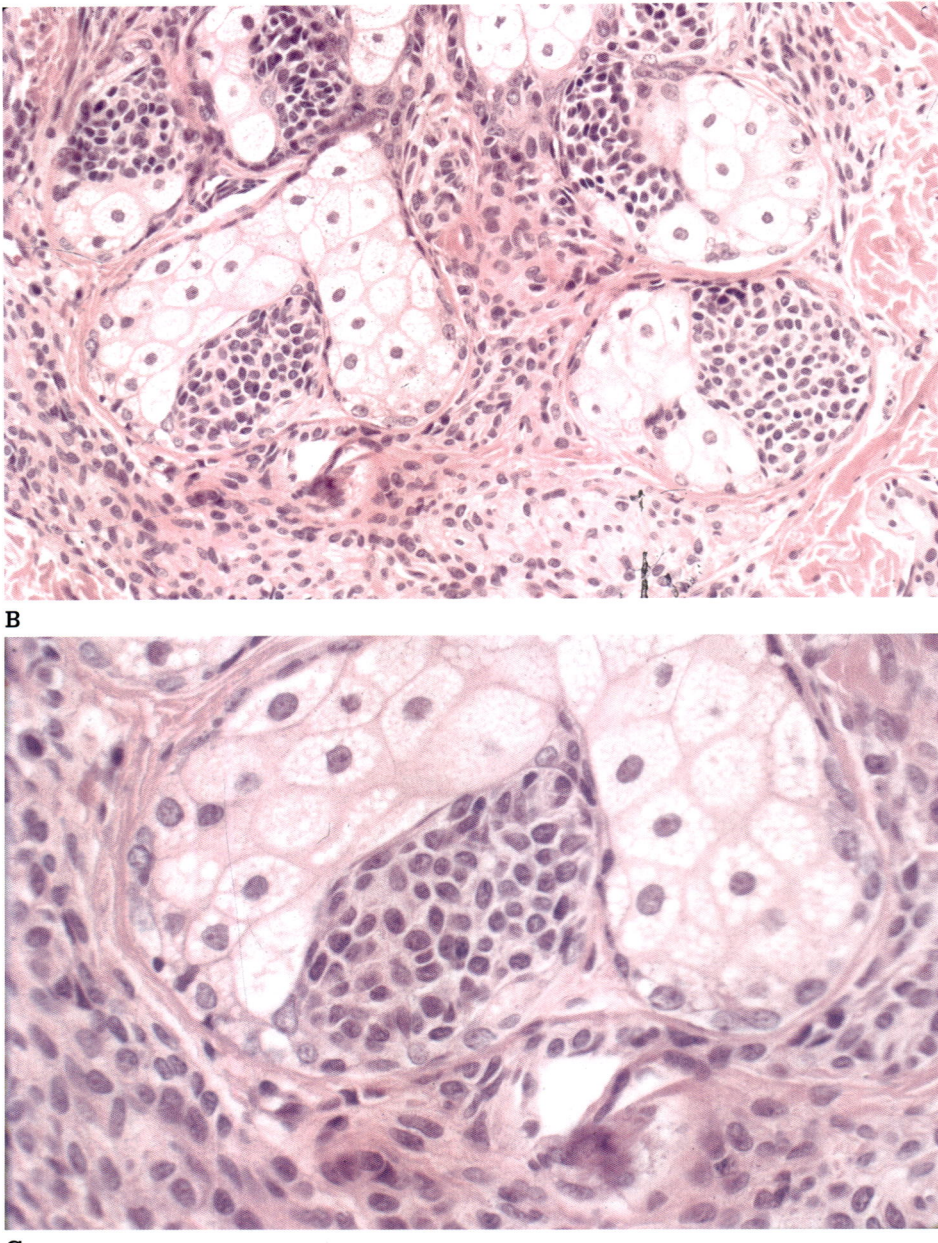

FIGURE 6-3 *Continued.* **B,** Nests of nevus cells within the sebaceous lobules. **C,** Higher magnification of panel B.

TABLE 6-7 Frequency distribution of atypia versus size of CMN in infants <1 year of age.[a]

Atypia	Small[b]	Medium[b]	Large[b]	Total[b]
No atypia	16 (14.6)	36 (32.7)	16 (14.6)	68 (61.8)
Atypia	8 (7.3)	30 (27.3)	4 (9.5)	42 (38.2)
Total	24 (21.8)	66 (60.0)	20 (18.2)	110 (100.0)

[a] According to χ^2 analysis, atypia was not significantly associated with size of the congenital nevus ($p > .1$).
[b] Percent is given in parentheses.

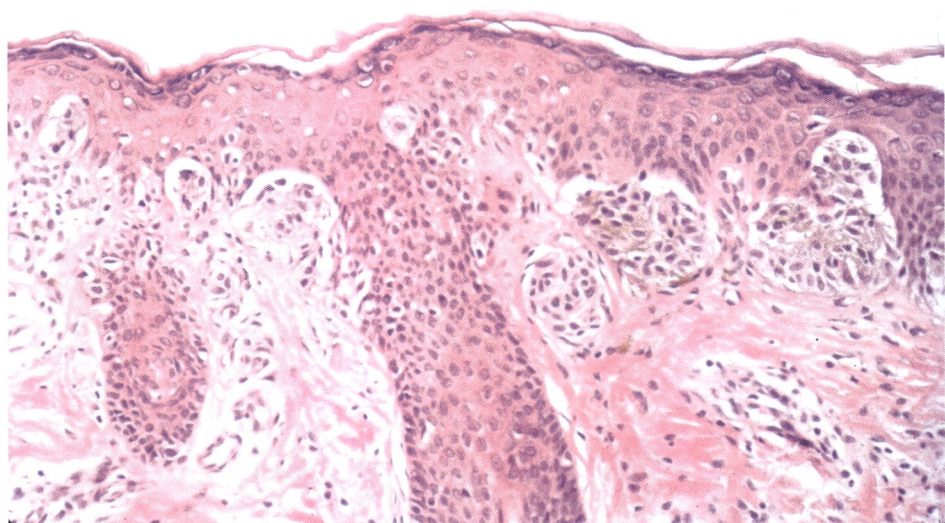

FIGURE 6-4 Small congenital nevus showing a prominent junctional component with only limited involvement of the papillary dermis.

in common acquired nevi. Occasional junctional nests of nevus cells are also observed. Foci of hypercellularity are also noted to a variable extent within the dermal population of cells (39) (Fig. 6-5). Both hair follicles and appendageal smooth muscle bundles may be enlarged (5,39).

A subset of large/giant CMN is also characterized by spindle cell or neuroidal differentiation resembling the histologic pattern of a neurofibroma (neuroid CMN) (7,37). In the latter instance, the constituent cells have a wavy configuration and are embedded in a delicate stroma. Neural differentiation resembling neural tubules or pseudo-Meissnerian structures are also typical histologic features (1,7,37) (Fig. 6-6). Rarely such variants may simulate desmoplastic melanoma because of neural differentiation and fibroplasia. However such lesions show maturation and lack appreciable atypia and mitoses. Such nevi may be associated with congenital anomalies such as club foot and spina bifida (37).

Large CMN may also show a variety of other patterns, suggesting that they are indeed hamartomas of neural crest differentiation (8). Such nevi may contain heterologous elements such as cartilage, bone, adipose tissue, vascular malformation, hemangioma, lymphangioma, mastocytoma, and schwannoma (1,7,8,9,37). Foci resembling blue nevus, cellular blue nevus, and spindle and epithelioid cell nevus are occasionally noted. The latter histologic picture thus may qualify as a combined nevus if found in the context of an otherwise typical CMN.

Epidermal Changes The epidermal changes in CMN are not distinctive and vary from almost no change to florid papillomatous or polypoid configurations (1,5,7,45).

TABLE 6-8 Distribution of nevus cell involvement in acquired and congenital nevi by size.

		Congenital[a]		
Distribution	Acquired[a]	< 1.5 cm	1.5–19.9 cm	Giant[a]
Junctional nesting	++	++	+	+
Papillary dermis	++	++	+	+
Upper reticular dermis				
Interstitial	+	++	++	++
Appendageal and/or neurovascular	±	++	++	++
Lower reticular dermis				
Interstitial	−	±	++	++
Appendageal and/or neurovascular	−	±	++	++
Subcutaneous	−	±	++	++

[a] ++, frequent; +, common; ±, may occur; −, usually not present.

TABLE 6-9 Histologic patterns of congenital melanocytic nevi.

Pattern	CMN
Acquired nevus	Mostly small
Patchy periadnexal, perivascular	Small to large
Diffuse infiltration of reticular dermis, subcutis	Mostly large/giant
Neuroid, resembling neurofibroma	Mostly large/giant
Spindle and epithelioid cell nevus	Mostly large/giant
Blue nevus, both ordinary and cellular blue nevus	Mostly large/giant

Lentiginous epidermal and melanocytic hyperplasia are possibly more common in CMN than acquired nevi.

Distinction of Relatively Small CMN from Acquired Nevi The distinction of small or any type CMN from acquired nevi is important only if small CMN are proved to have greater risk for the development of melanoma than acquired nevi (5). At present, there is no conclusive proof that there is a significant difference in melanoma risk between the latter two types of nevi. However, some authors do believe that there is sufficient circumstantial evidence for a difference in melanoma risk (23,24).

As was mentioned, because of histologic overlap between small CMN and acquired nevi, there are no features with 100% specificity and 100% sensitivity for recognition of CMN (5). Thus some CMN will be indistinguishable from common acquired nevi. Nonetheless, the presence of nevus cells in the lower half of the reticular dermis, in an appendageal/neurovascular pattern, or both enable one to detect a majority of small CMN (5,45). It should be emphasized that absence of the latter features does not preclude a congenital origin (5,45).

Congenital Nevi with Atypical Features

Architectural Disorder and/or Cytologic Atypia As with other types of melanocytic nevi, all varieties of congenital nevi may exhibit some degree of architectural and cytologic atypia of both the intraepidermal and dermal components (8,39) (Table 6-10). Perhaps one of the most common findings in congenital nevi is the presence of lentiginous melanocytic proliferation associated with or without some variation in junctional nesting pattern and generally low-grade cytologic atypia of the intraepidermal melanocytes (39). The latter changes are comparable to those seen in acquired atypical (dysplastic) nevi.

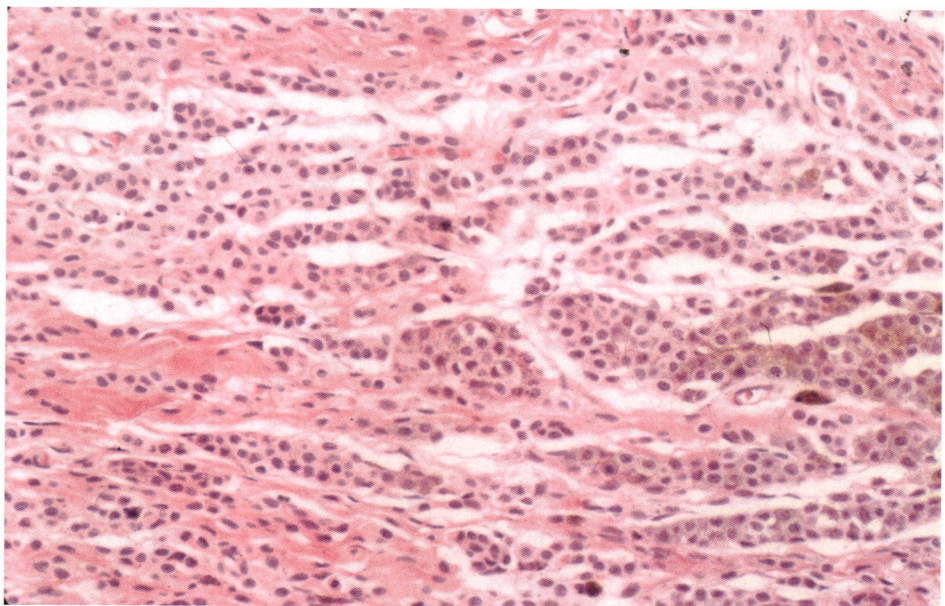

FIGURE 6-5 Large congenital nevus showing an area of increased cellularity in the reticular dermis. Such foci are common in large CMN.

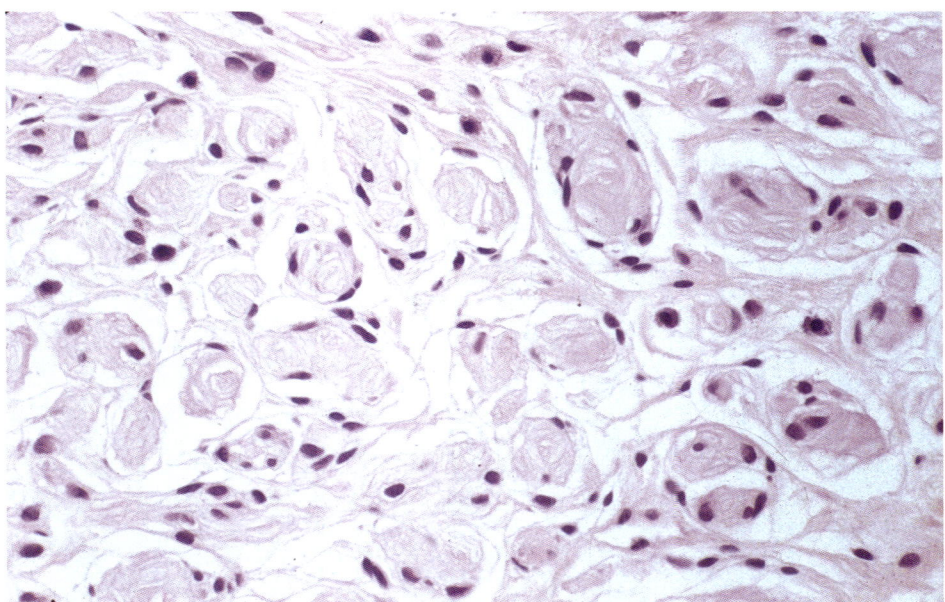

FIGURE 6-6 Large congenital nevus showing prominent neurotization of nevus cells in the dermis. The nevus cells form structures resembling Meissner-Wagner corpuscles.

Intraepidermal Pagetoid Spread of Melanocytes Another common finding, particularly in congenital nevi in individuals < 10 years of age and especially in the 1st year of life, is the pattern of upward migration of intraepidermal melanocytes (39,40,46–48) (Fig. 6-7A). Although the latter changes may be alarming, the proliferation is usually orderly and often confined to the lower half of the epidermis; and cytologic atypia is absent or low grade (39). It should be emphasized that one may encounter a spectrum of atypicality within the intraepidermal component, ranging from little or no atypia to frank melanoma in situ (Fig. 6-7B).

Dermal Nodular Proliferations

Large/giant CMN (or rarely melanocytic nevi, congenital or acquired, of any size) may give rise to intradermal nodular melanocytic proliferations (8,39,46–48) (Figs. 6-8 to 6-12; Tables 6-10 and 6-11). Such proliferations may occur in the superficial or deep reticular dermis and are characterized by the formation of cellular nodules. The constituent cells in these nodules may be epithelioid, spindled, or small cell in nature (8,39,46–48). The degree of melaninization may range from little or none to heavy. Varying degrees of cytologic atypia, mitotic activity, and occasionally necrosis may be observed. Most of these cellular aggregates tend to blend with the surrounding background nevus (Fig. 6-8B). The vast majority of such proliferations, particularly in the neonatal period, are biologically benign, despite atypical histologic features (Figs. 6-8–6-10). Nonetheless, all patients should receive close follow-up for evidence of recurrence. Small round cell tumors should be evaluated especially carefully for malignancy (Figs. 6-8 and 6-10). Many of these nodular proliferations are composed of enlarged epithelioid (Fig. 6-9) or spindled cells containing an increased cellular content of granular melanin. Usually the melanin does not have the finely divided ("dusty") character observed in melanoma cells. The nuclei in these cells also tend to show an overall uniformity and an evenly dispersed chro-

---

TABLE 6-10 Atypical variants of congenital nevi and atypical proliferations arising in congenital nevi.

Intraepidermal proliferations
   Congenital nevus with atypical features
      Lentiginous melanocytic proliferation
      Variation in junctional nesting
      Slight to severe nuclear atypia
   Congenital nevus with pagetoid spread
      Variant in children with little or no cytologic atypia
      Simulant of pagetoid melanoma
Dermal proliferations
   Atypical cellular proliferations
      Mainly spindle cells
      Mainly epithelioid cells
      Mainly small cells
      Blend with surrounding congenital nevus (maturation), variable degrees of cytologic atypia
   Tumors composed of above cell types and associated with indeterminate biologic behavior

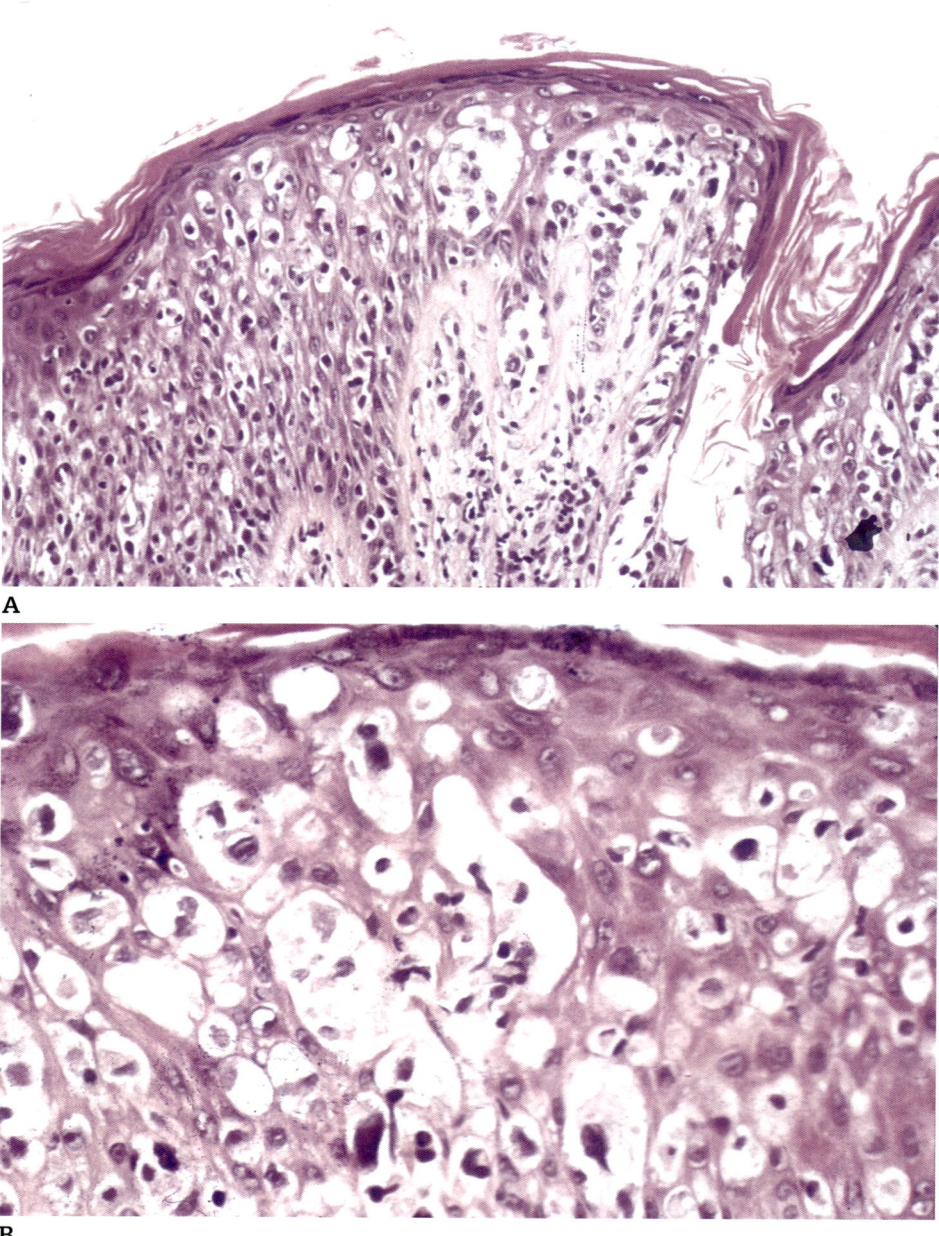

FIGURE 6-7 Congenital nevus with intraepidermal pagetoid spread. **A,** The epidermis overlying a small congenital nevus showing extensive pagetoid spread. **B,** Atypical epithelioid melanocytes scattered throughout epidermis. The findings qualify as melanoma in situ.

matin pattern, compared to the more striking pleomorphism and clumped chromatin of melanoma cells (39) (Fig. 6-9).

Neurocutaneous Melanosis Neurocutaneous melanosis (NCM) is defined by the proliferation of benign "melanotic cells" (a term used to avoid a more precise designation such as melanocyte or melanoblast) in the meninges (17–19). This melanosis may involve the convexities and the base of the brain; the ventral surfaces of the pons, medulla, and upper cervical; and the lumbosacral spinal cord.

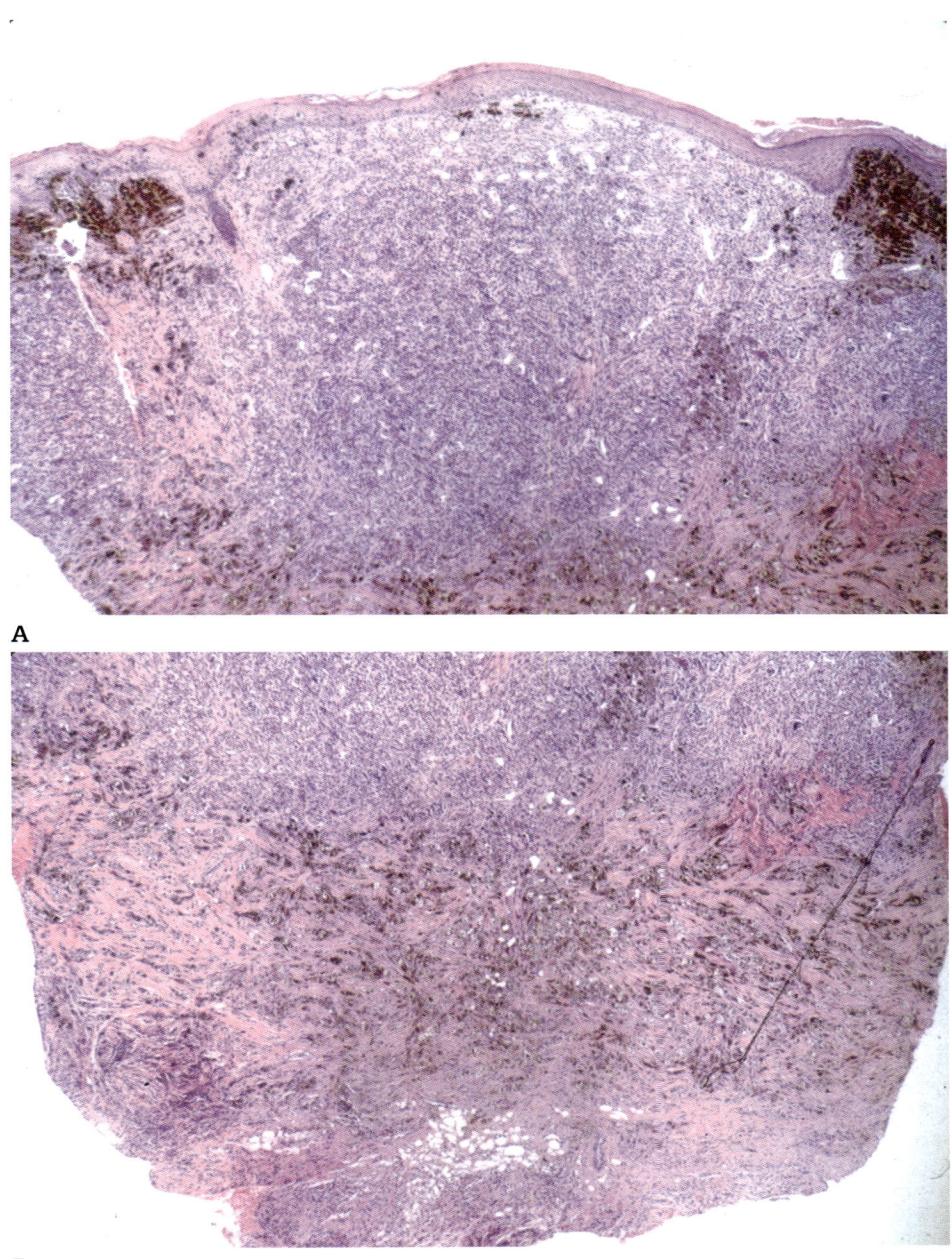

FIGURE 6-8 Superficial dermal atypical nodular proliferation in a medium congenital nevus of newborn. **A,** Large compact cellular nodule in the superficial and middle dermis resulting in an elevated surface. **B,** Deep reticular dermis showing maturation of the nevus in panel A. The nevus cells are dispersed among collagen bundles in an orderly pattern.

Melanoma Developing in Congenital Nevi

Conventional melanoma originating from an intraepidermal site is most commonly observed in relatively small CMN (25,46) (Fig. 6-13; Table 6-12). Such melanomas are usually of the conventional pagetoid or nodular type. However, such melanomas are uncommonly observed in large/giant CMN (46,47). The great majority of melanomas developing in the latter setting are dermal and composed of epithelioid cells, spindle cells, or small round cells resembling a small round ("blue") cell malignant tumor (7,8,46–48) (Fig. 6-14; Table 6-13). Some melanomas may have the character-

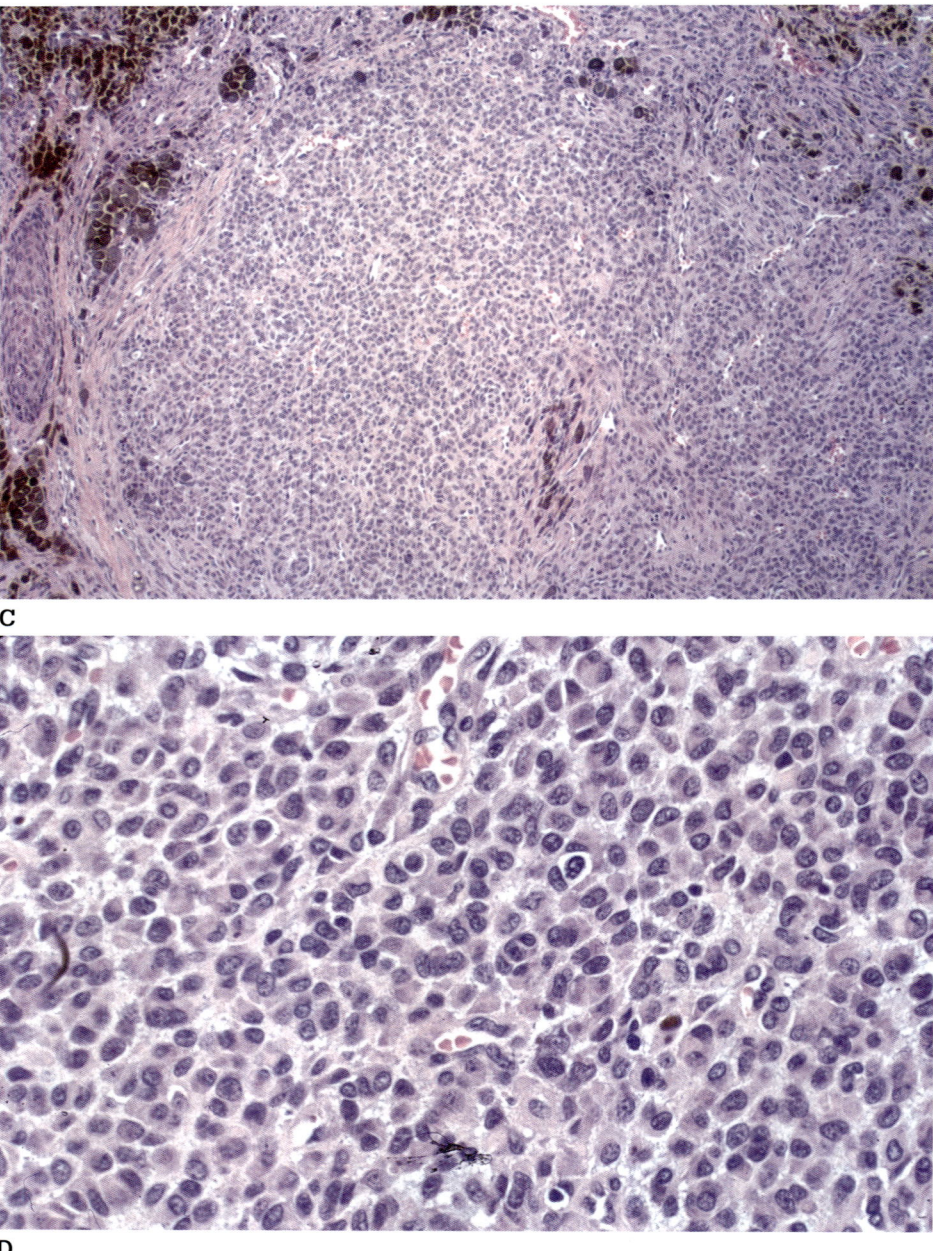

FIGURE 6-8 *Continued.* **C,** Compact cellular nodule composed of relatively small monotonous cells. **D,** Higher magnification of panel C showing a cohesive nodule of cells exhibiting low-grade atypia. Such a proliferation is often misdiagnosed as melanoma. The patient had no evidence of recurrence on follow-up.

istics of malignant blue nevus, or malignant epithelioid schwannoma (46,49). Such tumors usually manifest cohesive cellular nodules that are distinctly different from the surrounding nevus, substantial nuclear pleomorphism, necrotic cells, mitotic activity, and striking cellularity (46–48). Interpretation of such tumors may be exceedingly difficult, and it may not always be possible to arrive at a final diagnosis of benign or malignant tumor. As mentioned, melanoma in newborns and infants < 1 year of age is rare and must always be seriously questioned (47,48). Furthermore, the vast majority of epithelioid and spindle cell nodular proliferations de-

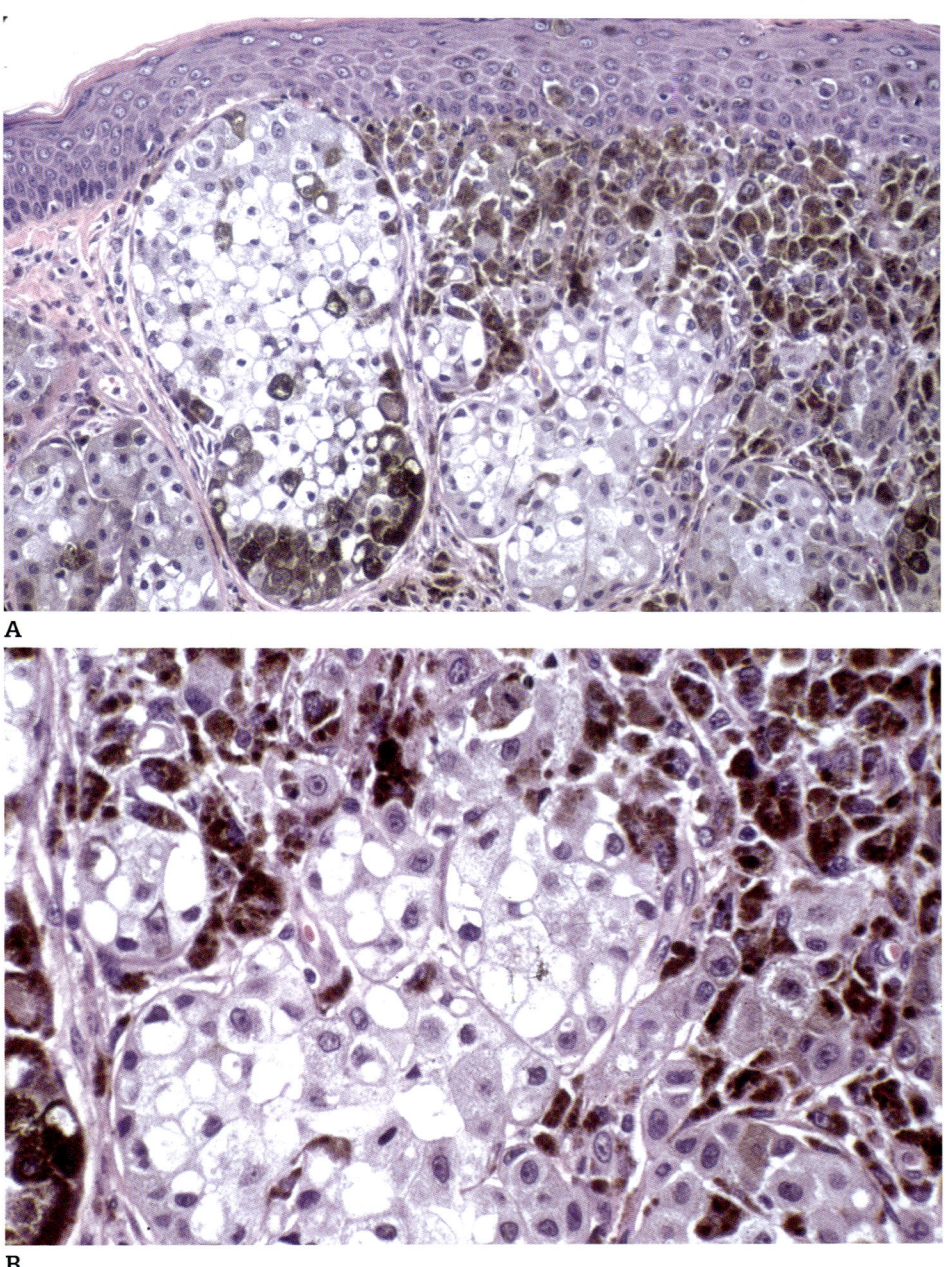

FIGURE 6-9 Atypical nodular proliferation in a congenital nevus of a newborn. **A,** Superficial nodule containing atypical epithelioid cells simulating melanoma. The nevus exhibited maturation with descent into the dermis. No evidence of recurrence was observed in this patient. **B,** Higher magnification of panel A showing epithelioid cells with some pleomorphism of nuclei. Many nuclei have fairly uniformly dispersed chromatin.

veloping in CMN, particularly in young individuals, are benign or not aggressive (39,47,48) (Figs. 6-8 to 6-12). Thus the pathologist should be cautious in rendering a diagnosis of melanoma in the latter circumstances. A prudent approach is to ensure complete surgical removal of such nodular lesions and to carefully monitor the patient for recurrence or metastasis. On the other hand, many of the true biologic forms of melanoma arising in giant CMN are of the small cell type (7,8,46–48) (Fig. 6-14). The cells forming such melanomas are disposed in sheets in a delicate myxoid stroma (8,46). The cells are closely crowded, have minimal cytoplasm, and

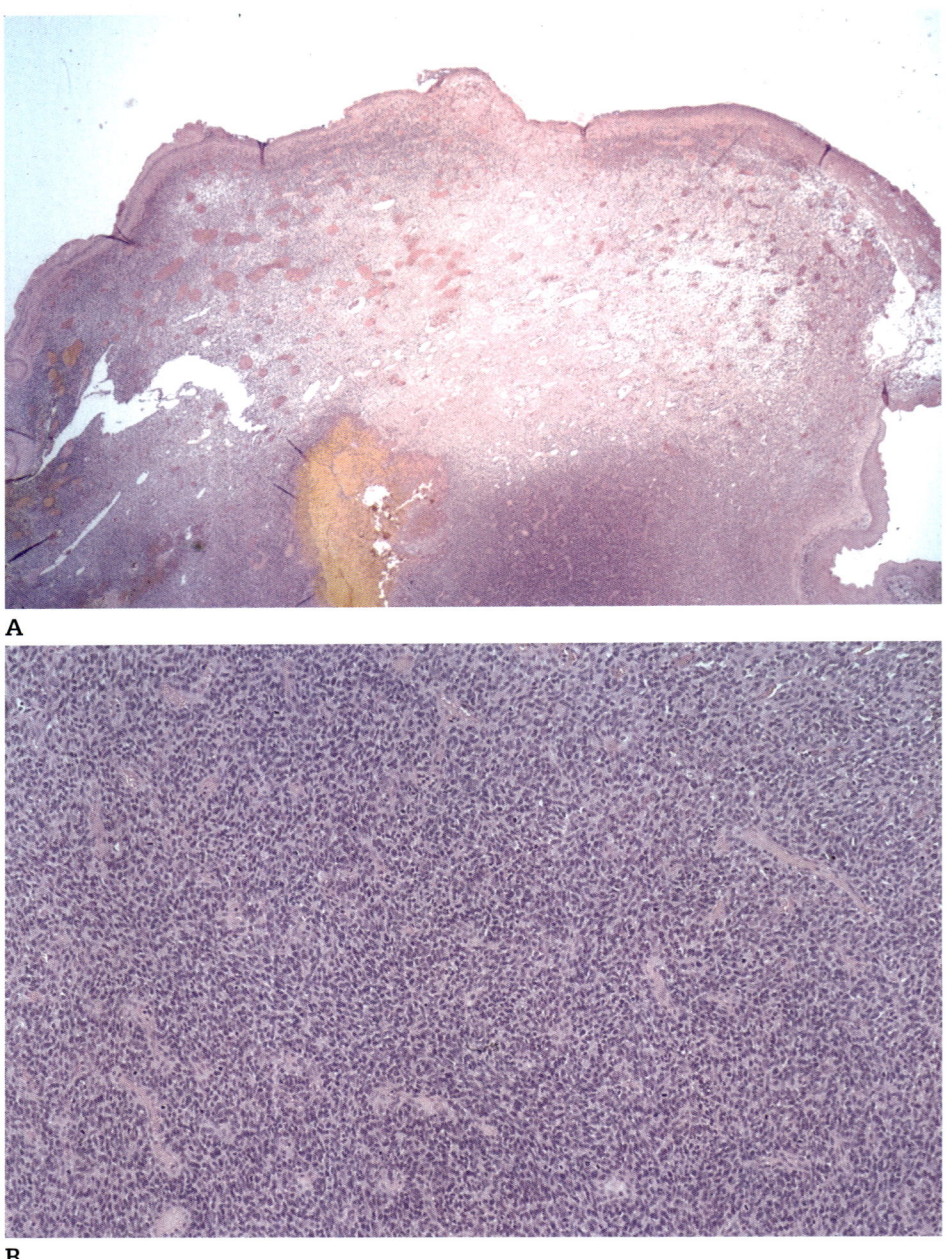

FIGURE 6-10 Atypical nodular proliferation in a giant congenital nevus of a newborn. The child was alive and well at the 6-years follow-up. **A,** Polypoid ulcerated nodule containing highly cellular aggregates of relatively small cells suggesting malignancy. **B,** Note the diffuse proliferation of the small melanocytes with scant cytoplasm.

contain small round or slightly oval nuclei with dense, uniformly dispersed chromatin. The cells take on the appearance of lymphoblastic lymphoma or comparable "blastic" tumors (Fig. 6-14B). Mitotic figures and nuclear debris are also commonly observed.

Leptomeningeal melanoma have been reported to arise in about two thirds of patients with NCM (19). These melanomas are intracranial in approximately 50% of cases and most commonly involve the frontal and temporal lobes. They prove to be rapidly fatal in almost all cases, with a median age of 3 years at death in one study.

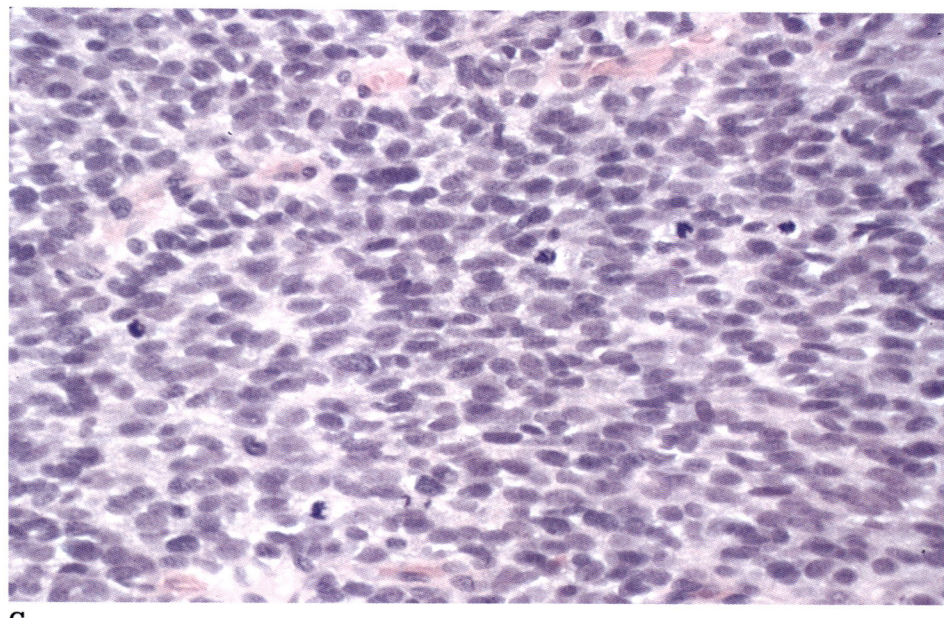

FIGURE 6-10 *Continued.* **C,** Higher magnification of panel B showing sheets of monomorphous small cells. The mitotic rate is high (26 mitoses/mm^2).

Other Mesenchymal Tumors and Aggregates

As delineated by Hendrickson and Ross (46), giant CMN may exhibit specific mesenchymal differentiation and rarely give rise to hamartomatous mesenchymal tumors containing cartilage, vascular channels, and other elements. Rarely liposarcoma, rhabdomyosarcoma, ganglioneuroblastoma and other primitive sarcomas have been reported to arise in giant congenital nevi (8,46,50).

There have been occasional reports of melanocytic lesions or satellites identified in the skin (Fig. 6-15), placenta, and lymph nodes of patients with large/giant CMN (51–55). Explanations for these peculiar lesions have included arrested or aberrant migration of neural crest elements during embryogenesis and benign metastases from the large CMN. There is evidence supporting both hypotheses. Further investigation is needed to establish the pathogenesis of these lesions.

Differential Diagnosis

The differential diagnosis for small CMN < 1.5 cm in diameter is primarily that of acquired melanocytic nevi (AMN) and atypical (dysplastic) nevi. Since there are no specific features for small CMN histologically, the distinction from acquired nevi often rests on documentation at birth. AMN are superficial proliferations that often involve the papillary dermis, resulting in a compound nevus.

One particular problem associated with CMN is the presence of prominent upward migration of melanocytic cells throughout the epidermis in congenital nevi of children and particularly neonates. These proliferations suggest melanoma in situ or even invasive melanoma (Fig. 6-7). However, in general, the pattern within the epidermis has an orderly character and many of the cells do not reach the granular layer. Furthermore, careful examination will reveal low-grade or no cytologic atypia of these cells. In our experience and in the experience of others, virtually all of these proliferations are benign.

Another diagnostic difficulty is the distinction of tumoral dermal nodules in large CMN from melanoma. Relatively small nodules generally measuring < 1 cm in greatest diameter are common in giant CMN. These nodules exhibit compact cellularity and the constituent cells are usually larger and exhibit variable degrees of cytologic atypia (Figs. 6-8 to 6-12). The distinction from melanoma relates to the gradual blending of the cellular nodule with the surrounding nevus cells in the dermis. The presence of an abrupt margin between the tumor nodule and the surrounding nevus is abnormal and suggests melanoma. The presence of necrotic cells, significant cytologic atypia, and easily found mitotic activity also suggest melanoma. Age is a significant factor to be considered in the evaluation of these proliferations. A diagnosis of melanoma should be made with extreme caution in individuals under the age of 1 year (39,47,48).

Risk Factors

Established risk factors for the development of melanoma in CMN include (a) large size (> 20 cm), (b) posterior

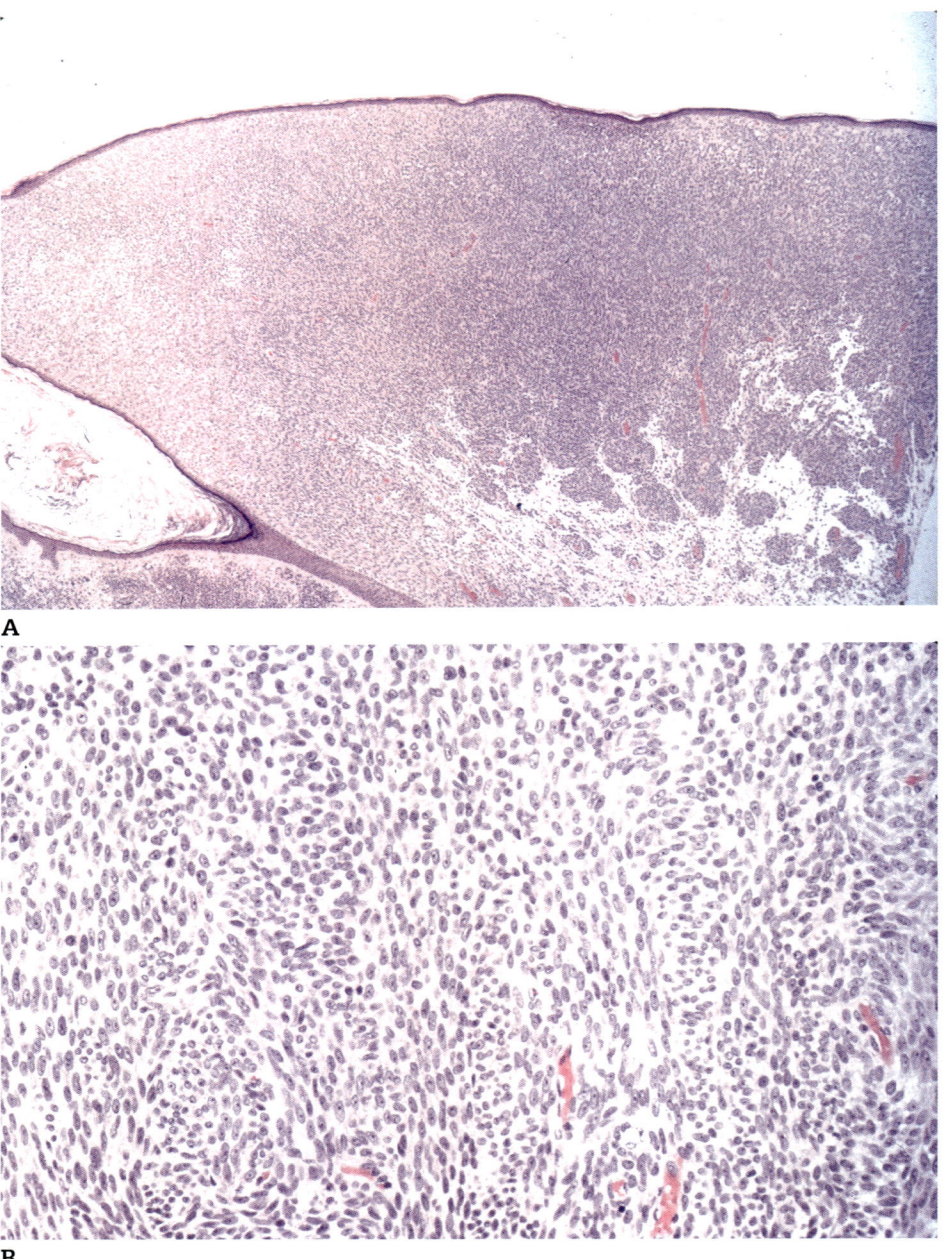

FIGURE 6-11 Atypical nodular proliferation in a congenital nevus. **A,** The lesion is raised and pedunculated. There is some maturation with depth. **B,** The papillary dermis is expanded by a nodular proliferation of relatively uniform fusiform cells.

axial location (i.e., the head, neck, back, buttock, or any combination), and (c) evidence of NCM. Other variables potentially relevant for melanoma risk might include evidence of hypopigmentation or regression, intraepidermal or dermal melanocytic proliferations with architectural disorder and cytologic atypia, DNA aneuploidy, and patterns of gene and protein expression assessed through tissue microarray technology (56–58). Atypical melanocytic proliferations would seem to correlate with increased melanoma risk but have not been sufficiently investigated as markers of elevated melanoma risk.

Recent data show that atypical melanocytic proliferations are characterized by numerical aberrations of whole chromosomes (59). These abnormalities are not

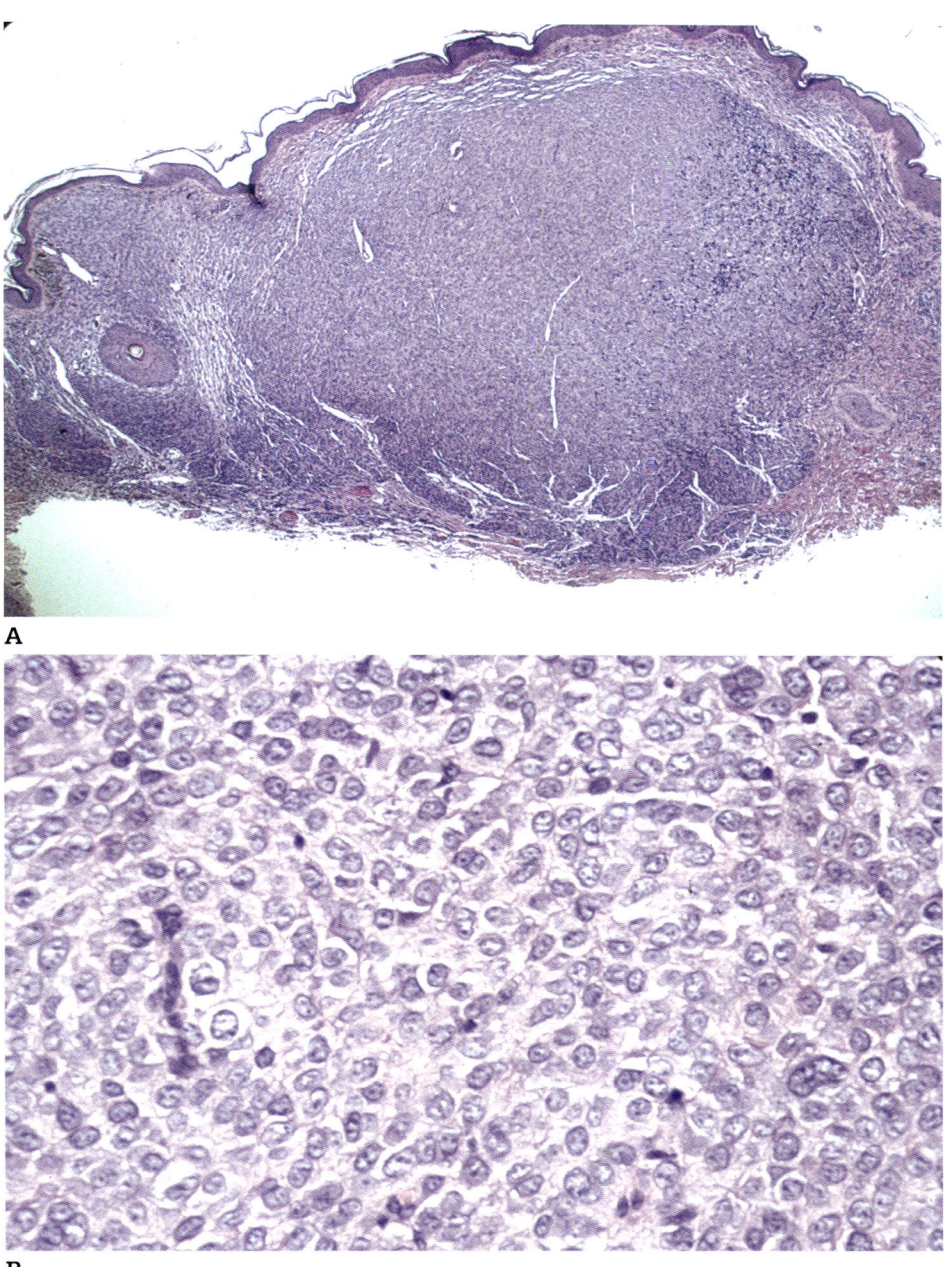

FIGURE 6-12 Atypical nodular proliferation in a congenital nevus. **A,** Compact nodule in the superficial dermis. **B,** Higher magnification of panel A showing monotypic cells with relatively little cytoplasm. This proliferation simulates nevoid melanoma. Patients with such lesions require careful monitoring.

observed in melanomas arising in CMN and suggest that atypical melanocytic proliferations are associated with a genomic instability due to a mitotic spindle check-point defect. Abnormal DNA content has been reported in CMN and has a higher prevalence in large/giant CMN than in small CMN (56–58,60). However, whether DNA aneuploidy is associated with elevated melanoma risk in CMN has not been established. The expression of two or more cell surface (progression-associated melanoma) antigens in CMN has been correlated with progression to melanoma in a series of 36 CMN (58). Activating point mutations in the N-*ras* gene have been detected at high frequency both in congenital melanocytic nevi and melanoma, suggesting that activated N-*ras* oncogene may

TABLE 6-11 Intraepidermal and dermal proliferations developing in large/giant congenital nevi.

Benign	Indeterminate/Malignant
1. Epithelioid cell	Pagetoid melanoma
Intraepidermal	
Pagetoid spread in nevi	
Dermal	
Expansile nodule of epithelioid cells	Melanoma, epithelioid cell type
Epithelioid schwannoma	Malignant epithelioid schwannoma
2. Pigmented spindle cell	
Dermal	
Expansile nodule of spindle cells	Melanoma, pigmented spindle cell type
3. Spindle cell with schwannian/perineurial differentiation	
Dermal	
Neurofibroma-like tumor	Malignant peripheral nerve sheath tumor
Schwannoma	
4. Small round cell	
Dermal	
Expansile nodule of small cells	Small cell melanoma ("lymphoblastic" type melanoma)
5. Specific mesenchymal ("ectomesenchymal") differentiation	
Cartilage	Rhabdomyosarcoma
Lipoma	
Hemangioma	
6. Neuronal elements	
Ganglioneuroma	Ganglioneuroblastoma
7. Unclassified or undifferentiated neoplasms	Undifferentiated sarcoma

Source: Adapted from Hendrickson and Ross (1981).

constitute a potential risk factor for melanoma formation within CMN (61).

CONGENITAL MELANOMA
With Alain Spatz*

The presence of malignant melanoma at birth is exceedingly rare and may be classified into three varieties (62–65) (Table 6-14). The first type, of which only five cases have been reported (63), is characterized by maternal melanoma metastatic to the fetus (63,66). Neonates usually present at birth with widespread visceral metastases and four of the five reported cases died within days to months. The placenta usually shows gross and histopathologic evidence of metastatic melanoma in such cases. Because of the theoretical risk of transmission from the mother to the fetus, the placentas should be examined for gross and histopathologic evidence of metastatic melanoma when the maternal melanoma is more > 1 mm in thickness. Even when present these placental metastases only rarely lead to congenital melanoma; some of the latter placental deposits also appear to be benign and may represent developmental arrests or "benign seeding" of the placenta (55). Nonetheless the finding of placental involvement by melanocytic deposits warrants careful examination and follow-up of the newborn.

Among > 350 women reported in the literature to have developed melanoma during pregnancy, 20 patients demonstrated placental metastases. Among the latter patients, fetal involvement was observed in 5 instances as mentioned above. Primary congenital melanoma is also vanishingly rare and may develop de novo or in association with a giant congenital nevus. Only 8 cases of de novo congenital melanoma have been reported (63,64,68–75) (Table 6-14). Among this small group of patients, only 2 succumbed to the melanoma. Congenital melanoma developing in giant congenital nevi with or without neurocutaneous melanosis has also been described in a small number of patients and probably constitutes the largest group of patients with congenital melanoma (46,61,71–82) (Table 6-14). Only 5 such patients have died from disseminated melanoma.

Because of the small number of primary congenital melanomas reported and only very limited descriptions of their histopathologic features (or none at all), it is not possible to make any definitive statements about primary congenital melanoma. However, it should be emphasized that because of the extreme rarity of these lesions, a diagnosis of congenital or neonatal melanoma must be viewed with considerable skepticism (39). However as noted, histopathologic distinction between atypical nodular proliferation developing in congenital nevi

*Institute Gustave-Roussy, Villejuif, France

Chapter 6: Congenital Melanocytic Nevi and Associated Neoplasms, Congenital and Childhood Melanoma

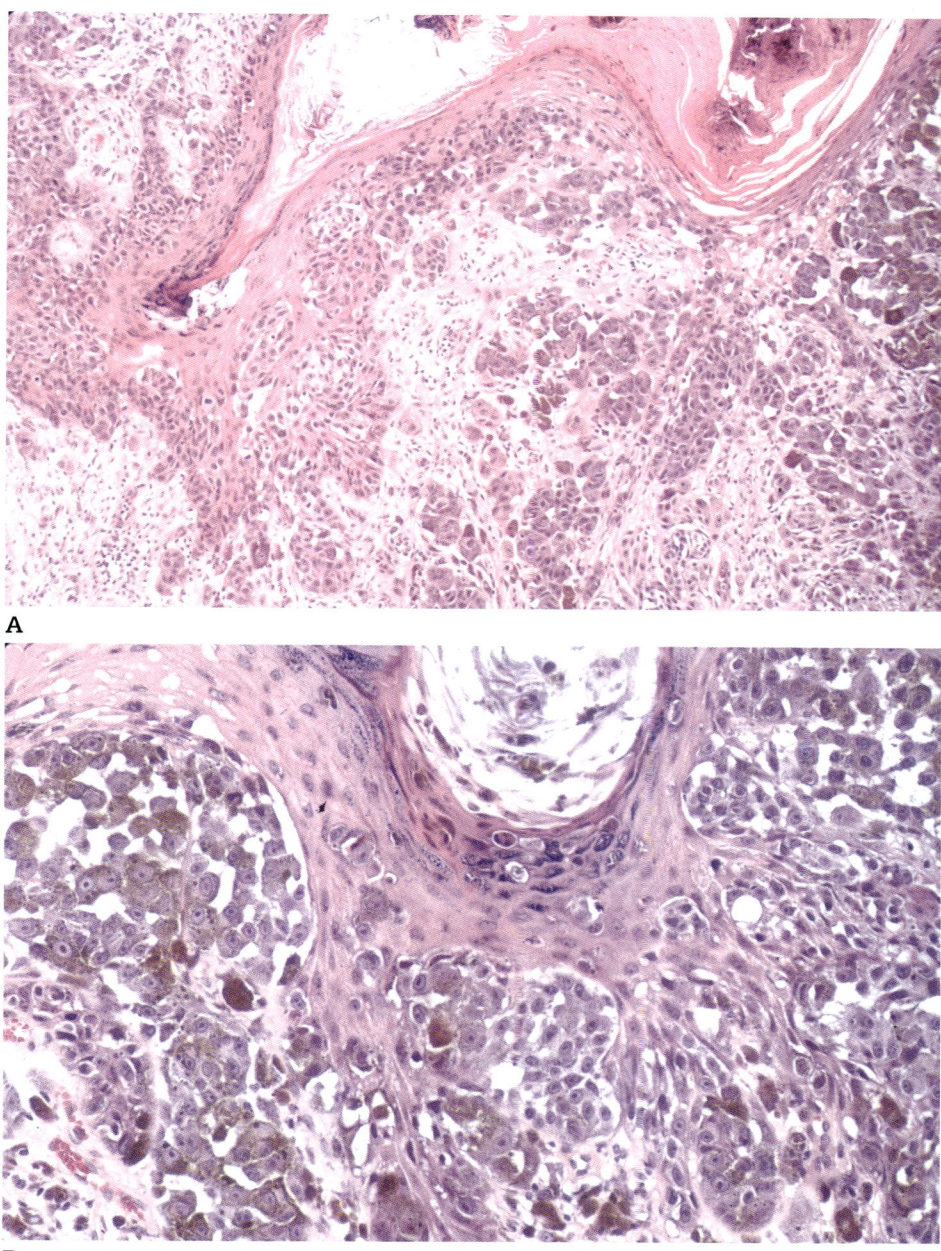

FIGURE 6-13 Melanoma arising from the intraepidermal component of a small congenital nevus. **A,** The lesion exhibits pagetoid spread and invasion of dermis. **B,** Higher magnification of panel A showing large intraepidermal nests of melanoma cells with pagetoid spread.

TABLE 6-12 Melanoma originating in relatively small congenital nevi (<10 cm).

Clinical features	Histopathological features
Onset after puberty	Virtually all melanomas have intraepidermal origin
Peak ages, 20–30 and 50–60 years	Pagetoid and "nodular" melanomas most common types
Melanoma often develops at periphery of CMN	CMN mostly involve upper two thirds or half of dermis
CMN relatively flat	

with benign evolution and melanoma may be extremely difficult or impossible. In rare instances, large or giant congenital nevi are associated with contiguous involvement of lymph nodes that must be distinguished from nodal metastasis.

Virtually all such congenital atypical proliferative lesions are biologically benign. Examination of these highly atypical tumors with reference to karyotype, expression of cell-surface antigens, growth in soft agar, and other parameters has shown that they have the properties of an immature proliferative but benign tumor (47,80). DNA image analysis of a similar congenital tumor associated with a CMN failed to show any evidence of abnormal DNA content (Schmidt BS, Barnhill RL, observations, 1992).

CHILDHOOD MELANOMA

The incidence of melanoma increases with age but is exceptionally rare in prepubertal individuals (estimated incidence approximately 0.4% among all melanomas) (83,84) and uncommon under the age of 20 years (incidence approximately 2%) (85). Recent epidemiologic studies confirmed that the incidence of melanoma in the population aged 15–19 years has doubled in 10 years. (86,87) This is not the case for melanomas in children younger than 15 years, the incidence of which is unchanged. Melanoma in children younger than 10 years of age is extremely rare. Less than 80 well-documented cases of melanoma in children younger than 10 years have been recorded in the literature over a period of 30 years. As in

FIGURE 6-14 Melanoma arising in the dermal component of a large congenital nevus in an adult. **A,** Biopsy showing the well-defined nature of the melanoma nodule in the dermis and subcutis. **B,** Note the abrupt sharply circumscribed margin of melanoma relative to the overlying congenital nevus remnant in the subsequent excision.

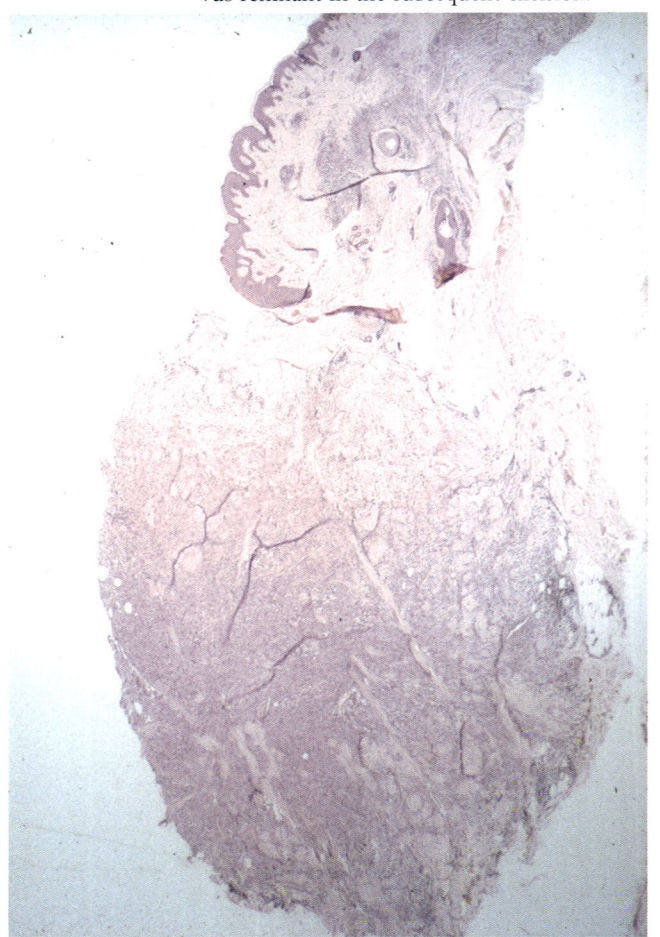
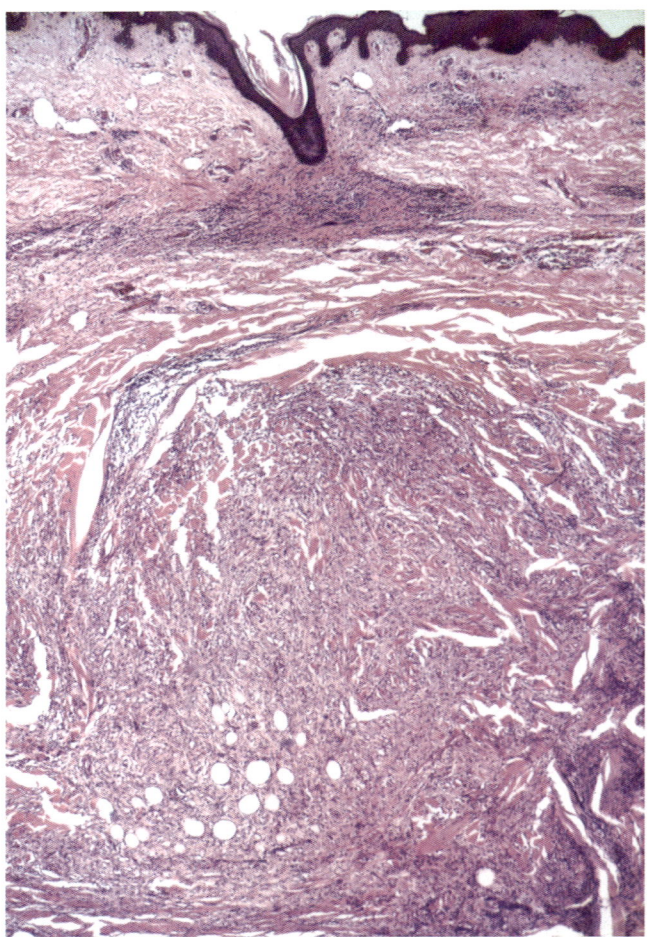

A B

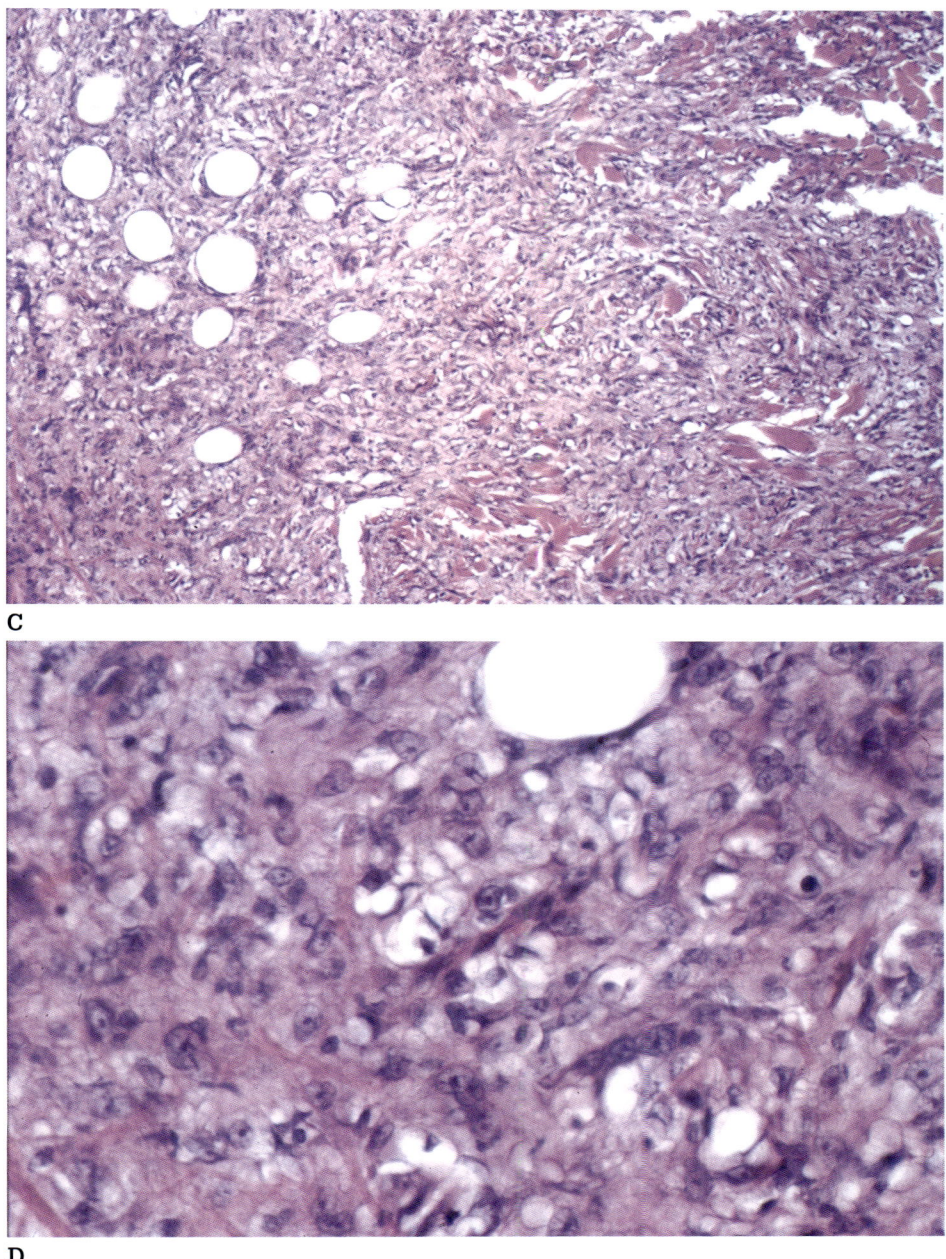

FIGURE 6-14 *Continued.* **C,** Diffuse sheet of polygonal cells in the melanoma nodule. **D,** Higher magnification of panel B.

adults, childhood melanomas affect mainly the white population. Several clinical features differentiate melanomas in children and in adults (88). These are summarized in Table 6-15.

With the realization that many cases of childhood melanoma in the past had been considered spindle and epithelioid cell (Spitz) nevi, it has become evident that malignant melanoma is much less common and has no better prognosis in children than in adults (89–102). Analysis of melanomas in individuals under the age of 20 shows fairly similar clinical and histologic features compared to melanomas in adults (Tables 6-15 and 6-16) (85,93). Features favoring a melanoma in a pigmented lesion are rapid increase in size, bleeding, color

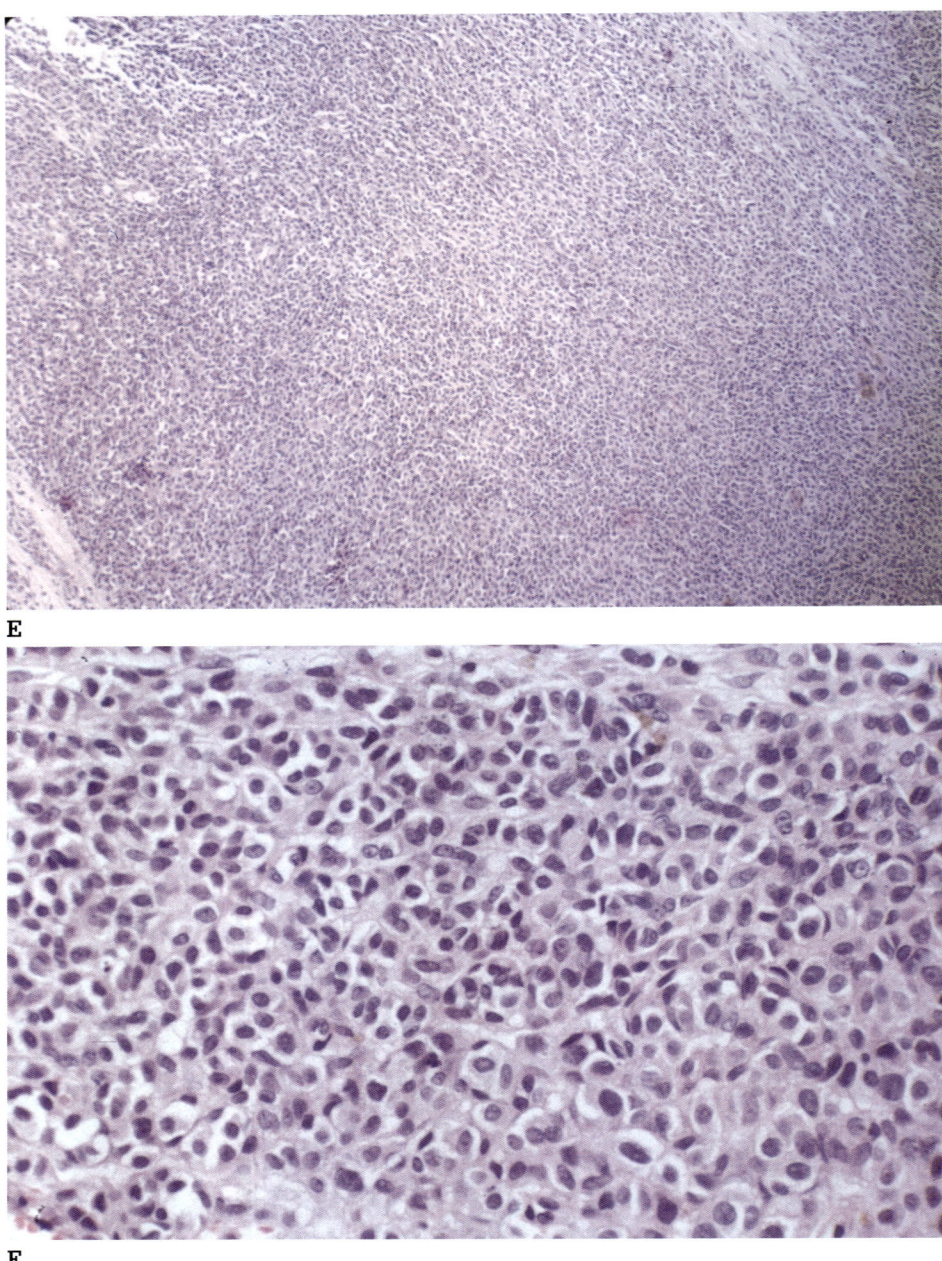

FIGURE 6-14 *Continued.* **E,** Small cell melanoma arising in the dermis and subcutis of large congenital nevus. The lesion proved to be fatal for the patient. **F,** The small melanoma cells have a monomorphous appearance with minimal cytoplasm. The tumor resembles other small round cell malignancies.

change of a nodular lesion; surface changes, such as ulceration; and loss of clearly defined margins. Recognition of melanoma appearing de novo requires a high degree of clinical suspicion, especially if the lesion is amelanotic. Following the classical ABCD criteria (asymmetry, ill-defined borders, irregular color, and large diameter) used for the clinical detection of melanoma in adults, all such lesions in children should be considered for removal and submitted for histopathologic examination. Melanoma in children can also be associated with pain or pruritus. It should be emphasized that thickness is the main prognostic parameter in childhood melanoma and that early diagnosis is also crucial in this population (65,86,88,95–102).

TABLE 6-13 Melanoma originating in large/giant congenital nevi.

Clinical features
- Onset most commonly in 1st decade (~ 60%), but at any age
- Median age, 5 years
- Mean age, 8.6 years
- True biologic melanoma rare or almost nonexistent < 1 year of age
- Development of or enlarging cutaneous nodule
- Darkening or lightening of skin

Histopathological features
- Majority originate in dermis
- Expansile tumors composed of epithelioid cells, spindle cells, or small round cells

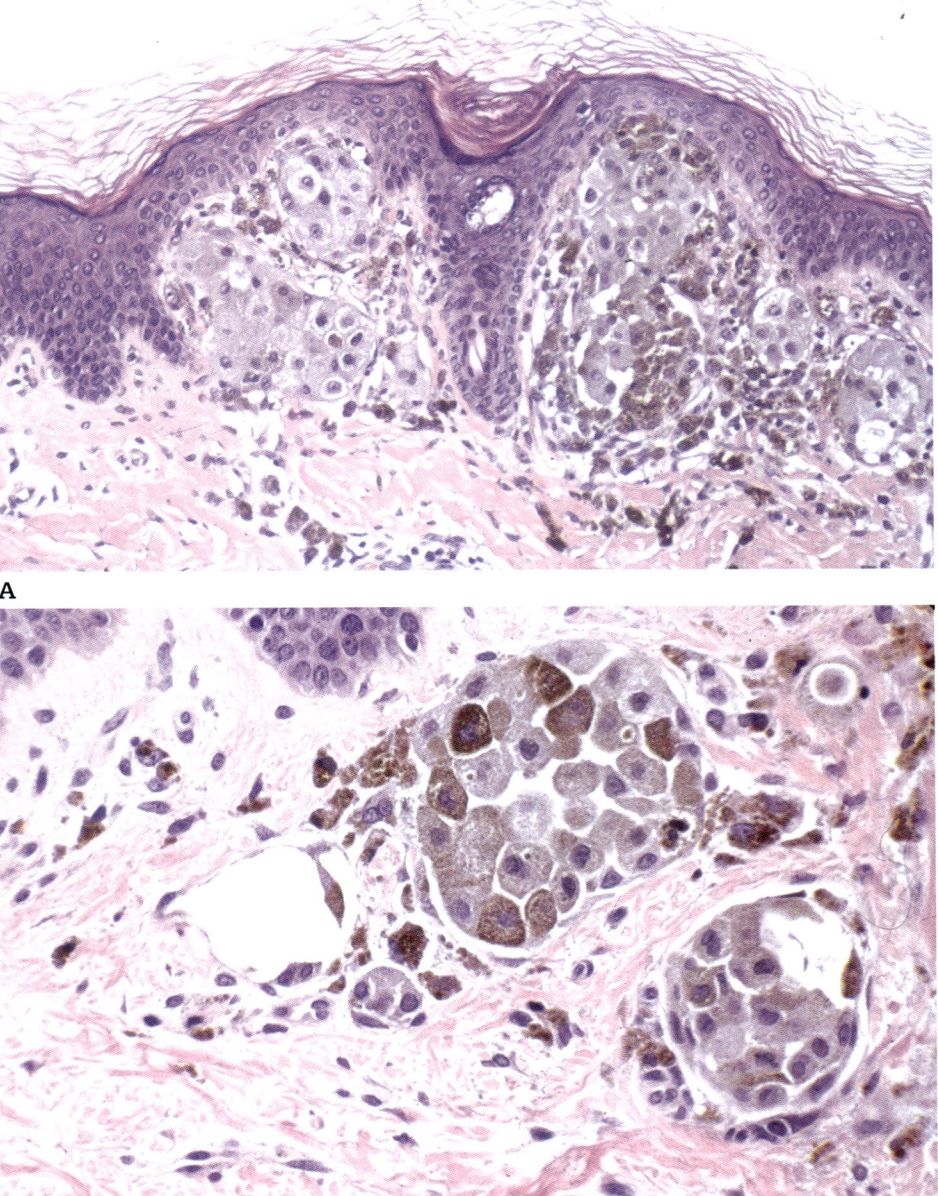

FIGURE 6-15 Cutaneous satellite lesion in a newborn with medium congenital nevus and atypical nodular proliferation. **A,** Well-circumscribed nodular aggregate of atypical epithelioid cells in the papillary dermis suggesting metastasis. **B,** Another satellite lesion in the papillary dermis. Such lesions are possibly explained by benign metastases or aberrant migration of neural crest–derived cells.

TABLE 6-14 Variants of congenital melanoma and summary of patients reported.

Variant	Number of patients	Sex	Location of melanoma	Outcome
Transplacental metastatic melanoma from maternal source	5	4M[a]	Widespread visceral metastases	4 dead (within 1 year) 5 mothers dead from metastatic melanoma
De novo melanoma	8	7M, 1F	Head and neck (3); trunk (2); extremities (3)	2 dead (4–7 months); 6 alive (follow-up 1–18 years)
Melanoma arising in large/giant congenital nevus	12	6M, 6F	Trunk (10); genitalia (1); head (1)	5 dead, 6 alive, 1 unknown

[a]Sex not reported for one neonate.

Etiology and Risk Factors

Melanoma Associated with Giant Congenital Nevus
It has been estimated that about half of the cases of melanoma associated with giant congenital nevus (GCN) occur in the first decade of life and if prophylactic removal of GCN is undertaken, it should be performed in early life (see above). As mentioned, the vast majority of nodular proliferations developing in GCN, particularly in young children, are benign or not aggressive. On the other hand, many of the true biologic forms of melanoma arising in GCN are of the small-cell type and can lead to a false diagnosis of benignity.

Melanoma Arising in Small Congenital Nevi The risk of melanoma developing in a small congenital nevus (SCN) is the greatest after puberty, with peak ages at 20–30 and 50–60 years (see above). In our experience, only 6 melanomas out of 145 diagnosed in childhood arose in a SCN (96). Clinical signs of malignant transformation are the same as those for melanomas associated with common nevi.

Melanoma Arising in Atypical Nevi and the Atypical Nevus Phenotype The relationship between number of nevi and the presence of atypical (dysplastic) nevi (AN) to the risk of melanoma has been demonstrated in many epidemiologic studies of adults (see Chapter 5) (103). Children affected with the AN phenotype are apparently normal at birth but may develop large numbers of morphologically common nevi in early childhood. These become more numerous and acquire atypical clinical features after 5–7 years. New lesions may continue to develop. There is no consensus about the minimum essential criteria for the AN phenotype—for example, 50 or 100 or more clinically atypical nevi. AN may be either familial or sporadic. In a study of 23 melanoma-prone families, a family history of melanoma and the presence of AN identify children with a high risk of melanoma developing at an early age (101). Among 125 patients under 20 years of age at the time of first clinical evaluation, 5 invasive melanomas were diagnosed before the age of 17 years in 4 patients, all of them occurring within a precursor nevus. In a population-based study conducted in Queensland, the presence of at least 1 large nevus increased the crude risk of melanoma under 15 years of age by 2.5 times, and the presence of more than 10 large nevi conferred a 10-fold increase in risk (97).

Melanoma Arising in Other Nevi The risk of melanoma in children is elevated with increased numbers of nevi, whatever their size.

Lichen Sclerosus and Melanoma An association between lichen sclerosus and melanoma in children of both sexes has been reported (104). The biologic basis for this association has not been established.

Risk factors for the development of melanoma in childhood reported in the literature include family history of melanoma and the atypical nevus phenotype, xe-

TABLE 6-15 Sex-ratio and anatomic site for childhood and adult melanomas.

Clinical features	Children (0–16 years)	Adults
Sex ratio (female/male)	1	1.9
Anatomic site (%)		
Trunk	50	F, 15; M, 40
Head/neck	15	F, 20; M, 25
Upper limbs	15	F, 15; M, 12
Lower limbs	20	F, 50; M, 23

TABLE 6-16 Melanoma in individuals younger than 20 years of age.

Clinical features
  Males = females
  Mean age, 16 years
  Very few cases < 10 years/puberty
  Distribution similar to adults
    Head and neck, 21.8%
    Extremities, 39.7%
    Trunk, 37.2%
  Clinical characteristics similar to adult patients
Histopathology
  Similar to adult melanomas
    Solar, 1.5%
    Pagetoid, 67.2%
    Nodular, 23.4%
    Acral, 7.8%
  Ulceration, 14.1%
  Tumor thickness, mean 1.76 mm (range 0.32–5.22 mm)
Differential diagnosis
  Spitz nevus
  Other melanocytic nevi
Prognosis
  Similar to adults
  5-year actuarial survival, 76%

Source: Reintgen et al. (1989).

roderma pigmentosum, immunosuppression, and sun exposure (64,94,95,96,98).

Prognosis

Because of the rarity of melanomas in children, few data are available in literature concerning prognosis. Moreover, it is obvious that the survival rate has been overestimated in the past by the inclusion of many cases of Spitz nevi that have been considered childhood melanoma. The reported 5-year survival rates range from 76 to 87.3%. As for adult melanomas, tumor thickness is the most important prognostic indicator (93,96,102). It has been suggested that a subset of lesions histologically similar to Spitz nevi could be associated with regional lymph node metastases without adverse prognostic significance (see Chapter 7). Additional multicenter studies are needed to address the latter issue.

Histopathological Features

Despite the justifiable reluctance of pathologists to diagnose melanoma in childhood without compelling evidence, virtually the same histopathologic criteria should be used for diagnosis as have been developed for adult melanomas (94–96,98,99) (see Chapter 10). However, clinical information must be strongly considered, particularly age; for example, cutaneous melanoma is almost nonexistent under the age of 2 years and especially so near the time of birth. Furthermore, the important stimulants of melanoma must be excluded: (a) atypical proliferations developing in CMN in infants and young children and (b) Spitz nevi. In fact 40% of lesions initially diagnosed as melanoma were reclassified after review as benign nevi in a large European multicenter study (96). On the other hand, several cases of melanoma associated with death or widespread metastases were initially diagnosed as Spitz nevus. Whatever the histologic type, features appearing to be most useful for distinguishing melanomas from nevi are large size (> 7 mm), ulceration, high mitotic activity (> 4 mitoses/mm^2), mitoses in the lower third of the lesion, asymmetry, poorly demarcated lateral borders, lack of maturation, dusty melanin, and marked nuclear polymorphism (94,96,99). Melanomas in children can be categorized into three principal groups based on the predominant cellular population. Although somewhat artificial, these categories are nonetheless associated with particular differential diagnoses and potentially different prognoses (94,96,99).

Epithelioid-Cell Type (Conventional Melanomas)

About 40–50% of melanomas in children are histologically similar to those in adults (94,96). The tumor thickness in this category of lesions varies, with a median ranging from 1.2 to 3.8 mm (89–96). It is likely that this reflects the level of awareness among clinicians for the risk of childhood melanoma. In a similar manner, the proportion of in situ melanomas among all childhood melanomas varies from 0 to 30%, according to the country and population studied. The diagnostic value of a prominent pagetoid intraepidermal component in adult melanomas is considerably diminished in children, since a significant proportion of nevi in children display this feature. As in adults, melanoma cells often proliferate as aggregates that are frequently large and have diminished cellular cohesion. "Nodular" melanomas (NM) are defined by an almost exclusively bulky or cohesive invasive component and little or no associated lateral intraepidermal component (see Chapter 10). Melanomas of glabrous skin are exceedingly rare in childhood (94,96). It cannot be overemphasized that lentiginous melanocytic proliferation and upward migration of melanocytes are features commonly observed in childhood nevi, particularly in glabrous skin. These changes must not be overinterpreted, unless architectural disorder is prominent and cytologic abnormalities are present throughout the breadth of the lesion. Among 145 European cases of childhood melanomas, only 3 cases involved the soles of white patients (96). Solar (so-called lentigo maligna) melanomas do not occur in childhood (see Chapter 10). However, melanomas diagnosed in patients with xeroderma pigmentosum (XP) are histologically often similar to solar

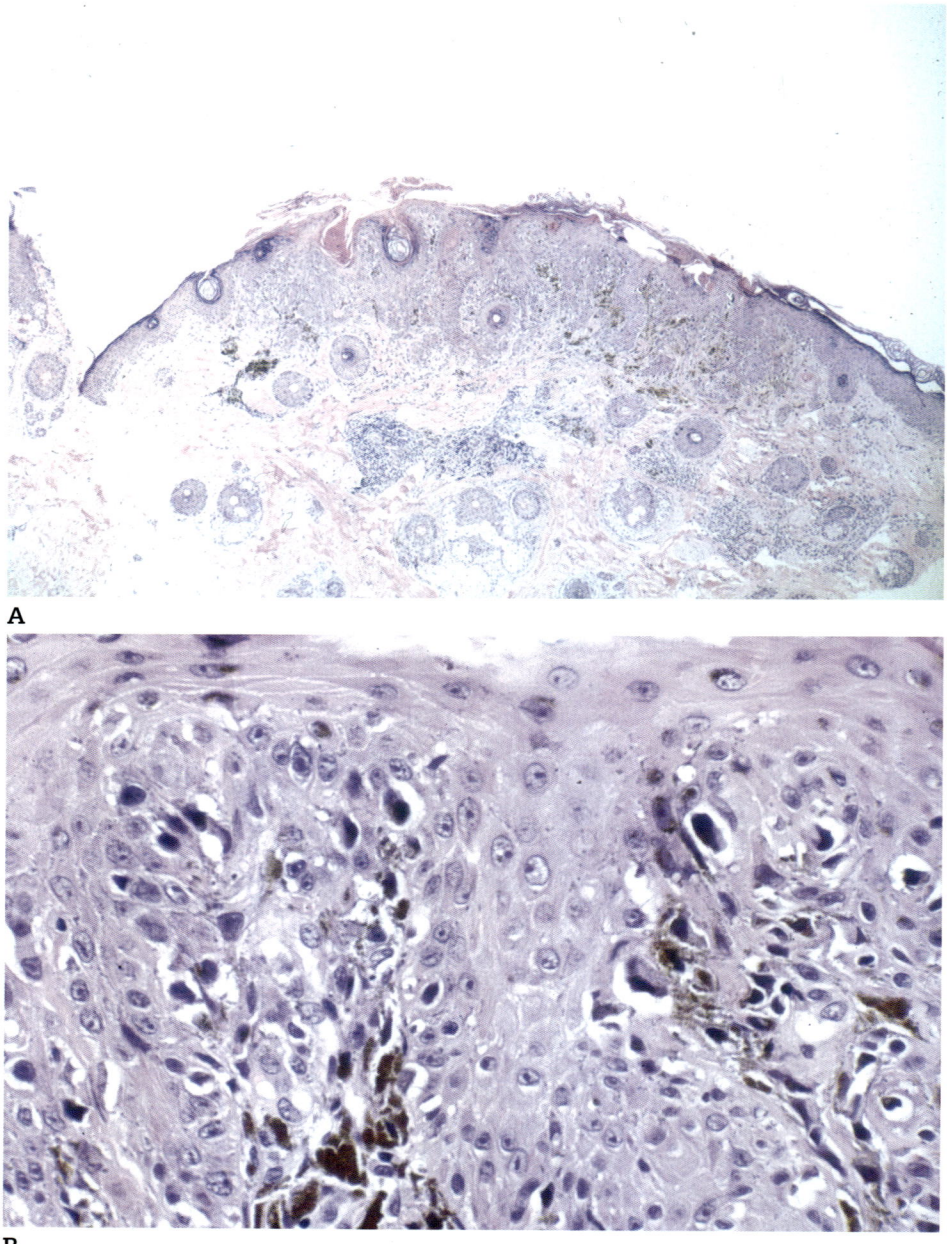

FIGURE 6-16 Lentiginous microinvasive melanoma developing in a child with xeroderma pigmentosum. **A,** The lesion shares features with solar melanomas (lentigo maligna variants) that occur in adults. This lesion is relatively small in diameter and demonstrates epidermal hyperplasia, in contrast to usual pattern of epidermal effacement in solar melanomas. **B,** Note lentiginous proliferation of pleomorphic melanocytes.

melanomas, except that the actinic damage characteristic of adult tumors is absent (94,96) (Fig. 6-16).

Small Cell Melanomas Small cell melanomas are composed of monomorphous small cells, reminiscent of small round cell malignancies such as lymphoma or a melanocytic nevus (94,96,99) (Fig. 6-17) (see below and Chapter 10). These cells are arranged in sheets or in organoid configurations. They contain basophilic round nuclei and condensed chromatin. The high cellular density and lack of maturation are features suggesting melanoma (Fig. 6-17). Mitotic figures are usually numerous. Rosettes and

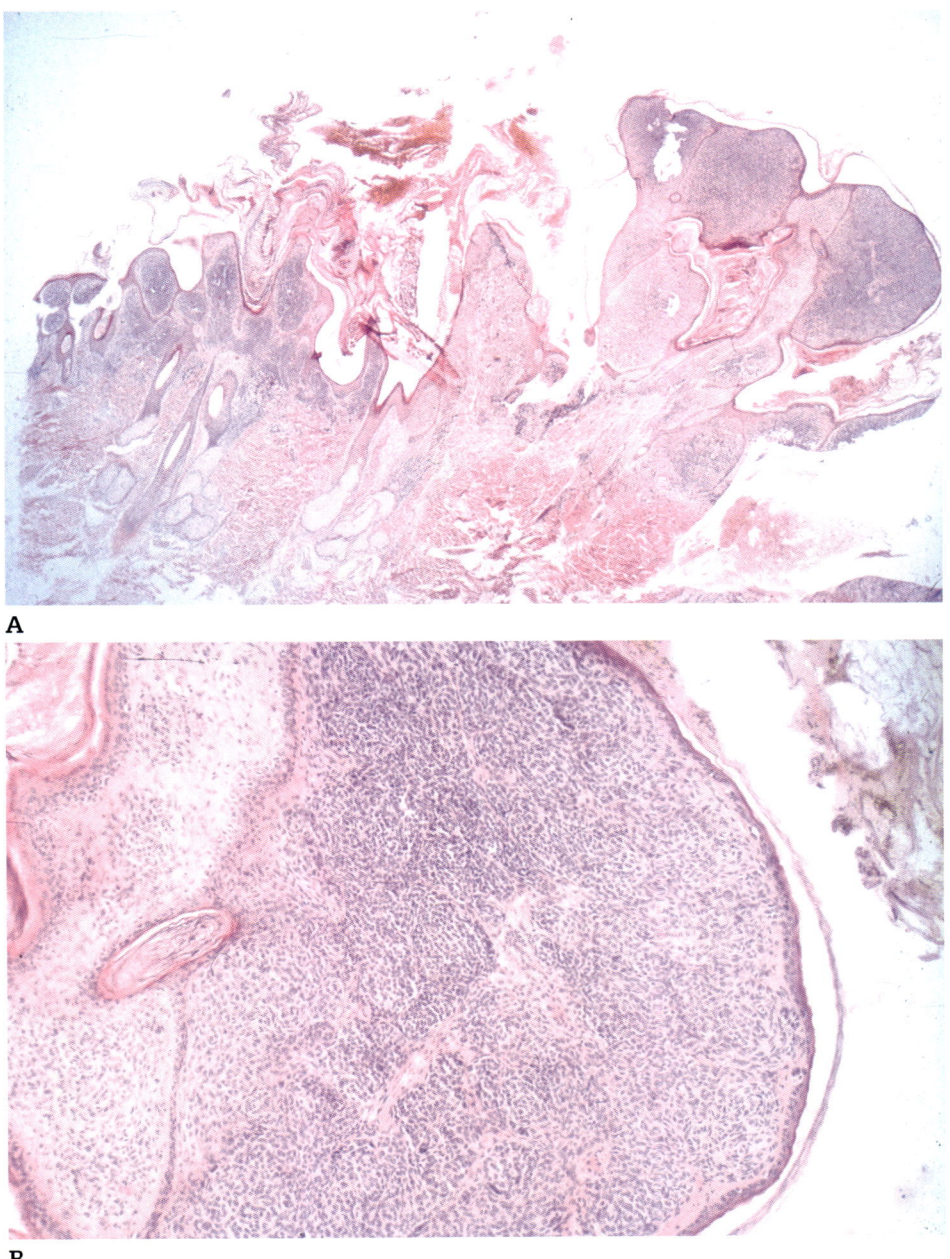

FIGURE 6-17 Small cell (verrucous) melanoma developing on the scalp of a child. This lesion resulted in metastases and death of the patient. **A,** The lesion has a papillomatous (verrucous) surface profile, suggesting a papillomatous melanocytic nevus. **B,** The melanocytes are arranged in a sheet-like pattern in the papillary dermis.

necrosis are often absent. In children, small cell melanomas may appear de novo or develop in association with a CMN. There are few reports of the clinical outcome of these lesions. The five childhood melanomas with small cell phenotypes described by Barnhill et al. (94) were characterized by localization to the scalp, striking Breslow thicknesses, and fatal outcome in all patients. Three out of the six cases reported from Europe (EORTC series) led to metastases (96). Only one melanoma was located on the scalp. These data support the proposal to place these lesions in a separate category because of their likely distinctive clinicopathologic presentation (94,96,99).

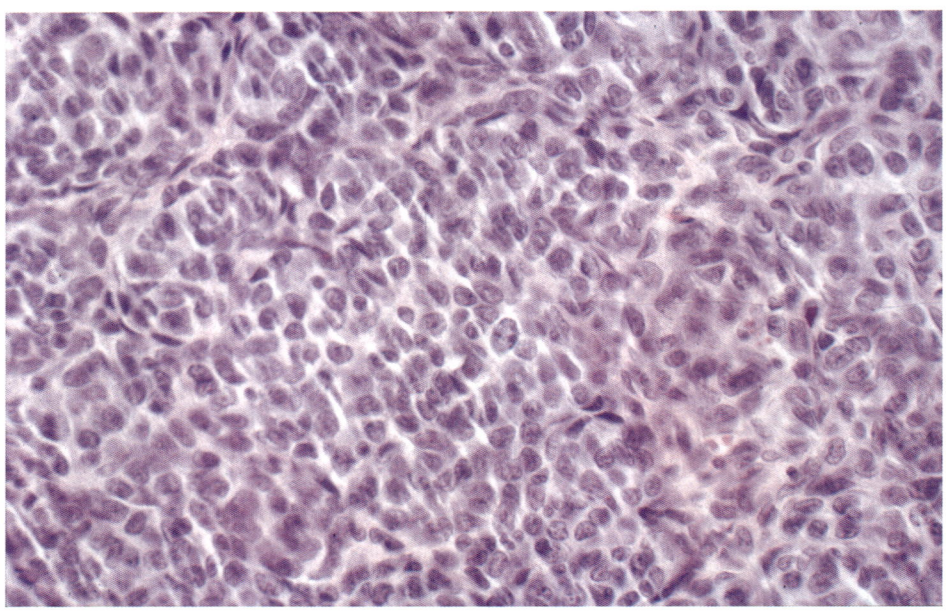

FIGURE 6-17 *Continued.* **C,** Small monotonous cuboidal melanocytes contain only scant cytoplasm and demonstrate high cellular density. Note nuclear pleomorphism; the cytomorphological appearance suggests a small round cell malignancy, such as lymphoma or neuroendocrine carcinoma.

Melanomas Simulating Spitz Nevus On occasion melanomas may exhibit features strongly suggesting a Spitz nevus. These features include both architectural and cytologic attributes, such as epidermal hyperplasia, wedge-shaped configuration, epidermal clefting about intraepidermal nests, large epithelioid cells, and spindle cells arranged in fascicles (94,96,99) (see Chapters 7 and 10).

Many studies have attempted to define the most useful criteria for distinguishing Spitz nevi from melanomas (see Chapters 7 and 10). Some of these criteria may be qualified as major, as they appear highly discriminating in most of the studies. These include deep mitoses (i.e., more than three mitoses in the lower third), high mitotic activity (i.e., $> 4/mm^2$), and marked nuclear atypia. Other criteria favoring melanoma are ulceration, asymmetry, deep extension, large size, abnormal mitoses, high cellularity, lack of maturation, and dusty melanin (94).

In addition to conventional melanomas and typical Spitz nevi (see Chapter 7), there is also an intermediate group of Spitz-like lesions that demonstrate not only some features of Spitz nevi but also varying degrees of atypicality. For these atypical Spitz tumors there is no set of criteria that can predict clinical outcome with certainty. Therefore, a grading system for the categorization of Spitz tumors in children and adolescents has been developed (see Chapter 7). As discussed in Chapters 7 and 10, much remains to be learned about the biologic nature of Spitz tumors in general and especially those showing overlap with melanoma.

For the differential diagnosis, see Chapters 7 and 10 for extensive discussions.

REFERENCES

1. Mark GJ, Mihm MC, Liteplo MG, et al. Congenital melanocytic nevi of the small and garment type. Hum Pathol 1973;4:395–418.
2. Walton RG, Jacobs AH, Cox AJ. Pigmented lesions in newborn infants. Br J Dermatol 1976;95:389–96.
3. Cramer SF. The melanocytic differentiation pathway in congenital melanocytic nevi: theoretical considerations. Pediatr Pathol 1988;8:253–65.
4. Stenn KS, Arons M, Hurwitz S. Patterns of congenital nevocellular nevi. J Am Acad Dermatol 1983;9:388–93.
5. Rhodes AR, Silberman RA, Harrist TJ, Melski JW. A histologic comparison of congenital and acquired nevomelanocytic nevi. Arch Dermatol 1985;121:1266–73.
6. Everett MA. Histopathology of congenital pigmented nevi. Am J Dermatopathol 1989;11:11–12.
7. Reed WB, Becker SW Sr, Becker SW Jr, Nickel WR. Giant pigmented nevi, melanoma, and leptomeningeal melanocytosis. Arch Dermatol 1965;91:100–18.
8. Reed RJ. Giant congenital nevi: a conceptualization of patterns. J Invest Dermatol 1993;100(Suppl):300S–12S.
9. Rhodes AR. Neoplasms: benign neoplasias, hyperplasias, and dysplasia of melanocytes. In: Fitzpatrick TB, Eisen AZ,

Wolff K, et al., eds. Dermatology in General Medicine. 4th ed. New York: McGraw-Hill, 1993;1026–37.
10. Pers AFM. Naevus pigmentosus giganticus: indikationer for operative Behandling. Ungeskrift Laeger 1963;125:613–9.
11. Lorentzen M, Pers M, Bretteville-Jensen G. The incidence of malignant transformation in giant pigmented nevi. Scand J Plast Reconstr Surg 1977;71:163–7.
12. Lanier VC Jr, Pickrell KL, Georgiade NG. Congenital giant nevi: clinical and pathological considerations. Plast Reconstr Surg 1976;58:48–54.
13. Greeley PW, Middleton AG, Curtin JW. Incidence of malignancy in giant pigmented nevi. Plast Reconstr Surg 1965;36:26–37.
14. Pilney FT, Broadbent TR, Woolf RM. Giant pigmented nevus of the face: surgical management. Plast Reconstr Surg 1967;40:469–74.
15. Kopf AW, Bart RS, Hennessey P. Congenital nevocytic nevi and malignant melanoma. J Am Acad Dermatol 1979; 1:123–30.
16. NIH Consensus Conference. Precursor to malignant melanoma. J Am Med Assoc 1984;251:1864–6.
17. Fox H, Emery JL, Goodbody RA, et al. Neurocutaneous melanosis. Arch Dis Child 1964;39:508-16.
18. Hoffman HJ, Freeman A. Primary malignant leptomeningeal melanoma in association with giant hairy nevi: report of two cases. J Neurosurg 1967;26:62–71.
19. Kadonaga JN, Frieden IJ. Neurocutaneous melanosis: definition and review of the literature. J Am Acad Dermatol 1991;24:747–55.
20. DeDavid M, Seth JO, Provost N, et al. Neurocutaneous melanosis: clinical features of large congenital melanocytic nevi in patients with manifest central nervous system melanosis. J Am Acad Dermatol 1996;35:529–38.
21. Kaplan EN. The risk of malignancy in large congenital nevi. Plast Reconstr Surg 1974;53:421–8.
22. Rhodes AR, Wood WC, Sober AJ, Mihm MC Jr. Nonepidermal origin of malignant melanoma associated with a giant congenital nevocellular nevus. Plast Reconstr Surg 1981;67:782–90.
23. Rhodes AR, Sober AJ, Day CL, et al. The malignant potential of small congenital nevocellular nevi. An estimate of association based on a histologic study of 234 primary cutaneous melanomas. J Am Acad Dermatol 1982;6:230–41.
24. Rhodes AR, Melski JW. Small congenital nevocellular nevi and the risk of cutaneous melanoma. J Pediatr 1982;100:219–24.
25. Illig L, Weidner F, Hundeiker M, et al. Congenital nevi less than or equal to 10 cm as precursors to melanoma. 52 cases, a review, and a new conception. Arch Dermatol 1985;121:1274–81.
26. Swerdlow AJ, English JSC, Qiao Z. The risk of melanoma in patient with congenital nevi: a cohort study. J Am Acad Dermatol 1995;32:595–99.
27. Dawson HA, Atherton DJ, Mayou B. A prospective study of congenital melanocytic naevi: progress report and evaluation after 6 years. Brit J Dermatol 1996;134:617–623.
28. Shpall S, Frieden I, Chesney M, Newman T. Risk of malignant transformation of congenital melanocytic nevi in blacks. Pediatr Dermatol 1994;11:204-208.
29. Sahin S, Levin L, Kopf AW, et al. Risk of melanoma in medium-sized congenital melanocytic nevi: a follow-up study. J Am Acad Dermatol 1998;39(3):428–33.
30. Castilla EE, da Graca Dutra M, Orioli-Parreiras IM. Epidemiology of congenital pigmented naevi: I. Incidence rates and relative frequencies. Br J Dermatol 1981;104:307–15.
31. Marghoob AA, Schoenback SP, Kopf AW, et al. Large congenital melanocytic nevi and the risk for the development of malignant melanoma. A prospective study. Arch Dermatol 1996;132:170–5.
32. DeDavid M, Orlow SJ, Provost N, et al. A study of large congenital melanocytic nevi and associated malignant melanomas: review of cases in the New York University Registry and the world literature. J Am Acad Dermatol 1997;36(3):409–15.
33. Kroon S, Clemmensen OJ, Hastrup N. Incidence of congenital melanocytic nevi in newborn babies in Denmark. J Am Acad Dermatol 1987;17:422–6.
34. Hamming N. Anatomy and embryology of the eyelids: a review with special reference to the development of divided nevi. Pediatr Dermatol 1983;1:51–8.
35. Rhodes AR, Slifman NR, Korf BR. Familial aggregation of small congenital nevomelanocytic nevi. Am J Med Genet 1985;22:315–26.
36. Pack GT, Davis J. Nevus giganticus pigmentosus with malignant transformation. Surgery 1961;49:347–54.
37. Solomon L, Eng AM, Bené M, Loeffel D. Giant congenital neuroid melanocytic nevus. Arch Dermatol 1980;116:318–20.
38. Albert VA Barnhill RL, Sober AJ. Leukoderma in association with giant congenital nevi: report of 2 cases. Dermatology 1992;185:140–2.
39. Barnhill RL, Fleischli M. Histologic features of congenital melanocytic nevi in infants less than a year of age. J Am Acad Dermatol 1995;33:780–5.
40. Silvers DN, Helwig EB. Melanocytic nevi in neonates. J Am Acad Dermatol 1981;4:166–75.
41. Zitelli JA, Grant MG, Abell E, Boyd JB. Histologic patterns of congenital nevocytic nevi and implications for treatment. J Am Acad Dermatol 1984;11:402–9.
42. Nickoloff BJ, Walton R, Pregerson-Rodan K, et al. Immunohistologic patterns of congenital nevocellular nevi. Arch Dermatol 1986;122:1263–8.
43. Rhodes AR. Congenital nevomelanocytic nevi. Histologic

patterns in the first year of life and evolution during childhood. Arch Dermatol 1986;122:1257–62.
44. Clemmensen OJ, Kroon S. The histology of "congenital features" in early acquired melanocytic nevi. J Am Acad Dermatol 1988;19:742–6.
45. Walsh MY, MacKie RM. Histologic features of value in differentiating small congenital melanocytic nevi from acquired naevi. Histopathology 1988;12:145–54.
46. Hendrickson MR, Ross JC. Neoplasms arising in congenital giant nevi: morphologic study of seven cases and a review of the literature. Am J Surg Pathol 1981;5:109–35.
47. Mancianti ML, Clark WH, Hayes FA, Herlyn M. Malignant melanoma simulants arising in congenital melanocytic nevi do not show experimental evidence for a malignant phenotype. Am J Pathol 1990;136:817–29.
48. Clark WH Jr, Elder DE, Guerry D IV. Dysplastic nevi and malignant melanoma. In: Farmer ER, Hood AF, eds. Pathology of the Skin. Norwalk, CT: Appleton & Lange, 1990;684–756.
49. Weidner N, Flanders DJ, Jochimsen PR, Stamler FW. Neurosarcomatous malignant melanoma arising in a neuroid giant congenital melanocytic nevus. Arch Dermatol 1985; 121:1302–6.
50. Zúniga SR, Las Heras J, Benvenisto S. Rhabdomyosarcoma arising in a congenital nevus associated with neurocutaneous melanosis in an neonate. J Pediatr Surg 1987;22: 1036–38.
51. Demian SDE, Donnelly WH, Frias JL, Monif GRG. Placental lesions in congenital giant pigmented nevi. Am J Clin Pathol 1974;61:438–42.
52. Sotelo-Avila C, Graham M, Hanby DE, Rudolph AJ. Nevus cell aggregates in the placenta. A histochemical and electron microscopic study. Am J Clin Pathol 1988;89: 395–400.
53. Jauniaux E, de Meeus M-C, Verellen G, et al. Giant congenital melanocytic nevus with placental involvement. Long-term follow-up of a case and review of the literature. Pediatr Pathol 1993;13:717–21.
54. Hara K. Melanocytic lesions in lymph nodes associated with congenital naevus. Histopathology 1993;23:445–51.
55. Ball RA, Genest D, Sander M, et al. Congenital melanocytic nevi with placental infiltration by melanocytes: a benign condition that mimics metastatic melanoma. Arch Dermatol 1998;134:711–4.
56. Stenziger W, Suter L, Schumann J. DNA aneuploidy in congenital melanocytic nevi: suggestive evidence for premalignant changes. J Invest Dermatol 1984;82:569–72.
57. Newton JA, Camplejohn RS, McGibbon DH. The flow cytometry of melanocytic skin lesions. Br J Cancer 1988;58: 606–10.
58. Steijlen PM, Hamm H, van Erp PEJ, et al. Immunohistologic evidence for the malignant potential of congenital melanocytic nevi. J Invest Dermatol 1989;92:366–70.
59. Bastian BC, Xiong J, Frieden IJ, et al. Genetic changes in neoplasms arising in congenital melanocytic nevi: differences between nodular proliferations and melanomas. Am J Pathol 2002;161(4):1163–9.
60. Fromont HG, Fraitag S, Wolter M, et al. DNA content and cell proliferation in giant congenital melanocytic naevi (GCMN). An analysis by image cytometry. J Cutan Pathol 1998;25(8):401–6.
61. Papp T, Pemsel H, Zimmermann R, et al. Mutational analysis of the N-ras, p53, p16INK4a, CDK4, and MC1R genes in human congenital melanocytic naevi. J Med Genet 1999;36(8):610–614.
62. Skov-Jensen T, Hastrup J, Lambrethsen E. Malignant melanoma in children. Cancer 1966;19:620–6.
63. Trozak DJ, Rowland WD, Hu F. Metastatic malignant melanoma in prepubertal children. Pediatr 1975;55:191–204.
64. Roth ME, Grant-Kels JM, Kuhn K, et al. Melanoma in children. J Am Acad Dermatol 1990;22:265–74.
65. Richardson SK, Tannous ZS, Mihm MC, Jr. Congenital and infantile melanoma: review of the literature and report of an uncommon variant, pigment-synthesizing melanoma. J Am Acad Dermatol 2002;47(1):77–90.
66. Potter JF, Schoeneman M. Metastasis of maternal cancer to the placenta and fetus. Cancer 1970;25:380–8.
67. Baergen RN, Johnson D, Moore T, Benirschke K. Maternal melanoma metastatic to the placenta: a case report and review of the literature. Arch Pathol Lab Med 1997;121: 508–11.
68. Coe HE. Malignant pigmented mole in an infant. Northwest Med 1925;24:181–5.
69. Lyall D. Malignant melanoma in infancy. J Am Med Assoc 1967;202:1153–63.
70. Oldhoff J, Koudstall J. Congenital papillomatous malignant melanoma of the skin. Cancer 1968;21:1193–7.
71. Conn A, Nicolescu F, Popescu G. Malignant melanoma developing in intrauterine life. Rom Med Rev 1971;15:41–2.
72. Voinov EA, Semskov VS, Maleskina LA. Case of congenital skin melanoma. Arch Patol 1973;35:78–80.
73. Stromberg BV. Malignant melanoma in children. J Pediatr Surg 1979;14:465–7.
74. Hayes FA, Green AA. Malignant melanoma in childhood: clinical course and response to chemotherapy. J Clin Oncol 1984;2:1229–34.
75. Prose NS, Laude TA, Heilman ER, Coren C. Congenital malignant melanoma. Pediatr 1987;79:967–70.
76. Fish J, Smith EB, Canby JP. Malignant melanoma in childhood. Pediatr Surg 1966;59:309–15.
77. Sweet LK, Connerty HV. Congenital melanoma. Report of a case in which antenatal metastasis occurred. Am J Diseases Child 1941;62:1029–40.
78. Borges AF, Lineberger AS. Malignant melanoma without metastasis in a giant nevus. Ann Plast Surg 1984;12: 454–60.

79. Schneiderman H, Wu AY-Y, Campbell WA, et al. Congenital melanoma with multiple prenatal metastases. Cancer 1987;1371–7.
80. Angelucci D, Natali PG, Amerio PL, et al. Rapid perinatal growth mimicking malignant transformation in a giant congenital melanocytic nevus. Hum Pathol 1991;22:297–301.
81. Baader W, Kropp R, Tapper D. Congenital malignant melanoma. Plast Reconstr Surg 1992;90:53–6.
82. Workman ML, Kaye VN, Anderson PM, Cunnningham BL. Malignant melanoma with evidence of maturation arising from a giant congenital nevocellular nevus. Ann Plast Surg 1992;28:381–5.
83. Mahre E. Malignant melanomas in children. Arch Pathol Microbiol Scand 1963;59:184–93.
84. Boddie AW, Smith L, McBride CM. Malignant melanoma in children and young adults. South Med J 1978;71:1074–8.
85. Bader JL, Li FP, Olmstead PM, et al. Childhood malignant melanoma. Incidence and etiology. Am J Pediatr Hematol Oncol 1985;7:341–5.
86. Hoang MT, Eichenfield LF. The rising incidence of melanoma in children and adolescents. Dermatol Nurs 2000;12(3):188–93.
87. Berg P, Lindelof B. Differences in malignant melanoma between children and adolescents. A 35-year epidemiological study. Arch Dermatol 1997;133(3):295–7.
88. Prosdocimo T, Smith M, Polack EP. The diagnosis and treatment of childhood melanoma. W V Med J 2002;98(4):149–51.
89. Malec E, Lagerlöf B. Malignant melanoma of the skin in children registered in the Swedish Cancer Registry during 1959–1971. Scand J Plast Reconstr Surg 1977;11:125–9.
90. Pratt CB, Palmer MK, Thatcher N, Crowther D. Malignant melanoma in children and adolescents. Cancer 1981;47:392–7.
91. Moss ALH, Briggs JC. Cutaneous malignant melanoma in the young. Br J Plast Surg 1986;39:537–41.
92. Partoft S, Sterlind A, Hou-Jensen K, Drzewiecki KT. Malignant melanoma of the skin in children (0 to 14 years of age) in Denmark, 1943–1982. Scand J Plast Reconstr Surg 1989;23:55–8.
93. Reintgen DS, Vollmer R, Seigler HF. Juvenile malignant melanoma. Surg Gyn Obstet 1989;168:249–53.
94. Barnhill RL, Flotte T, Fleischli M, Perez-Atayde AR. Childhood melanoma and atypical Spitz-tumors Cancer 1995;76:1833–45.
95. Ceballos PL, Ruiz-Maldonado R, Mihm MC. Melanoma in children. N Engl J Med 1995;332:656-63.
96. Spatz A, Ruiter D, Hardmeier T, et al. Malignant melanoma in childhood: An EORTC-MCG multicenter study on the clinico-pathological aspects. Int J Cancer 1996;68:317–24.
97. Milton GW, Shaw HM, Thompson JF, McCarthy WH. Cutaneous melanoma in childhood: incidence and prognosis. Australas J Dermatol 1997;38(Suppl 1):S44–8.
98. Ruiz-Maldonado R, de la Luz Orozco-Covarrubias M. Malignant melanoma in children. Arch Dermatol 1997;133:363–71.
99. Barnhill RL. Childhood melanoma. Semin Diag Pathol 1998;15:189–94.
100. Saenz NC, Saenz-Badillos J, Busam K, et al. Childhood melanoma survival. Cancer 1999;85(3):750–4.
101. Conti EM, Cercato MC, Gatta G, et al. Childhood melanoma in Europe since 1978: a population-based survival study. Eur J Cancer 2001;37(6):780–4.
102. Schmid-Wendtner MH, Berking C, Baumert J, et al. Cutaneous melanoma in childhood and adolescence: an analysis of 36 patients. J Am Acad Dermatol 2002;46:874–9.
103. Green MH, Clark WH Jr, Tucker MA, et al. High risk of malignant melanoma in melanoma-prone families with dysplastic nevi. Ann Intern Med 1985;102:458–65.
104. Carlson JA, Mu XC, Slominski A, et al. Melanocytic proliferations associated with lichen sclerosus. Arch Dermatol 2002;138:77–87.

CHAPTER 7

Spitz Nevus and Variants

Raymond L. Barnhill and Klaus J. Busam

Spitz nevus is also known as Spitz tumor, spindle and epithelioid cell nevus of large spindle and/or epithelioid cells, spindle cell nevus, juvenile melanoma, and benign juvenile melanoma. The Spitz nevus is a benign melanocytic neoplasm usually acquired with a distinct histopathologic appearance. The characteristic that sets this lesion apart from other nevi is the presence of large epithelioid and/or spindle cells in varying proportions. The lesion is frequently misdiagnosed as malignant melanoma.

TERMINOLOGY

Examples of melanocytic tumors resembling malignant melanoma on gross and microscopic appearance but behaving clinically in a benign manner were first described by Darier and Civatte (1) in 1910 and Miescher (2) in 1933. The discrepancy between histologic features that were at that time thought to represent melanoma and the benign clinical behavior was noted especially in children. This led Pack and Anglem (3) to develop the concept of *prepubertal melanoma*. They used this term for melanocytic tumors that histologically mimicked melanoma but failed to metastasize. Spitz's (4) major contribution was to establish histologic criteria to distinguish such lesions, which she termed *juvenile melanoma*, from true metastasizing melanoma. In her original series of childhood melanomas, the presence of giant cells was highlighted as the single most distinctive feature favoring the diagnosis of a juvenile tumor.

Subsequently, it became apparent that lesions clinically and histologically similar to those described by Spitz occurred also in adults, although less frequently (5,6). The concept of a distinct type of benign melanocytic tumor, which was different from other known nevi thus emerged. The original term used by Spitz, *juvenile melanoma,* and its modification by Kopf and Andrade (7) to *benign juvenile melanoma* were ultimately abandoned, because the word *melanoma* indicates malignancy and the lesion could also be found in adults (6). A variety of alternative terms has been proposed to name this lesion. Helwig (8) suggested spindle and epithelioid cell nevus, which emphasizes the distinct cell types of this nevus and is widely accepted. The term *nevus of large spindle and/or epithelioid cells* (9) was proposed as a more precise name, since the spectrum of cytologic appearances of this nevus includes not only an admixture of both cell types but also exclusively spindle or epithelioid cells. However the term is too long and cumbersome for routine diagnostic use. *Spitz nevus* is now preferred by many because of its simplicity. This nondescriptive term allows one to include a spectrum of similar albeit variable histomorphology and does not carry misleading connotations.

Nonetheless, the biologic nature of the Spitz nevus has not been sufficiently defined and is often controversial owing to its striking resemblance to melanoma in some proportion of cases and rare instances of metastases emanating from lesions diagnosed as Spitz nevus. The reasons for the latter quandary are the lack of long-term follow-up information concerning a sufficiently large group of well-characterized Spitz nevi, which would facilitate the development of reliable criteria (clinical, histopathologic, cytogenetic, etc.) for distinction of atypical variants of Spitz nevi and "Spitzoid" melanomas. Thus we prefer the term *Spitz tumor* to give recognition to the unusual nature of these lesions and to the idea that they may possess neoplastic properties beyond those of ordinary nevi. We contend that although Spitz tumors indeed share features in common with conventional melanocytic nevi, they also may potentially constitute a neoplastic continuum with melanoma or a Spitz-like malignant tumor. There are some emerging data to support the latter idea. Although we prefer the term Spitz tumor, Spitz nevus is currently the favored term in the literature and is used interchangeably with Spitz tumor in this chapter.

Since the early descriptions of Spitz nevi, it has become apparent that variants exist that share certain features with Spitz nevi but are distinct enough to justify a separate terminology. Of these, a number of variants, including the desmoplastic Spitz nevus and pigmented spindle cell nevus (tumor), are discussed in this chapter.

The terms *spitzoid*, *spitzian*, and *Spitz-like* are often used when lesions resemble Spitz tumors in one way or another but lack sufficient other features needed for diagnosis as Spitz nevus. Spitzoid features have been described in melanomas as well as in congenital and other nevi.

EPIDEMIOLOGY

Spitz nevi are relatively uncommon and may account for about 1% of melanocytic lesions surgically removed. Epidemiologic data regarding their incidence, age distribution, sex preference, geographic or ethnic predilection are scarce. Their annual incidence in Queensland, Australia, was estimated to be 1.4 cases/100,000 people compared to 25.4 cases/100,000 people for cutaneous melanoma (10). Most cases are diagnosed in children or adolescents. In a series of 262 patients with Spitz nevi in 1960, 85% were infants and children (11). In later series reported in the 1970s, the proportion of adult patients over 20 years of age was larger, reaching 20–30% of the cases (9,10,12). However, in these later series, there is probably a referral bias leading to an overrepresentation of adult patients (13). Although most Spitz nevi are acquired, congenital Spitz nevi occur (14,15) and may account for as many as 7% of cases. Spitz nevi are uncommon but do occur in individuals beyond the age of 40–50 years (12).

There is no obvious sexual predilection, although most reports indicate a slight female preponderance, especially in young adults (13). It has been suggested that the female preponderance of Spitz nevi in this age group may reflect the greater likelihood of their removal for cosmetic purposes (9). Most published cases of Spitz nevi have been described primarily in whites (13). Spitz nevi are thought to be rare in blacks and Asians (9,13).

Familial aggregation of Spitz nevi has been reported in identical twin boys (7), but the role of genetic factors has not been investigated systematically. It is believed that the great majority of Spitz nevi are sporadic with unknown cause.

CLINICAL FEATURES

Anatomic Site

Spitz nevus may occur anywhere on the body. However, there is a predilection for the face, especially the cheeks, and the lower extremities (6,11,16). In a large series of solitary Spitz nevi (17), 30% of 652 lesions were located on the lower extremities, 26% on the head, and 25% on the upper extremities. Most series report a female preponderance for lesions from the lower extremities (13).

Appearance and Presentation

In general, Spitz tumors are not sufficiently distinctive to be clinically recognized with any degree of reliability. They may present in a number of different ways. The most common form, typically observed in children, is that of a solitary; asymptomatic; red, pink, or flesh-colored; hairless; dome-shaped nodule (13,18). Some lesions may be tan, brown, or even black in color. Pigmentation tends to be seen more often in adolescents and adults (16,19). The surface appearance is usually smooth, but may be verrucous. Pedunculated and polypoid forms occur (7), and telangiectasia may be noted (7). Scale-crust, erosion, and ulceration are uncommon and, when present, generally reflect exogenous trauma (10). In children, the nodules tend to be slightly soft, but in adults, they are more often firm (9,18). Borders are usually sharp but may be irregular. In one series, 73% of lesions measured < 0.6 cm; and in 94%, the lesions were < 1 cm in size (10), although sizes up to 3 cm have rarely been reported (11). Some Spitz nevi are pruritic and tender (13). The duration of solitary Spitz nevus is usually < 9 months (13) but may vary from 1 month to more than 20 years.

Biologic Course

The natural history of Spitz nevi has not been clearly delineated. A small percentage of these lesions are present at birth, and some acquired ones are long-standing. Although there has been speculation that these lesions involute as do conventional nevi (20), or possibly evolve to conventional nevi, these outcomes have not been documented. Spitz nevi occurring in children are often compound and richly cellular, whereas those in adults are commonly dermal (or predominately dermal) and often show sclerosis (desmoplasia) of collagen, suggesting involution over time. However, the latter observations are only cross-sectional at best.

In most instances, there is a clinical history of recent onset and rapid growth or change. The vast majority of lesions with characteristics of Spitz nevi are benign. However, because of the histologic resemblance of Spitz nevi to some melanomas, the presence of atypical variants, and rare metastases from such lesions, there is some justification for the belief that uncommonly or rarely some Spitz tumors are capable of aggressive behavior and that some may progress to malignancy (21–23). The exact nature and classification of these lesions awaits definitive study. An aggressive variant termed malignant Spitz tumor or metastasizing Spitz tumor has been reported to result in regional lymph node metastases (see below) (21). On the other hand, such lesions must be considered to be melanomas until proved otherwise.

Multiple Spitz Nevi

Multiple Spitz nevi have been reported to occur either in a grouped (agminate) or disseminated pattern (24–27). The disseminated type is characterized by numerous, up to hundreds of Spitz tumors all over the body, typically

FIGURE 7-1 Spitz nevus. **A,** Note small size, dome-shaped morphology, striking symmetry, and sharp lateral demarcation. **B,** Higher magnification of panel A showing the overall symmetry of the lesion. There is moderate epidermal hyperplasia with a smooth surface topography.

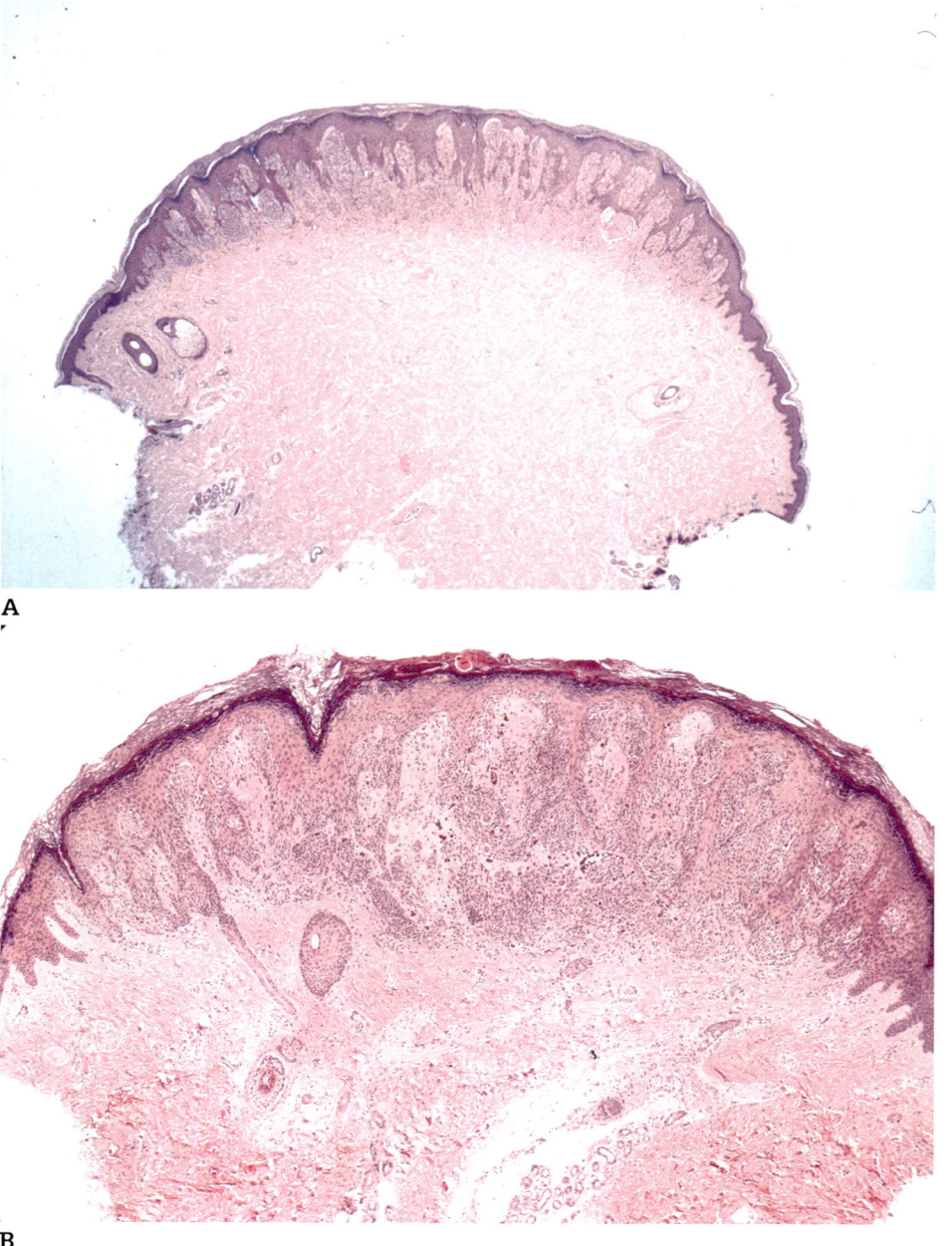

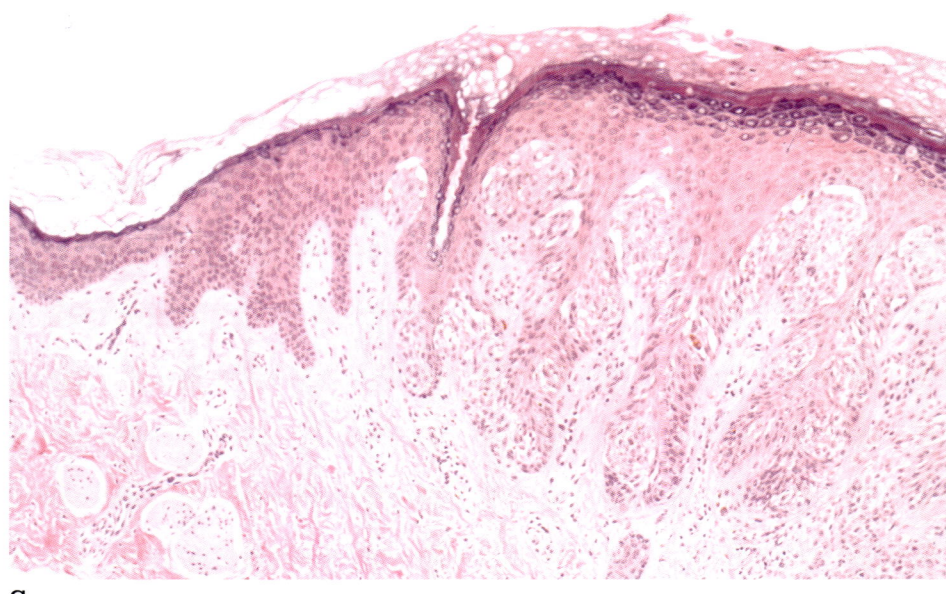

FIGURE 7-1 *Continued.* **C,** Sharp lateral demarcation of nevus.

sparing the palms, soles, and mucous membranes. Only a few cases have been reported to date, primarily affecting adults. In a review of 33 cases from the literature, 11 instances were reported in which multiple agminate Spitz nevi arose within a congenital circumscribed area of hyperpigmentation, most often described as a café-au-lait macule (27). In two instances, agminated Spitz nevi were reported to develop within a congenital speckled lentiginous nevus (28–31). Multiple agminate Spitz nevi affect women nearly twice as often as men, tend to occur on average earlier in life (76% younger than 6 years of age) than solitary Spitz nevi, and show a predilection for the face (50% of the cases), most often the cheeks. Some congenital forms have been reported (15,30) and may mimic melanoma clinically (31). Agminate Spitz nevi have been reported to follow trauma, such as previous excision of a solitary Spitz nevus, sunburn, and radiation therapy (32).

Clinical Differential Diagnosis

As the variety of presentations suggests, the clinical features of Spitz nevus are usually not distinctive enough to allow a correct diagnosis on clinical grounds alone. Weedon (10,13) reported that a correct clinical diagnosis is made in only about 20% of childhood cases and in < 10% of adult lesions. The most frequent clinical diagnosis is that of a common acquired melanocytic nevus. In about 10% of cases, malignant melanoma is suspected. Other lesions that may be mimicked by Spitz nevi on gross appearance and have been mentioned in the differential diagnoses of various series include pyogenic granuloma, juvenile xanthogranuloma, dermatofibroma, verruca vulgaris, insect bite granuloma, molluscum contagiosum, neurofibroma, adnexal tumors, and mastocytoma (13).

Histopathological Features

The histopathologic criteria for Spitz nevi have evolved from a body of published work reflecting individual series of Spitz nevi collected and reported by individual authors, often without long-term follow-up information (see Table 7.2) (1–46). In effect, the criteria for diagnosis have usually been based on circular reasoning and often have contradicted the criteria proposed by other authors (23). Nonetheless, from this collective body of work there has emerged perhaps an idealized depiction of the Spitz nevus that is currently described in most textbooks. In contrast, many Spitz nevi encountered on a regular basis in routine practice may deviate from this textbook image of what a Spitz nevus should be. A population-based study with long-term follow-up would help better refine criteria for Spitz nevi.

Spitz nevi may be junctional, compound, or intradermal (Figs. 7-1 to 7-7). The majority (about two thirds or more) are compound lesions (Fig. 7-1). Approximately 5–10% of the cases are junctional (13,33) (Fig. 7-7). Intradermal Spitz nevi account for 12–20% of the lesions and are mainly seen in adults (13,33,34) (Fig. 7-2).

The most distinctive histologic feature of Spitz nevus and an absolute prerequisite for its diagnosis is the presence of large epithelioid and/or spindle-shaped melanocytes or an admixture thereof (13) (Fig. 7-3). A number of other features in addition to cell type, however, need

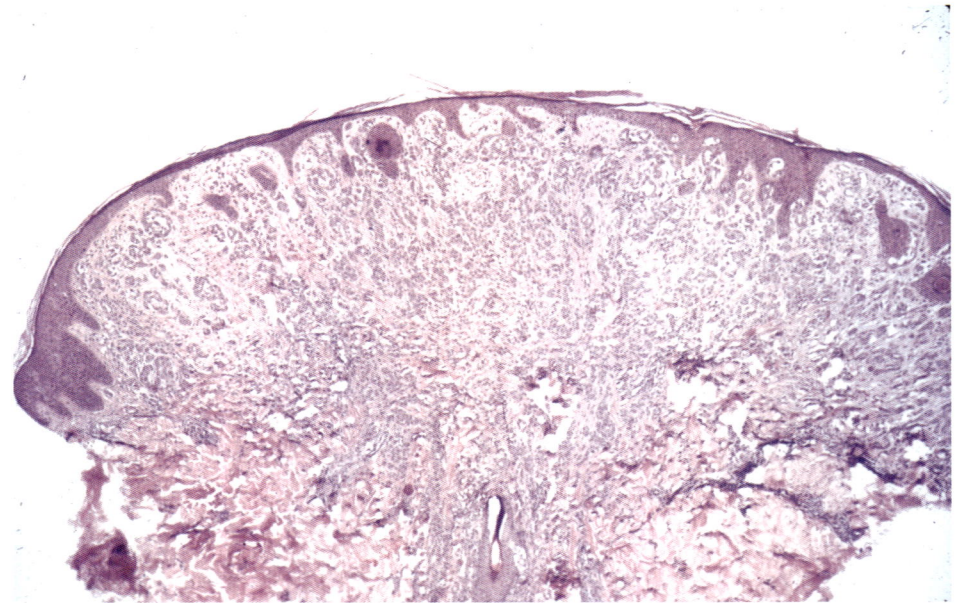

FIGURE 7-2 Spitz nevus, mainly dermal type. The lesion is notable for its dome-shaped profile, symmetry, and wedge-like extension into the dermis.

FIGURE 7-3 Spitz nevus. **A,** There are large intraepidermal nests of large spindle and epithelioid cells. Note the "raining down" pattern. **B,** Higher magnification of panel A showing junctional nest of spindle cells and epithelioid cells. Within the epidermis above the dermal papilla is a coalescent aggregate of eosinophilic globules (Kamino bodies).

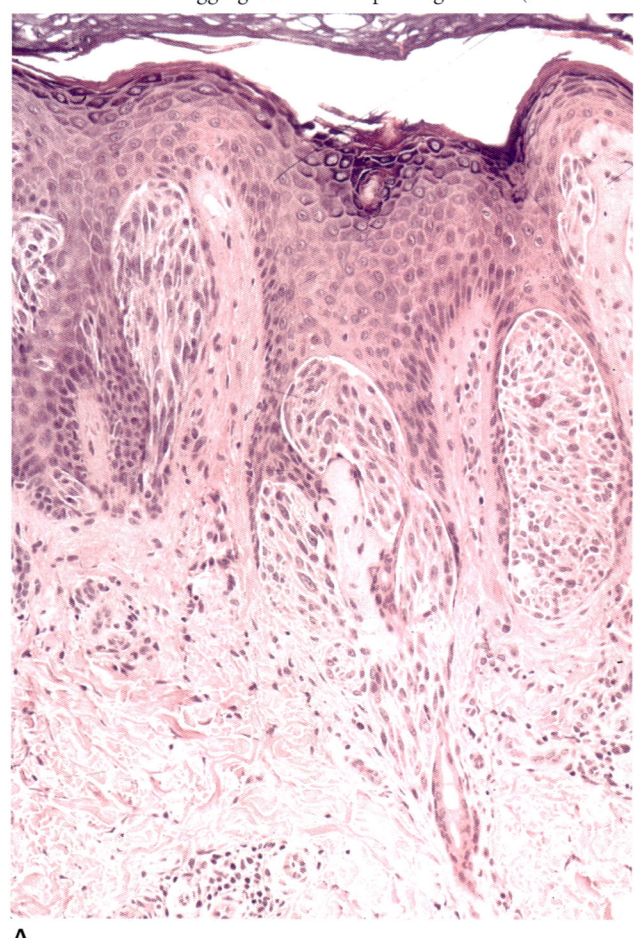
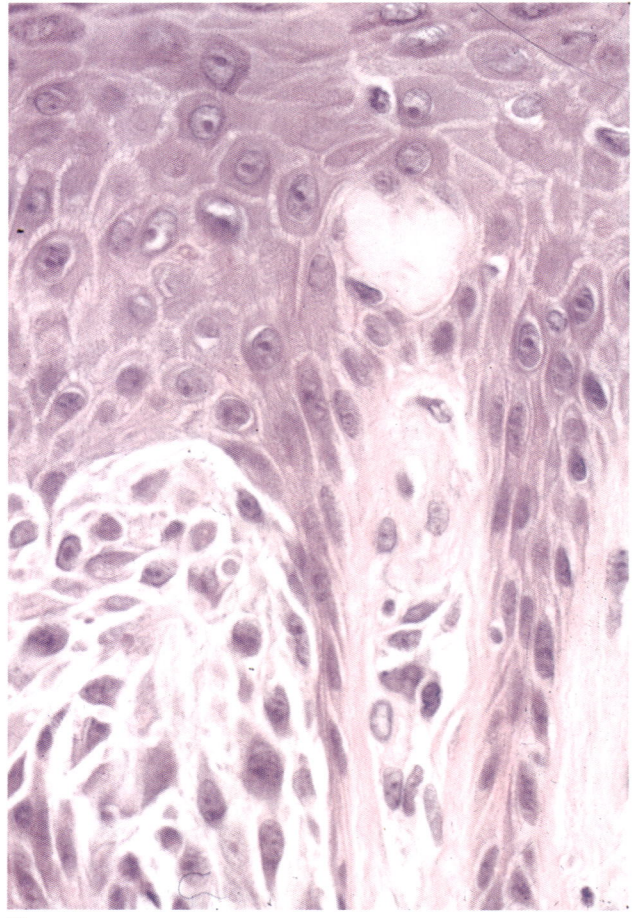

A   B

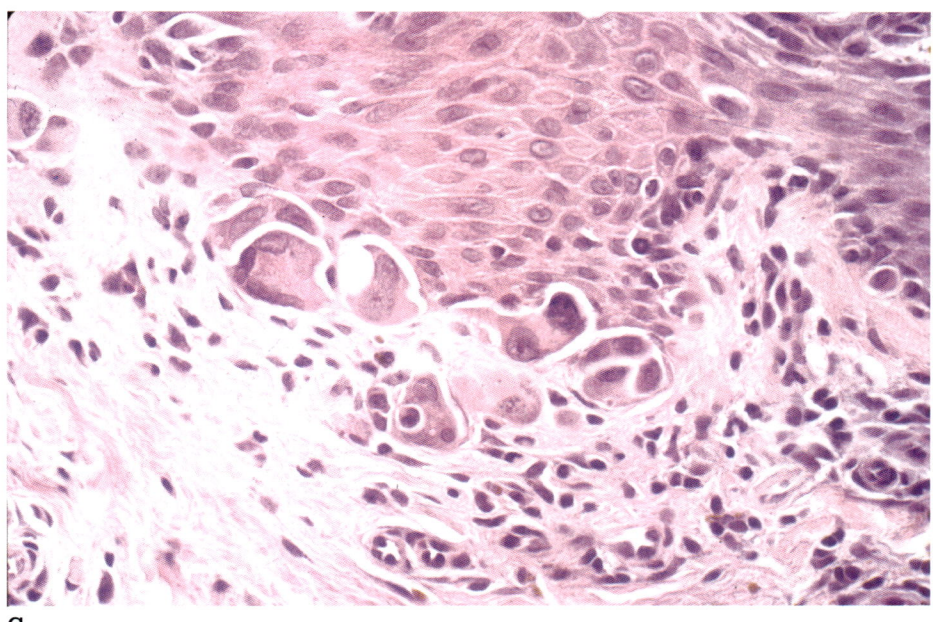

FIGURE 7-3 *Continued.* **C,** Nevus giant cells along the dermoepidermal junction.

to be assessed before a final diagnosis of Spitz nevus can be rendered (9,10,13). Some of these features, such as symmetry and sharp lateral demarcation, bear more weight than others, such as retraction spaces and perivascular distribution of lymphocytic infiltrates. These features are summarized in Table 7-1.

Spindle and/or Epithelioid Cell Type *Spindle cell melanocytes* in Spitz nevi are elongated fusiform, and often plump (Figs. 7-3B and 7-4A,C). Occasional tapered cytoplasmic processes resembling dendrites may be observed. They possess centrally located nuclei, comparable in size to or even larger than nuclei of keratinocytes (Fig. 7-4C). Nuclear contours are typically smooth and regular. The chromatin pattern is usually finely dispersed or slightly vesicular. Typically, a distinct, single, centrally located, round eosinophilic or amphophilic nucleolus is present. The cytoplasm is usually well developed with recognizable cytoplasmic borders. In most cases, the cytoplasm appears eosinophilic but may be bluish.

At the dermoepidermal junction, the spindle cells are arranged in fascicles or elongated nests, characteristically in vertical orientation to the epidermal surface and often adjacent to elongated rete ridges (Fig. 7-3A). In some instances, the spindle cells have whorled or concentric arrangements within nests. Both the overall size of the nests and the size of the individual melanocytes within them are variable and tend to decrease in the deeper parts of the lesion. Melanocytes may be tightly packed or loosely aggregated within their nests and fascicles. In the dermis, the spindle cell melanocytes of Spitz nevi are also arranged in fascicles but may be more angulated in their orientation to the epidermal surface (Fig. 7-4B,C).

Their plumper appearance, their nuclear features, and their arrangement in vertically streaming fascicles make spindle cell melanocytes of Spitz nevi quite distinct from spindle cells of other nevi, such as the slender dendritic cells of blue nevi or the melanocytes with schwannian features (type C melanocytes) of common acquired nevi.

Epithelioid melanocytes in Spitz nevi are large, round, oval, polygonal, rhomboidal, or polyangular cells with distinct cellular borders (Fig. 7-5). Their nuclei are enlarged, round, oval, and sometimes irregularly shaped or lobulated. The nuclei have similar chromatin patterns as the spindle cell forms and also frequently show one large centrally placed nucleolus. In some cases, the cytoplasmic and/or nuclear contours may become very irregular, leading to a pleomorphic appearance. This is particularly pronounced when large multinucleated forms are present (Fig. 7-3C). Such pleomorphism may be more striking than in melanoma but usually affects only a minority of cells. Some nuclei may appear hyperchromatic but close inspection reveals uniformly dispersed basophilia. Often such basophilia results from tissue crush artifact. Multinucleated cells are often seen when epithelioid forms constitute the predominant cell type of a Spitz nevus. Both mononuclear and multinucleate epithelioid cell forms may be strikingly large and bizarre on occasion. The

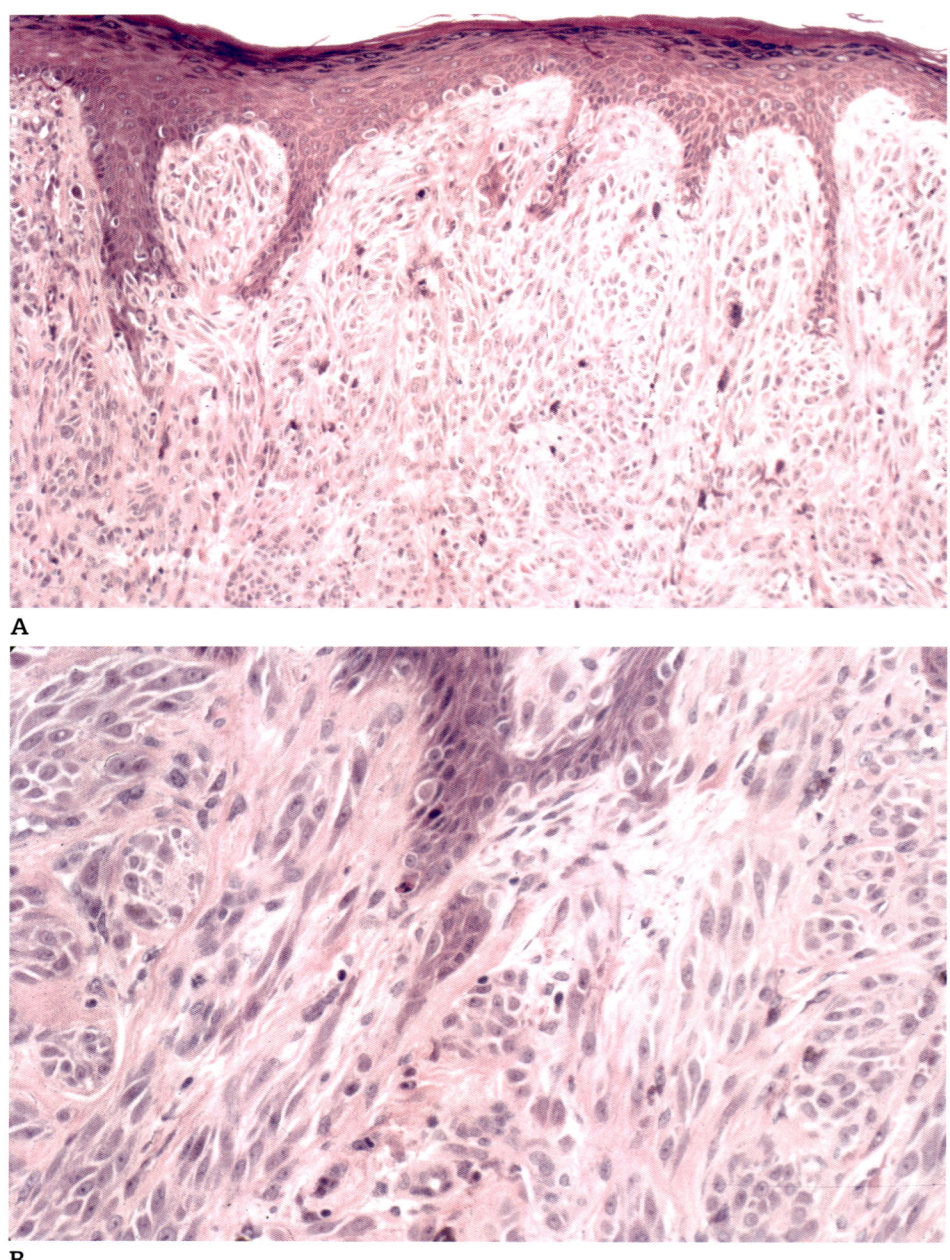

FIGURE 7-4 Spitz nevus. **A,** Diffuse sheet of spindle cells in the upper dermis. **B,** Fascicles of large spindle cells with abundant cytoplasm.

cytoplasm of epithelioid cells is usually abundant with a homogeneous eosinophilic or bluish, and often ground glass or opaque appearance. Melanin is typically absent or scarce.

The two cell types may be admixed in varying proportions, but either may occur alone. Regardless of the proportion of spindle and epithelioid cells, one of the most characteristic features of Spitz nevus is the uniformity of the cells and nuclei. From side to side in horizontal zones, the cells tend to show a strikingly uniform appearance and size. However, from top to bottom, despite maintaining a monotonous appearance, the cells and nuclei usually diminish in size (discussed later) (Fig. 7-6). In all age groups, Spitz nevi with predominant spindle cell morphology are the most common type and are especially prevalent in adults (35). Spitz nevi of the epithelioid cell type are observed mainly in childhood. In one study, 89% of the tumors contained predominantly spindle cells and

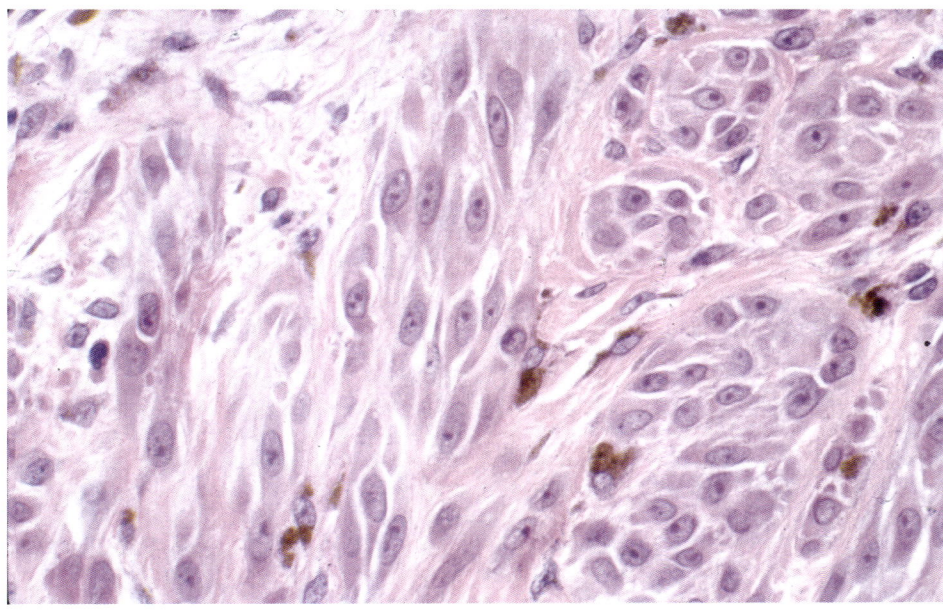

C

FIGURE 7-4 *Continued.* **C,** Note the striking uniformity of the spindle cells, which have abundant pink cytoplasm. Also note the uniformity of the nuclei. The chromatin is evenly dispersed, and one or two nucleoli are present.

11% primarily epithelioid cells (10). Compound epithelioid-type Spitz nevi show usually small junctional nests, often consisting of only a few cells. In contrast, large junctional nests are often observed in predominantly spindle cell Spitz nevi.

While the presence of spindle and/or epithelioid cells is a prerequisite for the diagnosis of Spitz nevus, they must appear in an appropriate architectural arrangement before a final diagnosis of Spitz nevus can be made. The major architectural criteria are symmetry and sharp lateral demar-

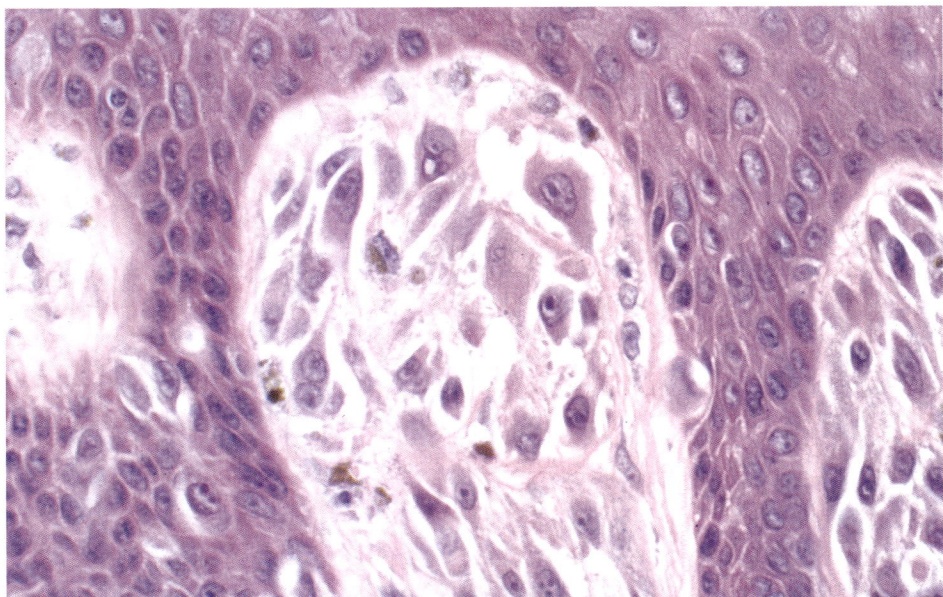

FIGURE 7-5 Large epithelioid cells and spindle cells in the papillary dermis within a Spitz nevus. Note the angular contours of cells; some are triangular, rhomboidal, and polygonal in morphology. The cytoplasm is pink with a ground glass appearance. Many nuclei contain prominent nucleoli.

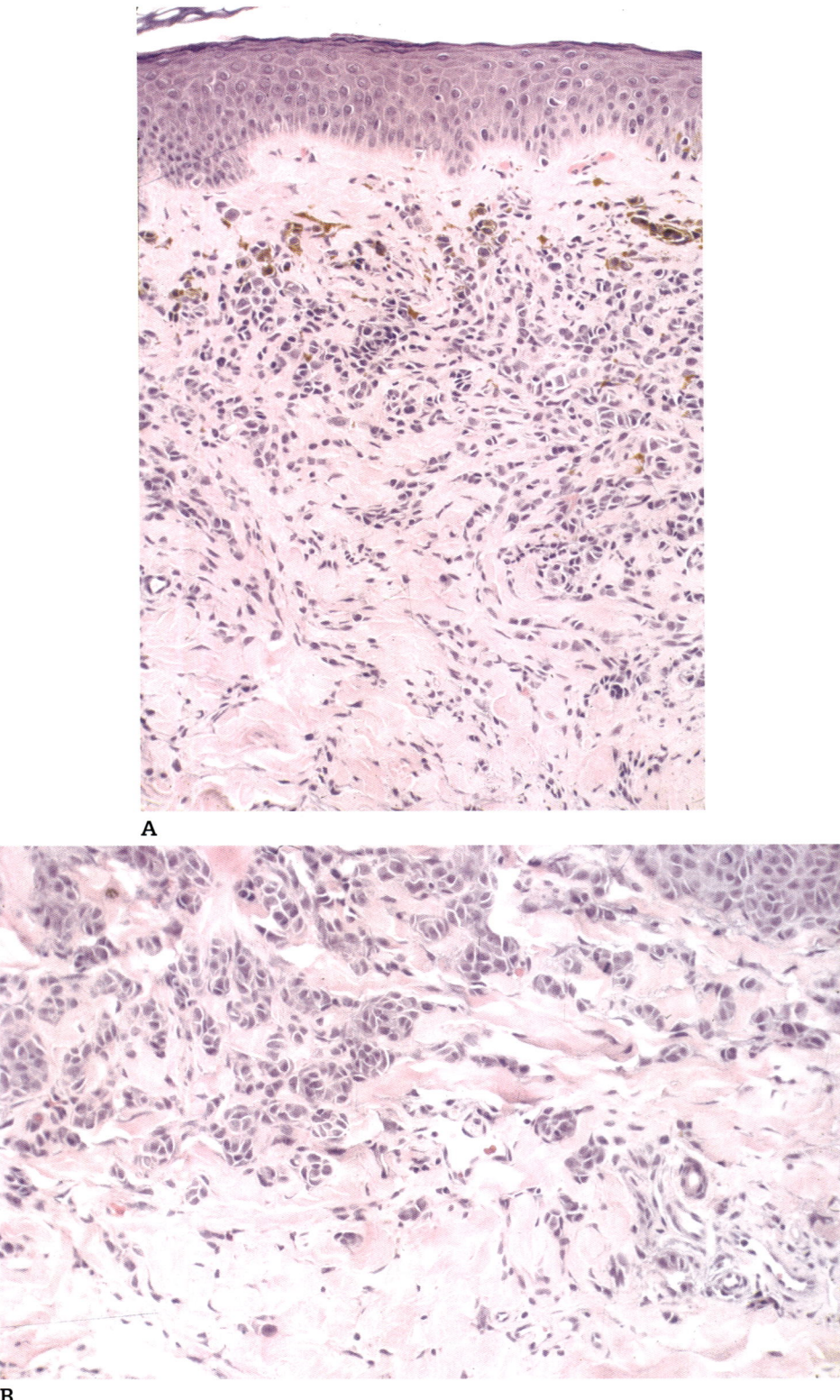

FIGURE 7-6 Spitz nevus. **A,** The lesion shows maturation from top to bottom. The overall cellularity is reduced near the base of the lesion. The cells infiltrate the collagen as cords of cells and individual cells. The stroma is slightly sclerotic. **B,** Higher magnification of panel A.

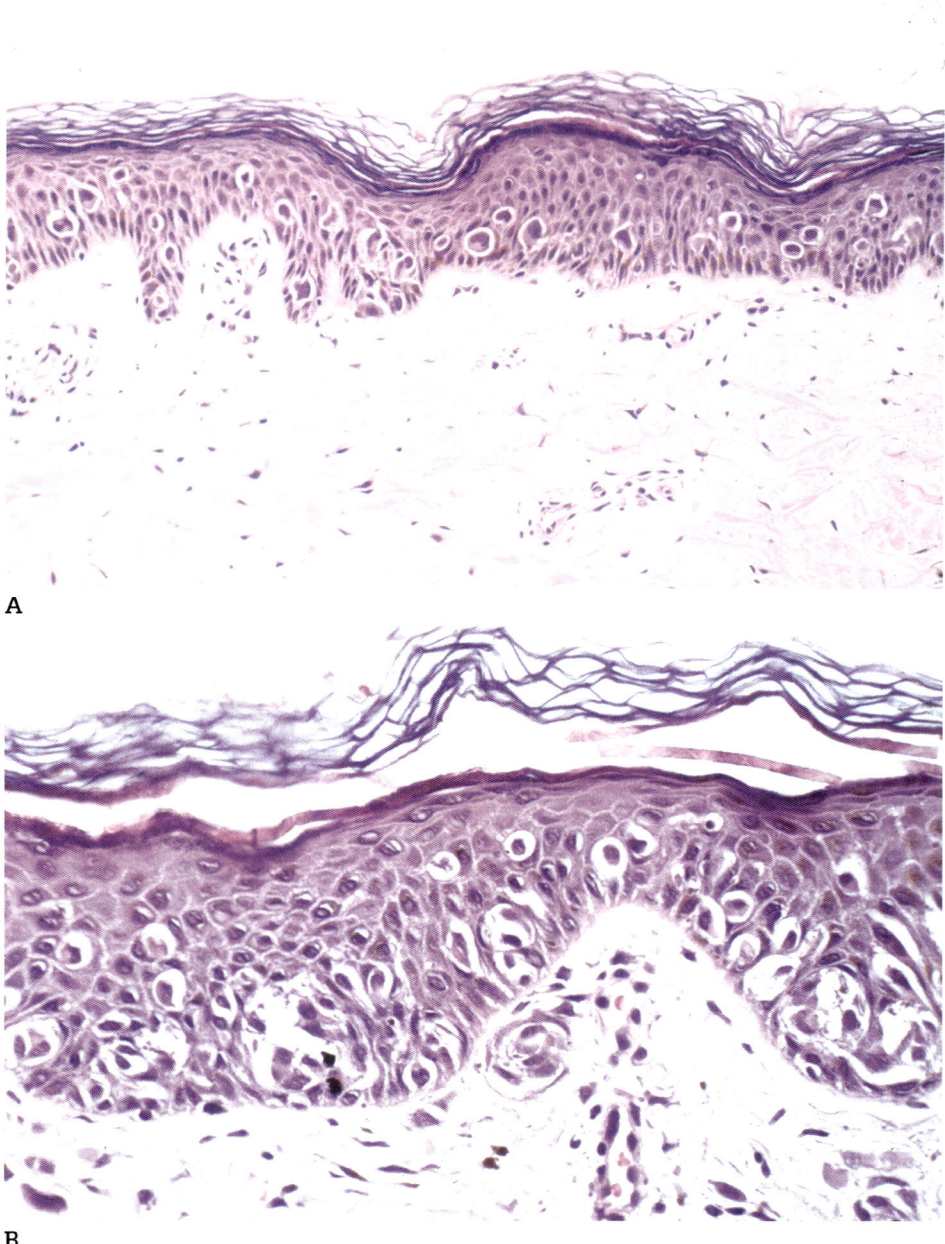

FIGURE 7-7 Pagetoid (intraepidermal) Spitz nevus. **A,** Pagetoid spread suggesting melanoma in situ. **B,** Note the characteristic cytologic details of Spitz nevus cells. The cells are polyangular and contain abundant ground glass cytoplasm, and the nuclei have dispersed chromatin.

cation. These criteria, which are thought to reflect ordered growth and favor benignancy, are not unique to Spitz nevi and also apply to the evaluation of other melanocytic nevi.

Symmetry Symmetry is a feature assessed on scanning magnification (Figs. 7-1A and 7-2). Symmetry in Spitz nevi is a symmetry from "side to side"—that is, the halves of the lesion around a central vertical axis are similar to one another. Common architectural appearances on histologic sections that convey symmetry are those of a semicircle with the epidermal surface as convexity and of a trapezoid, whose width decreases from epidermal "top to bottom" in the dermis (Fig. 7-2). The presence of symmetry is an important feature distinguishing Spitz nevus

TABLE 7-1 Spitz nevus.
Clinical features
Papule or nodule, often dome-shaped
Small (usually < 1 cm)
Smooth surface topography
Pink/red; pigmented forms occur
Majority in children and adolescents
Face and extremities, most common
Usually solitary; rare multiple forms occur
Commonly asymptomatic; rarely pruritic
History of growth in months; usually < 1 year
Histopathological features[a]
Cytologic features
Spindle and/or epithelioid cell type*
Overall monomorphous population of cells*
Striking pleomorphism in a minority of cells, occasional
Architectural features
Symmetry*
Sharp lateral demarcation*
Zonation with depth (e.g., maturation)*
Diminished cellular density with depth
Diminished cellular and nuclear sizes with depth
Wedge-shaped configuration in dermis, often
Orderly nondisruptive infiltration of collagen by Spitz nevus cells*
Other helpful diagnostic features
Absent or rare, but not atypical, mitoses in deep parts*
Giant nevus cells
Irregular contours of growth at deep margin*
Kamino bodies
Paucity or absence of single-cell upward spread (in central part of lesion if present)
Junctional clefts
Loss of cohesion between cells (retraction spaces)
Perivascular or diffuse inflammatory infiltrate
Superficial distribution of pigmentation
Telangiectasia and edema
Epidermal hyperplasia
Differential diagnosis
Malignant melanoma
Atypical (dysplastic) nevi with features of Spitz nevus
Variants of nevi with spindle and/or epithelioid cells
Pigmented spindle cell nevus
Desmoplastic Spitz nevus
Plexiform spindle cell nevus/deep penetrating nevus
Cellular blue nevus
Various "combined" nevi
Nonmelanocytic lesions
Paget's disease
Bowen's disease
Dermatofibroma
Epithelioid histiocytoma
Reticulohistiocytoma
Cellular neurothekeoma

[a]*, most helpful features.

from melanoma, in which uneven lateral and/or deep growth is common.

Sharp Lateral Demarcation Sharp lateral demarcation is a characteristic feature of the junctional component of Spitz nevi (Figs. 7-1A,B and 7-2). The impression of sharp demarcation is conveyed by the presence of nests rather than single cells at the lateral borders and by an abrupt transition from an epidermis with a high density of nested or single melanocytes to an adjacent area of epidermis devoid of melanocytic proliferation (Fig. 7-1C). The lateral borders become poorly circumscribed when there is lateral intraepidermal melanocytic growth that gradually diminishes without an abrupt termination. Also, marked variation in the position of nevus nests at the periphery with intervening "skip areas" devoid of nests and lentiginous junctional growth at the periphery that extends beyond the lateral borders of the dermal component (lateral extension, or "shoulder phenomenon") contribute to a loss of lateral demarcation at the dermoepidermal junction.

Zonation

Zonation in Spitz nevi is conveyed by the appearance of layers of differing morphology from top to bottom. Several features can give the appearance of zonation. Epithelioid giant cells, if present in a Spitz nevus, typically form a superficial cell layer at the dermoepidermal junction and are rarely seen deeper, thereby contributing to a zonal structure (13). The cytologic features of the spindle and/or epithelioid cells may change from above downward, leading to a gradient in cell size and shape, such as from large plump cells at the top to smaller or slender cells at the bottom (Fig. 7-6). This phenomenon of cytologic alteration or involution, in which the melanocytes of Spitz nevi progressively come to resemble melanocytes of conventional nevi in deeper parts of the lesions (or least demonstrate diminished nuclear and cellular sizes), has also been termed *maturation* (13). The frequency of maturation in Spitz nevi varies considerably among published accounts of Spitz nevi. Kernen and Ackerman (6) found maturation in only 4 of their 27 cases. In Weedon and Little's (10) review of 211 cases, maturation was present in 25%. Out of 41 compound and intradermal Spitz nevi, 31 showed maturation in a recent report by Binder et al. (33). Architectural features may also show a gradient, such as the transition from larger nests at the dermoepidermal junction to smaller nests near the deep margin of the nevus. With this transition from top to bottom, the cellular elements exhibit a nondisruptive insinuation among collagen bundles without induction of new stroma (Fig. 7-6). Finally, the distribution of pigment may be zonal. If melanin is present in Spitz nevi, it is largely confined to cells immediately subjacent to the epidermis in the majority of cases (13). In contrast to zonation in Spitz nevi, melanoma characteristically displays a more disorderly and disruptive growth pattern.

Although maturation is thought to reflect growth control and is an important feature favoring benignancy, it does not necessarily equate with benignancy. Features suggesting maturation occur in melanomas (pseudomaturation).

Irregular Contours of Growth at Deep Margins

Spitz nevi typically display a single-cell or single-file infiltrative growth pattern at their base (13). However, the deep parts of the nevus still appear to merge with, but not distort, the normal dermal architecture. Although melanocytes stretch fingerlike into the dermis, they seem to separate and ease apart, but not destroy, dermal collagen bundles (33) (Fig. 7.6). The impression of merging may be emphasized by a gradual decrease in the size of dermal fascicles or nests of melanocytes, ultimately to single cells. Isolated single melanocytes with fairly regular spacing at the base of a Spitz nevus is characteristic. The latter melanocytes often have an ameboid appearance with polyangular contours, abundant uniform ground glass cytoplasm, and a round or oval nucleus with uniform crystal-like chromatin. The end result is diminished cellular density and the orderly cellular infiltration at the deep margin of a Spitz nevus (Fig. 7-6). The latter finding is one of the most important histologic features distinguishing Spitz nevi from melanoma and cannot be overemphasized. On the other hand, the presence of compact nodules with pushing margins raises suspicion for malignant melanoma.

Absent or Rare Mitoses in Deep Parts

Mitoses are a variable finding in Spitz nevi. Binder et al. (35) reported mitoses in 7 out of 43 Spitz nevi, while according to Weedon (13), they may be found in more than half of the cases. In an individual lesion, they may be numerous, rare, or absent. Mitoses most commonly occur in the upper portion of the lesion and are usually bipolar. Although an occasional mitosis in the deeper parts of the lesion or a rare atypical mitosis may be observed in benign Spitz nevi, they should nonetheless prompt careful evaluation of the lesion for melanoma.

Giant Nevus Cells

The presence of nevus giant cells was emphasized by Spitz (4) in her original report. They are found in at least 50% of the cases (13). Giant cells may be multinucleate or contain only one nucleus. They are typically located near the dermoepidermal junction (Fig. 7-3C) and are rarely found in the deep parts of a Spitz nevus.

Kamino Bodies

Kamino et al. (36) reported the presence of eosinophilic amorphous or dull pink globules, either singly or in aggregates, at the dermoepidermal junction in 60% of their 293 Spitz nevi (Fig. 7-3B). They constitute an important diagnostic feature since they are found less frequently in malignant melanoma. However in our experience, their presence cannot be used as evidence to rule out melanoma.

In Kamino's original report, only 2% of malignant melanoma were found to have eosinophilic globules. Arbuckle and Weedon (37) found them in 86% of Spitz nevi, 12% of malignant melanomas, and 8% of benign compound nevi in their examination of 50 cases of each entity. They studied 10 sections from each case and reported that Kamino bodies were found in only 15% of Spitz nevi, if only a single section is examined (13).

Eosinophilic globules in Spitz nevi often coalesce to form irregular masses, while in melanomas, if present, they are usually smaller and rarely coalesce (13). Kamino et al. (36) noted that the eosinophilic globules stained positively with the periodic acid-Schiff (PAS) and trichrome stains in Spitz nevi, but not in malignant melanoma. However, others could not confirm this finding and questioned the reliability of these staining methods for distinguishing melanomas from Spitz nevi (13).

Ultrastructurally, Kamino bodies are composed of amorphous masses and bundles of filaments (37). Immunohistochemically, they contain basement membrane components, including collagen types IV and VII and laminin (38–40), which are probably synthesized by melanocytes, basal keratinocytes, or both. The globules show no reaction with antibodies against vimentin, cytokeratin, or S-100 protein (40). A recent study examining the eosinophilic globules for evidence of apoptosis with the TdT-mediated dUTP-x nick end-labeling (TUNEL) method failed to show any labeling (41). Thus from the latter studies eosinophilic bodies appear to be distinct from colloid or Civatte bodies and not derived from apoptosis. Degenerate material derived from melanocytes and keratinocytes may nonetheless also be present (36).

Paucity or Absence of Single-Cell Upward Spread

Pagetoid spread of single melanocytes is frequently found at all levels of the epidermis in malignant melanoma. This process can occur in Spitz nevus; however, usually to a lesser extent (Fig. 7.7) and is often focal and involves the central part of the lesion. In one study of 43 Spitz nevi, scattered suprabasal melanocytes were seen in 16% (35). When upward migration of melanocytes is present in Spitz nevus, if often takes the form of nests of two or more cells extending toward the stratum corneum (13). Such transepidermal elimination of nests is especially common in childhood lesions but may be found at any age. Pagetoid spread of melanocytes and transepidermal elimination of nests in Spitz nevus are characteristically limited to the epidermis overlying the junctional and/or dermal nevus component. If upward migration is found peripheral to the central part of the nevus, the lesion should be carefully scrutinized to rule out melanoma (13).

Junctional Cleavage (Clefting)
At the dermoepidermal junction, the fascicles of spindle cells in Spitz nevi, typically following the course of elongated rete ridges, are often separated by a cleft-like retraction space from the adjacent epidermis, a result of tissue shrinkage during processing (13) (Fig. 7-1C). This feature is present in about half of the cases of Spitz nevi but is probably less common in malignant melanomas. Because it seems a useful feature that can help in the differential diagnosis from melanoma, the phenomenon of junctional cleavage has been called a meaningful artifact.

Loss of Cohesion
Loss of cohesion may be seen within fascicles or nests of melanocytes, which is reflected by the presence of spaces between individual cells. This allows a loosely packed appearance of melanocytes within the confines of a nest. Loss of cellular cohesion can be seen in both spindle and epithelioid cell nevi but may be particularly prominent in the latter (13).

Adnexal Involvement
Spitz nevi and its variants have a striking propensity to involve hair follicles and eccrine ducts. In most instances, intraepidermal fascicles of cells track along the adventitial sheaths of appendageal structures into the papillary dermis and often into the reticular dermis. Knowledge of the prevalence of this morphologic feature in Spitz nevi and their variants is important, since such a finding might otherwise raise undue concern about melanoma.

Perivascular or Diffuse Inflammatory Infiltrates
The distribution of the inflammatory infiltrate in Spitz nevi can be a helpful diagnostic feature. It tends to be perivascular but may diffusely infiltrate the dermal component of some Spitz nevi, often in a symmetrical pattern. On the other hand, in melanomas the inflammatory infiltrate is usually at the base, has a patchy asymmetrical disposition, and is not uncommonly associated with tumor regression (13).

Other Features
A number of other features have been suggested as helpful in the distinction of Spitz nevi from malignant melanoma, such as the type or distribution of pigment, epidermal hyperplasia, edema, and telangiectasia (34,35,42). As part of the overall constellation of findings, these features may be helpful. However, their diagnostic usefulness is limited. Although they appear more common in Spitz nevi, they are observed frequently enough in melanoma to preclude their diagnostic value.

Pigmentation Spitz nevi are usually only slightly pigmented or amelanotic. Pigment is prominent in only about 10% of cases (13). When it is present, it is typically superficial, especially near the dermoepidermal junction. While the texture of the pigment is typically fine and dusty in melanomas, it is said to be coarser in Spitz nevi.

Epidermal Hyperplasia Epidermal hyperplasia is a common finding in Spitz nevi (Fig. 7-1B). In one study, acanthosis was seen in 58% of Spitz nevi and pseudoepitheliomatous hyperplasia in 74% of the cases (35,43).

Telangiectasia and Edema A zone of telangiectatic fibrous tissue, typically in the superficial dermis, partly or completely separating the epidermis from the upper melanocytes, is observed in about 50% of Spitz nevi. Edema is less common and prominent in only about 10% of Spitz nevi (13).

Vascular and Lymphatic Invasion, Angiotropism, and Neurotropism Invasion of lymphatic spaces, which has been demonstrated in 7 out of 49 Spitz nevi in children, may be a histologic curiosity and is not in itself a predictor of metastasis (even if benign). No evidence of metastasis was found during a follow-up period of up to 14 years (44). We have observed both angiotropism and neurotropism in Spitz nevi. The biologic significance of the latter findings is unclear and has not yet been correlated with increased risk of recurrence or aggressive behavior.

SPITZ TUMOR WITH ATYPICAL FEATURES (ATYPICAL SPITZ TUMOR)

The concept of Spitz nevi with atypical features (or atypical Spitz nevi) is controversial at present and is not universally accepted (23). The reasoning behind the reluctance to acknowledge atypical variants is the perspective that all melanocytic lesions can hypothetically be classified into discreet categories, such as Spitz nevus and melanoma, leaving no room for controversial or intermediate lesions that are difficult to classify precisely (Tables 7-2 to 7-5). The use of such terminology as *atypical Spitz nevus* acknowledges the extraordinary difficulty posed by some lesions. Fundamental questions relate to the biologic nature of such lesions:

- Do Spitzoid lesions constitute a biologic spectrum of neoplasia with behavior ranging from low to high

TABLE 7-2 Contrasting criteria for the Spitz nevus from reports in the literature.

Criterion	Kernen and Ackerman (1960)(6)	Reed et al. (1975)(46)	Weedon and Little (1977)(10)	Paniago-Pereira et al. (1978)(9)
Pagetoid spread	Not stated	Not stated	Occasional	Sparse
Nuclear atypia	Absent	Minimal	Present	Not important
Giant cells	Occasional	Present	Present	Not helpful
Epidermis	Thinned	Hyperplastic	Hyperplastic	Hyperplastic
Cell type	Mostly spindled	No comment	Mostly spindled	Mostly spindled
Dermal mitoses	Rare	Variable (rarely high)	Common	Occasional
Atypical mitoses	Rare	Not stated	Uncommon	Rare
Maturation with descent	Mostly absent	Present	Mostly absent	Prominent
Deep dermal margin	Pushing	Infiltrative	Infiltrative	Pushing

grade and showing a correlation with histomorphologic and other characteristics? (There is some evidence for this, but additional study is needed.)
- Does malignant Spitz tumor exist and is it biologically different (less aggressive than) from conventional melanoma? (There is no clear evidence for this, but further study is needed.)
- Are all Spitzoid lesions that can be categorized as Spitz nevus benign, regardless of atypical features? (Probably not, but this requires further study.)
- Are metastasizing Spitzoid lesions simply melanomas that have been misclassified by pathologists or are they melanomas that are too difficult to recognize as such by conventional microscopy? (The answer may be yes to both questions for selected lesions, but more study is needed.)

Another issue is the lack of consensus about which features should be considered aberrant or atypical, and

TABLE 7-3 Assessment of atypical Spitz tumors in children and adolescents for risk for metastasis

Parameter	Score
Age (years)	
0–10	0
11–17	1
Diameter (mm)	
0–10	0
> 10	1
Involvement of subcutaneous fat	
Absent	0
Present	2
Ulceration	
Absent	0
Present	2
Mitotic Activity (mm^2)	
0–5	0
6–8	2
> 9	5

Note: Total score and risk for metastasis: 0–2, low risk; 3–4, intermediate risk; 5–11, high risk.

TABLE 7-4 Spitz nevus/pigmented spindle cell nevus with atypical features.

Intraepidermal variant
  Architectural disorder
    Disordered intraepidermal melanocytic proliferation:*
      Lentiginous or single-cell pattern*
      Disordered junctional nesting*
        Variation in size, shape, orientation, spacing, cellular cohesion of nests
        Horizontal confluence and bridging of nests
      Pagetoid spread over large front or at periphery
    Asymmetry
    Poor circumscription
    Lateral extension of intraepidermal component (shoulder phenomenon)
  Cytologic atypia beyond that acceptable for a Spitz nevus*
    Nuclear pleomorphism
    Variation in nuclear chromatin patterns
    Nuclear enlargement
    Variation in nucleoli
  Host response
    Patchy to band-like mononuclear infiltrates in papillary dermis
    Fibroplasia
Dermal variant
  Architectural abnormalities*
    Expansile nodules
    Increased cellularity
    Loss of cellular cohesion
    Asymmetry
    Deep extension (into subcutaneous fat)
    Lack of maturation or orderly infiltration of collagen
    Ulceration
    Necrosis
  Cytologic atypia (as above)
  Mitotic activity
    Numerous mitoses
    Mitoses at base of lesion
    Atypical mitoses
  Host response
    Prominent mononuclear cell infiltrates with plasma cells
    Formation of tumor stroma

[a]*, essential criteria for diagnosis.

TABLE 7-5 Comparison of Spitz nevus, Spitz nevus with atypical features, and melanoma.

Feature	Spitz nevus	Spitz nevus with atypical features[a]	Melanoma
Size	Usually < 1 cm	Often > 1 cm	Usually > 1 cm
Symmetry	Symmetry	Often asymmetric	Asymmetric
Lateral borders	Sharply demarcated	Often poorly defined	Often poorly defined
Lateral extension	Uncommon	Common	Common
Lentiginous melanocytic proliferation	Uncommon	Variable	Common
Irregular nesting	Uncommon	Common	Frequent
Upward migration	Common in children; nests > single cells	Variable, prominent on occasion	Frequent, usually as single cells
Ulceration	Uncommon	Variable	Common
Kamino bodies	Common	Less common	Uncommon
Cell type	Monomorphous	Often pleomorphic	Pleomorphic
Deep extension	Uncommon	Common	Variable
Expansile nodules	Uncommon	Common	Frequent
Maturation/zonation	Common	Uncommon or absent	Uncommon
Deep border	Orderly infiltrating pattern	Often rounded, "pushing"	Irregular
Cellularity	Variable	Prominent	Prominent
Cytologic atypia	Uncommon	Common	Prominent
Cellular cohesion	Diminished	Diminished	Variable
Mitoses, deep	Uncommon	Common	Frequent
Atypical mitoses	Uncommon	Variable	Common
Mononuclear infiltrates	Perivascular	Patchy	Bandlike, patchy

[a]Atypical Spitz tumor, Spitz tumor with indeterminate biologic potential.

this returns full circle to the problem of defining what is a prototypic Spitz nevus. As one can see from Table 7-2, there are striking discrepancies among authors as to the basic criteria for a conventional Spitz nevus (23). As already mentioned, there has been an evolution of criteria over time as to what is now considered to be the prototypic Spitz nevus. In our experience, Spitz nevi with morphologic (abnormal or atypical?) features that deviate from the idealized version are in fact encountered on a regular basis (23,45).

The term *atypical Spitz tumor* was first used, to our knowledge, in 1975 by Reed et al. when illustrating a Spitz nevus (in a photomicrograph) that differed from conventional Spitz nevi by exhibiting confluent and densely cellular fascicles of spindle cells that "crowded and compressed their stroma" (46). In a subsequent report of 32 cases Smith et al. (21) introduced the term "spindle and epithelioid cell nevus with atypia and metastasis (malignant Spitz nevus)" (see below) to describe a series of Spitz-like melanocytic tumors characterized by large size (> 1 cm), frequent ulceration, deep extension into subcutaneous fat with bulbous "pushing" margins, prominent cellular density, lack of maturation, cytologic atypia greater than that expected for a Spitz nevus (large and pleomorphic cells, prominent nucleoli), significant numbers of mitoses (up to five in a single high-power field), and focal necrosis. These tumors developed in relatively young individuals (41% < age 14 years and 82% < 29 years of age), and virtually all were located on the head and neck and extremities (71%). Six patients were also observed to have regional lymph node metastases with involvement of the sinuses and parenchyma by tumor identical to the primary cutaneous lesion. According to the authors, there was no subsequent progression of disease; however, long-term follow-up of these patients has not been reported. Furthermore, there were no distinctive features that predicted the development of metastases.

We (22) reported a series of 12 atypical Spitz-like melanocytic tumors in children and adolescents. There were 3 tumors (classified as melanoma) among the 12 cases that were associated with metastases and the death of 1 patient. Of the latter, 2 patients had only single lymph node metastases and have been disease-free with long-term follow-up. These 2 tumors also could be described under the rubric of metastasizing Spitz tumor. In general, all 12 tumors were characterized by many of the same features as reported by Smith et al.—large size, ulceration, significant depth, prominent cellular density, lack of maturation, a pushing border, variable but often frequent and deep mitosis, and prominent cellular pleomorphism.

Based on these and other reports, we caution against using the term *metastasizing* or *malignant Spitz tumor* once metastases have developed from these atypical variants of Spitz tumor; such lesions should be designated as melanoma until definitive data are available to suggest an alternative diagnosis.

The recent application of the sentinel lymph node (SLN) biopsy to assess atypical Spitz-like tumors provides a means of obtaining more information about the biologic characteristics of such lesions. We have observed that such atypical Spitz-like melanocytic tumors may have apparent metastatic deposits in the parenchyma of sentinel lymph nodes (47). Although the finding of tumor deposits in SLN is de facto evidence for melanoma, only the study of sufficient numbers of cases with long-term follow-up will determine which atypical Spitz-like tumors are prone to metastases, if they are inherently different from conventional melanomas, and if they potentially have better prognoses. In the few cases studied thus far by SLN biopsy, such Spitz tumors have not necessarily had the degree of abnormality (size > 1 cm, ulceration, involvement of subcutaneous fat, high mitotic rate) as such tumors that result in macroscopic metastases (Table 7-3) (47). However, tumor deposits in SLNs may possibly have a different biology or significance than metastases in conventional lymph nodes. It is apparent that many questions remain to be answered about the significance of SLN involvement by tumor deposits, particularly microscopic metastases.

Atypical Features of the Intraepidermal Component

Spitz nevi (and pigmented spindle cell nevi) may show abnormal morphologic features of the intraepidermal component, and the immediate question usually is whether melanoma in situ or intraepidermal melanoma is present or not. It is controversial as to whether the intraepidermal abnormalities encountered in Spitz nevi have any relationship or analogy to those in conventional atypical (dysplastic) nevi (Table 7-4). The latter question requires further study. However, it is reasonable to conclude that all melanocytic nevi or tumors may demonstrate a spectrum of abnormality intermediate to the benign and malignant ends of a continuum, until proved otherwise. Abnormal features include (a) variable epidermal thickness vs. a uniform epidermal thickness from side to side; (b) presence or absence of epidermal thinning and dermoepidermal separation; (c) significantly disordered architectural patterns of the intraepidermal component—that is, lentiginous melanocytic proliferation and/or significant variation in junctional nesting (variation in size, shape, orientation, and spacing of junctional nests; horizontal confluence and bridging of nests; diminished cellular cohesion of nests) beyond that expected for a Spitz nevus; (d) prominent pagetoid spread as described above (Fig. 7-7) and not simply transepidermal elimination of large nests of melanocytes; and (e) unequivocal cytologic atypia of melanocytes (Fig. 7-8). The features of such Spitz nevi are outlined in Table 7-4.

Pagetoid Spitz Nevus: Intraepidermal or Mainly Intraepidermal Spitz Nevi with Prominent Pagetoid Spread

A distinctive variant of Spitz nevus that has received little attention in previously published series is the mainly intraepidermal or junctional subtype with a prominent pagetoid pattern (48,49). This variant may occur anywhere but is most commonly encountered on the lower extremities of young women. The most important reason for recognizing this lesion is its frequent misdiagnosis as in situ or radial growth phase melanoma. The clinical findings are often unremarkable. Most lesions measure < 5–6 mm and are diagnosed as a nevus or atypical nevus.

Scanning magnification usually discloses a mainly intraepidermal proliferation of enlarged epithelioid cells typically devoid of melanin (Fig. 7-7A). The proliferation commonly has an overall symmetry from side to side and is often fairly well demarcated. However, some lesions have ill-defined margins. Many of these lesions show a combination of both a single-cell and nested proliferation of epithelioid melanocytes. The single-cell proliferative pattern is often both basilar and pagetoid and commonly varies within the lesion (Fig. 7-7B). Typical junctional nests of epithelioid cells with associated clefting are also usually present and may be quite small in size. Nests of cells or single Spitz nevus cells may or may not be present in the papillary dermis. Often the degree of pagetoid spread is focal or limited; however, it may be prominent in some lesions, raising the possibility of melanoma in situ (Fig. 7-7B).

Differential Diagnosis

The intraepidermal or junctional variants of Spitz nevi must first of all be discriminated from in situ or early invasive melanoma. These intraepidermal Spitz nevi often show relatively small size, symmetry, a uniformity of the epidermis and stratum corneum throughout (e.g., a uniform degree of epidermal hyperplasia from side to side), limitation of pagetoid spread to the lower half of epidermis (common), often only focal pagetoid spread or sparsely cellular upward migration, evidence of growth control, and sharp circumscription compared to melanoma. Of particular importance are the cytologic characteristics of the epithelioid cells; they tend to be fairly monotypic with abundant pinkish cytoplasm that has a ground glass appearance, rather than the granular cytoplasm often observed in melanoma cells. The nuclei of Spitz nevus cells are also fairly uniform with evenly dispersed chromatin versus the pleomorphism of melanoma cells.

As discussed above and in Chapter 5, atypical forms of plaque-type Spitz nevi may show features of conventional atypical (dysplastic) nevi. Distinction from con-

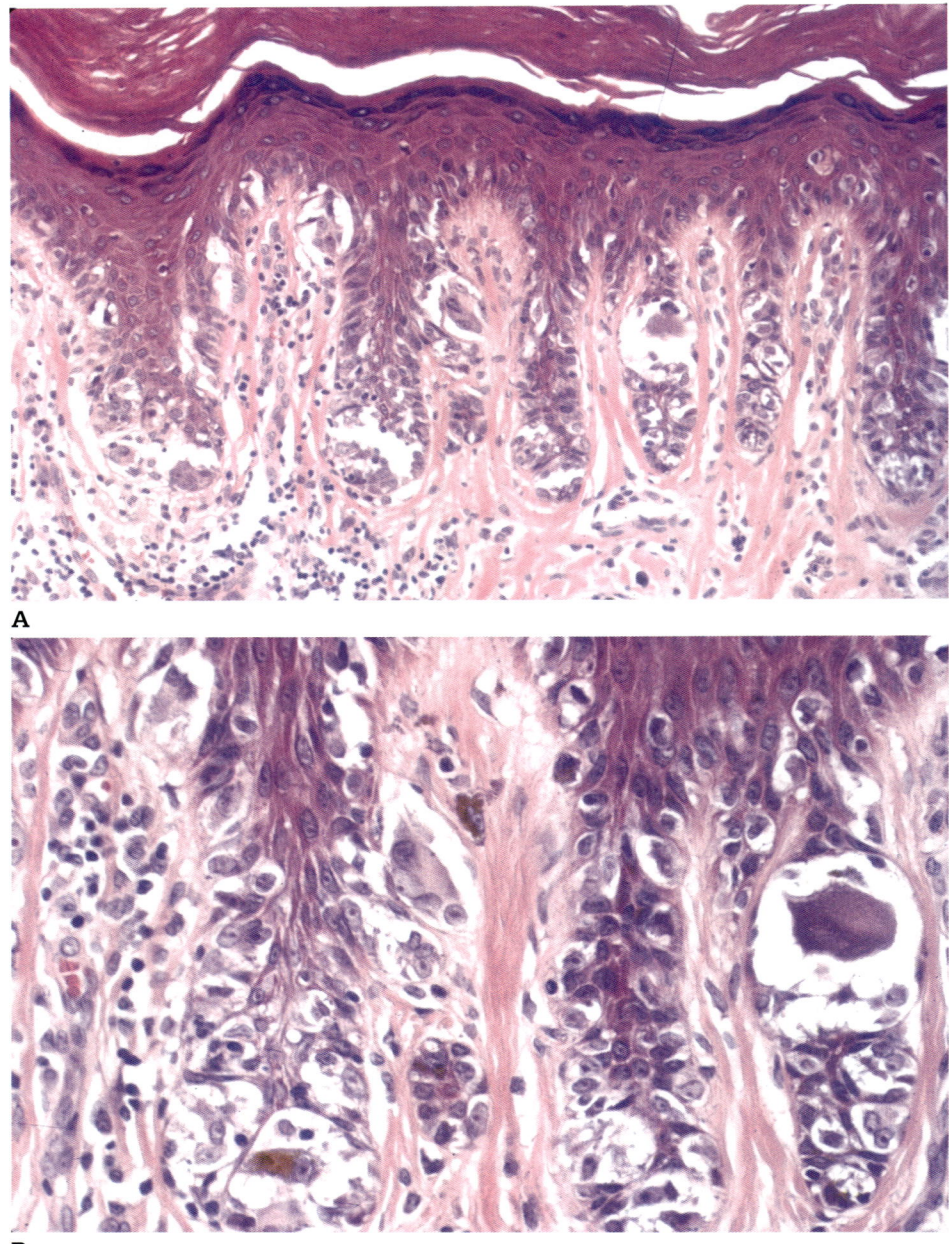

FIGURE 7-8 Spitz nevus with atypical features (atypical Spitz tumor). **A,** The lesion demonstrates prominent lentiginous melanocytic proliferation and variation in the junctional nesting pattern. **B,** Higher magnification of panel A showing disordered and atypical intraepidermal melanocytes. The cells also exhibit the features of Spitz nevus cells: abundant ground glass cytoplasm, angulated contours, and characteristic multinucleate giant cells.

ventional atypical nevi is primarily based on the presence of the characteristic cell types of Spitz nevi.

Rarely, exclusively intraepidermal or junctional Spitz nevi may mimic *Paget's disease* or *Bowen's disease,* both of which can be distinguished from Spitz nevus by immunoreactivity for cytokeratins (50).

Atypical Features of the Dermal Component

As outlined in the second part of Table 7-4, certain Spitz nevi may demonstrate prominent atypicality of the dermal component. These various features include (as already mentioned above) the presence of cohesive cellular nodules, increased cellularity, diminished cellular

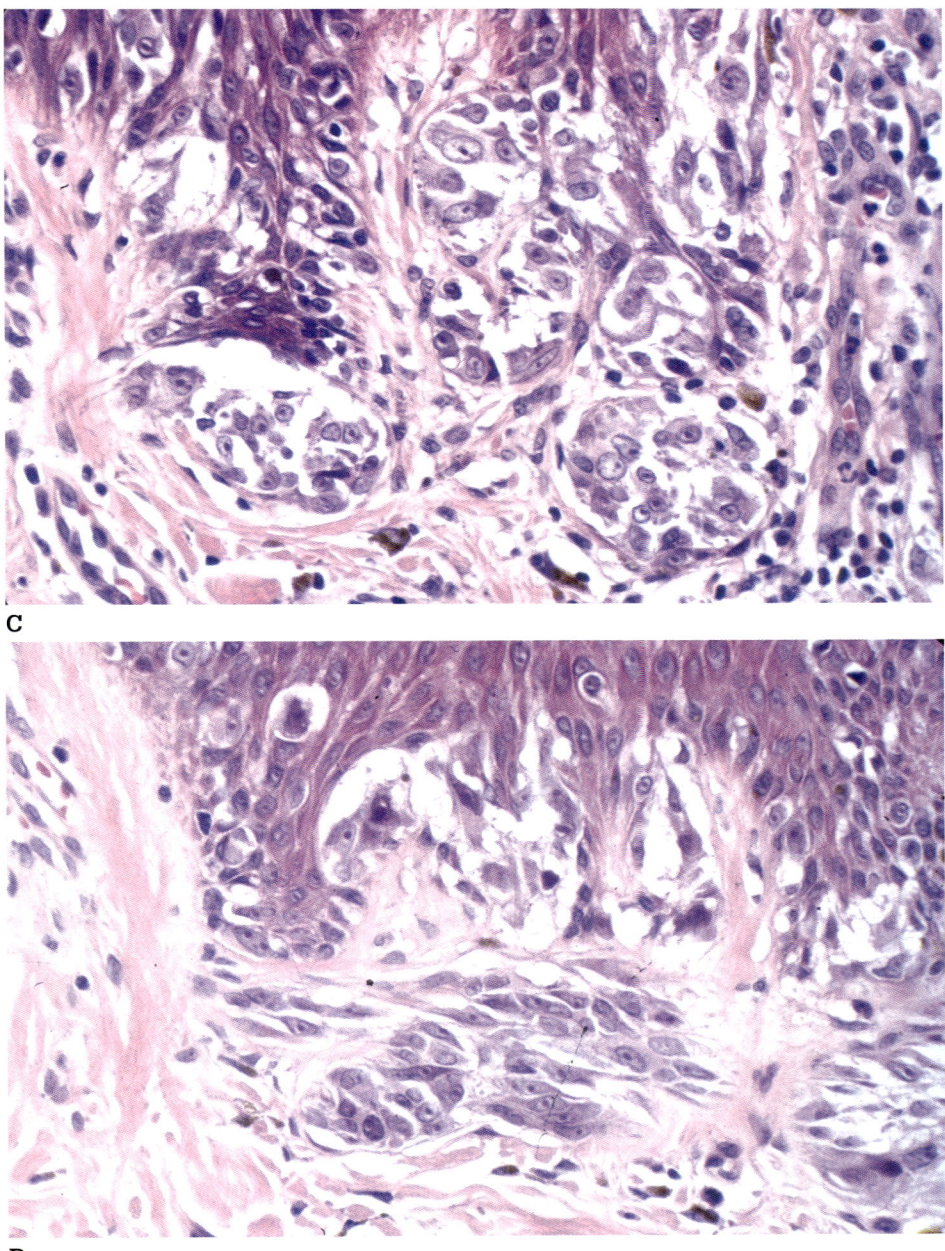

FIGURE 7-8 *Continued.* **C,** Variation in the nesting of enlarged epithelioid cells. These cells show features of Spitz nevus cells but also display nuclear atypia. **D,** Note the horizontal confluence of enlarged fusiform cells typical of Spitz nevus. The cells have a monotonous appearance and contain nuclei with evenly dispersed chromatin.

cohesion, asymmetry, deep extension into the lowermost dermis or subcutis, lack of maturation or orderly infiltration of collagen, substantial cytologic atypia, a significant mitotic rate that is especially deep, and mononuclear infiltrates (Figs. 7-9 and 7-10). One potential caveat in regard to the idea that cohesive dermal nodular components are abnormal in Spitz nevi is that we have observed such nodular components rather commonly in Spitz nevi of children under 10 years of age. However, no other significant abnormalities should be present in such lesions.

Approach to the Problem of Spitz Tumors with Atypical Features Assuming that a priori melanoma can be

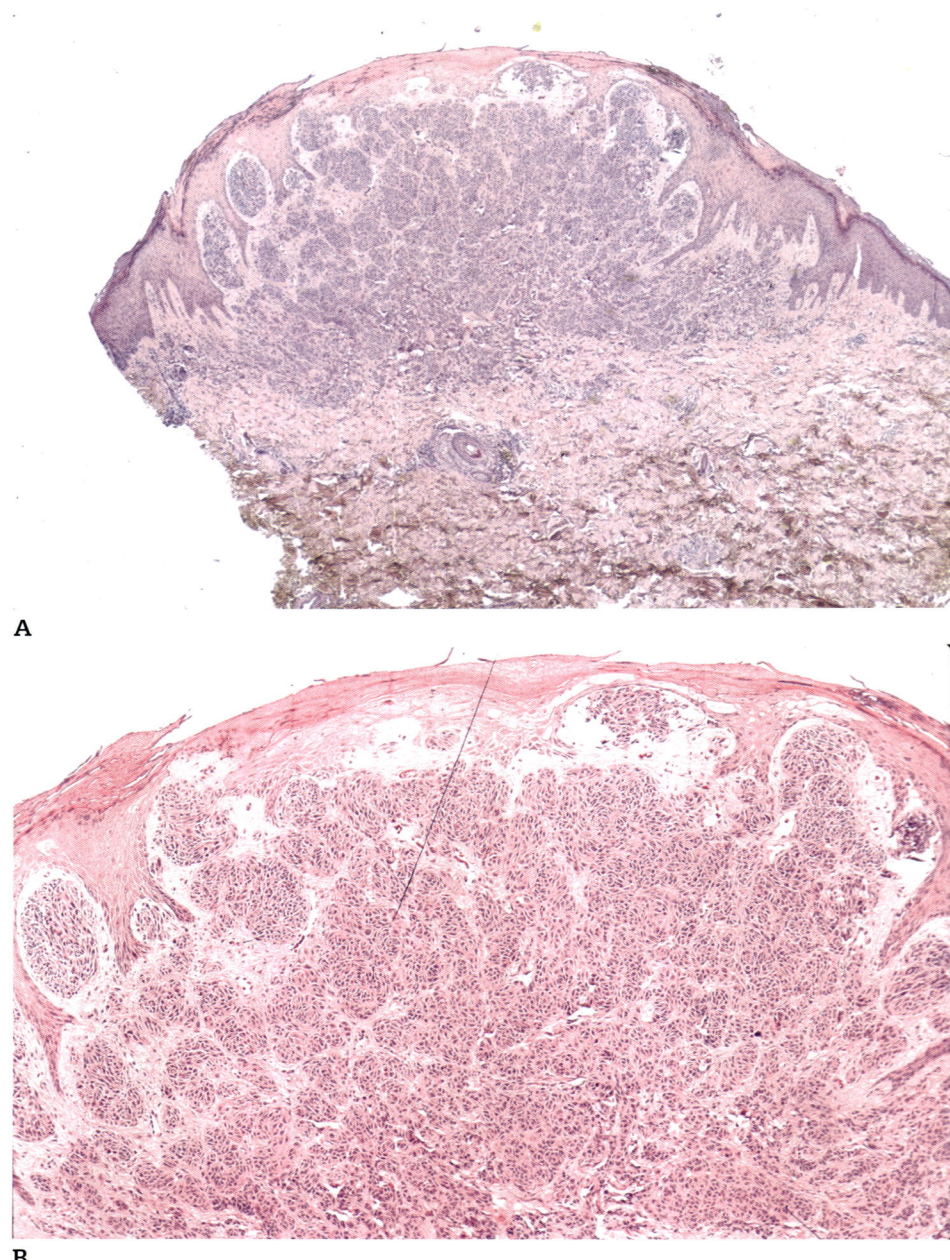

FIGURE 7-9 Atypical variant of Spitz nevus (atypical Spitz tumor). **A,** The lesion is dome shaped and fairly symmetric but is characterized by an expansile cellular nodule with only slight maturation. These are the atypical features. **B,** The nodule is characterized by a monotonous cellular appearance, which is acceptable from side to side but not from top to bottom.

ruled out, the approach of some pathologists is to consider that such aberrant features are within a spectrum of what is allowable or acceptable (within normal limits) for a Spitz nevus. The latter philosophy is a logical one; however, one is left with the problem of how to deal with a percentage of cases that simply defy dichotomous classification. The latter problem has been underscored by a published blinded review of 30 melanocytic lesions exhibiting features of Spitz nevus (the cases included typical Spitz nevi, Spitz nevi with atypical features, biologically indeterminate Spitz-like lesions, and unequivocal melanomas) by 10 pathologists, demonstrating that this group could not reach consensus about diagnosing such Spitz lesions or distinguishing them from melanoma (23).

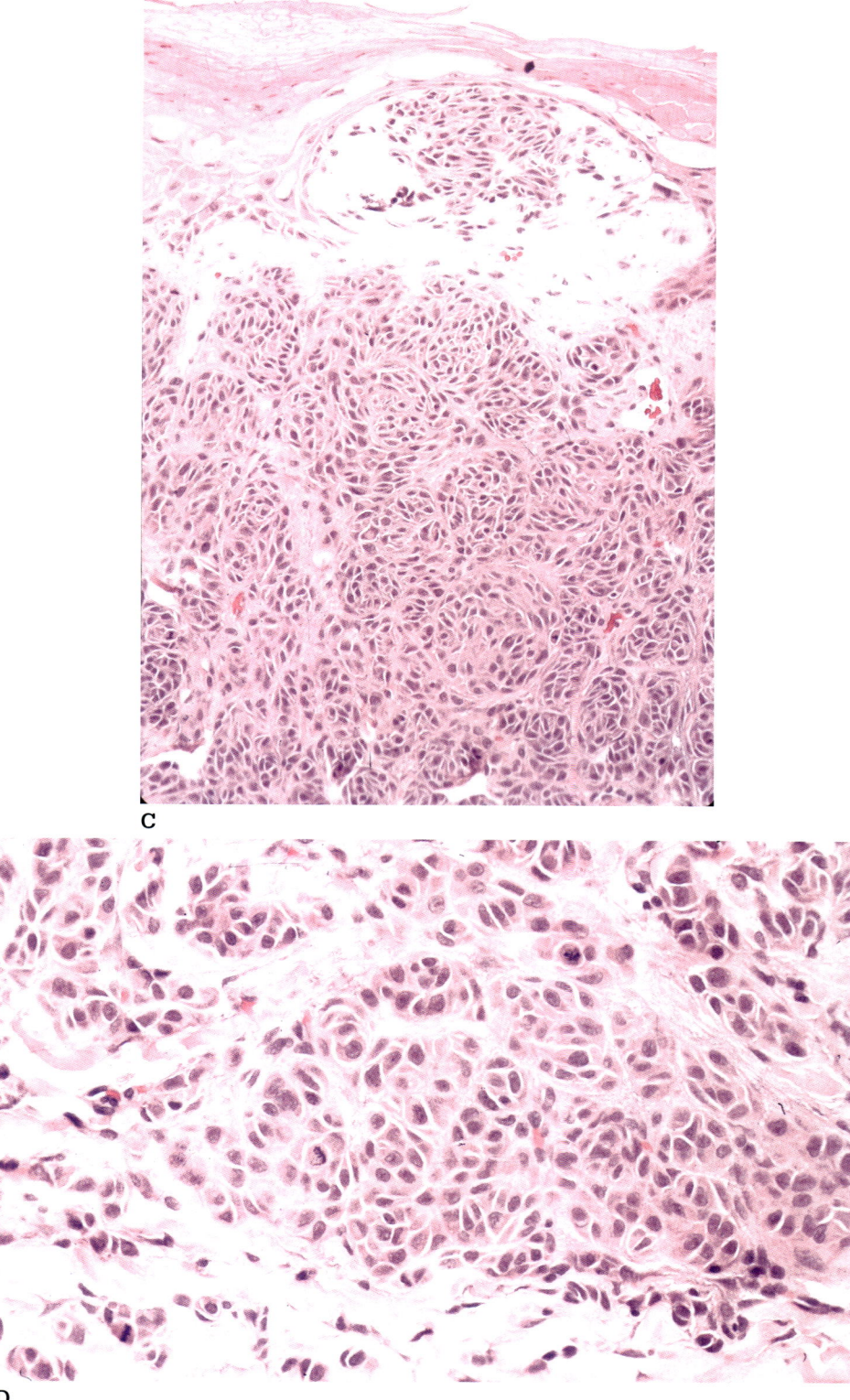

FIGURE 7-9 *Continued.* **C,** Dyscohesion of the junctional nest. The cells have the cellular attributes of Spitz nevus cells—monotonous, angular, and abundant pink cytoplasm. **D,** Nests of epithelioid cells at base of lesion.

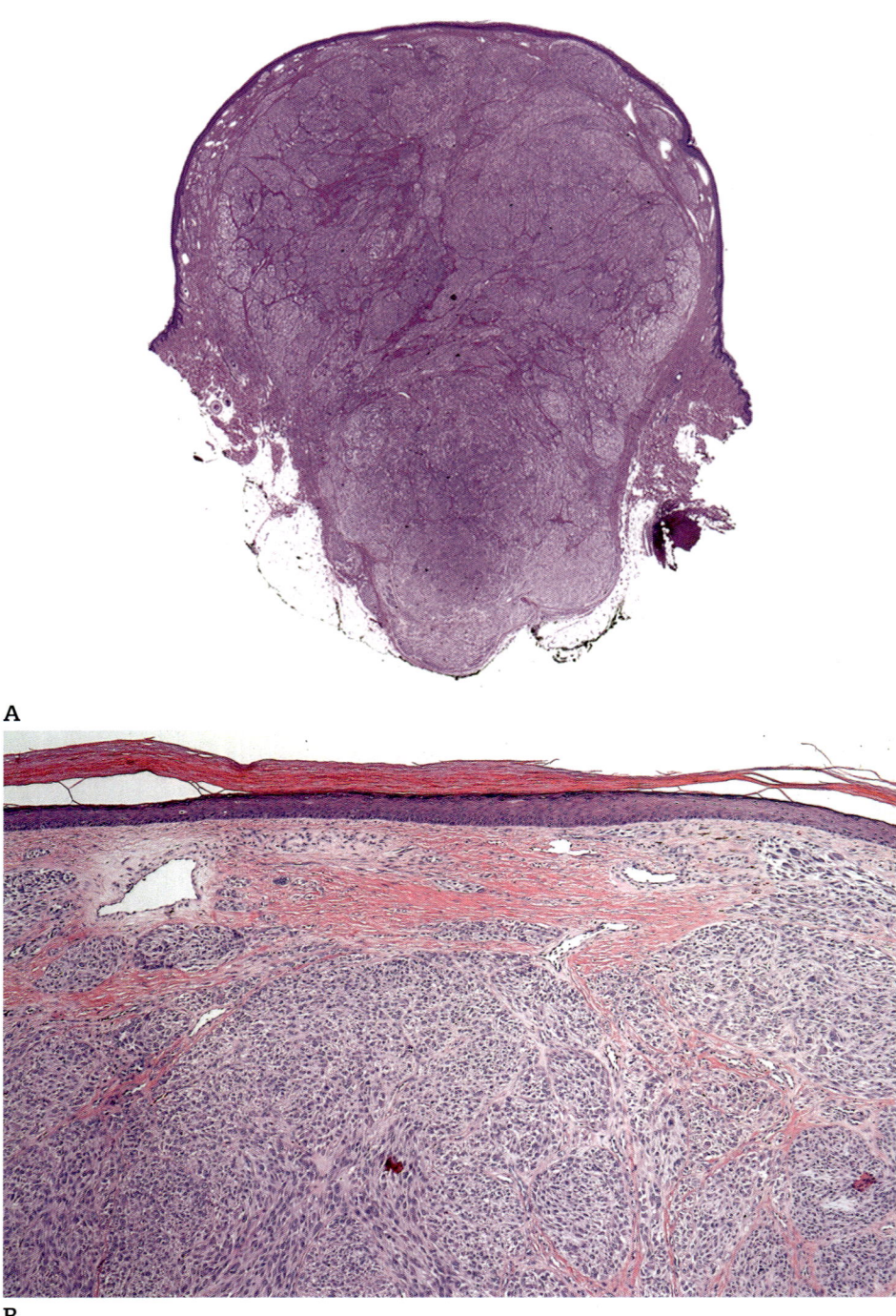

FIGURE 7-10 Atypical variant of Spitz nevus (atypical Spitz tumor). The lesion is characterized by large size, extension into subcutaneous fat, prominent cellular density and confluence, the lack of maturation, and dermal mitoses. **A,** The lesion is large and dome shaped. **B,** Note large aggregates of melanocytes in dermis exhibiting significant cellular density and confluence.

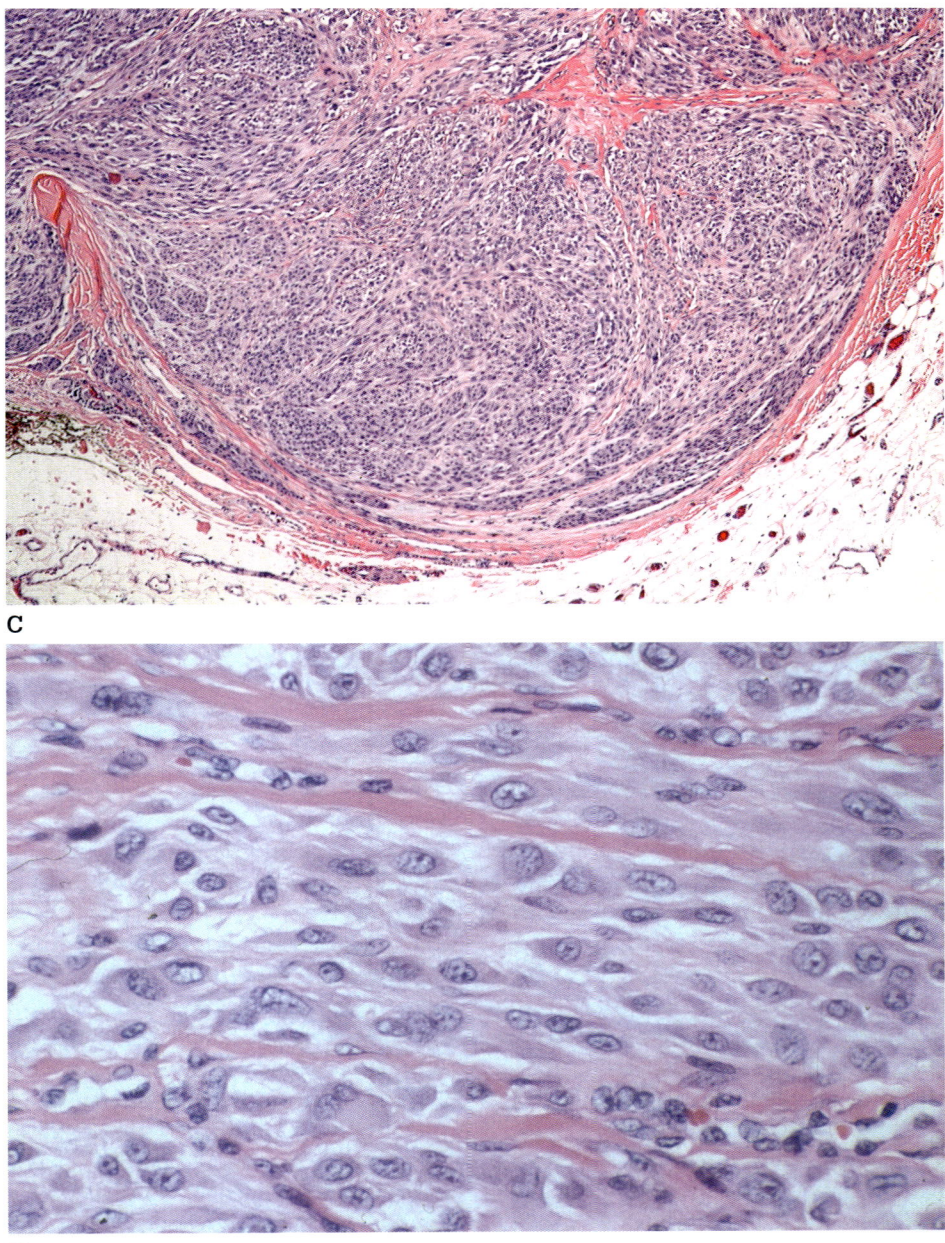

FIGURE 7-10 *Continued.* **C,** The tumor demonstrates a protuberant interface with the subcutaneous fat. **D,** The melanocytes have the cellular attributes of cells in a Spitz tumor—monotonous, angular, and abundant pink cytoplasm. There are confluent fascicles of spindle cells in the dermis.

Particular problems again illustrated by this study are that published criteria for Spitz nevi have often been formulated from circular reasoning and the lack of long-term follow-up. Thus criteria for recognizing and assessing Spitzoid lesions and discriminating them from melanoma are still not standardized or universally accepted.

Until objective data become available, we recommend a pragmatic approach to this problem. In practical terms, the initial evaluation should be to determine whether an obvious melanoma or prototypic Spitz nevus is present. If *clear-cut* melanoma can be excluded (which is often not possible for some proportion of lesions), we next recommend that such Spitz-like tumors be systematically examined for particular attributes, some of which can be quantified (51) (Table 7-3). These attributes may involve the epidermis, the dermis/subcutis, or both. (a) Determine diameter in millimeters; increasing size > 1 cm (although arbitrary) is generally considered abnormal. (b) Measure tumor thickness in millimeters and determine whether the subcutaneous fat is involved or not. (c) Record presence or absence of ulceration. (d) Determine mitotic rate per millimeter squared. (e) Record presence or absence of maturation (zonation), as described above. (f) Note symmetry or asymmetry. (g) Record presence or absence of prominent cellular density and confluence of dermal melanocytes. (h) Note deep mitoses in the dermal component. (i) Record atypical mitoses. (j) Determine significant cytologic atypia beyond that appropriate for a Spitz nevus. (k) Note pagetoid spread in terms of a large front, the upper half of the epidermis, as single cells, and lateral to the central part of the lesion. (l) Note sharp peripheral demarcation of the tumor.

In evaluating such lesions, a number of other factors, including those listed in Table 7-3 should be weighed in the final interpretation. Clinical factors such as the age of the patient, location of the tumor, clinical appearance, history of recent change in a long-standing stable lesion, and family history of melanoma should be considered carefully. The older the patient, especially individuals older than 30 years, the much greater the likelihood of malignancy. As a general rule, one's threshold for diagnosing melanoma in such lesions should correlate inversely with the age of the patient—that is, high threshold for very young individuals and a lower threshold for elderly individuals. However, it should be stressed that there are many exceptions. The location of atypical tumors on sites less commonly involved by Spitz nevus, such as the back, is also another such factor suggesting careful scrutiny of the lesion for melanoma.

Because of the lack of objective data and sufficient follow-up, the significance of the various features mentioned above has not been elucidated. The absence or incomplete development of major diagnostic features, such as symmetry or sharply demarcated lateral borders, are of concern and should prompt a careful search for features of melanoma. Even if symmetry and sharp lateral demarcation are observed, the presence of extensive pagetoid spread, the lack of maturation in depth, the presence of prominent cellularity of the dermal component, nuclear pleomorphism of more than a small proportion of cells, cohesive cellular nodules in the dermis, or deeply located (albeit rare) mitoses are worrisome (Figs. 7-9 and 7-10).

There is little question that the presence of these abnormalities in any given lesion is highly worrisome for melanoma and that as these features increase in number and severity, the likelihood of melanoma increases. The grading protocol outlined in Table 7-3 was developed to aid in the assessment of metastatic risk of Spitz tumors with abnormalities of the dermal component in children and adolescents (51). In an evaluation of 30 atypical Spitz-like melanocytic tumors, we found an increasing score resulted in greater risk for the development of metastases. We recognize the limitations of such an approach; nonetheless, it provides the first objective evaluation of such lesions and is a work in progress.

Ancillary techniques (see below)—such as immunohistochemisty, cytogenetic studies (comparative genomic hybridization, fluorescence in situ hybridization), loss of heterozygosity, and sentinel lymph biopsy—may provide additional objective information in this systematic evaluation of a particular lesion. The goal of such an exercise is to record (or quantify as best one can) the number of abnormal features present to classify a tumor as follows:

- Conventional Spitz tumor with relatively little or low risk for recurrence (few or no abnormal features present).
- Spitz-like melanocytic tumor with atypical features and indeterminate biologic potential (increased risk for recurrence and metastasis based on one or more or several atypical features).
- Malignant melanoma.

These factors help determine the appropriate management. Correlation of such abnormal findings with clinical outcomes from long-term follow-up will ultimately provide the data for the more precise classification of such problematic Spitzoid tumors. If after weighing these factors a clear-cut diagnosis of melanoma cannot be made, a practical approach is to communicate the situation to the clinician and patient. We consider it appropriate to indicate in a comment whether the lesion shows only slight atypicality or whether its features approach melanoma. Depending on the severity of the atypia, we state that the diagnosis of malignant melanoma cannot completely be excluded. A diagnosis of malignancy should not be made unless there is sufficient histologic evidence, so that overtreatment and undue psychologic burden for the patient can be avoided. We advise that such highly atypical tumors are designated as Spitz-like melanocytic tumors with indeterminate biologic potential and that they be completely excised with surgical margins of approximately 1 cm, and that the patient be carefully monitored as for melanoma (i.e., regular examinations) for evidence of recurrence or metastasis. Recently sentinel lymph node (SLN) biopsy has been performed for such markedly atypical Spitz-like melanocytic tumors. However, the use of the latter technique remains controversial for such lesions. Although the finding of large deposits meeting established criteria for malignancy in lymph nodes provides confirmatory evidence for true metastatic disease, the biological significance of small, often bland cellular aggregates in SLNs from such Spitzoid lesions has not been established and requires further study. Thus we urge caution in the recommendation of SLN biopsy for patients with such Spitzoid lesions and also in its interpretation if performed. Lymph node dissections should be considered for palpable and persistent lymphadenopathy. It must be stressed that all such lesions be managed on an individual basis.

Aside from melanoma and atypical (dysplastic) nevi, Spitz nevus needs to be distinguished from its variants desmoplastic Spitz nevus, pigmented spindle cell nevus, as well as other melanocytic nevi with features shared by Spitz nevi. The characteristics of these nevi are discussed throughout this book.

A number of nonmelanocytic, primarily histiocytic lesions may also simulate Spitz nevus and need to be considered in the differential diagnosis. Juvenile or adult xanthogranuloma lacks a junctional component and typically has Touton giant cells (52). In a lesion with rare or no giant cells, the finding of histiocytes with foamy cytoplasm or the presence of eosinophils is helpful. In contrast to Spitz nevi, the cells in juvenile xanthogranuloma are typically not immunoreactive with S-100 protein and Mart-1. Epithelioid cell histiocytoma (53) is another lesion that can mimic Spitz nevus. It primarily occurs as a solitary nodule in adulthood (mean age, 42 years), most commonly on the lower limbs. It lacks a junctional component, often has an epidermal collarette, and is composed of a proliferation of large epithelioid cells with polygonal or triangular outlines, which do not show a gradient in size from above downward to the base. Epithelioid histiocytomas usually show prominent vascularity with clustering of epithelioid cells around the blood vessels. A small number of cells may be S-100 protein positive, but the majority are not. Staining for factor XIIIa, however, is common, for which melanocytes in Spitz nevi are said to be negative.

Reticulohistiocytoma of the skin is characterized by the presence of giant cells with abundant ground glass eosinophilic cytoplasm (52). These cells often have large hyperchromatic nuclei. They are usually more densely aggregated than melanocytes in Spitz nevi and may have an accompanying mixed inflammatory infiltrate of lymphocytes, plasma cells, and eosinophils. The cytoplasm of the giant cells is PAS positive and diastase resistant. If no intraepidermal melanocytes can be found, then melanin stains and immunoreactivity S-100 protein and Mart-1 may be of help. Melanin stains are negative and the cells in reticulohistiocytoma lack immunoreactivity for S-100 protein and other melanocytic markers, such as Mart-1.

Spitz nevi differ from cellular neurothekeoma (54) by the presence of junctional nests, maturation, or melanin pigment; by the feature of individual cells infiltrating the dermis at the base of the lesion; and by the expression of melanocytic markers, such as S-100 protein and Mart-1. The stroma in cellular neurothekeoma is usually slightly myxoid.

Metastasizing Spitz Tumor

As already mentioned, melanocytic lesions classified as Spitz nevi have been reported to spread to regional lymph nodes without alleged subsequent disease progression (5,7,21,55,56). The concept of localized, presumably "benign" metastases has been proposed to explain this rare phenomenon. However, some of these metastasizing melanocytic lesions, albeit resembling in many ways Spitz nevi, are generally unusually large (i.e., > 1 cm), are often deep and involve the subcutaneous fat, are ulcerated, and have high mitotic rates or showed other uncommon features (see above) (21–23,51) (Figs. 7-11 and 7-12). An alternative explanation is that these tumors are simply unusual melanomas with Spitzoid features, which may or may not have a less aggressive potential for spread beyond regional lymph nodes. More definitive characterization is needed before any conclusions can be drawn about the latter group of tumors. Suffice it to say that there are no convincing data available at present to suggest that there exists a unique variant of melanoma with less aggressive behavior.

SPECIAL TECHNIQUES FOR DIAGNOSIS

The diagnosis of Spitz nevus still rests on light microscopic morphologic features. A number of additional techniques have been used in an attempt to facilitate the distinction between Spitz nevus and malignant melanoma. Ultrastructurally, a distinct type of cell was reported to be characteristic of Spitz nevus. This cell was described to contain a large number of premelanosomes, oriented around the Golgi complex, without melanin synthesis (57). However, the applicability of electron microscopy to the routine diagnostic work-up of Spitz nevi appears limited.

Silver-Staining Nucleolar Organizer Region

A difference in numbers of silver-staining nucleolar organizer regions (AgNORs) between Spitz nevi and melanomas was suggested (58). However, there was overlap in the results, which questions the usefulness of this technique to resolve diagnostic dilemmas.

Immunohistochemistry

Spitz nevi have been evaluated with a variety of melanocytic markers. S-100 protein is probably the most sensitive marker, and Mart-1 may be somewhat less consistent. The antibodies to these show diffuse expression throughout Spitz nevi in contrast to the characteristic diminished expression of HMB-45 and tyrosinase toward the base of the lesion (59,60). Spitz nevi have low prolif-

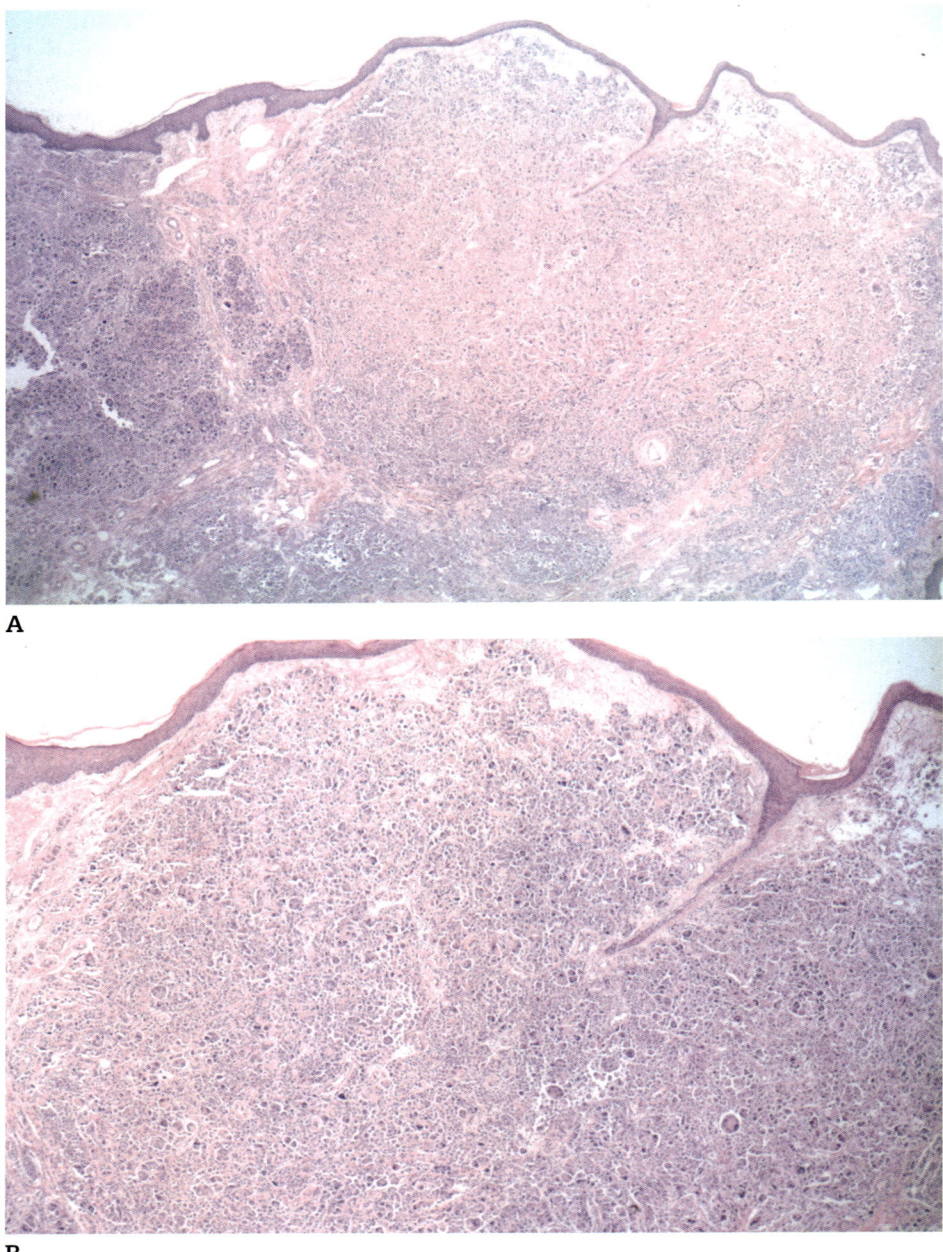

FIGURE 7-11 Metastasizing Spitz tumor (malignant melanoma). This tumor developed on the arm of a 2-year-old girl and resulted in a single axillary lymph node metastasis and no subsequent progression of disease at the 3-year follow-up. **A,** Superficial portion of lesion measuring > 1 cm in diameter. The tumor showed ulceration in other fields. **B,** Higher magnification of panel A showing sheets of enlarged epithelioid melanocytes.

eration rates (in the range of 1–2%) when assessed with Ki-67 compared to much higher rates in melanoma. In addition, there is a gradient of diminished proliferation with increasing depth of the dermal component paralleling mitotic rate and cyclin D1 expression (61–65). Spitz nevi also appear to exhibit lower rates of both p53 and Bcl-2 expression compared to melanoma (61). Although many of these studies are of interest, they are usually not very helpful when the pathologist encounters a difficult Spitzoid lesion that suggests melanoma.

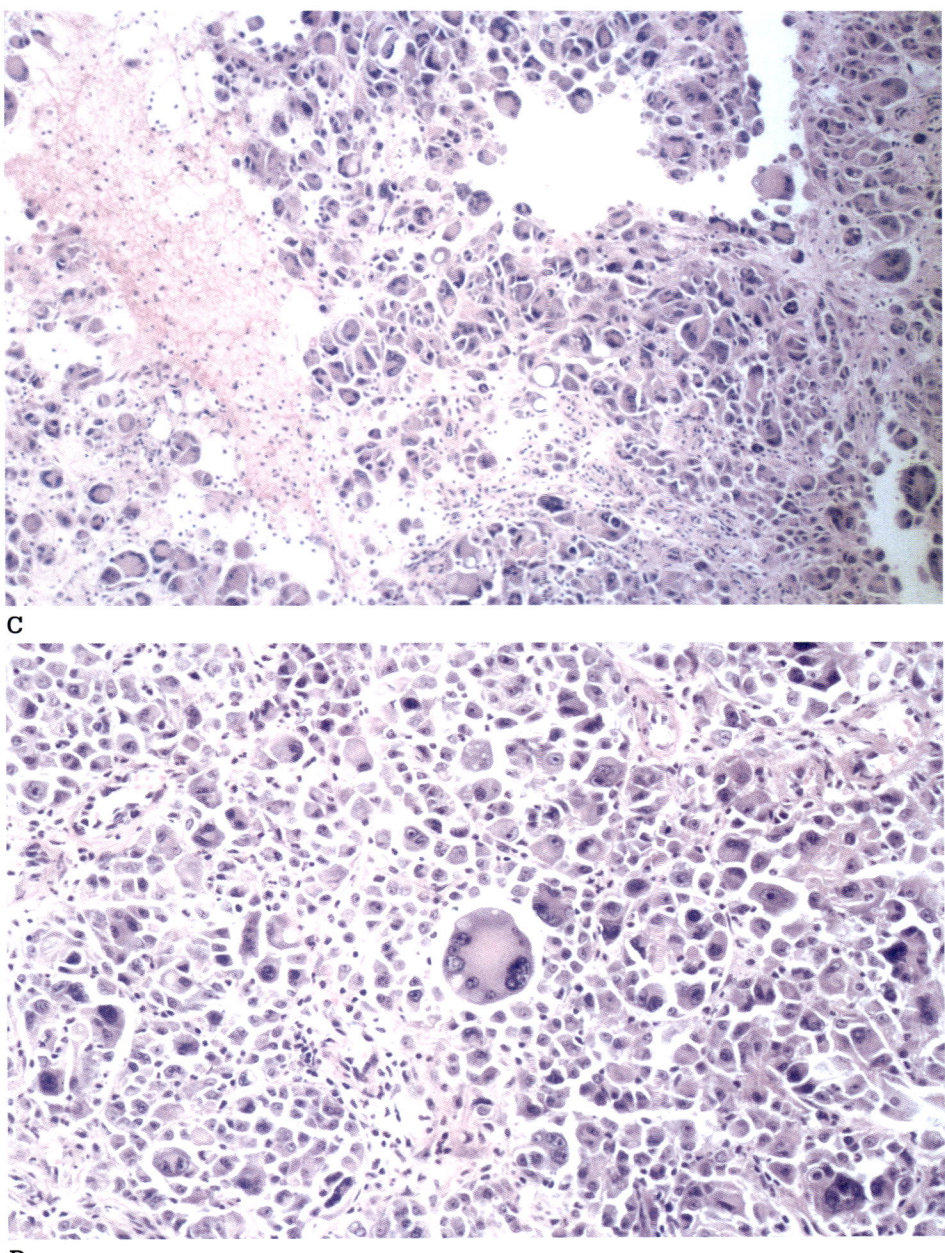

FIGURE 7-11 *Continued.* **C,** Dyscohesive aggregates of melanocytes in the dermis without maturation. **D,** Note the pleomorphism of cells and bizarre multinucleate giant cell.

DNA-Ploidy

The cells in Spitz nevi show a normal diploid pattern in the majority of cases (59). Several investigators using a variety of techniques to determine DNA-ploidy have not been able to discriminate between Spitz nevi and malignant melanoma (66,67).

Volume-Weighted Mean Nuclear Volume

Volume-weighted mean nuclear volume, a stereologic technique, indicates that Spitz nevi tend to have significantly smaller mean nuclear volumes, especially toward the base of the lesion, compared to melanomas (68).

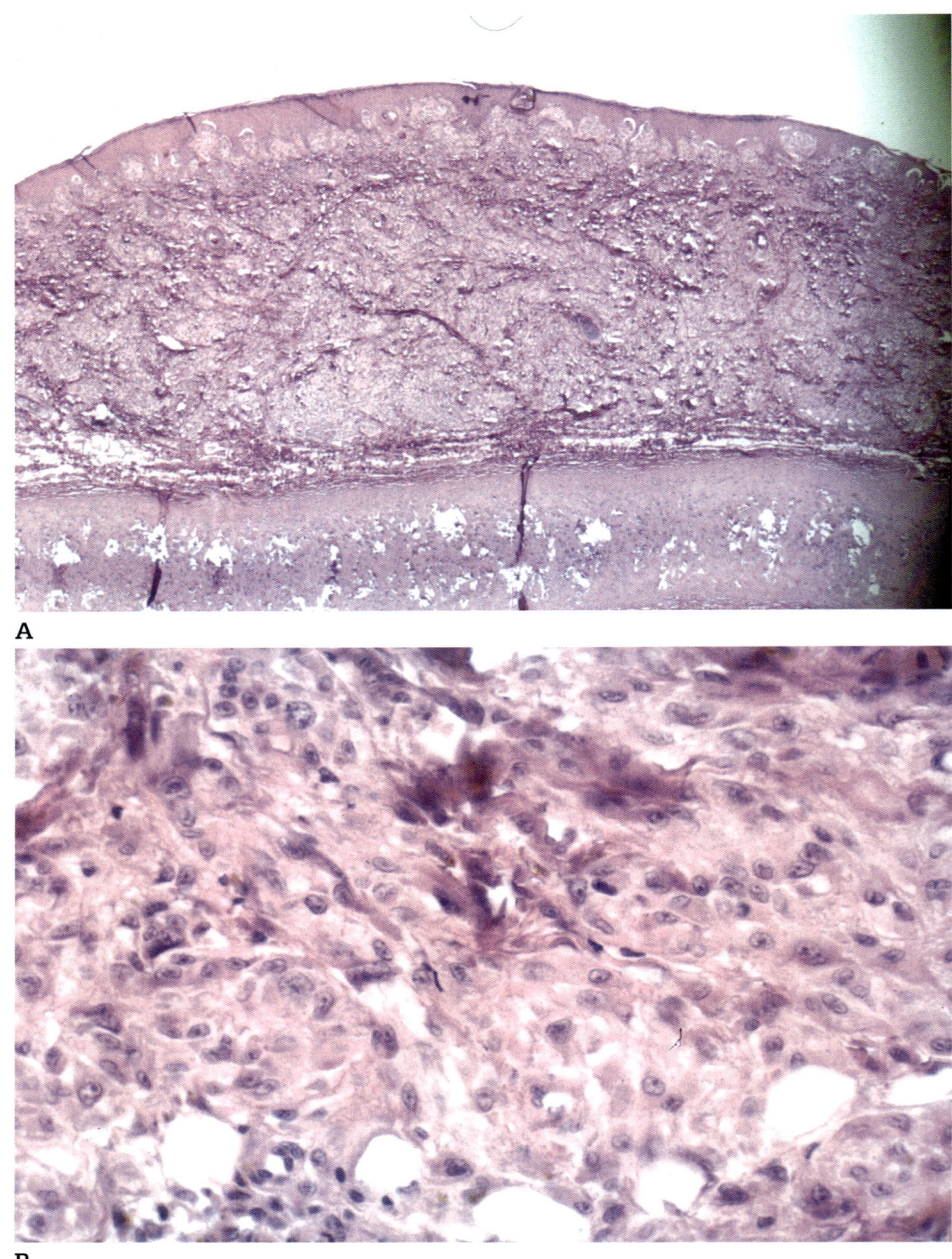

FIGURE 7-12 Metastasizing Spitz tumor (malignant melanoma). This tumor developed on the ear of a 7-year-old boy and resulted in a single cervical lymph node metastasis; the patient remains healthy after 9 years' of follow-up. **A,** There is a broad, dome-shaped, melanocytic tumor overlying the elastic cartilage of the ear. **B,** Confluent nests of enlarged epithelioid melanocytes are present in the deep dermis and lack maturation.

Comparative Genomic and Fluorescence in situ Hybridizations

The recent application of comparative genomic hybridization (CGH) and fluorescence in situ hybridization, to study both the biological nature of Spitz nevi and the potential distinction from melanoma has demonstrated that the majority of Spitz nevi studied by CGH had no chromosomal abnormalities (69,70). On the other hand, amplification of chromosome 11p has been observed in a subset of cases and was found to correlate with Spitz nevi that were often larger in size, were dermal based, were desmoplastic, had vesicular nuclei in melanocytes, and exhibited dermal infiltrating features. Further study of Spitz nevi with gains of chromosome 11p has shown an increase in copy number of and mutations in the *HRAS* gene by fluorescence in situ hybridization. The latter abnormalities do not usually occur in melanoma, thus suggest that such findings (and the absence of chromosomal aberrations in most Spitz nevi) may aid in the distinction of Spitz nevi from melanoma. Other conclusions from the latter studies are that Spitz nevi are probably clonal proliferations, the majority of melanocytes are diploid with some large nuclei being polyploid, and Spitz nevi may be cytogenetically distinct from melanoma (70). While those findings are of considerable interest, they require confirmation.

Loss of Heterozygosity

Two independent studies have demonstrated loss of heterozygosity on chromosome 9p with DNA polymorphic markers in 2 of 27 and 5 of 5 Spitz nevi studied (71,72). The latter findings provide additional evidence for the close relationship between Spitz nevi and melanoma.

DESMOPLASTIC SPITZ NEVUS (SCLEROSING SPITZ NEVUS, DESMOPLASTIC NEVUS)

Clinical Features

Although the desmoplastic Spitz nevus is considered by many to be an unusual variant of Spitz nevus (73,74), some authors maintain that this lesion is a distinct entity (termed simply "desmoplastic nevus") (74,75). The basis for considering such desmoplastic nevi to be a nevus sui generis is the absence of an intraepidermal component typical of Spitz nevus in many instances and the frequent presence of a somewhat smaller cell type, often spindled, with relatively scant cytoplasm. In fact both perspectives are correct and simply indicate the heterogeneity of nevi and how strict or relaxed are the criteria applied for Spitz nevus or another type of nevus. Such sclerosing nevi (and many nevi in general) are commonly heterogeneous with respect to the phenotype of melanocytes present. The final decision to designate a particular nevus as Spitz or not must be based on whether most of the cellular population has characteristics of Spitz melanocytes or not. Therefore, a nevus potentially could be categorized as a desmoplastic Spitz nevus, a desmoplastic nevus not otherwise specified, or a desmoplastic nevus with Spitz and non-Spitz components, etc.

Desmoplastic Spitz nevus typically presents as a firm dome-shaped papule or nodule, measuring up to 1 cm or more in greatest diameter, and most often located on the extremities (9,73,74) (Table 7-6). In many instances, the lesion is flesh colored, erythematous, or slightly pigmented with reddish hues and suggests a dermatofibroma. This variant of Spitz nevus primarily affects adults with a peak incidence in the 3rd decade. However, it may also be encountered in children. Usually, the patient gives a history that the lesion has been present for months or even years.

Histopathological Features

The desmoplastic Spitz nevus is characterized by a poorly circumscribed growth of large polygonal or elongated melanocytes in a collagen-rich stromal background (9,73–75) (Fig. 7-13; Table 7-6). It is usually a wholly intradermal lesion, although minor junctional components may be present (Fig. 7-13A,B). It should be noted that the desmoplastic changes in Spitz nevi may affect the entire lesion or any portion of it. As with other Spitz nevi, epidermal hyperplasia is often present but there may be central effacement of the epidermis with hyperplasia at the peripheries. In the superficial dermis, melanocytes may be grouped in nests or aggregates, whereas in the deeper parts of the lesions, they tend to infiltrate singly between typically thickened collagen bundles, often keloidal in appearance (Fig. 7-13C). The latter phenomenon is maturation, as in other Spitz nevi. Scattered multinucleated giant cells or large pleomorphic forms may be present. Cytologically, the melanocytes of desmoplastic Spitz nevi are characterized by nuclei that are often hyperchromatic with clumped or finely dispersed chromatin (Fig. 7-10D). Nucleoli are commonly inconspicuous but may be prominent, especially in larger cells. The size of the nuclei tends to diminish as melanocytes approach the base of the lesion, which is usually ill-defined. Mitoses are rare (usually < 1/20 HPF) (26). A lymphohistiocytic infiltrate may be present, but is generally sparse. As described for other variants of Spitz nevi, HMB-45 immunoreactiviy if present is observed in the most superficial portion of the lesion and diminishes with depth. Ki-67 expression as an indicator of proliferation rate is low versus much the higher rates in melanoma.

Angiomatoid Spitz Nevus

The angiomatoid variant of desmoplastic Spitz nevus is notable for prominent numbers of microvessels, often clustered, distributed throughout the lesion (76). Five women (19–28 years of age) have been reported with solitary lesions; the extremities were involved in four cases.

Differential Diagnosis

The major differential diagnostic problem with desmoplastic Spitz nevus is its distinction from desmoplastic melanoma, but it also includes other sclerosing dermal

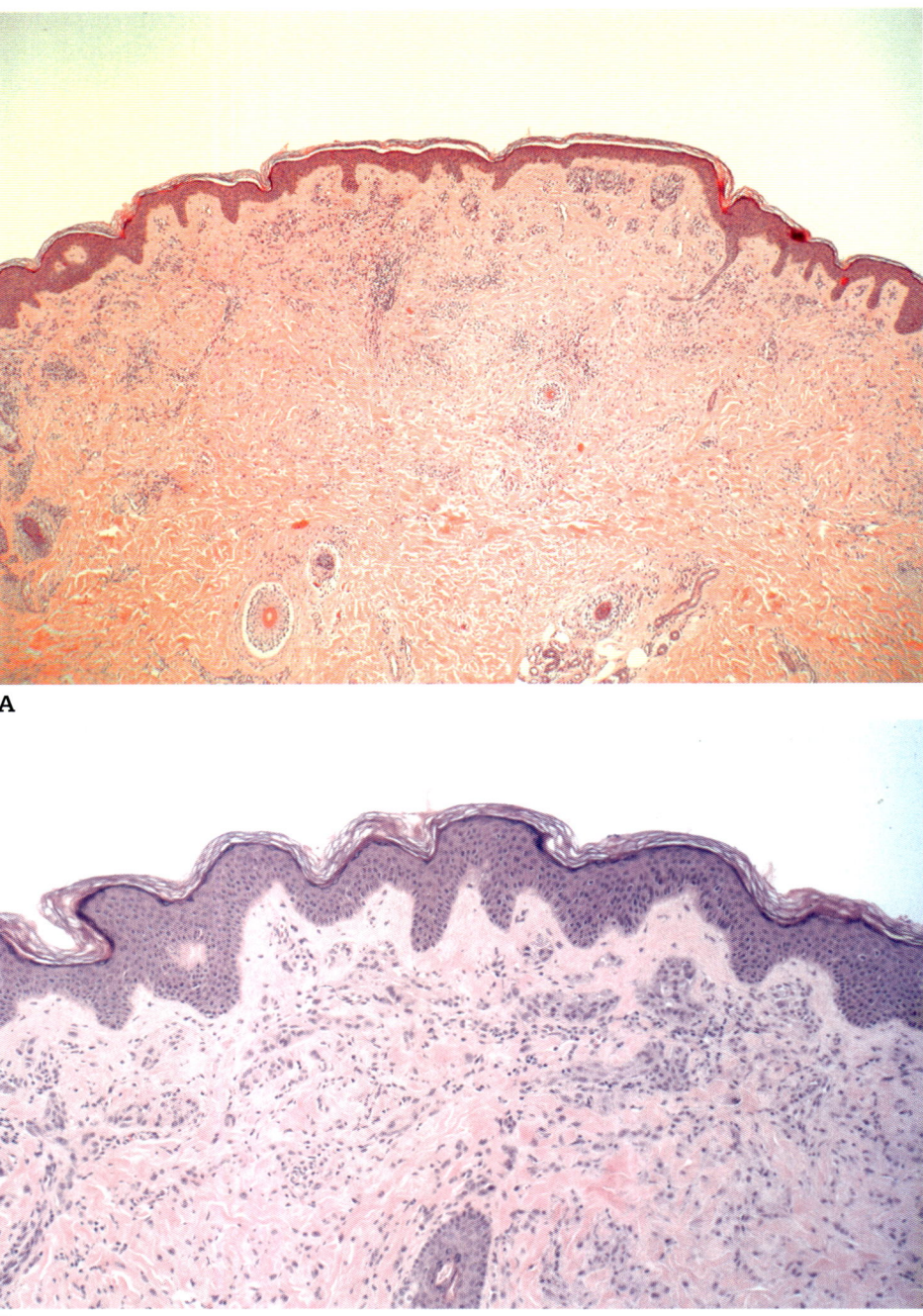

FIGURE 7-13 Desmoplastic Spitz nevus. **A,** The lesion is entirely intradermal and characterized by a nondescript appearance at this magnification. Nonetheless, the tumor exhibits symmetry and an orderly pattern. **B,** Nests, cords, and individual cells dispersed in sclerotic dermis.

tumors, such as sclerosing (hypomelanotic) blue nevi, dermatofibromas, cellular neurothekeomas, and scars (73–75). A number of features help distinguish desmoplastic Spitz nevus from desmoplastic melanoma (Table 7-7). The desmoplastic Spitz nevus may present in a similar fashion to desmoplastic melanoma—that is, an indurated amelanotic or slightly pigmented nodule. However, in other respects, the desmoplastic Spitz nevus is strikingly different from desmoplastic melanoma. There is a predilection for the extremities of young individuals

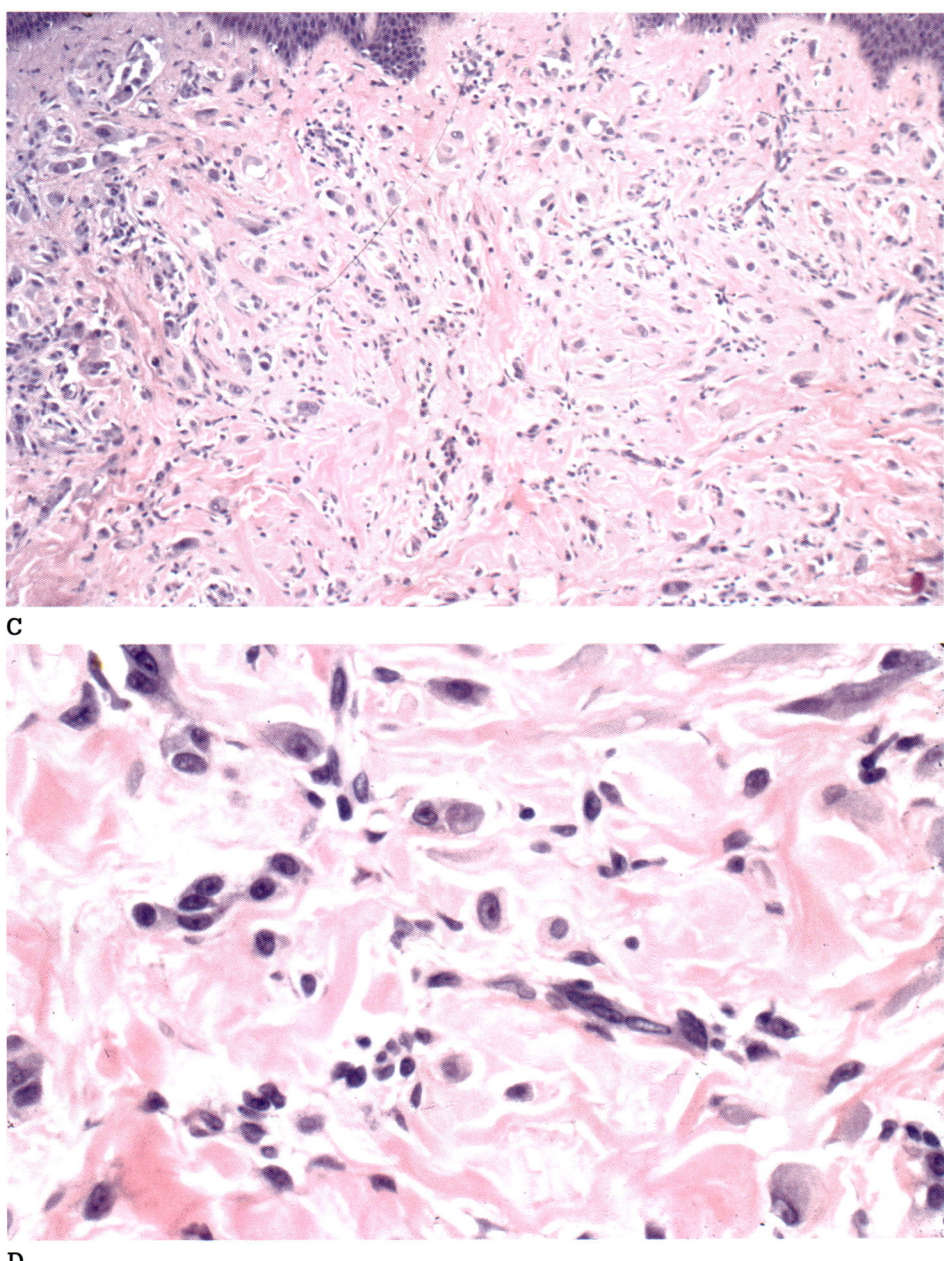

FIGURE 7-13 *Continued.* **C,** Typical epithelioid cells of Spitz nevus scattered throughout sclerotic dermis. **D,** Note the pink homogenous quality of the collagen. The Spitz nevus cells infiltrate the collagen without disruption.

but for the head and neck in elderly persons in desmoplastic melanoma. Histologically, desmoplastic Spitz nevi tend to be small, well-circumscribed, superficial lesions, whereas desmoplastic melanomas are often larger, poorly demarcated, and characterized by deep involvement of the dermis or subcutis. The desmoplastic variant of Spitz nevus also shows maturation (isolation of individually smaller cells with increasing depth) versus little or no such transition in desmoplastic melanoma. As outlined above, the cell types in the two processes tend to be rather different. Desmoplastic Spitz nevi contain typical large epithelioid or fusiform cells, whereas desmoplastic melanoma is notable for pleomorphic spindle cells, often with hyperchromatic nuclei.

TABLE 7-6 Desmoplastic Spitz nevus.

Clinical features
- Firm papule or nodule
- Adults (peak incidence in 3rd decade)
- Women > men
- Most commonly located on extremities (especially proximal arm)

Histopathological features
- Spindle and/or epithelioid cells
- Predominantly intradermal location of melanocytes
- Junctional component, sometimes
- Dermal stroma with increased collagen
- Well circumscribed, usually
- Vaguely wedge shaped, often
- Diffuse distribution of cells with low cell density, usually
- Small nests and single melanocytes, typical
- Maturation often present
- Mitoses absent or rare
- Multinucleate giant cells not uncommon (usually superficial)
- Melanin usually sparse or absent
- Angiomatoid Spitz nevus
    - Prominent number of microvessels, often clustered, throughout lesion

Differential diagnosis
- Desmoplastic melanoma
- Sclerosing blue nevus
- Dermatofibroma, largely regressed
- Epithelioid cell (fibrous) histiocytoma
- Cellular neurothekeoma
- Multinucleate cell angiohistiocytoma

A benign melanocytic lesion that may be confused with this variant of Spitz nevus is the sclerosing often hypomelanotic blue nevus. Although blue nevus may have pronounced sclerosing features, it is usually a more ill-defined melanocytic lesion than desmoplastic Spitz nevus and is composed of a more slender and more diffusely pigmented melanocytic population than the plumper cells of Spitz nevi. Blue nevi in general are often oriented about skin appendages and neurovascular bundles in a lobular organoid configuration.

Nonmelanocytic dermal spindle cell lesions that may share morphologic features of desmoplastic Spitz nevus are dermatofibroma, reticulohistiocytoma, cellular neurothekeoma, and epithelioid cell histiocytoma (see above).

OTHER VARIANTS OF SPITZ NEVUS

Combined Spitz Nevus (Spitz Nevus with Phenotypic Heterogeneity)

As discussed in detail in Chapter 9, Spitz nevi may demonstrate heterogeneity of the melanocytic populations resulting in the concomitant presence of other components such as ordinary nevus, nevus spilus, or blue nevus.

Hyalinizing Spitz Nevus

Suster (77) reported a dermal variant of Spitz nevus, probably closely related to desmoplastic Spitz nevus, that is characterized by a strikingly hyalinized or collagenized stroma. The five cases occurred in adults (ages 23–45 years) and possibly represent an involutional or regressing form of Spitz nevus. These nevi demonstrate sparse numbers of melanocytes, epithelioid and/or spindled, disposed as single cells or in small nests. Because of the retraction of the melanocytes from the surrounding hyalinized stroma, these lesions raise a differential diagnosis of tumors with chondroid differentiation, such as a mixed tumor (chondroid syringoma), metastatic carcinoma, and melanoma. The collagenous nature of the stroma has been confirmed by Masson trichrome stain; some mucin may be present as evidence by Alcian blue positivity.

Plexiform Spitz Nevus

Analogous to plexiform pigmented spindle cell nevi, rare dermal forms of Spitz nevus may demonstrate spindle and epithelioid melanocytes arranged in lobules and bundles with a plexiform configuration in the dermis (78). We reported two men, aged 17 and 52 years, with

TABLE 7-7 Desmoplastic Spitz nevus versus desmoplastic melanoma.

Characteristic	Desmoplastic Spitz nevus	Desmoplastic melanoma
Preferred site	Extremities (arm)	Head and neck
Preferred age group	Early adulthood	Late adulthood
Size	< 1 cm, often	>1 cm, often
Symmetry	Usually present	Usually absent
Melanocytic atypia		
Intraepidermal	Rare	Common
Dermal	Not uncommon but usually slight	Common, often more than slight
Mitoses	Rare	Variable, usually low mitotic rate
Necrosis	Absent	Occasional
Maturation	Common	Uncommon

solitary lesions on the lower leg and back, respectively. The two lesions measured 4.8 and 6.2 mm in diameter, were dome shaped, exhibited no intraepidermal component or detectable melanin pigment, and showed melanocytes with abundant eosinophilic cytoplasms disposed in fascicular or whorled arrangements with a slightly myxoid stroma (Fig. 7-14). The nuclei were ovoid and vesicular with small nucleoli. A single superficial mitosis was noted in the second case. The tumor cells were positive with S-100 protein (Fig. 7-14B) and negative with HMB-45, desmin, and actin. The differential diagnosis includes melanoma, plexiform pigmented spindle cell nevus, deep penetrating nevus, blue nevus, some congenital nevi, and plexiform peripheral nerve sheath tumors including neurofibroma, schwannoma, and cellular neurothekeoma.

FIGURE 7-14 Plexiform Spitz tumor. **A,** The melanocytic elements are arranged in plexiform aggregates throughout the dermis. **B,** S-100 protein immunostain highlights the plexiform nature of the tumor.

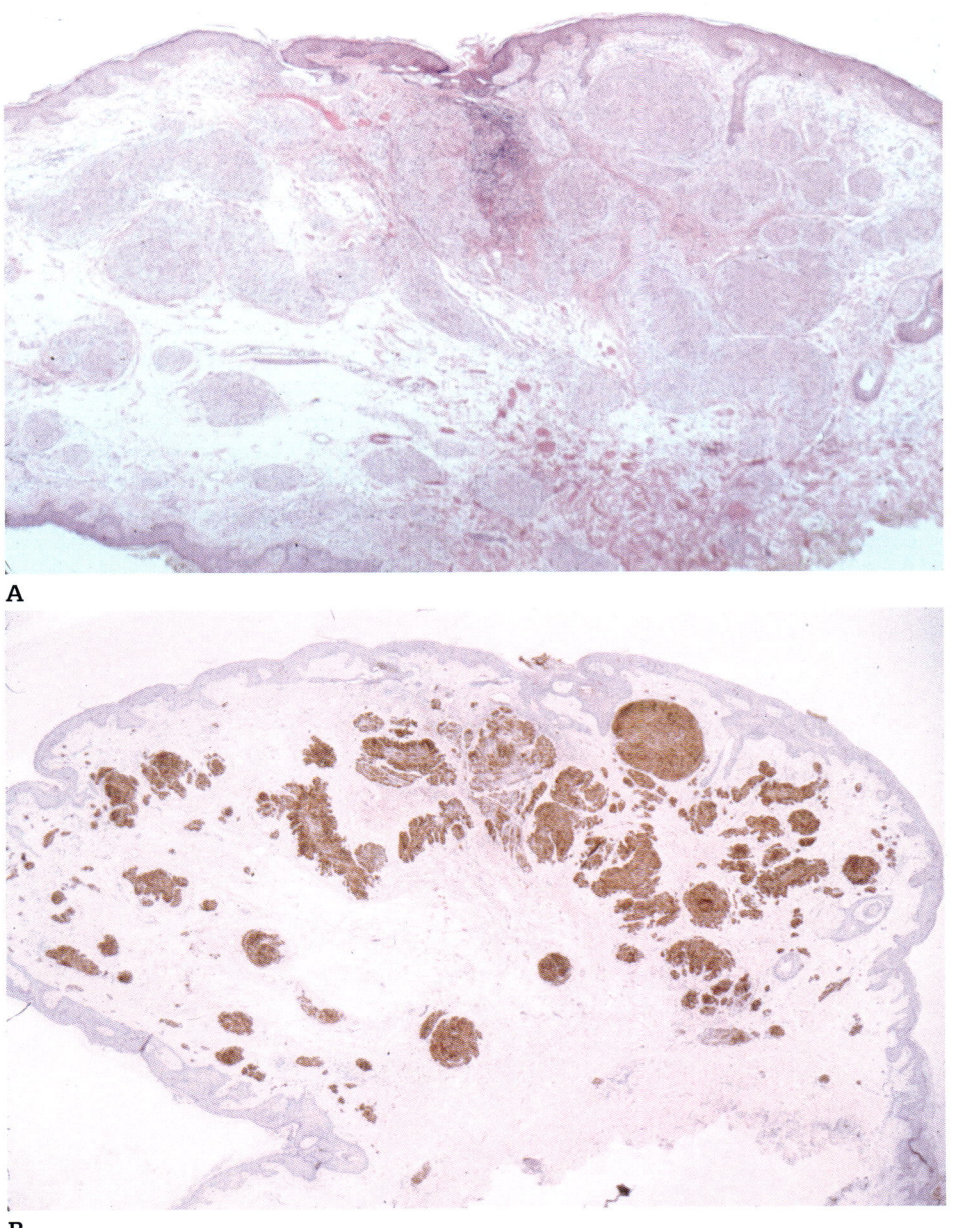

Spitz Nevus with Halo Reaction

In addition to the typical perivascular lymphocytic infiltrates observed in Spitz nevi, a small minority of these nevi may exhibit dense lymphoid infiltrates (halo reaction) comparable to such infiltrates in conventional melanocytic nevi (79,80). The concomitant occurrence of a clinical halo however is much less common. The presence of a halo reaction in a Spitz nevus adds another level of complexity to an already difficult diagnostic problem, vis-à-vis, the distinction of a Spitz nevus from melanoma.

A description of 17 Spitz nevi with halo reaction revealed that an additional nevus component, either a conventional acquired or superficial congenital pattern nevus component, was frequently present (in 9 cases) and were designated combined Spitz nevus with halo reaction (80). One must consider that the Spitz-like epithelioid cytologic features may be induced by the inflammatory reaction rather than necessarily being de novo Spitz nevi, combined or otherwise.

Such Spitz nevi display a diffuse permeation of dermal melanocytes by the lymphocytic infiltrate to the level of the dermoepidermal junction. These nevi often demonstrate features consonant with typical Spitz nevi: small diameter, symmetry, sharp circumscription, and wedge-shaped configuration. However, as stated above, such lesions are more diagnostically challenging than ordinary Spitz nevi because of the halo reaction. The maturation of dermal melanocytes may be disrupted and obscured by the infiltrate. In addition, aberrant cytologic alterations of melanocytes, such as prominent eosinophilic cytoplasm and nuclear degenerative changes, may make diagnostic interpretation more problematic.

The presence of an additional nevus component in a Spitz nevus with halo reaction (so-called combined Spitz nevus) introduces another dimension of complexity. Such lesions are thus often asymmetrical and may suggest the focal development of melanoma. The approach to such lesions is the systematic study of each component separately, which will commonly reveal a symmetrical and orderly character of each individual part.

Differential Diagnosis

The major challenge is the discrimination of Spitz nevi with halo reaction from melanomas with prominent lymphoid infiltrates mimicking halo nevi (80). The general approach to this problem of Spitz nevus versus melanoma has been extensively discussed above. However, a few points merit some attention. The inflammatory infiltrates in such Spitz nevi are often well defined, symmetrical, and permeate the entire dermal portion of the Spitz nevus as compared to the patchy, asymmetrical, and poorly defined infiltrates in melanoma. Furthermore, the lymphoid infiltrates in melanoma are commonly present at the base or infiltrate only the lower half to two thirds of the invasive tumor. Since maturation may be absent in both lesions, this is not a discriminatory feature. Other features that may favor melanoma include confluent aggregates of melanocyes toward the base of the lesion that are also often large, asymmetrical, and hypercellular and the presence of deeply located mitoses.

Tubular Spitz Nevus

The occurrence of empty spaces or vacuoles within small dermal aggregates of epithelioid cells in a Spitz tumor has been reported as "tubular" Spitz nevus (81). However, this unusual phenomenon has been ascribed to an artifact from tissue processing—that is, diminished cellular cohesion and shrinkage, resulting in empty spaces that suggest lumina (82).

PIGMENTED SPINDLE CELL NEVUS (PIGMENTED SPINDLE CELL NEVUS OF REED, PIGMENTED SPINDLE CELL TUMOR)

Clinical Features

The pigmented spindle cell nevus (PSCN) is a distinctive clinicopathologic entity important to recognize because of its frequent confusion with melanoma. PSCN usually presents as a symmetric, sharply circumscribed, dark brown or black papule or nodule (46,83–88) (Table 7-8). It is typically a small lesion, often measuring < 0.6 cm in diameter. Hypopigmented halos surrounding the lesion have been described (83), but are rare. PSCN is preferentially located on the extremities, especially the thigh, and less often on the trunk or arm. The lesion is uncommon in the head and neck region. It appears to affect women slightly more than men (46,84). The peak incidence of the lesion is in the 3rd decade, but may occur in children as well as in late adult life. Occasionally PSCN are congenital. There is usually a history of recent onset.

Histopathological Features

The architectural profile of PSCN at scanning magnification tends to be rather characteristic and is quite helpful in their recognition (83–88) (Table 7-8). These lesions are usually relatively small; strikingly well circumscribed; and remarkable for a slightly elevated, flat-topped plaque-like appearance of the epidermis (Fig. 7-15). The epidermis is often of fairly uniform thickness throughout or may diminish in thickness at the margins. However, some variants of PSCN may show elongation of epidermal rete ridges, but this is not the usual case. Although the PSCN may be junctional or compound, many are almost entirely intraepidermal. If dermal involvement occurs, the

TABLE 7-8 Pigmented spindle cell nevus.

Clinical features
- Peak incidence in 3rd decade (mean age ~ 24 years)
- Most often located on extremities (especially thigh)
- Women > men
- Small (usually < 0.6 cm)
- Symmetric
- Pigmented (usually evenly, often heavily, dark brown or black)
- Sharply circumscribed
- Papule or nodule
- History of recent onset

Histopathological features
- Predominately junctional
- Predominantly spindle cells but occasional epithelioid cells
- Spindle cells more slender and delicate than in Spitz nevi
- Uniform population of cells from side to side
- Symmetrical configuration
- Predominance of junctional nests or fascicles
- Typically ovoid nests with fusiform cells oriented vertically
- Often confluence of nests leading to irregular shapes
- Sharp lateral borders, occasional lentiginous lateral spread
- Often some pagetoid spread
- Usually abundant coarse melanin
- Uniform nuclear features
- Inconspicuous or small nucleoli
- Decrease in cell size from top to bottom (maturation)
- Mitoses not uncommon in intraepidermal component
- Absent or rare dermal mitoses
- Uniform platelike hyperplasia of epidermis from side to side
- Plaquelike aggregates of spindle cells in papillary dermis (cells often smaller compared to intraepidermal component)

Differential diagnosis
- Solar melanoma
- Pagetoid melanoma
- Atypical nevus

---

spindle cell elements are usually confined to the papillary dermis.

The PSCN is also remarkable for the presence of uniform, delicate, spindle cells present in tightly packed fascicles in its most typical presentation (Fig. 7-15B). These fascicles of cells tend to have a fairly uniform and symmetric spacing and size within the epidermis. The fascicles are often vertically oriented (Fig. 7-16A) but may also form concentric arrangements (Fig. 7-16B) and be horizontally disposed.

The nests or fascicles vary in size and density. They are often closely apposed to each other and may be fused. They tend to be centered at or near the dermoepidermal junction and sometimes fill the majority of junctional space of the lesion. The predominant cellular growth pattern is within nests or fascicles. However, some PSCN, particularly in children, may show florid upward migration of single melanocytes, closely simulating melanoma in situ (Fig. 7-16D). Epithelioid cells may be present, but only as a minor cell population (83–88). The fusiform cells are often slightly more slender than the spindle cells of "classic" Spitz nevus (Fig. 7-16B). Their nuclei are equal in size or are smaller than the nuclei of adjacent keratinocytes (87,88). A decrease in nuclear size from top to bottom may or may not be present, but many PSCN are not sufficiently thick for such an assessment to be meaningful. The nuclear shape is typically oval and regular. The chromatin pattern is usually finely stippled. Nucleoli may be inconspicuous or prominent (87,88). A particularly important feature that is very useful in the recognition of PSCN is the uniformity of nuclei. Nuclear pleomorphism or anisochromasia is uncommon and, if present, need to be viewed as an atypical features.

Also in contrast to ordinary Spitz nevus, melanocytes of PSCN contain variable amounts of granular melanin. Heavy pigmentation may also involve the adjacent keratinocytes, cornified layer, and papillary dermis, giving the lesion a very dark color on gross appearance (46).

It must be clearly stated that there is a histologic continuum of Spitz nevus and PSCN (Table 7-9). One will encounter many nevi showing varying degrees of transition between the two poles of the spectrum. For example, some nevi may exhibit slender spindle cells typical of PSCN yet, at the same time, contain somewhat larger fusiform cells that are less heavily melaninized. The latter cells would be more suggestive of Spitz nevus.

The lesion grows in an expansile fashion. The lateral intraepidermal growth is usually sharply demarcated, with an abrupt transition from closely apposed nests to uninvolved epidermis. However, occasional lateral lentiginous proliferation of single melanocytes can be present and does not preclude the diagnosis of PSCN (see below).

In contrast to the infiltrative-appearing, often wedge-shaped deep portion of a Spitz nevus, the base of PSCN is typically broad with pushing borders if papillary dermal involvement is present (Fig. 7-16A). Compact rounded nests of relatively small cuboidal nevus cells often characterize the dermal component of PSCN. These cells often contain less pigment than intraepidermal spindle cells. The expansile nature of the papillary dermal nests may prompt scrutiny to rule out melanoma. However, the cytologic characteristics of such cells are usually unremarkable and one can observe a maturation from the intraepidermal cells to the lower-most nevus cells at the base of the lesion. Extension into the reticular dermis is much less frequent than in Spitz nevus (46).

As in Spitz nevus, shrinkage during tissue processing may lead to prominent clefts between fascicles of spindle

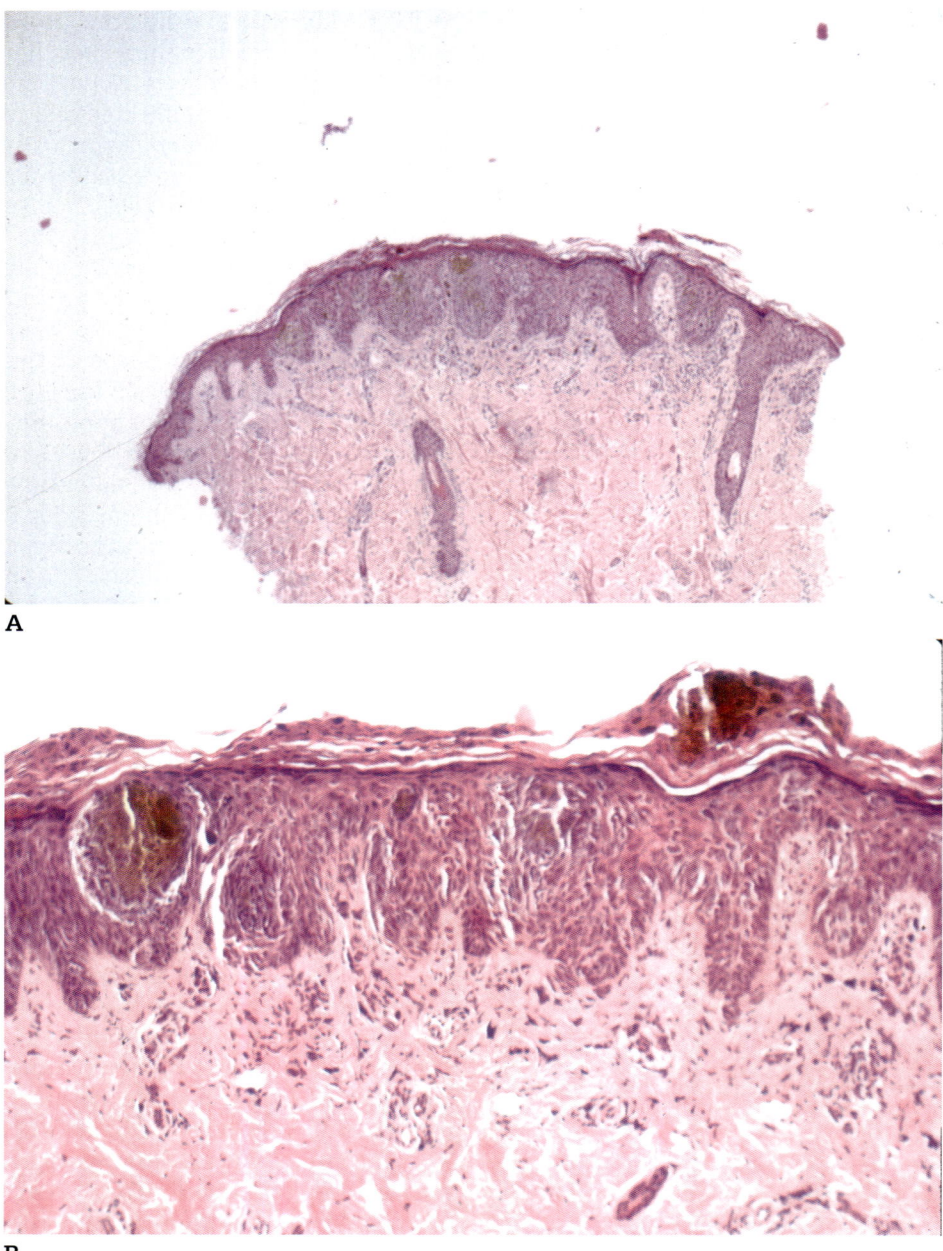

FIGURE 7-15 Pigmented spindle cell nevus. **A,** The lesion is small, symmetric, and well circumscribed. **B,** Scattered intraepidermal nests of spindle cells, some heavily pigmented.

cells from the adjacent epidermis. The same process leads also to retraction spaces separating melanocytes from each other and giving them a loosely aggregated appearance. As already mentioned, upward single cell extension of melanocytes toward the stratum corneum or transepidermal elimination of nests are not uncommon (88). However, lateral pagetoid melanocytic spread raises the suspicion for melanoma.

A rather characteristic feature of PSCN, also shared with Spitz nevus, is the proclivity of fascicles of spindle cells to track along skin appendages. One typically observes fascicles extending from the intraepidermal component to involve eccrine ducts or hair follicles, often following these structures into the reticular dermis. These nests or fascicles tend to be compact and commonly fusiform in shape. This striking feature may suggest

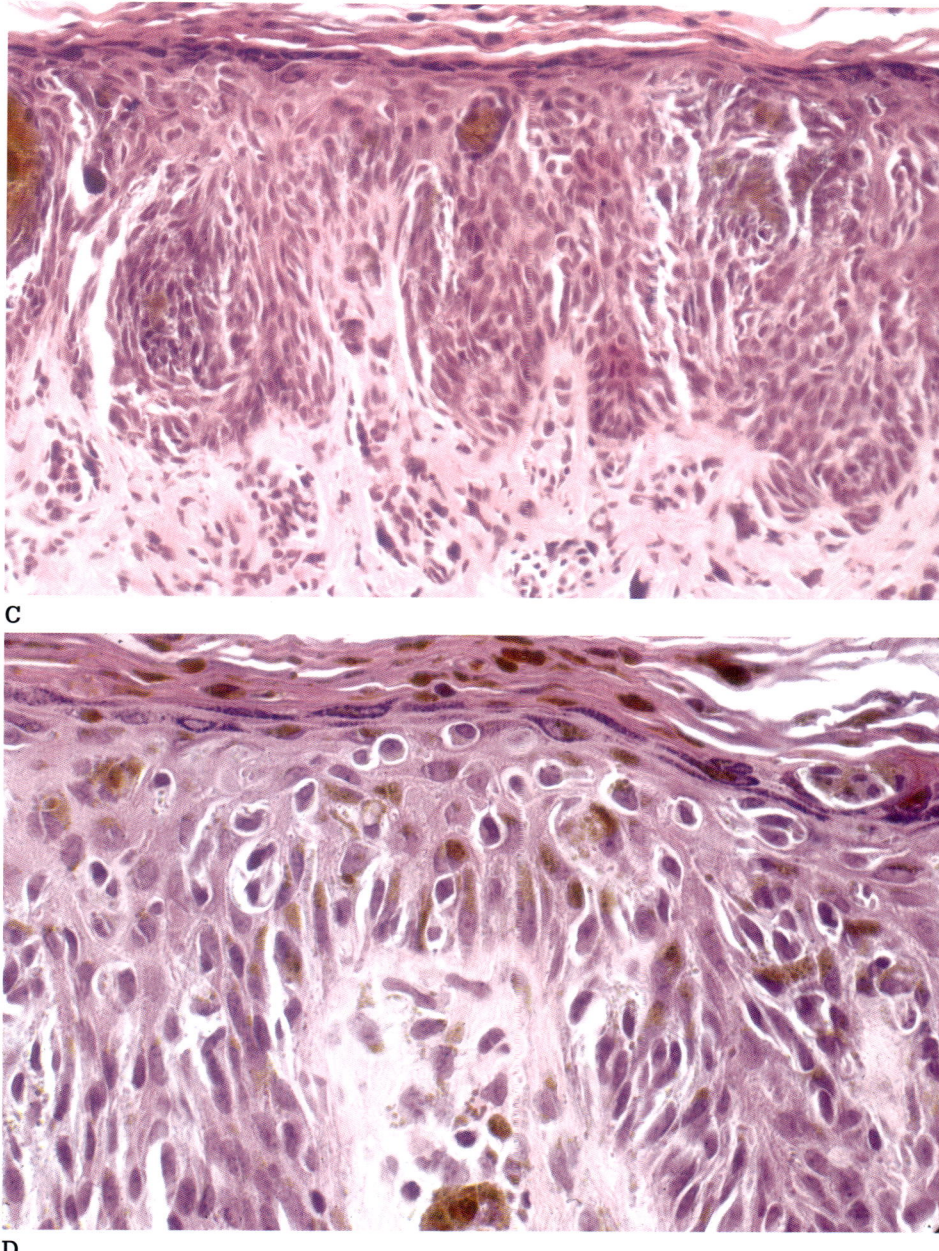

FIGURE 7-15 *Continued.* **C,** Fascicles of spindle cells are vertically disposed and seem to be part of the thickened epidermis. **D,** Prominent pagetoid spread simulating melanoma in situ. Nonetheless, the lesion has all the features of a benign process noted in panel A.

lentigo maligna, and the entire lesion should be carefully evaluated with this in mind.

Kamino bodies are less commonly seen than in Spitz nevus, but they can be found in the majority of cases, if serial step sections are examined (39). A patchy lymphocytic infiltrate with an admixture of melanophages is usually present at the base of the lesion, a feature that may cause confusion with melanoma.

Pigmented Spindle Cell Nevus with Atypical Features

The same discussion applies to the atypical variants of PSCN as previously elaborated for atypical forms of Spitz nevus (87,88) (Table 7-2). However, most atypical variants of PSCN are primarily intraepidermal. Substantial overlap may occur with conventional atypical nevi (Figs. 7-17 and 7-18).

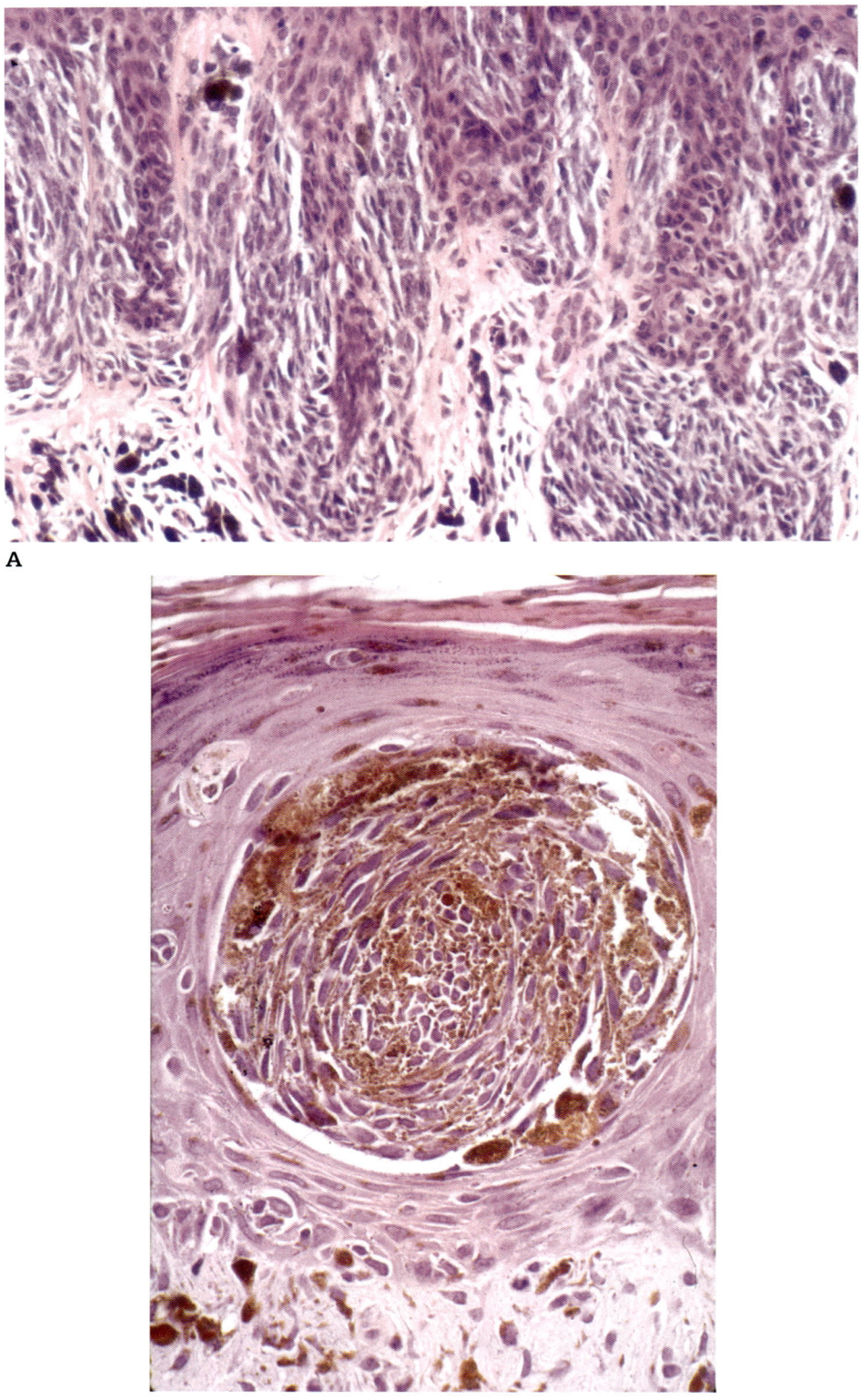

FIGURE 7-16 Pigmented spindle cell nevus. **A,** Vertically oriented fascicles of spindle cells and compact nest of cells in the papillary dermis. **B,** Uniform spindle cells in a concentric whorl.

TABLE 7-9 Comparison of Spitz nevus and pigmented spindle cell nevus.

Characteristic	Spitz nevus	Pigmented spindle cell nevus
Surface topography	Dome shaped	Plaquelike or gently elevated
Epidermal hyperplasia	Prominent, often almost pseudoepitheliomatous	Platelike
Pagetoid spread	Variable, may be focal	Common
Dermal architecture	Inverted wedge, often	Rounded nests of cells, usually confined to papillary dermis
Cell type	Enlarged epithelioid cells, spindle cells	Slender spindle cells; occasional transitional Spitz-like spindle cells; epithelioid cells, uncommon
Melanin content	Often minimal, prominent on occasion	Spindle cells contain granular melanin; epidermis and papillary dermis contain substantial melanin deposits

Note: This table lists features of the poles of what is a morphologic continuum.

Differential Diagnosis

Pigmented spindle cell nevus and its atypical variants must be distinguished from the the intraepidermal and microinvasive components of solar and pagetoid variants of melanoma and from atypical (dysplastic) nevus (87,88). Important features that distinguish PSCN from melanoma are listed in Table 7-10.

Pigmented spindle cell nevus (particularly atypical forms of PSCN) and solar melanoma (lentigo maligna) may show considerable similarity on occasion. Both are typically composed of pigmented spindle cells that may be arranged in junctional nests and may involve skin appendages to a striking degree. It is unusual for PSCN to occur on sun-exposed skin of the head and neck of older individuals, but this occasionally happens. Discrimination of the two is based on the usual small size, sharp circumscription, predominantly nested pattern, and uniformity of cell type in PSCN. Solar melanoma, on the other hand, tends to be broader, poorly circumscribed, and usually typified by a mainly basilar single-cell proliferation of pleomorphic melanocytes. Rare lesions may show such striking overlap that distinction may not be possible. In such circumstances, we recommend that such lesions are completely excised with a cuff of normal tissue, and that the lesion site be carefully monitored for aggressive behavior.

Pigmented spindle cell nevus and atypical variants of PSCN are often confused with the intraepidermal or microinvasive pagetoid variants of melanoma because of prominent pagetoid spread. This is one of the most commonly encountered problems in the pathology of melanocytic lesions. As discussed above, one must rely on clinical factors—young age, anatomic site (e.g., the extremities), and the overall morphologic appearance. PSCN are typically small, well demarcated, symmetric, and orderly. Even with striking pagetoid spread in some lesions, the latter features argue strongly in favor of a benign process, especially if present in a young individual and on a site such as the thigh. However, atypical forms of PSCN are extremely challenging, and all of the clinical and histologic features must be prudently weighed in the final interpretation. In many instances, a clear-cut diagnosis of melanoma cannot be made based on the constellation of findings. In such a situation, we often diagnose such lesions as PSCN (or melanocytic proliferation) with atypical features and recommend careful follow-up of the patient for recurrence. In our experience, recurrence of such lesions does not happen or seems to be extremely rare.

The same features characteristic of PSCN, such as cytologic uniformity and nuclear regularity, as well as its tendency to contain vertically disposed melanocytes (raining down) to the epidermal surface, help distinguish PSCN from conventional atypical (dysplastic) nevus, in which the melanocytes are oriented more parallel to the epidermal surface and show more cytologic variability and atypia. Atypical nevi are generally less cellular and often display a pronounced lentiginous melanocytic proliferation with elongation of the rete ridges and associated papillary dermal fibrosis, which are not typical features of PSCN. However, some atypical forms of PSCN show substantial overlap with conventional atypical nevi. Discrimination of the two lesions thus may not be reproducible. Such lesions may be designated as PSCN with atypical features or an atypical nevus with features of PSCN.

RECURRENT/PERSISENT SPITZ NEVUS

The recurrence of a Spitz nevus is by all accounts exceptionally rare (64,89–93). Harvell et al. (64) studied 22 cases, which is the largest series to date, and estimated an incidence of 0.9% (22 cases recurring among approximately 2400 Spitz nevi collected over an 11-year period). Since Spitz tumors are uncommon, this suggests an incidence of about 0.009% among all surgically removed melanocytic lesions. However, population-based data are not available;

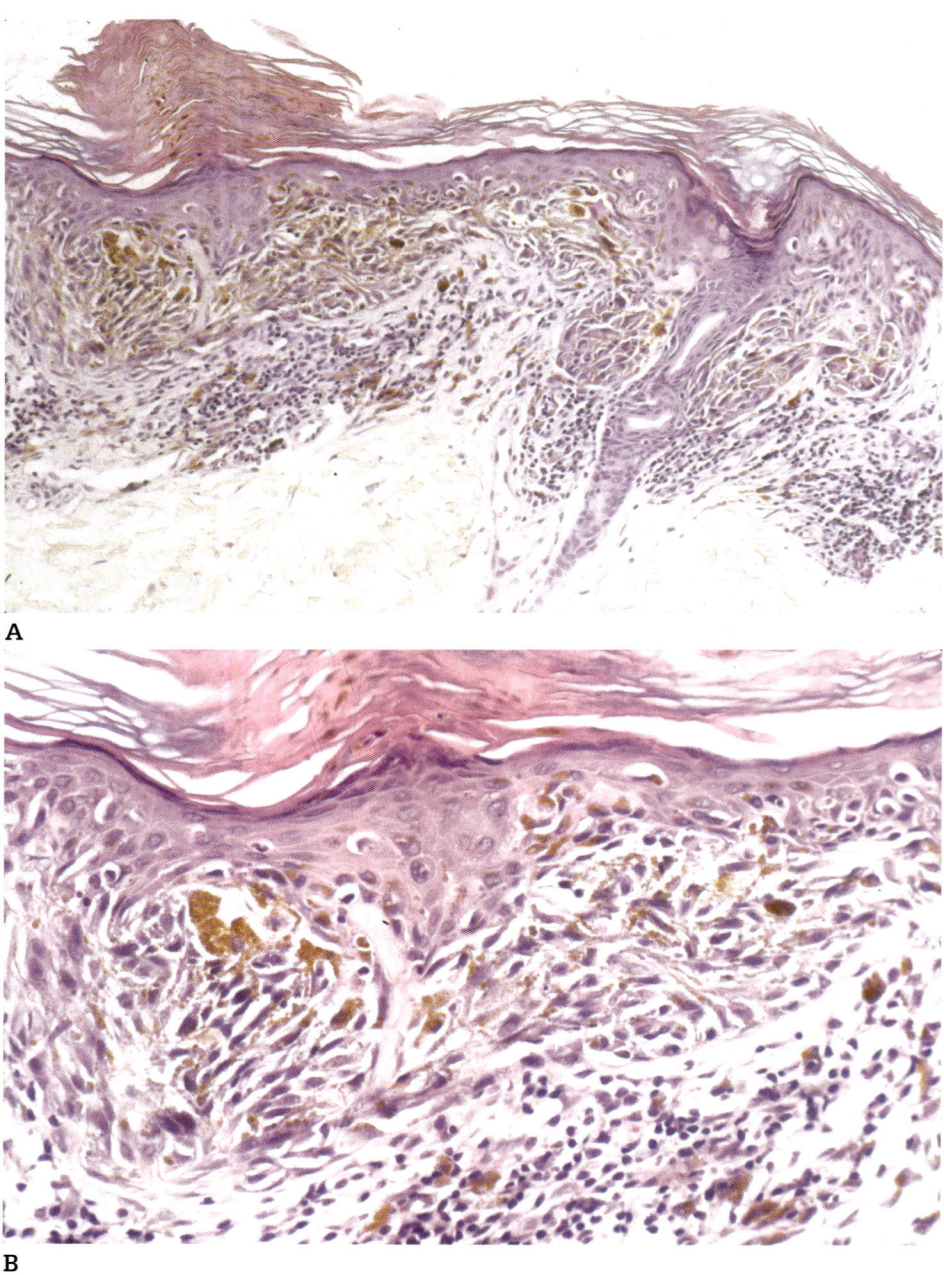

FIGURE 7-17 Pigmented spindle cell nevus with atypical features. **A,** Note the confluence of nests along dermoepidermal junction, an abnormal architectural feature. **B,** Higher magnification of panel A showing horizontal confluence. The nevus is recognizable as a PSCN because the cells are fusiform and contain melanin. Kamino bodies are also present in this field.

thus the latter estimates can be only tentative and are subject to significant referral bias and other factors, such as lack of consensus about standardized diagnosis.

Examining all published work to date, just over 50 cases of recurrent Spitz nevus have been reported (with varying degrees of detail). Given the extreme rarity of this phenomenon and the potential for confusion with melanoma, no meaningful information on this subject has been available until recently and is just beginning to emerge. The principal risk factor for recurrence identified thus far is involvement of the margins by the initial lesion (in at least 83% of cases). It is now well established that Spitz nevi recur after a much longer interval on average than do conventional melanocytic nevi (almost 1.5

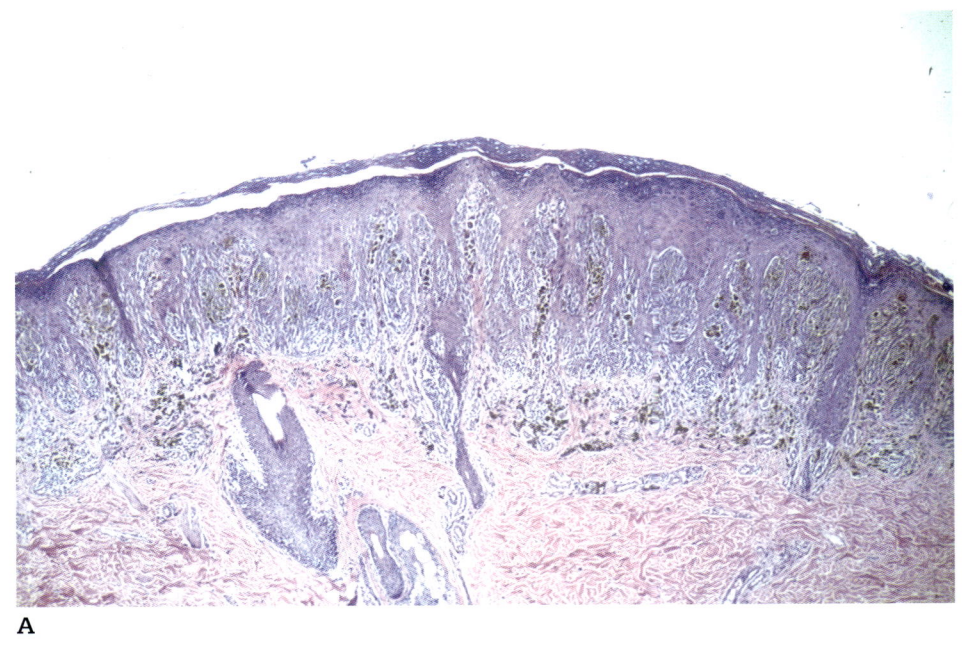

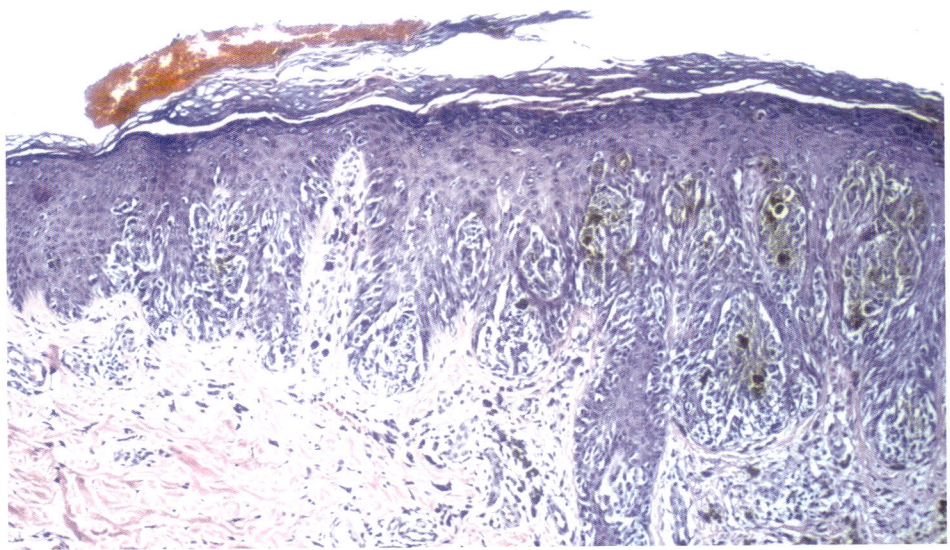

FIGURE 7-18 Pigmented spindle cell nevus with atypical features. **A,** The lesion is atypical because of rather broad size, irregular and confluent nesting along the dermoepidermal junction, pagetoid spread, and some nuclear pleomorphism. **B,C,** The lesion demonstrates fascicles of spindle cells along the dermoepidermal junction and some upward scattering of melanocytes.

years and up to 5 years, as compared to weeks to months for ordinary nevi). In addition, Spitz tumors may recur with greater size than the original Spitz nevus, as papular or nodular lesions, with extension beyond the surgical scar, and with more disturbing histologic features that suggest melanoma. Another important observation requiring further study is that, rarely, such recurrent tumors may eventuate in regional lymph node metastases and probable tumor progression to malignancy. We have reported a 12-year-old girl with a thigh lesion initially diagnosed as a typical Spitz nevus on shave biopsy (with positive margins) that resulted in two recurrences at the

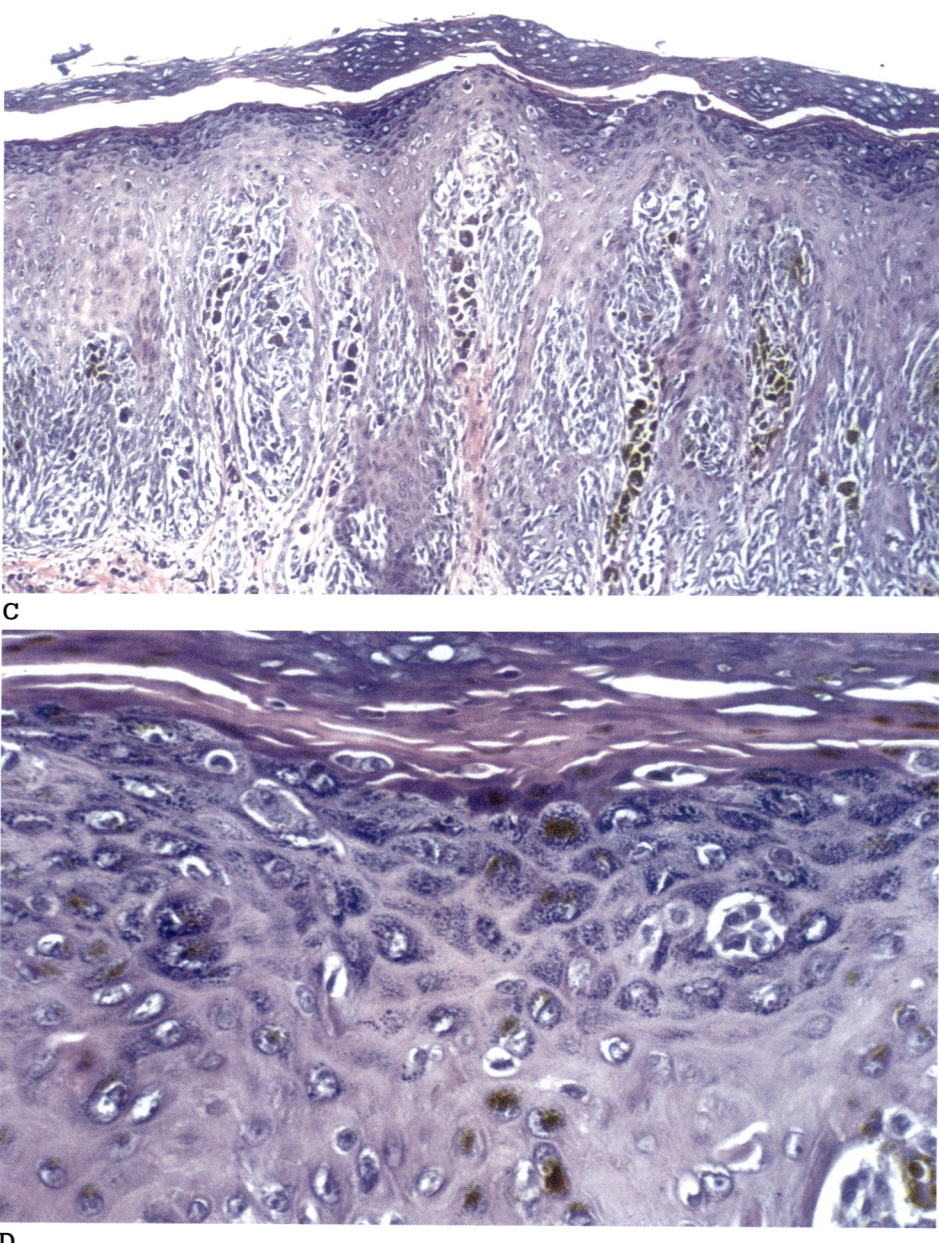

FIGURE 7-18 *Continued.* **D,** The pagetoid spread seen on higher magnification suggests melanoma; however, the other histopathologic features—including symmetry, the reasonably well-defined peripheral junctional component, and the lack of prominent cytologic atypia—argue against melanoma.

site, a deep satellite metastasis after 13 years, a regional lymph node metastasis the same year, and widespread metastases and death the following year (15 years after initial diagnosis) (23). It is clear that some of the attributes of recurrent Spitz nevi, such as interval to recurrence, parallel that of melanoma and again point out the many shared properties of Spitz nevi and melanoma in general.

Clinical Features

From the information currently available in the literature, recurrent Spitz nevi occur in young individuals with average age of 15.3 years (range 3–50 years) and suggest a close correspondence to the normal age distribution of individuals with Spitz nevi (64,87–93) (Table 7-11).

TABLE 7-10 Pigmented spindle cell nevus and atypical variants versus solar melanoma and pagetoid melanoma.

Characteristic	PSCN[a]	Atypical PSCN[a]	Solar melanoma (lentigo maligna)[a]	Pagetoid melanoma[a]
Symmetry	+	±	−	−
Sharp lateral borders	+	±	−	−
Cytologic uniformity	+	±	−	−
Regularity of nests	+	±	−	−
Maturation	+	±	−	−
Prominent vertical orientation of spindle cells	+	+	±	−
Involvement of appendages	+	+	+	±
Prominent coarse pigmentation	+	+	+	−

[a]+, usually present; ±, variably present; −, usually absent. Invariably there are exceptions to these guidelines.

TABLE 7-11 Recurrent (persistent) Spitz nevus.

Clinical features
  Extremely rare (estimated incidence 0.9% of Spitz nevi)
  Average age, 15.3 years (range 3–50 years)
  Females (59.6% of cases) > males
  Sites
    Extremities, most common site, 63.9% (especially individuals > 10 years)
    Head and neck (especially cheeks), 27.8% (especially children ≤ 5 years)
    Trunk, 8.3%
  Solitary papule or nodule at site of biopsy
  Occasional multiple lesions
  Time to recurrence, 1.4 years (range weeks to 5 years)
  Rare lymph node metastases and death reported
Histopathological features
  Size often about the same but may be larger and deeper than original lesion
  Conventional features of Spitz nevus commonly noted
    Spindle and/or epithelioid cells in all cases
    Maturation (zonation; dispersion, diminished cellularity of melanocytes with depth), often
    Clefting about junctional nests of melanocytes, often
    Low mitotic rate, usually
    Epidermal hyperplasia may be present
  Atypical features, present less commonly
    Some asymmetry
    Deep mitoses more common than in conventional Spitz nevi
    Extension into subcutaneous fat
    Prominent cytological atypia
  Patterns
    Resemblance to conventional recurrent melanocytic nevus: -disordered intraepidermal melanocytic proliferation (i.e., basilar single cell and nested proliferation of melanocytes along effaced epidermis), variable upward migration
    Resemblance to original Spitz nevus; association with scar
    Cohesive nodular aggregates of melanocytes in dermis
      Cytologic atypia may greater that original biopsy
      Maturation may be absent
      Mitotic rate may be greater than in original lesion
    Resemblance to desmoplastic Spitz nevus
      Predominantly intradermal location of melanocytes
      Dermal stroma with increased collagen
      Well circumscribed, usually
      Vaguely wedge shaped, often
      Diffuse distribution of cells with low cell density, usually
      Small nests and single melanocytes, typical
      Maturation, often
      Mitoses, absent or rare
      Multinucleate giant cells, not uncommon (usually superficial)
Differential diagnosis
  Melanoma, primary or metastatic
  Desmoplastic Spitz nevus
  Epithelioid cell (fibrous) histiocytoma
  Cellular neurothekeoma

There is predilection for the extremities (63.9%) followed by the head and neck, especially the central face (27.8%), and trunk (8.3%). Recurrent lesions are particularly prone to involve the cheeks and nose in children < 5 years of age, the extremities of patients > 10 years of age, and women in general (59.6% of recurrent lesions thus far reported).

The vast majority of lesions have been initially biopsied with the shave technique and at least 83%, perhaps almost all, have positive margins. The time to recurrence averaged 1.4 years (range weeks to 5 years). The recurrences generally present as slightly raised pink papules or nodules associated with or suggesting a scar, that on average are about the same size as the original lesion (usually < 5 mm). However, uncommonly, the recurrences may be strikingly nodular lesions that are larger that the antecedent tumor and may extend beyond the confines of the surgical scar.

Histopathological Features

Essential criteria for diagnosis include (a) review of the original biopsy from the site of recurrence to confirm a primary Spitz nevus and to exclude melanoma; (b) careful scrutiny of the margins of the antecedent biopsy for involvement or close proximity by the tumor suggesting persistence of the lesion at the site; and (c) histopathologic features consonant with a recurrent Spitz nevus and associated with a biopsy scar, corresponding to four general presentations (64,87–93) (Figs. 7-19 and 7-20; Table 7-11).

Conventional Recurrent/Persistent Melanocytic Nevus Pattern Disordered intraepidermal melanocytic proliferation overlies a dermal scar, as is observed in conventional recurrent nevi, and suggests melanoma in situ. The Spitz melanocytes are arranged as single cells and in small nests along the dermoepidermal junction of an effaced epidermis overlying the dermal scar (Fig. 7-19B,C). There may be some upward migration of melanocytes and possibly greater cytologic variation of melanocytes compared to the original biopsy. Often the original lesion is beneath or adjacent to the biopsy scar.

Original Spitz Nevus Pattern The recurrent tumor very closely resembles the antecedent lesion with the possible exception that the biopsy scar may introduce some distortion or asymmetry of the nevus architecture (Fig. 7-20).

Desmoplastic Spitz Nevus Pattern In his series of 16 cases, Stern (90) emphasized the striking resemblance of recurrent lesions to desmoplastic variants of Spitz nevi. However, Harvell et al. (64) found only 1 case among 22 to have this appearance. This discrepancy may be related to the patient populations in the series, the small numbers of cases, and other sources of bias.

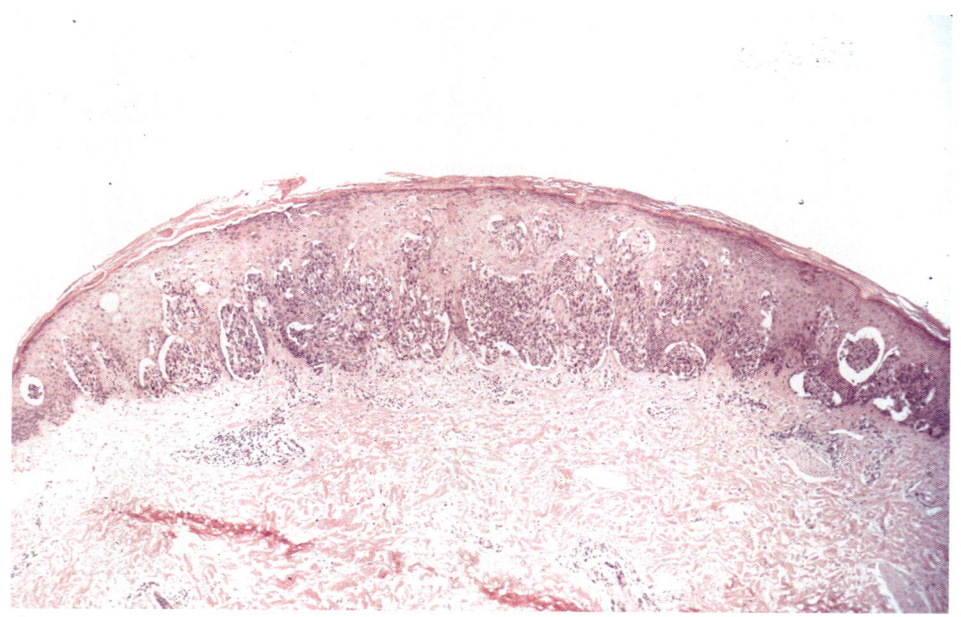

FIGURE 7-19 Recurrent/persistent Spitz tumor. **A,** The original lesion is characterized by a dome-shaped symmetrical profile, fairly sharp lateral demarcation, and cytologic features of a Spitz tumor. The lesion extended to a side margin.

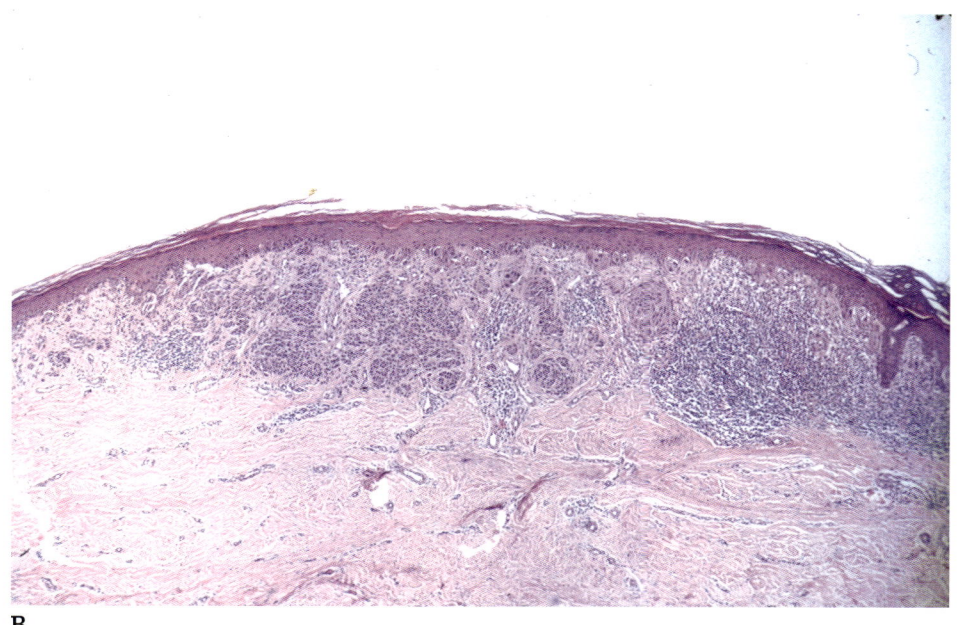

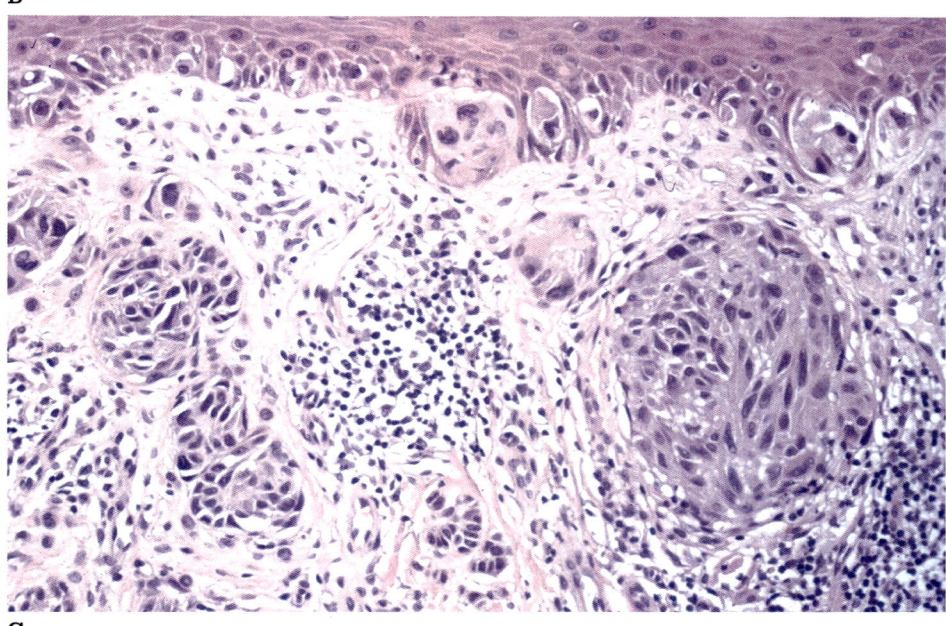

FIGURE 7-19 *Continued.* **B,** The recurrent lesion resected > 1 year later. This proliferation demonstrates asymmetry, shows effacement of the epidermis, is larger in size, shows a more voluminous dermal component, and displays variation in the arrangement of dermal nests. **C,** Note the asymmetry and variability in size and shape of both junctional and dermal nests of melanocytes. There are cohesive nests of melanocytes in the dermis without maturation. However, the cytologic features characteristic of the melanocytes in a Spitz tumor are present.

Dermal/Subcutaneous Tumoral Pattern A proportion of Spitz nevi seem to recur with confluent aggregates of melanocytes in the dermis and possibly subcutis that suggest melanoma (Fig. 7-20). The original and recurrent lesion must be carefully assessed to exclude melanoma.

Despite their unusual nature, recurrent Spitz nevi often demonstrate attributes characterisic of a primary Spitz nevus in a large proportion of cases: enlarged spindle and/or epithelioid melanocytes, typical maturation (i.e., dispersion of nests and melanocytes, diminished cellular

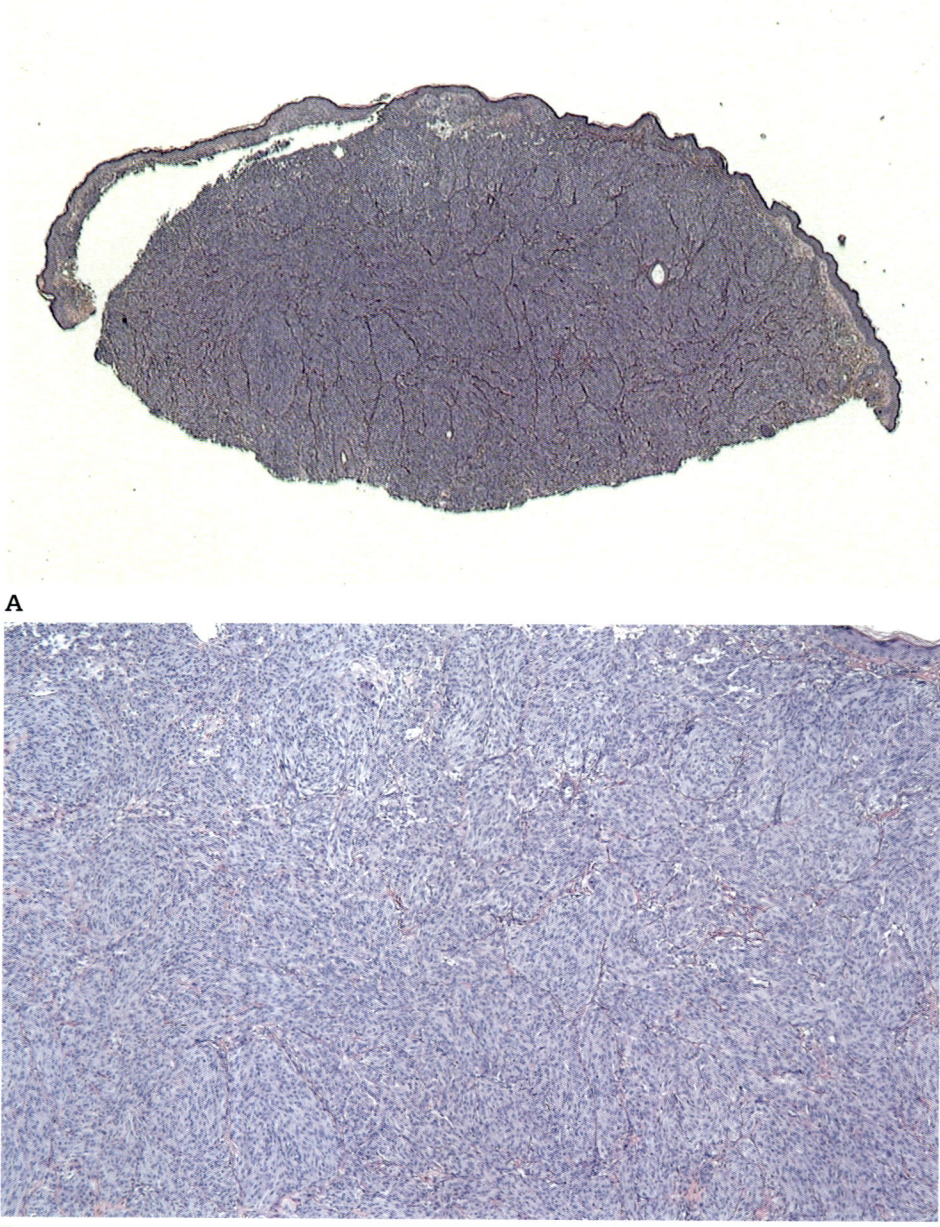

FIGURE 7-20 Recurrent/persistent atypical Spitz tumor. This lesion arose on the left cheek of a 6 year-old boy. **A–C,** Initial biopsy shows a dome-shaped tumor with strikingly high cellular density and confluence of melanocytes in dermis. Although there is some effacement of the epidermis, pagetoid spread is absent. There is no maturation. The mitotic rate is 9/mm². The lesion extends to all margins.

density, and diminished cellular and nuclear sizes with depth), clefting about nests of melanocytes in the epidermis, epidermal hyperplasia, symmetry, relatively low mitotic rate of the dermal component, superficial mitoses, infrequent pagetoid spread, and a perivascular disposition of a lymphocytic infiltrate (64).

However, based on our experience and reports from the literature, recurrent Spitz nevi have a propensity to be somewhat more asymmetrical, to be larger, to be more dermal based, to extend into subcutaneous fat, to demonstrate greater cellular density and confluence, to show some loss of maturation, to show perhaps greater cyto-

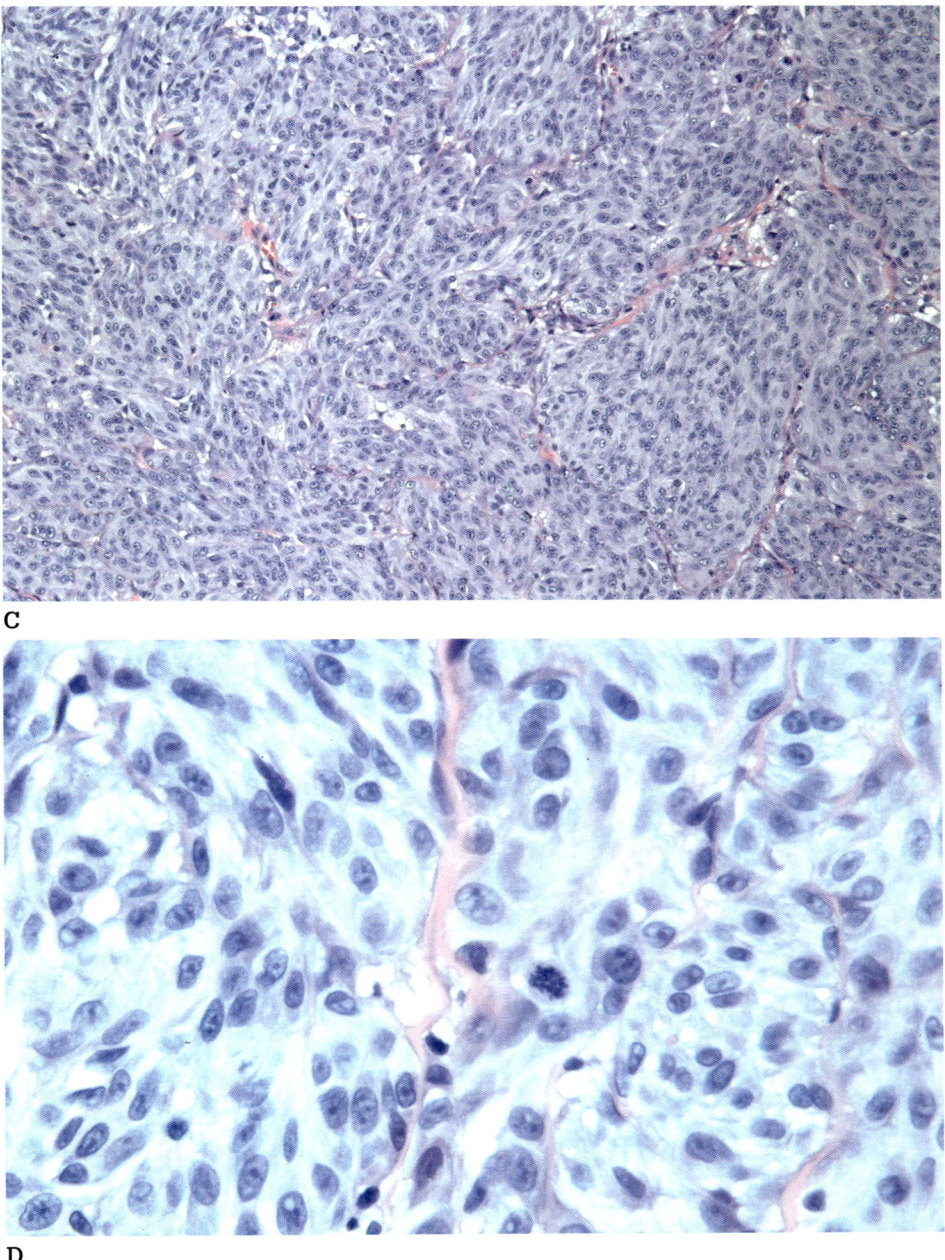

FIGURE 7-20 *Continued.* **D,** Note the uniformity of the spindle cells at higher magnification.

logic atypia, to possess higher mitotic rates, and to exhibit dermal fibrosis as compared to conventional Spitz nevi (64,90) (Figs. 7-19 and 7-20). The latter findings, however, may be found in only a minority of cases.

Ancillary Studies

In one study, 18 recurrent lesions showed typical staining patterns with HMB-45 and Ki-67, as observed in primary Spitz nevi. HMB-45 marked the junctional component only or possibly also the superficial portion of dermal component (64). The proliferation rate of recurrent tumors as assessed by Ki-67 was low—1–2%. Potential cytogenetic abnormalities have been studied in a small number of cases with comparative-genomic hybridization (CGH) and fluorescence in situ hybridization (FISH). Among 10 cases studied by CGH, 5 demonstrated no chromosomal abnormalities; 3 cases, an amplification of chromosome 11p; 1 case, a gain of

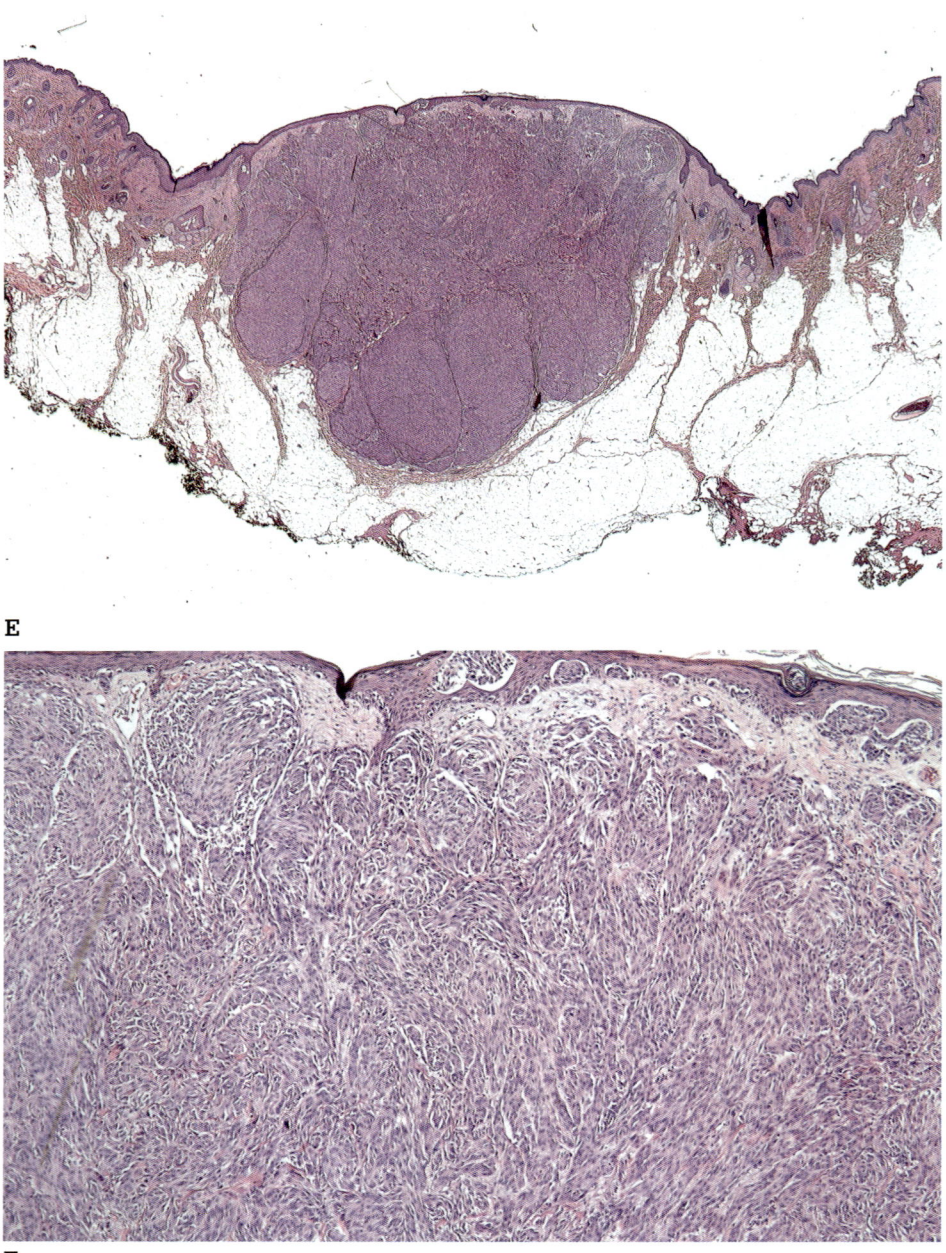

FIGURE 7-20 *Continued.* **E–H,** The recurrent/persistent tumor excised several months latter. Note the lobular symmetrical profile of the tumor; there is extension into subcutaneous fat without maturation (the tumor measures 4.80 mm in thickness). As in the initial biopsy, the tumor exhibits high cellular density and confluence of spindled melanocytes similar to the initial specimen. The mitotic rate is 9/mm^2 and mitoses are conspicuous at the base. Although demonstrating features of a Spitz tumor, this lesion is most appropriately considered as biologically indeterminate.

chromosome 1q and a loss of 9p; and 1 case, multiple chromosomal gains (3p, 6p, 11q, 17q) and losses (8q, 13q, 21q) (64). The chromosomal alterations in the latter two cases were consistent with melanoma. FISH showed no abnormal expression in 10 of 13 lesions, 2 cases showed an increase in 11p copies, and the case with multiple chromosome alterations by CGH showed variable 11p and 11q copy numbers.

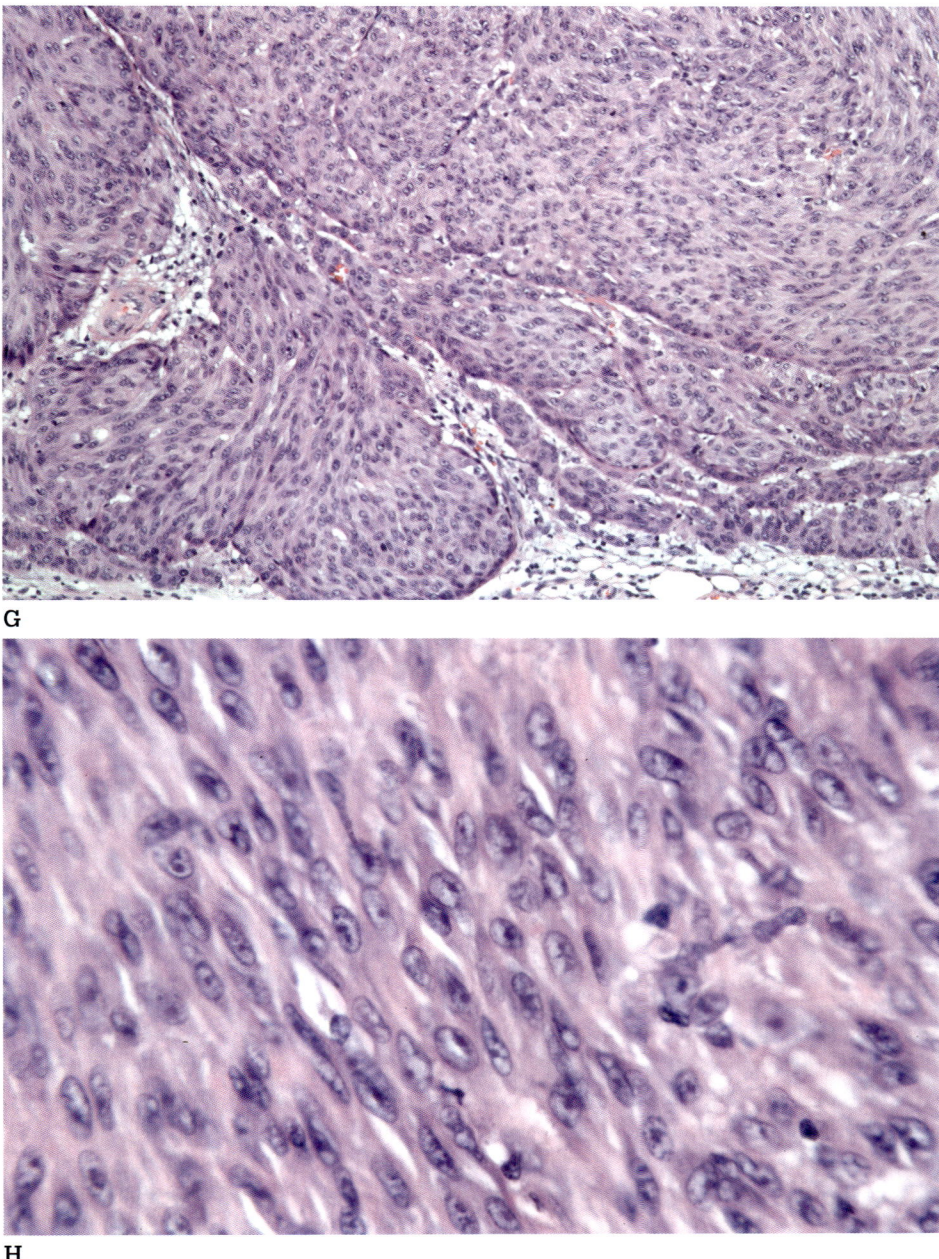

FIGURE 7-20 *Continued.*

Differential Diagnosis

The recurrent Spitz nevus must be distinguished from melanoma, atypical variants of primary Spitz nevi, desmoplastic Spitz nevus, and nonmelanocytic lesions such as epithelioid cell fibrous histiocytoma and cellular neurothekeoma (64,87–93). As with the conventional recurrent melanocytic nevus, it is necessary that the original biopsy be examined to establish a diagnosis of Spitz nevus and to determine if the initial lesion extended to the surgical margins. As has been mentioned previously, almost all recurrent Spitz nevi are associated with positive margins in the original lesion. Examination of the original specimen is also necessary to exclude melanoma, since recurrent Spitz nevi may exhibit histologic features suggesting melanoma to a greater extent than the initial lesion. Clinical presentation should also figure into the discrimination of recurrent Spitz nevus from melanoma—that is, younger age, location, and so on (discussed earlier). Although recurrent Spitz nevus may display unusual histologic features, careful examination should disclose in most instances maturation, typical cytologic characteristics of Spitz nevus, low mitotic rates, and absence of mitotic figures at the base of the lesion.

As discussed previously for atypical Spitz nevi, some recurrent Spitz nevi may be particularly difficult or impossible to distinguish from melanoma. Because of the rarity of recurrent Spitz nevus and the lack of sufficient data on long-term follow-up, we advise a similar management strategy as that outlined for markedly atypical Spitz tumors (discussed above). The possibility of aggressive behavior should be discussed with the clinician and patient. Such lesions should have adequate reexcision with surgical margins clearly free of tumor; sentinel lymph node biopsy may be considered for selected patients, although this remains controversial (see earlier discussion); and the patients followed carefully on a periodic basis for potential recurrence.

Clinical Course

Follow-up data for 14 reported cases of recurrent Spitz nevi suggest that the vast majority of patients (especially children < 10 years) have no further recrudescence or progression of disease (64). The mean follow-up was 4.8 years and ranged from 7 months to 9 years. Just 1 patient developed a single lymph node metastasis after 3 years, and, based on this event and CGH findings (loss of chromosome 9p and gain of 1q), was reclassified as melanoma. However, long-term follow-up with additional cases is needed since we have observed disease progression 13 years after two recurrences of a Spitz nevus that eventuated in a deep local metastasis followed by regional lymph node and widespread metastases and death (23). The detailed analysis of the biologic nature of such tumors throughout their natural history is of critical importance in understanding these neoplasms, risk factors for recurrence and tumor progression, and their relationship to melanoma.

REFERENCES

1. Darier J, Civatte A, Naevus ou naevo-carcinoma chez un nourisson. Bull Soc Franc Derm Syph 1910;21:61–3.
2. Miescher G. Faszikulaerer typus des pigmentzellennaevus. In: Jadassohn J, ed. Handbuck der Haut unde Geschlechtskrankheiten. Berlin: Springer-Verlag, 1933;12:1034–6.
3. Pack G, Anglem T. Tumors of soft somatic tissues in infancy and childhood. J Pediatr 1939;15:372–400.
4. Spitz S. Melanomas of childhood. Am J Pathol 1948;24:591–609.
5. Allen A, Spitz S. Malignant melanoma: a clinico-pathological analysis of the criteria for diagnosis and prognosis. Cancer 1953;6:1–45.
6. Kernen J, Ackerman L. Spindle cell nevi and epithelioid cell nevi (so-called juvenile melanomas) in children and adults: a clinicopathological study of 27 cases. Cancer 1960;13:612–25.
7. Kopf A, Andrade R. Benign juvenile melanoma. In: Kopf A, Andrade R, eds. Yearbook of Dermatology 1965–1966. Chicago Yearbook, 1966:7–52.
8. Helwig E. Seminar on skin neoplasms and dermatoses. In: Proceedings of the Twentieth Seminar of the American Society of Clinical Pathologists, Sept. 11, 1954. American Society of Clinical Pathology, 1955:63–7.
9. Paniago-Pereira C, Maize J, Ackerman A. Nevus of large spindle and/or epithelioid cells (Spitz's nevus). Arch Dermatol 1978;114:1811–23.
10. Weedon D, Little J. Spindle and epithelioid cell nevi in children and adults. A review of 211 cases of the Spitz nevus. Cancer 1977;40:217–25.
11. Allen A. Juvenile melanomas of children and adults and melanocarcinomas of children. Arch Dermatol 1960;82:325–35.
12. Coskey R, Mehregan A. Spindle cell nevi in adults and children. Arch Dermatol 1973;108:535–6.
13. Weedon D. The Spitz nevus. Clin Oncol 1984;3:493–507.
14. McWorther H, Woolner L. Pigmented nevi, juvenile melanomas, and malignant melanomas in children. Cancer 1954;7:564–85.
15. Palazzo J, Duray P. Congenital agminated Spitz nevi: immunoreactivity with a melanoma-associated monoclonal antibody. J Cutan Pathol 1988;15:166–70.
16. Peters M, Goellner J. Spitz nevi and malignant melanomas of childhood and adolescence. Histopathology 1986;10:1289–302.
17. Gartmann H, Ganser M. Der Spitz-Naevus. Spindelzellen und/oder epithelienzellennaevus. Eine klinische analyse von 652 tumoren. Z Hautkr 1985;60:22–8.
18. Rhodes A. Neoplasms: benign neoplasias, hyperplasias, and dysplasias of melanocytes. In: Fitzpatrick TB, Eisen AZ, Wolff K, et al., eds. Dermatology in General Medicine. New York: McGraw-Hill, 1993;1:996–1077.
19. Echevarria R, Ackerman L. Spindle and epithelioid nevi in the adult. Clinicopathologic report of 26 cases. Cancer 1967;20:175–89.
20. Allen A. Juvenile melanomas and malignant melanomas. Surg Gynecol Obstet 1957;104:735–54.
21. Smith K, Skelton H, Lupton G, Graham J. Spindle cell and epithelioid cell nevi with atypia and metastasis (malignant Spitz nevus). Am J Surg Pathol 1989;13:931–9.
22. Barnhill RL, Flotte T, Fleischli M, Perez-Atayde AR. Childhood melanoma and atypical Spitz tumors. Cancer 1995;76:1833–45.
23. Barnhill RL, Argenyi ZB, From L, et al. Atypical Spitz nevi/tumors: lack of consensus for diagnosis, discrimination from melanoma, and prediction of outcome. Hum Pathol 1999;30:513–20.

24. Lancer H, Muhlbauer J, Sober A. Multiple agminated spindle cell nevi: unique clinical presentation and review. J Am Acad Dermatol 1983;8:707–11.
25. Wallace H. Eruptive juvenile melanomata. Br J Dermatol 1974;91(Suppl 10):37–8.
26. Weimar V, Zuehlke R. Multiple agminate spindle and epithelioid cell nevi in an adult. Arch Dermatol 1978;114:1383–4.
27. Hamm H, Happle R, Broecker E. Multiple agminate Spitz nevi: review of the literature and report of a case with distinctive immunohistological features. Br J Dermatol 1987;117:511–522.
28. Dawe RS, Wainwright NJ, Evans AT, Lower JG. Multiple widespread eruptive Spitz nevi. Br J Dermatol 1998;138:872–4.
29. Onsun N, Saracoglu S, Demirkesen C, et al. Eruptive widespread Spitz nevi: can pregnancy be stimulating factor? J Am Acad Dermatol 1999;40:866–7.
30. Aloi F, Tomasini C, Pippione M. Agminated Spitz nevi occurring within a congenital speckeled lentiginous nevus. Am J Dermatopathol 1995;17:594–8.
31. Betti R, Inselvini E. Palvarini M, Crosti C. Agminated intradermal Spitz nevi arising on an unusual speckled lentiginous nevus with localized lentiginosis: a continuum? Am J Dermatopathol 1997;19:524–7.
32. Cramer Stewart F. The melanocyte differentiation pathway in Spitz nevi. Am J Dermatopathol 1998;20(6):555–70.
33. Zaenglein AL, Heintz P, Kamino H, et al. Congenital Spitz nevus clinically mimicking melanoma. J Am Acad Dermatol 2002;47:441–4.
34. Mooi W, Krausz T. Spitz naevus, desmoplastic Spitz naevus and pigmented spindle cell naevus. In: Mooi W, Krausz T, eds. Biopsy: Pathology of Melanocytic Disorders. London: Chapman & Hall, 1992:156–85.
35. Binder S, Asnog C, Paul E, Cochran A. The histology and differential diagnosis of Spitz nevus. Semin Diagn Pathol 1993;10:36–46.
36. Kamino H, Misheloff E, Ackerman A, et al. Eosinophilic globules in Spitz's nevi. New findings and a diagnostic sign. Am J Surg Pathol 1979;1:319–24.
37. Arbuckle S, Weedon D. Eosinophilic globules in the Spitz nevus. J Am Acad Dermatol 1982;7:324–7.
38. Havenith M, van Zandvoort E, Cleutjens J, Bosman F. Basement membrane deposition in benign and malignant nevomelanocytic lesions: an immunohistochemical study with antibodies to type IV collagen and laminin. Histopathology 1989;15:137–46.
39. Wistuba I, Gonzalez S. Eosinophilic globules in pigmented spindle cell nevus. Am J Dermatopathol 1990;12:268–71.
40. Skelton HG, Miller ML, Lupton GP, Smith KJ. Eosinophilic globules in spindle cell and epithelioid cell nevi: composition and possible origin. Am J Dermatopathol 1998;20:547–50.
41. Wesselmann U, Becker L, Brocker E, et al. Eosinophilic globules in Spitz nevi: no evidence for apoptosis. Am J Dermatopathol 1998;20(6):551–4.
42. Elder D, Murphy G. Spindle and epithelioid cell nevus (Spitz nevus). Atlas of tumor pathology. In: Elder D, Murphy G, eds. Melanocytic Tumors of the Skin. Washington DC: Armed Forces Institute of Pathology, 1990:40–57.
43. Scott G, Chen KTK, Rosai J. Pseudoepitheliomatous hyperplasia in spitz nevi: a possible source of confusion with squamous cell carcinoma. Arch Pathol Lab Med 1989;113:61–3.
44. Howat A. Variend S. Lymphatic invasion of spitz nevi. Am J Surg Pathol 1985;9:125–8.
45. Piepkorn M. On the nature of histologic observations: the case of the Spitz nevus. J Am Acad Dermatol. 1995;32,248–54.
46. Reed R, Ichinose H, Clark W, Mihm MC. Common and uncommon melanocytic nevi and borderline melanomas. Semin Oncol 1975;2:119–47.
47. Lohman CM, Coit DG, Brady MS, et al. Sentinel lymph node biopsy in paitents with diagnostically controversial spitzoid melanocytic tumors. Am J Surg Pathol 2002;26(1):47–55.
48. Busam KJ, Barnhill RL. Pagetoid Spitz nevus. Intraepidermal Spitz tumor with prominent pagetoid spread. Am J Surg Pathol 1995;19:1061-1067.
49. Han MH, Koh KJ, Choi JH, et al. Pagetoid Spitz nevus: a variant of Spitz nevus. Int J Dermatol 2000;39:555–7.
50. Guldhammer B, Norgaard T. The differential diagnosis of intraepidermal malignant lesions using immunohistochemistry. Am J Dermatopathol 1986;8:295–301.
51. Spatz A, Calonje E, Handfield-Jones S, Barnhill RL. Spitz tumors in children: a grading system for risk stratification. Arch Dermatol 1999;135:282–5.
52. Peters M. Histiocytic and Langerhans cell reactions. In: Farmer ER, Hood AF, eds. Pathology of the Skin. Norwalk, CT: Appleton & Lange, 1990:249–72.
53. Wilson-Jones E, Cerio R, Smith N. Epithelioid cell histiocytoma: a new entity. Br J Dermatol 1989;120:185–95.
54. Barnhill RL, Mihm MC. Cellular neurothekeoma. A distinctive variant of neurothekeoma mimicking nevomelanocytic tumors. Am J Surg Pathol 1990;14:113–20.
55. Reed R Malignant Spitz nevus. Paper presented at the Clinicopathology Conference of the Meetings of the American Academy of Pathology, New York, Dec 1980.
56. Delacretaz J. Melanoma juvenile (melanome de Spitz) a evolution maligne. Dermatologica 1969;139:79–83.
57. Ainsworth A, Folberg R, Reed R, Clark W. Melanocytic nevi, melanocytomas, melanocytic dysplasias, and uncommon forms of melanoma. In: Clark W, Goldman, Mastrangelo, eds. Human Malignant Melanoma. New York: Grune & Stratton, 1979:167–208.
58. Howat A, Giri D, Cotton D, Slater D. Nuclear organizer re-

58. gions in Spitz nevi and malignant melanomas. Cancer 1989;63:474–8.
59. Rode J, Williams R, Jarvis L, et al. S-100 protein, neuron-specific enolase, and nuclear DNA content in Spitz nevus. J Pathol 1990;161:41–5.
60. Bergman R, Dromi R, Trau H, et al. The pattern of HMB-45 antibody staining in compound Spitz nevi. Am J Dermatopathol 1995;17:542–6.
61. Kanter-Lewensohn L, Hedblad MA, Wejde J, Larsson O. Immunohistochemical markers for distinguishing Spitz nevi from malignant melanomas. Mod Pathol 1997;10:917–20.
62. Li LX, Crotty KA, McCarthy SW, et al. A zonal comparison of MIB1-Ki67 immunoreactivity in benign and malignant melanocytic lesions. Am J Dermatopathol 2000;22:489–95.
63. Bergman R, Malkin L, Sabo E, Kerner H. MIB-1 monoclonal antibody to determine proliferative activity of Ki-67 antigen as an adjunct to histopathologic differential diagnosis of Spitz nevi. J Am Acad Dermatol 2001;44:500–4.
64. Harvell JD, Bastian BC, LeBoit PE. Persistent (recurrent) Spitz nevi: a histopathologic, immunohistochemical, and molecular pathologic study of 22 cases. Am J Surg Pathol 2002;26(5):654–61.
65. Ewanowich C, Brynes RK, Medeiros J, et al. Cyclin D1 expression in dysplastic nevi. Arch Pathol Lab Med 2001;125:208–10.
66. Winokur T, Palazzo J, Johnson W, Duray P. Evaluation of DNA ploidy in dysplastic and Spitz nevi by flow cytometry. J Cutan Pathol 1990;17:342–7.
67. LeBoit P, Fletcher H. A comparative study of Spitz nevus and nodular melanoma using image analysis cytometry. J Invest Dermatol 1987;88:753–7.
68. Steiner A, Binder M, Mossbacher U, et al. Estimation of the volume-weighted mean nuclear volume discriminates Spitz's nevi from nodular malignant melanomas. Lab Invest 1994;70(3):381–5.
69. Bastian BC, Wesselman U, Pinkel D, LeBoit Molecular cytogenetic analysis of Spitz nevis shows clear differences to melanoma. J Invest Dermatol 1999;113:1065–9.
70. Bastian BC, LeBoit PE, Pinkel D. Mutations and copy number increase of HRAS in Spitz nevi with distinctive histopathologic features. Am J Pathol 2000;157:967–72.
71. Healy E, Belgaid C, Takata M, et al. Allelotypes of primary cutaneous melanoma and benign melanocytic nevi. Cancer Res 1996;56:589–93.
72. Bogdan I, Burg G, Boni R. Spitz nevi display allelic deletions. Arch Dermatol 2001;137:1417–20.
73. Barr R, Morales R, Graham J. Desmoplastic nevus. A distinct histologic variant of mixed spindle and epithelioid cell nevus. Cancer 1980;46:557–64.
74. MacKie RM, Doherty VR. The desmoplastic melanocytic naevus: A distinct histological entity. Histopathology 1992;20:207–11.
75. Harris GR, Shea CR, Horenstein MG, et al. Desmoplastic (sclerotic) nevus an underrecognized entity that resembles dermatofibroma and desmoplastic melanoma. Am J Surg Pathol 1999;23(7):786–94.
76. Diaz-Cascajo C, Borhi S, Weyers W. Angiomatoid Spitz nevus: a distinct variant of desmoplastic Spitz nevus with prominent vasculature. Am J Dermatopathol 2000;22:135–9.
77. Suster S. Hyalinizing spindle and epithelioid cell nevus. A study of five cases of a distinctive histologic variant of Spitz's nevus. Am J Dermatopathol 1994;16:593–8.
78. Spatz A, Peterse S, Fletcher CD, Barnhill RL. Plexiform Spitz nevus: an intradermal Spitz nevus with plexiform growth pattern. Am J Dermatopathol 1999;21:542–6.
79. Yasaka N, Furue M, Tamaki K. Histopatholgic evaluation of halo phenomenon in Spitz nevus. Am J Dermatopathol 1995;17:484–6.
80. Harvell JD, Meehan SA, LeBoit PE. Spitz's nevi with halo reaction: a histopathological study of 17 cases. J Cutan Pathol 1997;24:611–9.
81. Burg G, Kempf W, Hochli M, et al. "Tubular" epithelioid cell nevus: a new variant of Spitz's nevus. J Cutan Pathol 1998;25:475–8.
82. Ziemer M, Diaz-Cascajo C, Kohler G, Weyers W. Tubular Spitz's nevus an artifact of fixation? J Cutan Pathol 2000;27:500–4.
83. Gartmann H. Der pigmentierte Spindelzellentumor. Z Hautkrankh 1981;56:862–76.
84. Sagebiel R, Chinn E, Egbert B. Pigmented spindle cell nevus. Clinical and histologic review of 90 cases. Am J Surg Pathol 1984;8:645–53.
85. Sau P, Graham J, Helwig E. Pigmented spindle cell nevus. Arch Dermatol 1984;120:1615–22.
86. Smith N. The pigmented spindle cell tumor of Reed: An underdiagnosed lesion. Sem Diagn Pathol 1987;4:75–87.
87. Barnhill RL, Mihm MC. Pigmented spindle cell nevus and its variants: distinction from melanoma. Br J Dermatol 1989;121:717–26.
88. Barnhill RL, Barnhill MA, Berwick M, Mihm MC Jr. The histologic spectrum of pigmented spindle cell nevus: a review of 120 cases with emphasis on atypical variants. Human Pathol 1991;22:52-58.
89. Omura EF, Kheir SM. Recurrent Spitz's nevus. Am J Dermatopathol 1984:6(Suppl 1):207–12.
90. Stern JB. Recurrent Spitz's nevi: a clinicopathologic investigation. Am J Dermatopathol 1985;7(Suppl):49–50.
91. Tanaka K, Mihara M, Shimao S, et al. The local recurrence of pigmented Spitz nevus after removal. J Dermatol 1990:17:575-80.
92. Peters MS, Argenyi Z, Cerio R, et al. Friday evening slide symposium, case 1. J Cutan Pathol 1993;20:465–78.
93. Gambini C, Rongioletti F. Recurrent Spitz nevus: case report and review of the literature. Am J Dermatopathol 1994;16:409–13.

CHAPTER 8

Dermal Melanocytoses, Blue Nevi, and Related Conditions

Klaus J. Busam and Raymond L. Barnhill

The subject of this chapter is blue nevi and related proliferations of melanocytes, usually dendritic or spindled, primarily involving the reticular dermis. The nomenclature for this group of lesions is somewhat confusing and inconsistent. Some of this confusion is related to clinical description (*blue nevus*) for some entities and histologic characterization for others (*cellular blue nevus*). Inconsistency results from histologic overlap with other melanocytic lesions such as spindle and epithelioid cell nevi and pigmented peripheral nerve sheath tumors (see Chapter 9).

The classification of lesions within this general category is based on assessing a number of features: clinical appearance; anatomic site of lesion; localization in the reticular dermis, subcutis, etc.; the extent to which the lesion is made up of dendritic versus spindle-shaped melanocytes; degree of cellularity of lesion; degree of fibrosis (sclerosis); degree of melanization and accumulation of melanophages; overall architecture—fibrous nodule, cellular nodule, or nests; plexiform configuration; presence of other nevus components—junctional compound elements; and degree of cytologic atypia, and mitotic activity (Fig. 8-1).

The bluish appearance of these various lesions is primarily related to depth of melanin in the dermis and the Tyndall phenomenon. The longer wavelengths of visible light penetrate the reticular dermis and are absorbed by melanin. However, the shorter wavelengths, representing the bluish part of the color spectrum, do not penetrate as deeply and are reflected back from the superficial dermis and epidermis. The result is that the lesion appears blue to the observer.

HISTOGENESIS

The dermal melanocytoses and blue nevi are thought to result from the dermal arrest and accumulation of cells migrating from the neural crest (1–4). In contrast to ordinary nevi, it is believed that these migratory cells never reach the epidermis. The immediate origin of the cells making up the dermal melanocytoses and blue nevi has been postulated to be either melanocytes, melanogenic Schwann cells, or a common neural crest–derived precursor cell with differentiation along both melanocytic and schwannian lines (1–4). Since blue nevi are not uncommonly associated with ordinary nevi (combined nevi), they most likely represent nevomelanocytes with differentiating features similar to Schwann cells. On cytologic grounds alone—that is, in the absence of contextual architectural information—a reliable distinction between a blue nevus cell and a pigmented Schwann cell may not be possible, since there is significant overlap at the light microscopic and ultrastructural level (1–6). Both cell types may exhibit basal lamina, desmosome-like junctional structures, and compound melanosomes. As a general rule, the prominent presence of external lamina and the lack of premelanosomes favor a Schwann cell, but these criteria are not absolute, especially on a small biopsy sample. Immunohistochemistry is of some, albeit limited, help in the distinction of blue nevi from Schwann cell proliferations.

Immunostaining for melanocyte differentiation antigens gp100, tyrosinase and Mart-1/Melan-A is commonly seen in blue nevi, but usually absent in amelanotic Schwann cells (7–9). Pigmented Schwann cells on

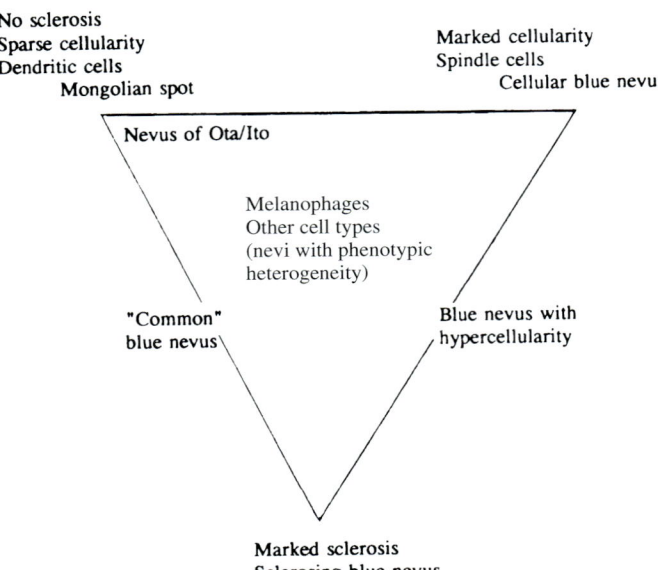

FIGURE 8-1 Histologic spectrum of blue nevus and related conditions. The particular disorder is defined by the degree of dermal sclerosis (none to marked), the degree of cellularity (sparse to marked), and the cell types present (mainly dendritic cells, mainly spindle cells, other cell types, and melanophages).

the other hand cannot be distinguished from melanocytes by means of immunohistochemistry, since they are usually positive for all melanocyte differentiation markers. The distinction of pigmented Schwann cell tumors from melanocytic tumors requires a complex analysis that integrates clinical, gross morphologic, light microscopic, immunohistochemical, and ultrastructural features.

DERMAL MELANOCYTOSES

- Mongolian spot
- Nevus of Ota (nevus fuscocaeruleus ophthalmomaxillaris)
- Nevus fuscocaeruleus zygomaticus (acquired nevus of Ota-like macules)
- Acquired dermal melanocytosis of the face and extremities
- Nevus of Ito (nevus fuscocaeruleus acromiodeltoideus)
- Dermal melanocyte hamartoma

These six entities are related because they are all essentially bluish macular lesions that histologically demonstrate scattered dendritic melanocytes in the reticular dermis with little or no stromal alteration (Table 8-1).

Mongolian Spot

Clinical Features Mongolian spots are oval or round, often poorly defined, macules varying in color from slight gray to blue-black or dark brown (10,11) (Table 8-1). There is no change in the skin texture. The lesions most often affect the lumbosacral region but may be seen in other (ectopic, or aberrant) locations. The size of Mongolian spots varies from < 1 cm to > 10 cm. These lesions are present at birth but usually spontaneously regress by age 3–4 years. However, some lesions may persist until the 2nd decade or even into adulthood. Mongolian spots have been observed in > 90% of blacks and American Indians, 81% of Asians, 70% of Hispanics, and 10% of white newborns (12). The development of malignant melanoma in typical Mongolian spot has to our knowledge not been reported yet.

Histopathological Features The Mongolian spot is characterized by widely spaced dendritic melanocytes localized to the lower half or two thirds of the reticular dermis. The dermis is unaltered, and melanophages are usually not present. The melanocytes are generally bipolar, with their axes oriented parallel to the skin surface and situated in low density between individual collagen bundles. The individual cells have slender, lengthy cytoplasmic processes (dendrites) that contain finely divided melanin granules. The nuclei are often obscured by melanin but when visible have clumped chromatin patterns.

Differential Diagnosis Mongolian spots are distinguished from other dermal dendritic lesions by location (sacral area), disappearance in infancy, and sparse number of dermal melanocytes without melanophages or fibrosis. Persistent ectopic Mongolian spots may be difficult to discriminate from nevus of Ota and Ito. It is likely that some previously reported examples of ectopic Mongolian spots are in fact nevus of Ota or Ito.

Nevus of Ota (Nevus Fuscocaeruleus Ophthalmomaxillaris)

Nevus of Ota usually presents at birth or in childhood as a unilateral speckled bluish macule involving the periorbital region, forehead, temple, cheek, or nose (13,14). The areas correspond to the distribution of the first two branches of the trigeminal nerve. Examination may also disclose involvement of the sclera, conjunctiva, cornea, retina, or oral and nasal mucosa. Brownish lentigo-like lesions and bluish papules or nodules are occasionally associated with nevus of Ota. About 13% of cases are bilateral. The natural history of nevus of Ota is persistence with slight extension of the process.

TABLE 8-1 Differential features of dermal melanocytoses.

Feature	Mongolian spot	Nevus of ota	Nevus of ito	Blue nevus
Onset	Birth or soon after	Birth or soon after	Birth or soon after	Birth or later in life
Size	5 cm	5 cm	5 cm	1.5 cm
Color	Gray-tan, slate blue	Brown, slate blue	Brown, slate blue	Bluish black
Surface	Macular	Macular, rarely discrete papules	Macular, rarely discrete papules	Papular
Hair	Normal for site	Normal for site	Normal for site	Normal for site
Distribution	Midline	Unilateral	Unilateral	Unilateral
Number	Single, can be multiple	Single	Single	Single, rarely multiple
Site	Lumbosacral	First and second division trigeminal nerve	Shoulder and upper arm	Extensors of extremities: dorsa of hands and feet, buttocks, face
Racial incidence	Asians and dark-skinned peoples	Asians and dark-skinned peoples	Asians and dark-skinned peoples	More common in dark-skinned peoples
Familial incidence	Common	Rare	Rare	None
Sex	No difference	80% in females	80% in females	60% in females
Age of appearance	At birth	60% at birth	60% at birth	At or just after birth
Spontaneous fate	Usually disappears during first few years of life	Persist; rarely disappear	Persist; rarely disappear	Persist
Tendency to malignancy	Never reported	Rare	Rare	Rare
Histologic features	Scattered dermal melanocytes in lower half of dermis, in low concentrations	Moderate number of dermal melanocytes in upper dermis	Moderate number of dermal melanocytes in upper dermis	Common form has high concentration of dermal melanocytes in middle and lower third of dermis; melanophages usually present; cellular form also contains bundles of spindle cells
Ultrastructure	Fully developed melanocytes with only mature melanosomes; virtually no premelanosomes	Fully developed melanocytes with only mature melanosomes; virtually no premelanosomes	Fully developed melanocytes with only mature melanosomes; virtually no premelanosomes	Fully developed melanocytes with only mature melanosomes; virtually no premelanosomes

The development of malignant melanoma in association with nevus of Ota has been recorded in only a few instances (15). However, patients with involvement of the eye have also been observed to develop melanoma of the choroid, iris, orbit, and brain.

Nevus Fuscocaeruleus Zygomaticus (Acquired Nevus of Ota-Like Macules; Sun's Nevus)

The development of bilateral bluish macules in the zygomatic areas of the face has primarily been reported in Chinese and Japanese women (16). The affected individuals have ranged in age from 19 to 69 years. In contrast to typical nevus of Ota, there is no involvement of either the eye or oral mucosa by the melanocytosis.

Acquired Dermal Melanocytosis of the Face and Extremities

Acquired dermal melanocytosis is associated with bilateral bluish or brownish discoloration of the face, somewhat similar to nevus of Ota, but also associated with involvement of the extensor surfaces of the upper extremities and possibly the palms (17). This particular entity is associated with onset in adults in a similar fashion to the acquired bilateral nevus zygomaticus.

Nevus of Ito (Nevus Fuscocaeruleus Acromiodeltoideus)

The nevus of Ito is closely related to the nevus of Ota but is distinguished by its unilateral distribution involving the supraclavicular, scapular, or deltoid regions (18). Similar to nevus of Ota, this lesion has a mottled appearance with bluish or brownish macules. Onset is noted at birth or later in childhood. The nevus of Ito may occur in association with the nevus of Ota. The development of malignant melanoma in nevus of Ito has been recorded (19).

Dermal Melanocyte Hamartoma

The term *dermal melanocyte hamartoma* has been used to describe a small number of developmental abnormalities usually present at birth and exhibiting extensive involvement of the skin (20).

Histopathological Features

The histologic changes of the entities described above are very similar for the bluish macules (10–20). Scattered dermal melanocytes with prominent dendritic processes are noted in the upper dermis without alteration of the dermal stroma (Fig. 8-2A). There may be involvement of the papillary dermis, and in some instances, there is aggregation of these cells about sebaceous glands, eccrine ducts, blood vessels, and cutaneous nerves. Uncommonly, there may be extension of these cells into the subcutaneous fat. As in Mongolian spot, the cells contain prominent deposits of fine melanin granules (Fig. 8-2B). Melanophages, in general, are uncommon. The density of melanocytes is generally greater than in Mongolian spot.

Based on the examination of 450 cases of Ota's nevus, Hirayama and Suzuki (14) have recently reported a new histopathologic classification of this entity. The classification is related to the location of melanocytes in the dermis: (a) superficial type (i.e., melanocytes present in the superficial dermis), (b) deep type, (c) diffuse type (melanocytes scattered throughout entire dermis), (d) superficial dominant type, and (e) deep dominant type. The authors also noted that cheek lesions tended to have a superficial pattern, whereas all other sites were typified by diffuse, deep, or deep dominant patterns.

The brownish macules demonstrate dermal melanocytes located very close to the epidermis. In these areas, slight basilar melanocytic hyperplasia and basal layer hypermelanosis may also be present. The slightly raised or papular lesions that may be seen in these lesions demonstrates an even greater concentration of dendritic melanocytes, resembling the findings seen in blue nevus.

BLUE NEVUS

Historically, the blue nevi have been classified based on their clinical appearance or various histologic findings. Degos (21) described three clinical variants: the common small solitary blue nevus (common blue nevus), the rare occurrence of multiple blue nevi, and the even rarer plaque-type blue nevus (naevus blue en nappe etendu). Histologically, many subtypes have been proposed, but the two main variants are the common blue nevus and cellular blue nevus. The common blue nevus, first described in detail by Tieche in 1906 (22) is, as implied by the name, the most frequent subtype 22–26). It is usually acquired, but may be congenital. It primarily involves the dorsal aspects of the hands and feet and has a relatively small diameter (<1 cm). Histologically, it is characterized by the presence of dendritic melanocytes with variable fibrosis (22–26). The less-prevalent cellular blue nevus has been defined primarily by its larger size, greater cellular density, and the presence of nests of relatively amelanotic spindle cells in addition to the dendritic melanocytic component (27).

However, examination of sufficient numbers of blue nevi reveals that there is a spectrum of histologic changes, and the typical common blue nevus and typical cellular blue nevus simply reflect the poles of a spectrum. Common blue nevi may become large, and the relative number and density of dendritic melanocytes, the number of melanophages, the degree of fibrosis, and the relative number and disposition of spindle cells may vary from lesion to lesion. The spindle cell component may consist of individually disposed spindle cells separated by collagenous stroma; the spindle cells are arranged in loose or compact fascicles. As the overall cellular density of the lesion increases, biphasic patterns usually become more pronounced, and typically, the silhouette of the tumor becomes nodular. For such cellular nodular lesions, the term *cellular nevus* is appropriate.

Not all nevi are homogeneous in their cytologic elements. Some nevi have phenotypically heterogenous components. In those nevi, a blue nevus–like component may be admixed with cellular elements of another type of nevus, such as an ordinary acquired nevus or Spitz nevus. Those lesions are discussed as nevi with phenotypic heterogeneity in Chapter 9.

The following classification of blue nevi is based on the predominant histologic changes:

Common Blue Nevus (Dendritic-Fibrotic Type)

Clinical Features The most common form of blue nevus usually presents as a well-demarcated, slightly raised or dome-shaped bluish papule (20–26) (Table 8-2). The color is usually a uniform slate gray, blue-black, or black appearance. The borders are generally regular and these nevi usually measure <1 cm in diameter. They are primarily located on the dorsal aspects of the hands and feet. They also commonly involve the face and scalp. Onset is

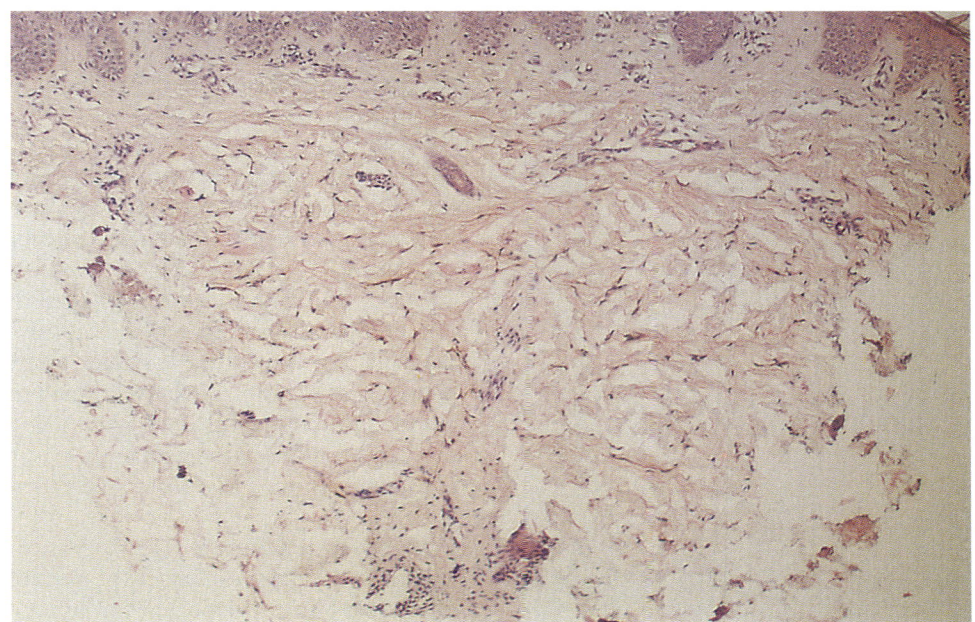

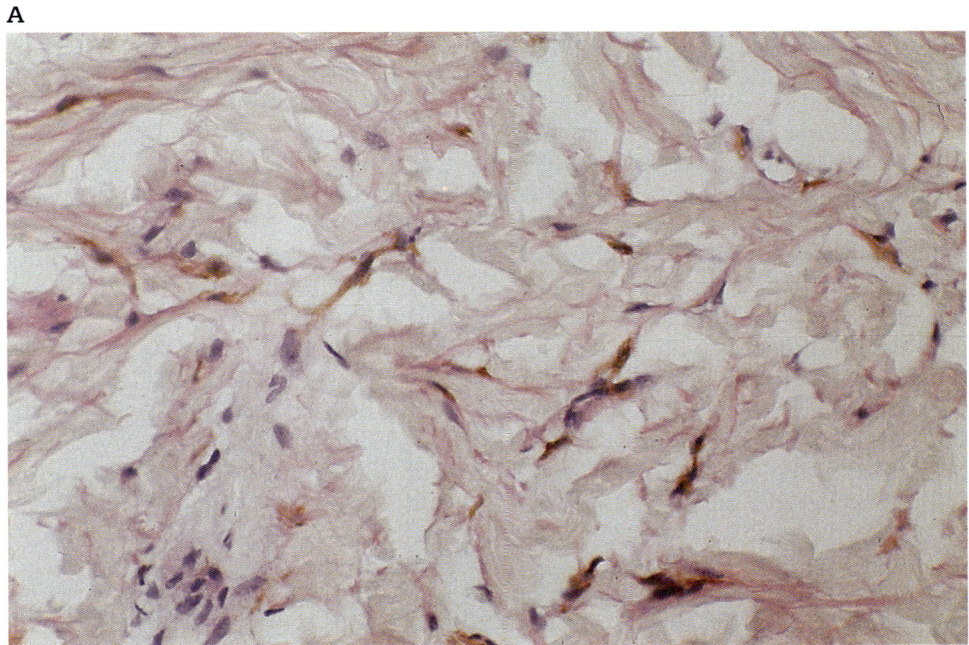

FIGURE 8-2 Nevus of Ito. **A,** A punch biopsy shows a largely unaffected dermis. There are increased numbers of pigmented dendritic cells in the mid reticular dermis scattered among collagen bundles. Neither fascicles of cells nor fibrosis is present as would be observed in blue nevus. **B,** Higher magnification showing scattered dendritic melanocytes with delicate cytoplasmic processes containing melanin.

generally in childhood but may occur later in life. Melanoma has only rarely been reported to originate from this type of blue nevus (28). Common blue nevi are usually solitary but may occur in multiple or agminated forms (29).

Histopathological Features This form of blue nevus is characterized by an aggregation of dendritic melanocytes, generally in the upper dermis with formation of a space-occupying mass that deforms the normal configuration of the dermis (20–26) (Fig. 8-3A; Table 8-2). The lesion

TABLE 8-2 Common blue nevus.
Clinical features
Onset, birth or later
Women > men
Located on face, dorsum of wrist or foot, buttock
2–10 mm or larger
Well circumscribed
Symmetric
Dome shaped, often
Uniform blue, blue-gray, blue-black
No alteration of skin markings
Regular borders
Histopathological features
Symmetry
Alteration of dermis by variable admixture of dendritic melanocytes (usually heavily melaninized), melanophages, and fibrosis
Dendritic cells, often in bundles
Periadnexal aggregation of dendritic cells, often
Infiltration of smooth muscle, nerves
Differential diagnosis
Other dermal melanocytoses
Desmoplastic melanoma
Regressed melanoma
Metastatic melanoma

may occur anywhere in the reticular dermis and even in the papillary dermis. In general, there are bundles of dendritic cells with frequent aggregation about appendages and neurovascular bundles (Fig. 8-3B). The cells are generally bipolar or stellate and characterized by lengthy dendritic processes (Fig. 8-3B and 8-4). Most cells contain a dense accumulation of relatively fine melanin granules. The nuclei are ovoid with uniform chromatin patterns. Melanophages are usually present and may be the principal cell type in some cases. These cells are distinguished from melanocytes by the lack of dendritic processes, their polygonal morphology, and the presence of coarser melanin granules. Variable degrees of fibrosis are also present (Fig. 8-3B).

Differential Diagnosis This type of blue nevus shares the common dendritic cell type noted in the dermal melanocytoses already discussed. The blue nevus differs from the above entities by a greater concentration of dendritic melanocytes that results in a deformation of the reticular dermis and is accompanied by varying degrees of fibrosis and melanophage accumulation. However, the papular and nodular lesions within nevus of Ota or Ito are indistinguishable from this variant of blue nevus. The most important differential diagnosis is its distinction from primary and metastatic melanoma (30). In general, blue nevi can be distinguished from melanoma by their overall symmetry, lack of cytologic atypia, usually lack of inflammatory reaction, and absence of mitotic activity and necrosis.

Sclerosing Blue Nevus

This histologic variant of blue nevus is distinguished from the other types based on a prominent fibrous or sclerotic stroma.

Histopathological Features The silhouette of a sclerosing blue nevus is typically that of a symmetric and fairly well circumscribed fibrous nodule occupying the superficial dermis (Figs. 8-5 and 8-6). The fibrous component is conspicuous relative to the cellular elements. The cellular elements generally consist of a relatively sparse number of dendritic melanocytes, variable numbers of melanophages, and occasional relatively small numbers of spindle or uncommonly epithelioid cells (Fig. 8-6). This variant may represent the later stages in the natural history of some blue nevi, although this has not been definitely confirmed.

Differential Diagnosis The relevance of the sclerosing variant of blue nevus lies in the possible confusion with other sclerosing melanocytic or nonmelanocytic lesions. Sclerosing blue nevus needs to be distinguished from dermatofibroma, particularly the hemosiderotic variant, sclerosing Spitz nevus, and desmoplastic melanoma (Table 8-3) (see Chapter 10). The type of dermatofibroma associated with prominent deposits of hemosiderin can closely mimic blue nevus. However, the typical epidermal changes resembling seborrheic keratosis are usually found with dermatofibroma as well as the typical infiltrating pattern of cells in dermatofibroma. Close inspection of the pigment granules in dermatofibroma will usually reveal the golden refractile character of hemosiderin. If necessary, special stains for iron and melanin can be used to help distinguish these two entities. The desmoplastic or sclerosing form of Spitz nevus is usually easily separated from blue nevus since there is typically no pigment in the Spitz variant and the cell type is normally epithelioid. Desmoplastic melanoma is distinguished from sclerosing blue nevus by the presence of an atypical lentiginous melanocytic proliferation, fascicles of markedly atypical spindle cells, mitoses, and the minimal pigment in the desmoplastic melanoma (Table 8-3). However, the distinction of early desmoplastic melanoma from sclerosing blue nevus may occasionally be quite difficult. Diagnosis must be based on weighing the degree of cellularity, the degree of cytologic atypia, the presence of necrotic cells, mitotic activity, and clinical presentation.

Amelanotic Blue Nevus

Blue nevi typically contain melanin pigment, which is readily recognizable on routine hematoxylin and eosin (H&E) stained sections. Amelanotic blue nevus refers to the fact that on occasion melanocytic proliferations with the growth pattern and cytologic typical of blue nevus may lack readily recognizable melanin pigment (31).

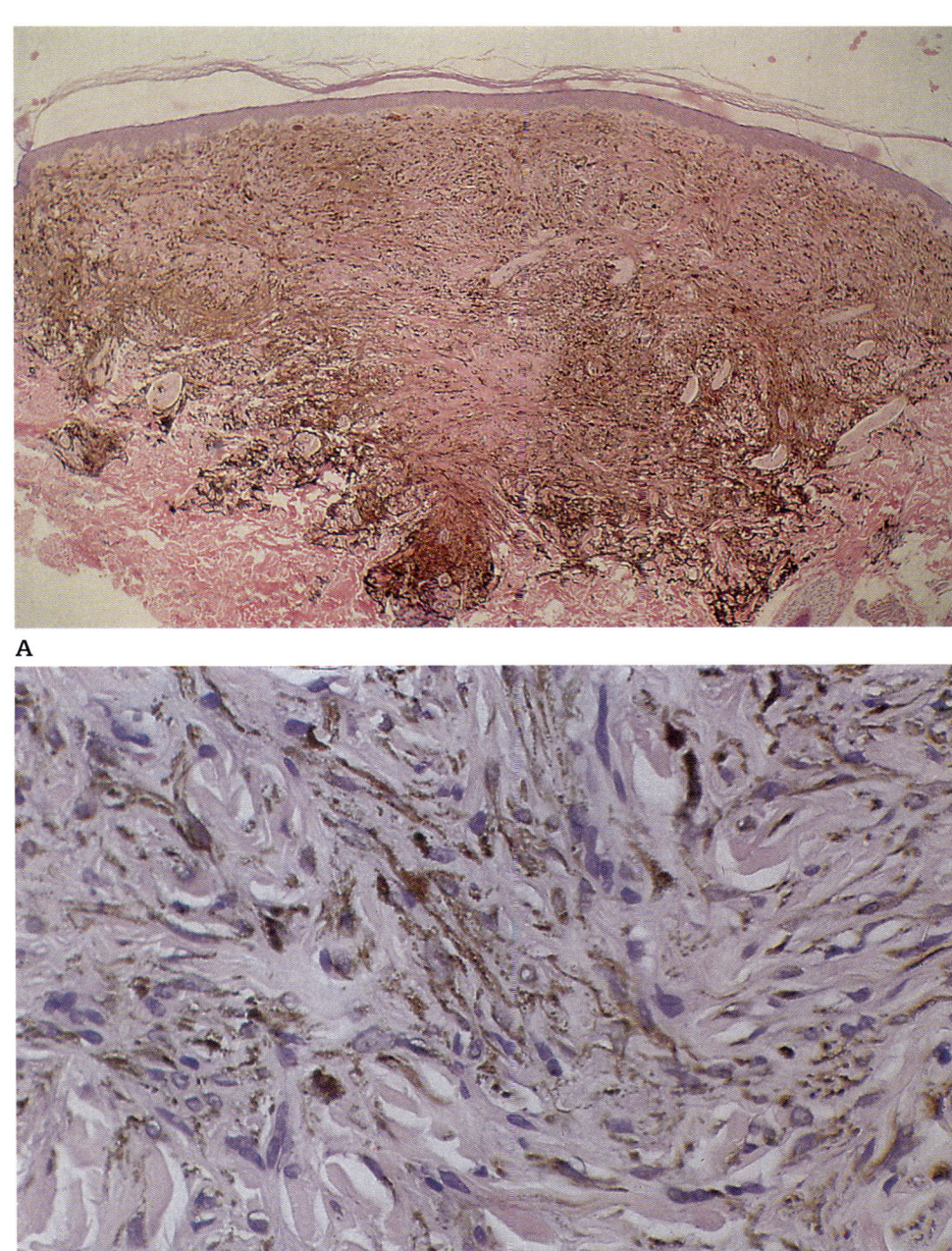

FIGURE 8-3 Blue nevus, ordinary type. **A,** The lesion is slightly raised and has an inverted wedge configuration in the reticular dermis. The nevus is composed of numerous pigmented dendritic cells in a slightly fibrotic matrix. **B,** The dendrites are easily identified by their melanin content.

Histopathological Features Any variant of blue nevus may be poorly pigmented, but it is most often found in sclerosing variants, for which the lack of pigment is also diagnostically most problematic.

Differential Diagnosis Amelanotic melanocytic proliferations are more difficult to be recognized as being melanocytic in origin. They may be confused with dermatofibroma, neurofibroma, a scar, or desmoplastic

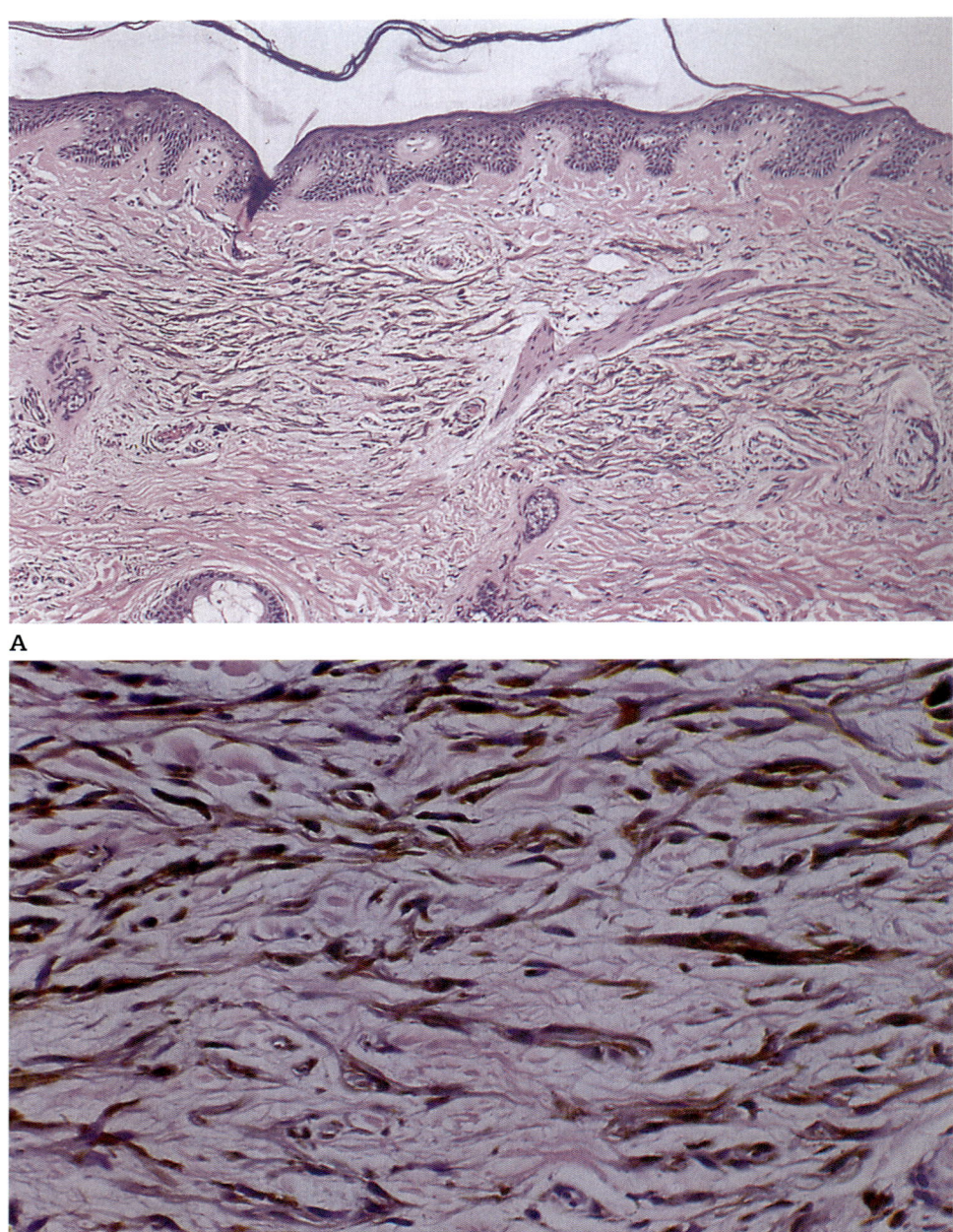

FIGURE 8-4 Blue nevus. **A,** The lesion is composed mainly of dendritic, horizontally disposed melanocytes in the upper dermis. **B,** Higher magnification of panel A.

melanoma. The melanocytic origin of a suspected nevus is usually made readily apparent by immunohistochemical studies for melanocyte differentiation antigens.

Blue Nevus, Epithelioid Cell Variant

The epithelioid cell variant of blue nevus is distinguished histologically by the relative prominence of epithelioid cell elements relative to dendritic cells and fibrous tissue (32–34). Epithelioid blue nevi may be associated with Carney complex, but many cases appear to be sporadic.

Histopathological Features In addition to the presence of variable numbers of dendritic melanocytes, melano-

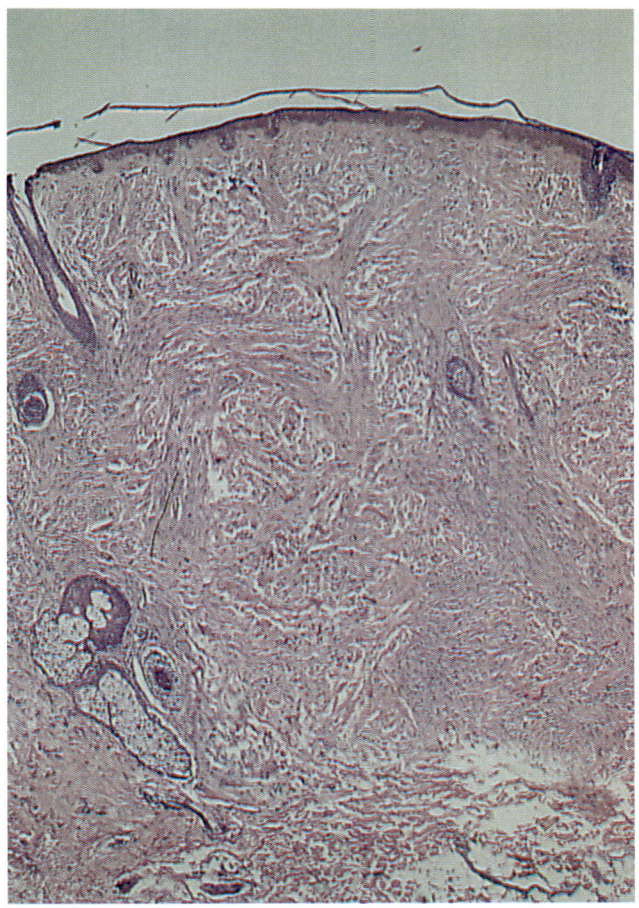
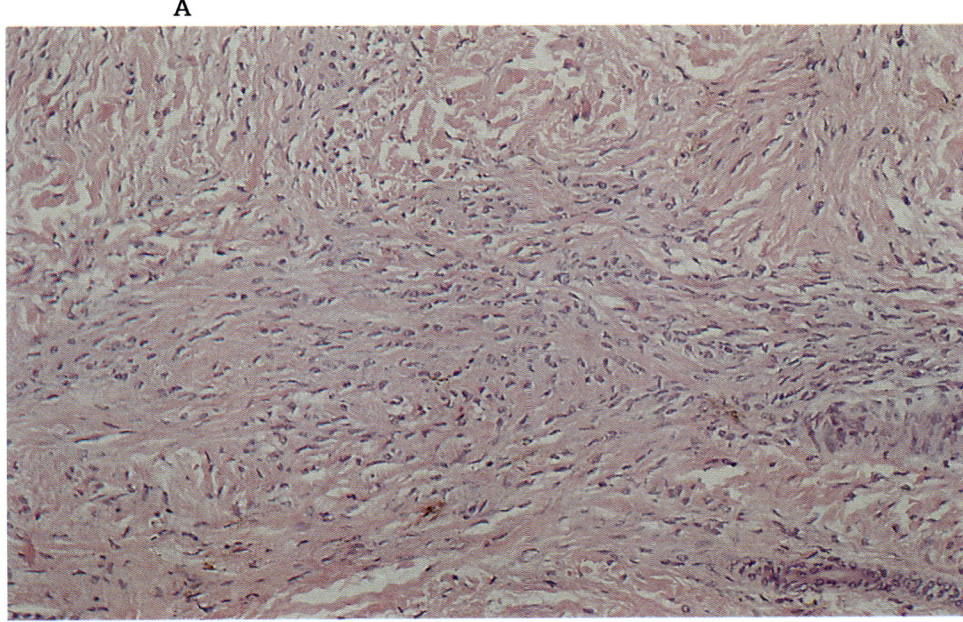

FIGURE 8-5 Blue nevus. **A,** The lesion contains almost no pigment and consists of a symmetric fibrotic nodule. **B,** Oval and fusiform cells disposed in fibrotic dermis. There is a resemblance to dermatofibroma.

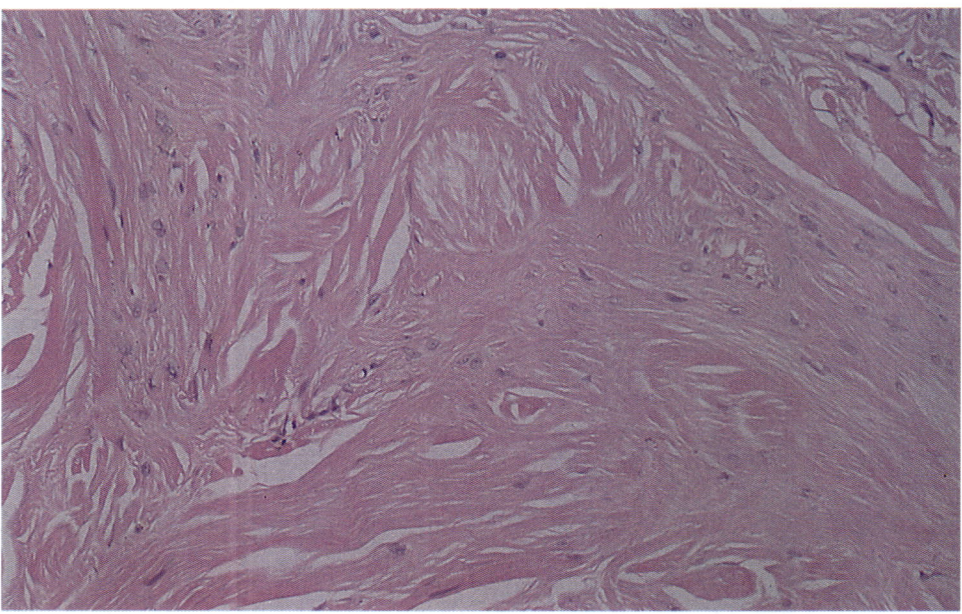

FIGURE 8-6 Blue nevus, sclerotic type. Note the markedly hyalinized collagen and dearth of cells.

phages, and fibrosis, this variant of blue nevus is characterized by conspicuous numbers of epithelioid cells (Fig. 8-7). In some instances, the lesions may have a plexiform configuration. They may be confined to the superficial and middle reticular dermis or extend into the subcutis.

Cytologically, the epithelioid cells are characterized by round or oval nuclei with relatively dispersed uniform chromatin patterns. Small distinct nucleoli are usually observed. Mitotic figures are absent or rare. Their presence should be cause for concern.

TABLE 8-3 Comparison of sclerosing blue nevus and desmoplastic-neurotropic melanoma.

Sclerosing blue nevus	Desmoplastic melanoma
Clinical features	
Common	Rare
Age, mean 38.6 years	Age, mean 60 years
Women > men	Men ≥ women
Dorsal hands, feet, face	Head and neck, sun-exposed skin
Blue, blue-black	Flesh-colored papule or nodule, may have tan or brown component
Histopathological features	
No intraepidermal component, usually	About two thirds have intraepidermal component, often lentigo maligna
Symmetry, common	Asymmetry, often
Superficial dermal, usually	Extending deep to subcutis, often
Pigmented, usually	Amelanotic, usually
Little or no atypia	Atypia common with hyperchromatic nuclei
Neurotropism, common	Neurotropism, common
Tropism for adnexal structures	No tropism for adnexal structures
No mitoses, usually	At least rare mitoses, usually
No mucin, usually	Mucinous stroma, on occasion
No inflammation, usually	Patchy lymphocytic aggregates, often
Immunohistochemistry	
S-100 protein+	S-100 protein+
HMB-45+	HMB-45− (in most cases)
Melan-A+	Melan-Ap− (in most cases)
Tyrosinase+	Tyrosinase− (in most cases)
MIB-1-staining absent or rare (0–< 5%)	MIB-1 staining is common but usually low (1–15%)

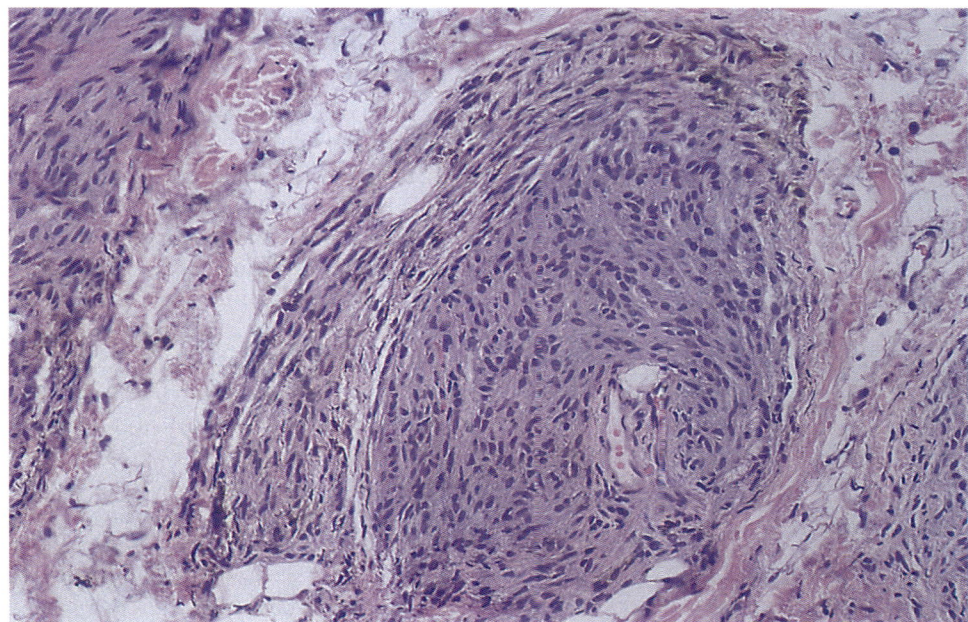

FIGURE 8-7 Blue nevus, spindle cell variant. The circumscribed cellular focus in the deep dermis resembles palisaded encapsulated neuroma.

Differential Diagnosis Epithelioid blue nevi need to be distinguished from melanoma arising in association with blue nevi or metastatic melanoma mimicking blue nevus (30). In general, presence of pleomorphism and/or mitoses, and the formation of expansile nodular aggregates of melanocytes within the lesion favor melanoma. Epithelioid blue nevi show overlap with the proposed entity of deep penetrating nevus (35,36) or may be a constituent of combined nevi (37).

Compound Blue Nevus

"Compound" blue nevus is a histologic variant of blue nevus defined by intraepidermal proliferation of dendritic melanocytes (38,39).

Clinical Features Only few cases have been reported (35,36). The most common site is the trunk. The lesions measured 2–4 mm in diameter and were described as blue-gray, blue-black, or black.

Histopathological Features The unique feature in these lesions is the presence of basilar epidermal proliferation of heavily pigmented dendritic melanocytes (35,36). Junctional nests are not present. The papillary and upper reticular dermis contains a fairly well circumscribed aggregate of spindle and dendritic melanocytes, usually heavily melanized with numerous melanophages.

Differential Diagnosis Compound blue nevus must be distinguished from a combined blue nevus, pigmented spindle cell nevus, variant of deep penetrating/plexiform nevus, melanoma, and regressed melanoma.

Cellular Blue Nevus

Clinical Features The cellular blue nevus (CBN) is less common than the typical dendritic and fibrotic variant (27,40–42). CBN are generally 1–2 cm in diameter with a blue, blue-black, or black coloration and most commonly involve the buttocks, sacral area, or scalp (Table 8-4). They are generally diagnosed between the ages of 10 and 40 years and are usually asymptomatic. The natural history is that of persistence but rarely these lesions may undergo transformation to malignant blue nevus. Incomplete excision of CBN is rarely associated with recurrence.

Histopathological Features As already mentioned, it is clear that there is a continuum from ordinary blue nevi to cellular blue nevi. Blue nevi are thus characterized by varying proportions of pigmented dendritic cells; oval, elongate, and fusiform cells arranged in various configurations and exhibiting varying degrees of melaninization; melanophages; and fibrosis (Figs. 8-8 and 8-9A; Table 8-4). Size, depth, and architecture also figure into this spectrum. No criteria have been established as to what proportion of a blue nevus should consist of fusiform cells

TABLE 8-4 Cellular blue nevus.

Clinical features
  Onset, birth, childhood, adolescence
  Age, mean 33 (range 6–85) years
  Buttocks, sacrococcygeal area, forearm/wrist,
    leg/ankle/foot, scalp, face
  Gray-blue to blue-black papule, nodule
  Well circumscribed, usually
  Regular borders
  0.3–3 cm

Histopathological features
  Symmetry
  Localization to reticular dermis
  Often deep extension with bulging, nodular
    configuration, rounded, well-
    demarcated inferior margin
  Heterogeneity of patterns
    Biphasic pattern most common
      Melanin-laden dendritic melanocytes and fibrosis
      Bundles of amelanotic fusiform cells
    Alveolar pattern
      Fascicles or nests of fusiform cells compartmentalized
        by fibrous trabeculae
    Fascicular pattern
      Fascicles of spindle cells often with clear cytoplasm
        and prominent
        schwannian differentiation
    Atypical cellular blue nevus
      Marked cytologic atypia
      Enlarged bizarre cells
      Multinucleate cells
  Lacunae containing melanophages
  Cystic degeneration in central part of nevus with loose
    edematous stroma
  Few or no mitotic figures
  Necrosis absent or uncommon

Differential diagnosis
  Malignant blue nevus
  Metastatic melanoma
  Clear cell sarcoma

to qualify as a cellular blue nevus. The heterogeneity of CBN is further discussed in Chapter 9.

The following criteria are proposed for diagnosis of CBN: The lesion should occupy the reticular dermis, at least a third to a half of the lesion should contain oval to fusiform cells, and the overall architecture should be multilobular or plexiform with deep extension, occasionally into subcutaneous fat.

Architecture of Cellular Blue Nevus

In general, CBN occupy a major portion of, if not the entire reticular dermis, and are notable for a rounded, well-demarcated lobular configuration (Fig. 8-9A). The lesion may show a single lobular mass with a well-defined horizontal inferior margin that parallels or bulges into the subcutaneous fat. Alternatively, there may be two or more lobules or digitate bulbous projections that extend into the deep reticular dermis or subcutaneous fat; these bulbous structures may also display a plexiform spatial arrangement (Figs. 8-8A and 8-9B).

Composition of Cellular Blue Nevus

Cellular blue nevus are remarkable for their heterogeneity, and it is apparent that the morphologic limits of CBN have not been clearly defined. For example, the distinction from common blue nevi, some pigmented peripheral nerve sheath tumors, and other unusual melancytic nevi may be problematic (see Chapter 9). Essential for the diagnosis are cellular foci of round, oval, elongate, or fusiform cells that constitute at least a third to a half, if not most of the tumor (Fig. 8-8C and 8-9C). These cells are arranged in a number of patterns and vary considerably as to melanin content. As opposed to the frequent diffuse distribution of melanin-laden dendritic melancytes in the ordinary type of blue nevus, the fusiform cells of CBN are usually disposed in variably organized nests or bundles (Figs. 8-9D,E). These bundles may or may not be encapsulated by fibrous tissue. In some instances, there are fascicles of fusiform cells oriented randomly in all directions without evidence of compartmentalization. However, a common pattern is that of compact highly cellular nests or fascicles separated by fibrous trabeculae. There may be linear or concentric arrangements of cells within these nests. Often pigmented dendritic melancytes and melanophages are present in the peripheral fibrous tissue surrounding the cellular fascicles (Fig. 8-9D). The sizes of the fascicles or nests may vary considerably. There may be large lobules of fusiform cells constituting much of the tumor without any intervening fibrous tissue. The presence of well-defined rounded nests of cells has been described as the "alveolar" pattern in CBN. In some CBN, fascicles of spindle cells may have striking Schwannian differentiation and may merge with and infiltrate cutaneous nerves.

The cells making up the cellular foci in CBN are most often fusiform or spindle-shaped but may also be round or oval (Fig. 8-8C and 8-9E). These cells are usually somewhat enlarged but may be relatively small on occasion. The cells' boundaries are often ill-defined; the cytoplasm is usually either clear, vacuolated, slightly eosinophilic or bluish. In many CBN, the fusiform cells do not contain readily apparent melanin pigment by conventional microscopy. Because of the paucity or absence of melanin, these cellular foci appear pale or clear on scanning magnification, in contrast to the often heavily pigmented areas containing dendritic melanocytes, melanophages, and sclerosis. The latter pale areas are quite helpful in recognizing CBN. However, the degree of melaninization may vary from barely visible fine granular melanin to heavy pigmentation obscuring cytologic detail. Usually, the dendritic melanocytes and melanophages contain the heaviest deposition of melanin. However, the latter cells are usually located in peripheral fibrous trabeculae or in areas of sclerosis.

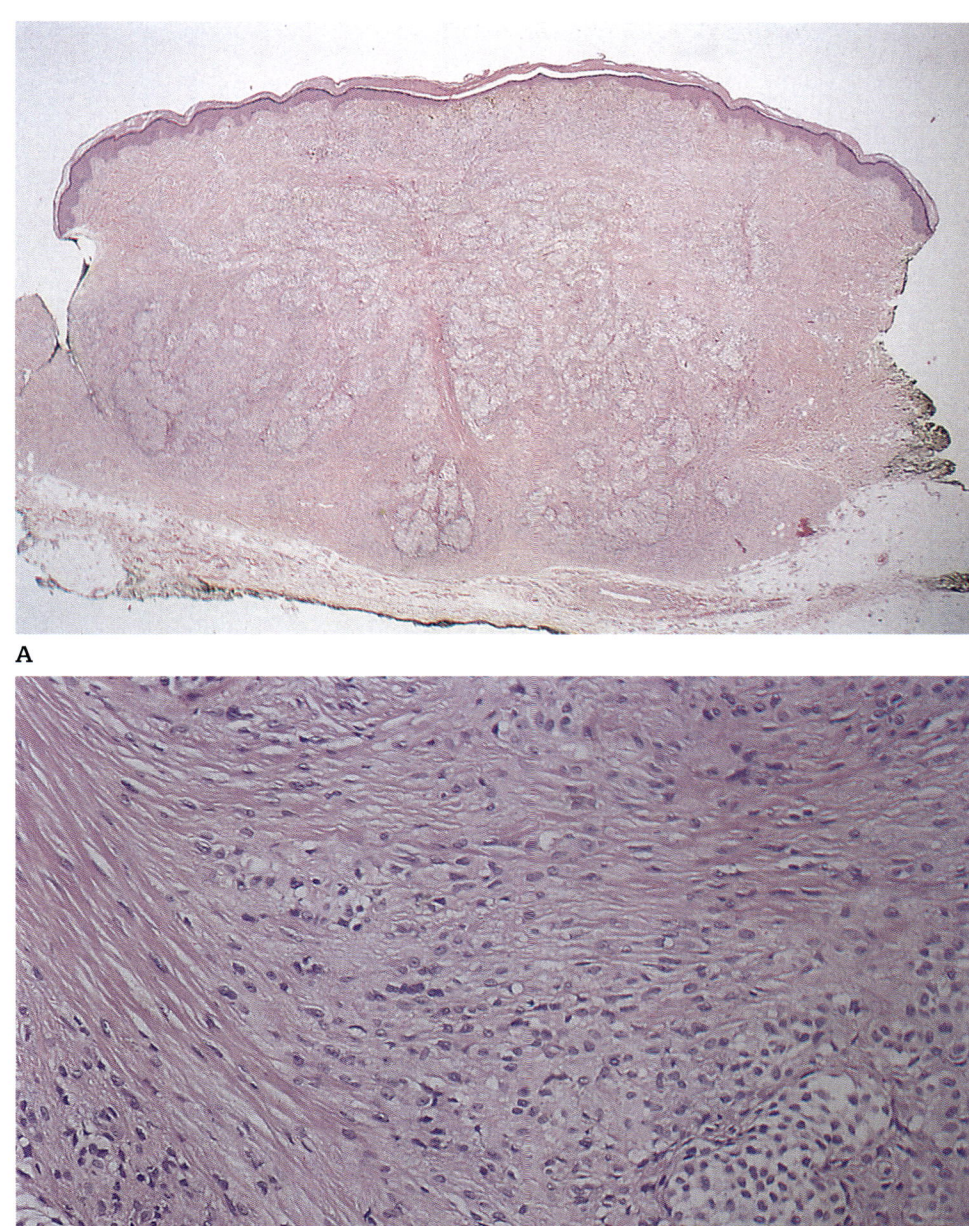

FIGURE 8-8 Blue nevus, cellular variant. **A,** This lesion occupies the entire dermis and displays a well-demarcated, slightly rounded deep margin. **B,** Fibrotic area containing scattered cells and little if any melanin.

The nuclei of these cells are usually round, oval, or fusiform and commonly somewhat enlarged (Fig. 8-9E). The chromatin tends to be evenly dispersed, and one or more small nucleoli are often observed. Minimal or low-grade nuclear pleomorphism is noted in many CBN. However, this should not be pronounced. Similarly, occasional mitoses are noted in many CBN. As a general rule, if two or more mitoses are present per square millimeter, the lesion should be carefully evaluated for other corroborating evidence of malignancy.

Multinucleate giant cells are occasionally noted in the cellular areas and may be numerous in some CBN. Such giant cells may also occur in areas of cystic degeneration.

Occasional CBN are composed of discreet nests of amelanotic round or oval cells, analogous to the usual

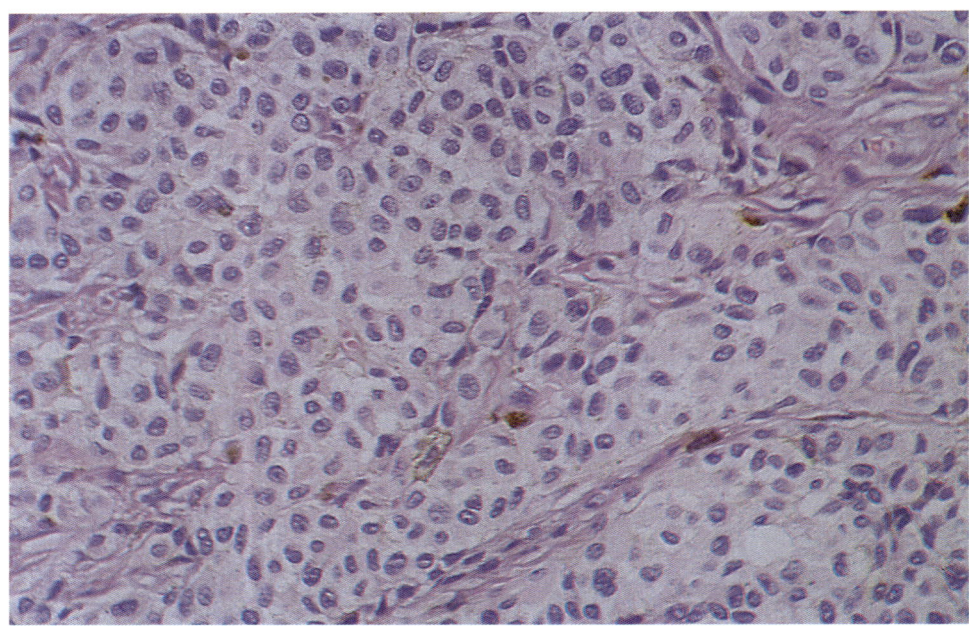

FIGURE 8-8 Continued. **C,** Discreet nests of round, oval, and slightly elongate cells with clear cytoplasm.

fusiform cells (Fig. 8-8C). Such nests are separated in the typical fashion by fibrous trabeculae that usually contain some dendritic melanocytes and melanophages. Recognition of other morphologic (e.g., lobular well-demarcated configuration) and clinical features are necessary for diagnosis as CBN. Such presentations point out the heterogeneity of CBN, relationships to other melanocytic nevi, and problems of proper nosology (see Chapter 9).

FIGURE 8-9 Cellular blue nevus. **A,** Pale-staining, central area corresponds to nests and fascicles of fusiform cells. Fibrosis and pigment are at the periphery of this area.

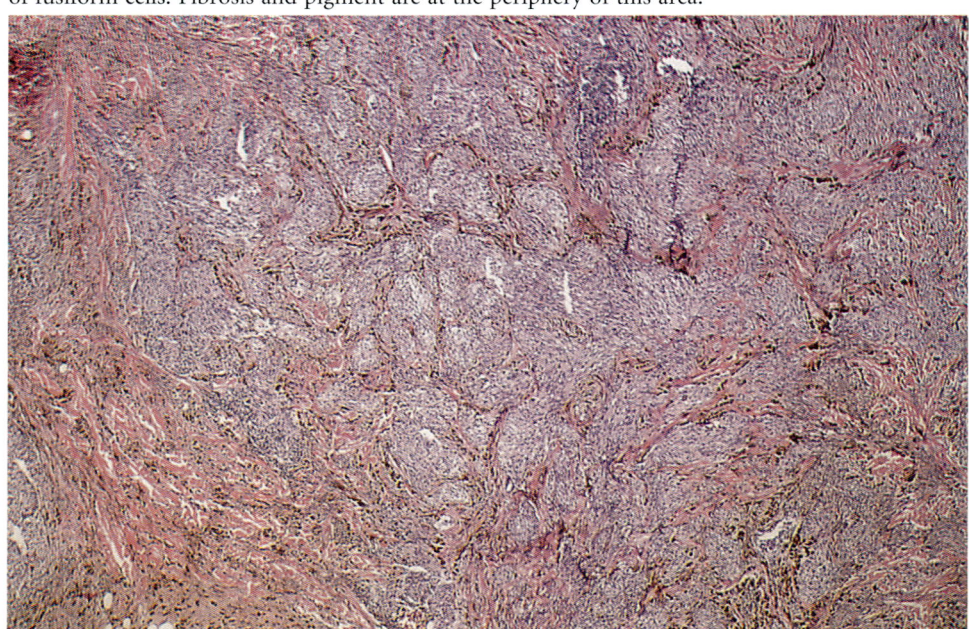

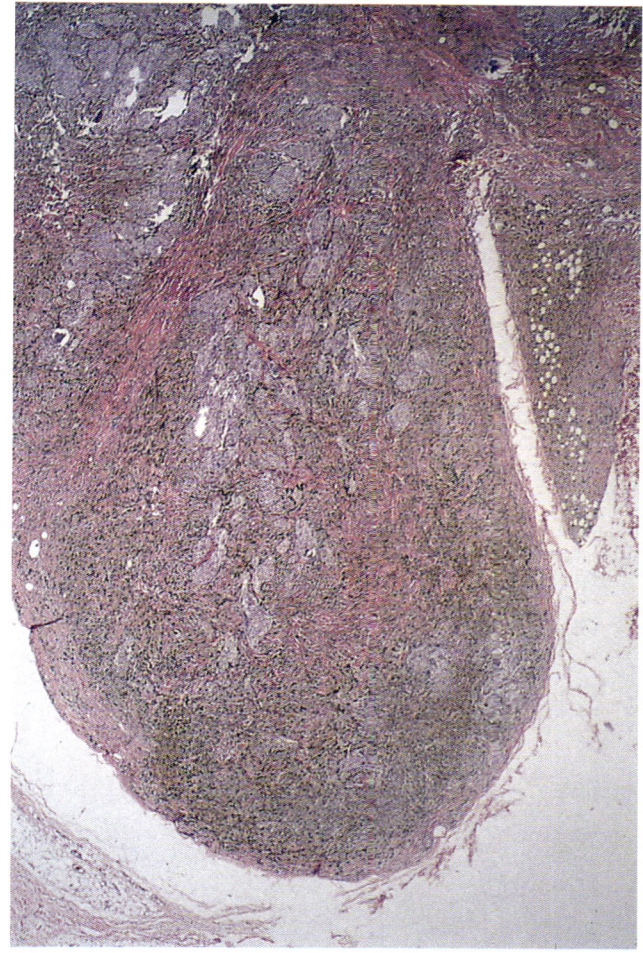

B

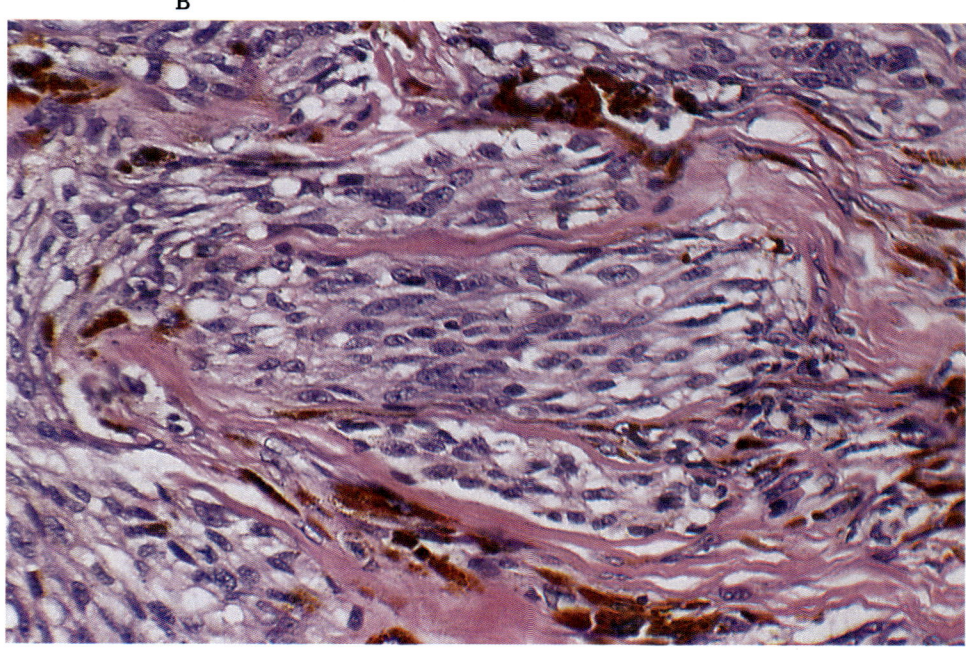

C

FIGURE 8-9 *Continued.* **B,** Characteristic bulbous configuration of cellular blue nevus extending into subcutis. **C,** Well-defined compact nests of fusiform cells with slightly eosinophilic or clear cytoplasm are bounded by fibrous tissue. Melanophages are present in fibrous trabeculae separating the cellular fascicles.

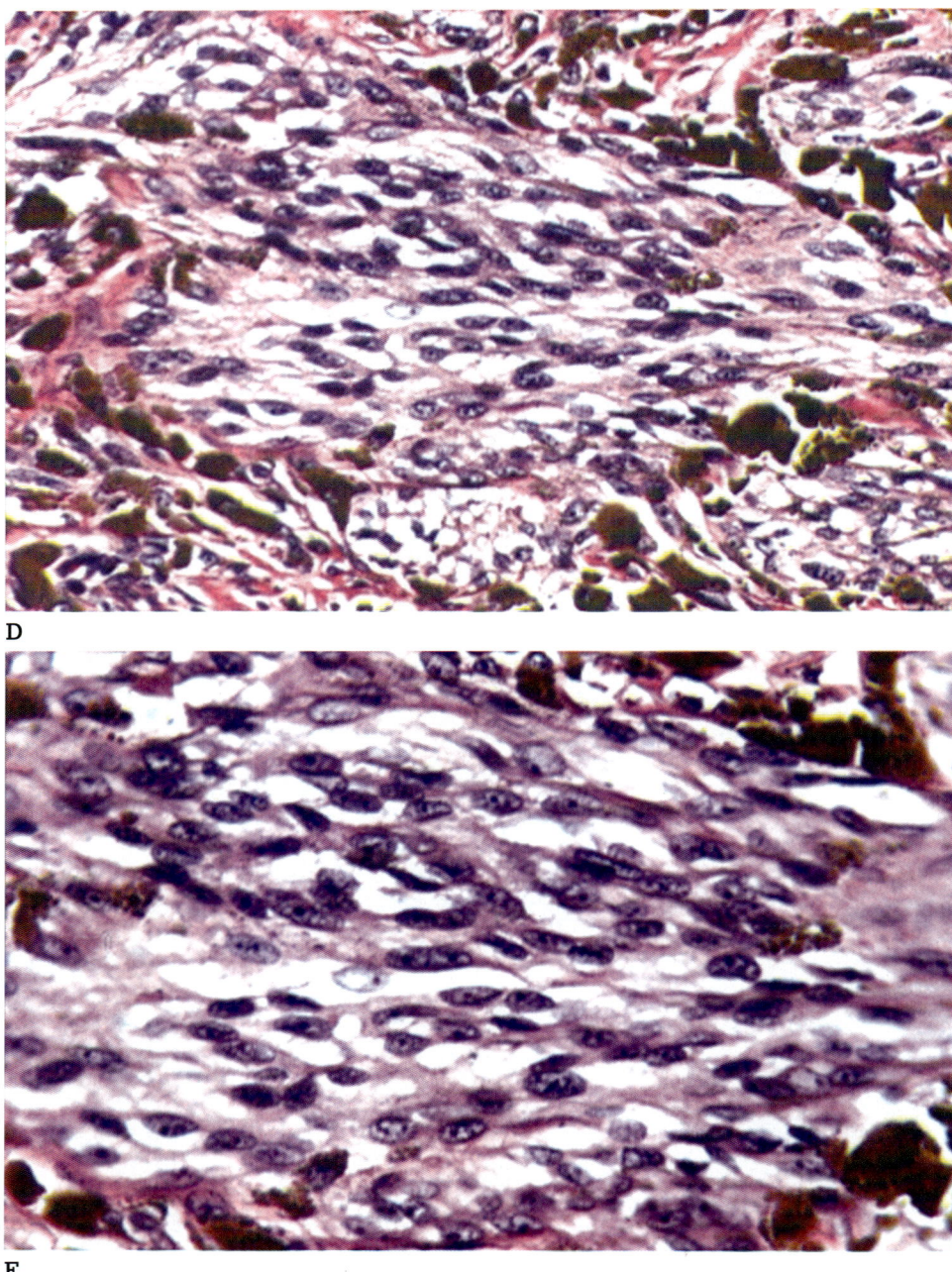

FIGURE 8-9 *Continued*. **D,** Fascicles of fusiform melanocytes with slightly eosinophilic or clear cytoplasms. **E,** The melanocytes have vacuolated cytoplasm and elongate nuclei. The nuclei have dispersed chromatin and occasional nucleoli are present. There is some resemblance to clear cell sarcoma.

Other Morphologic Features of Cellular Blue Nevus

Perhaps two thirds or so of CBN have a so-called biphasic pattern, which refers to a component of common blue nevus—that is, areas containing pigmented dendritic melanocytes, variable sclerosis, and melanophages. These areas are often in the superficial dermis overlying or at the periphery of cellular lobules. These areas are indistinguishable from ordinary blue nevus and provide evidence that all blue nevi are indeed on a continuum.

A rather characteristic feature of CBN is the presence of cystic degeneration (encystification), which is often centrally located (Fig. 8-10). The latter changes are probably indistinguishable from those occurring in ancient Schwannoma and may have an ischemic or traumatic basis. These degenerative changes are typified by edema, myxoid stro-

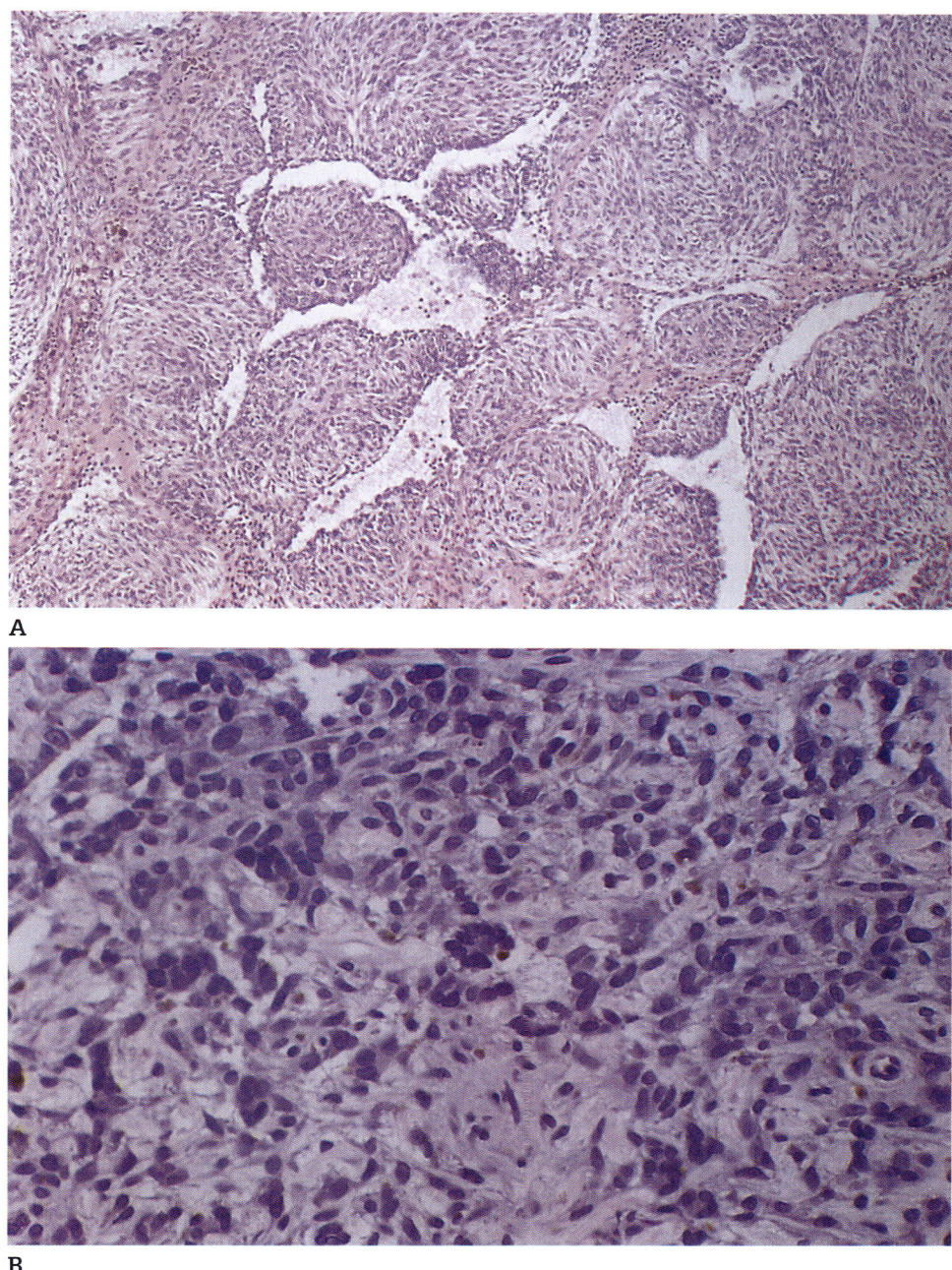

FIGURE 8-10 Cellular blue nevus with central cystic degeneration. **A,** Nests of cells are separated by edema and myxoid stroma. **B,** The cells exhibit pleomorphism occasional multinucleate giant cells are seen.

mal alteration, some degree of diminished cellularity, and scattered melanophages. Alterations of blood vessels also tend to be a prominent feature. Commonly ectatic blood vessels show hyalinization of their walls and thrombosis, features suggesting a component of ischemia.

Atypical Variants of Cellular Blue Nevus (Atypical CBN) There are variants of CBN that may be extremely difficult to distinguish from malignant blue nevus (MBN, melanoma) (43,44). The controversial term *atypical CBN* has been proposed to accommodate such lesions with features beyond what is considered acceptable for CBN. The problem is that the limits and biologic potential of CBN have not been sufficiently well characterized to define the latter spectrum. Therefore, until definitive criteria are formulated for the distinction of atypical CBN from typical

CBN and MBN, the use of such a term is likely to constitute a wastebasket for any unusual CBN. Thus we discourage the use of the term without qualification. An acceptable approach is to specify the features that are considered to be abnormal, for example: large size (e.g., > 2–3 cm), significant depth, presence of necrosis, mitotic rate (e.g., $6/mm^2$), asymmetry, ulceration, infiltrating features, high cellular density, confluence or sheetlike arrangements of melanocytes, and presence of pronounced cytologic atypia. The clinical history associated with such lesions is usually that of recent change or enlargement.

Histopathological Features

Atypical variants of CBN are generally characterized by large size (> 2–3 cm), deep extension, large expansile nests of spindle cells, focal infiltrative patterns, necrosis, and some asymmetry (43,44). These large tumoral aggregates of cells display greater cellularity than what is normally seen in CBN. There is also greater cellular pleomorphism with hyperchromatism and variation of nuclear characteristics. Nucleoli may be prominent as well. There may also be greater mitotic activity in such lesions. The distinction from melanoma may be quite difficult. Such discrimination is based on determining that a majority of the cells have a fairly uniform appearance, that necrosis is absent, and that there is no cytologically distinct and atypical tumor nodule present, which differs from the background blue nevus cells. Otherwise, a diagnosis of malignant melanoma must be carefully weighed.

Differential Diagnosis The differential diagnosis of CBN (and atypical and variants of CBN) includes malignant blue nevus (malignant melanoma arising in association with cellular blue nevus or mimicking cellular blue nevus) (45–48), metastatic melanoma, and clear-cell sarcoma (see Chapter 10). MBN is an extremely rare entity and thus this diagnosis should be made only after careful evaluation (Table 8.5).

The clinical history of a long-standing blue nevus with subsequent change or finding an associated benign blue nevus remnant (usually CBN) is critical for the diagnosis of MBN. Without the latter criteria, MBN cannot be distinguished from conventional melanoma, whether primary or metastatic. In general, MBN is discriminated from CBN and atypical variants by larger size, greater degrees of asymmetry, greater cellular density and confluence, more pronounced cytologic atypia, greater mitotic activity with atypical forms, and necrosis—but there are exceptions. In some MBN, the mitotic rate may be relatively low (e.g., $2/mm^2$) and thus comparable to many CBN. It is important to emphasize that there may be considerable heterogeneity within MBN and the diagnosis may be missed because of this histologic variation. The presence of a concomitant conventional blue nevus element favors a diagnosis of CBN. It cannot be overemphasized that although MBN is vanishingly rare, atypical variants of CBN should be completely excised and the patients monitored very carefully for recurrence. Metastases from such lesions have been observed after the passage of up to 20 years. Thus, because of the unusual nature of these lesions, their rarity, and the lack of long-term follow-up, the biologic potential of atypical forms of CBN is largely unknown and requires further study.

Clear-cell sarcoma may have a very similar appearance to CBN, but it has an infiltrative growth pattern, has greater cytologic atypia, has mitotic activity, and is generally centered in the deep soft tissue (subcutis, fascia) of the extremities. In contrast, CBN is usually centered in the deep dermis and typically involves the subcutis only superficially (see Chapter 10). In difficult cases, molecular studies for the EWS-ATF1 fusion transcript can be decisive (49).

Lymph Node Involvement by Blue Nevus

For some time, it has been recognized that blue nevi, including cellular foci of blue nevi, may be encountered on

TABLE 8-5 Comparison of cellular blue nevus and melanoma arising in or mimicking blue nevus (malignant blue nevus).

Cellular blue nevus	*Malignant blue nevus*
Clinical features	
Usually in the young or middle-aged	Usually seen in elderly
Women > men	Men > women
Buttock, sacrococcygeal area, extremities	Scalp but also other sites
1.8 cm (1–2 cm)	2.5 cm (1.3–4 cm or more)
Blue, blue-gray, blue-black nodule	Blue, blue-black nodule
Histopathological features	
Symmetry	Asymmetry
Lobular or multilobular pattern	Lobular or multilobular pattern
Fascicles or nests of melanocytes with associated ordinary blue nevus cells	Sheets of large epithelioid cells or sarcomatoid pattern of spindle cells
Cytologic atypia, mild or absent	Cytologic atypia, moderate to severe
Mitoses, usually < $1–2/mm^2$	Mitoses, usually > $2/mm^2$
Necrosis, usually absent (infarct-type necrosis may be seen in large lesions)	Necrosis, present in approximately on third of tumors
	Recognition is facilitated, if there is a distinctly different associated benign precursor

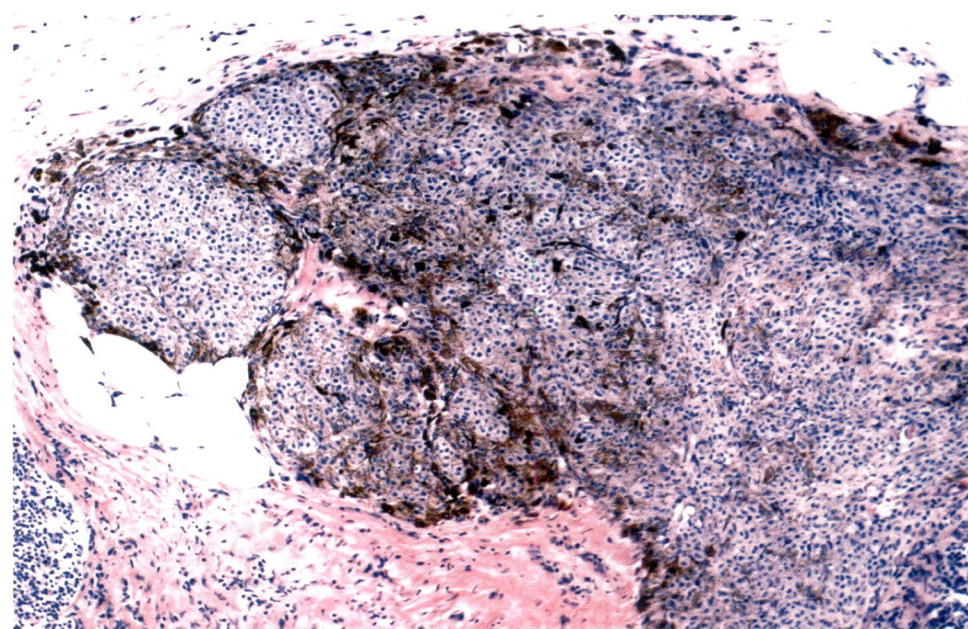

FIGURE 8-11 Cellular nodal blue nevus. Nested aggregates of pale epithelioid melanocytes are seen in a background of pigmented fusiform and dendritic nevomelanocytes. The lesion is entirely located in the lymph node capsule.

occasion in regional lymph nodes (50–52). These regional lymph nodes have almost always been axillary or inguinal lymph nodes proximal to a blue nevus on an extremity. Like other nodal nevi, nodal blue nevi, predominantly involve the lymph node capsule, but subcapsular extension and focal parenchymal involvement can also be seen. Because of the nodal localization of these cellular aggregates, explanations for this phenomenon have included dislodgement of benign nevus cells as well as aberrant migration of neural crest cells (50–52). An example of a cellular nodal blue nevus is shown in Figure 8-11.

The most important point regarding this phenomenon is that it is recognized and not misdiagnosed as metastatic melanoma or MBN. Similarly, it is important that a cutaneous lesion if present is not misdiagnosed as MBN simply because of the lymph node involvement. This is not to say that the distinction between CBN and MBN is not difficult or that MBN with metastasis does not exist. Thus it is incumbent on the pathologist to be certain that there are sufficient changes for malignancy in such a circumstance—cytologic atypia, necrosis, mitotic activity, and/or increased labeling index for Ki-67—before rendering a diagnosis of metastatic melanoma (or metastatic MBN) and primary MBN.

Patchlike Blue Nevus

Patchlike blue nevus is a macular area of blue-gray pigmentation, varying in size from 1 cm to several centimeters and clinically resembling a Mongolian spot (53). In contrast to Mongolian spot, this lesion contains a greater number of dendritic melanocytes in the dermis.

Plaque-Type Blue Nevus

Clinical Features The plaque-type variant of blue nevus is often congenital or its onset can be usually be traced back to early childhood. Clinically, this nevus is characterized by an area of blue-gray pigmentation and measures 1 cm to several centimeters in diameter (54–60). The plaque is either a single lesion or composed of multiple but distinct macules or papules. There is probably a close relationship of eruptive or agminated blue nevi, patchlike blue nevi, and plaque-type blue nevi (Table 8-6).

TABLE 8-6 Plaque-type blue nevus.
Clinical features
Congenital or later onset
Site, anywhere
Size 1–17 cm
Plaque, either confluent or composed of numerous macules and papules
Blue-gray to blue-black
May increase in size
Histopathological features
Features of ordinary to cellular blue nevus
Differential diagnosis
Melanoma
Melanotic neurocristic hamartoma

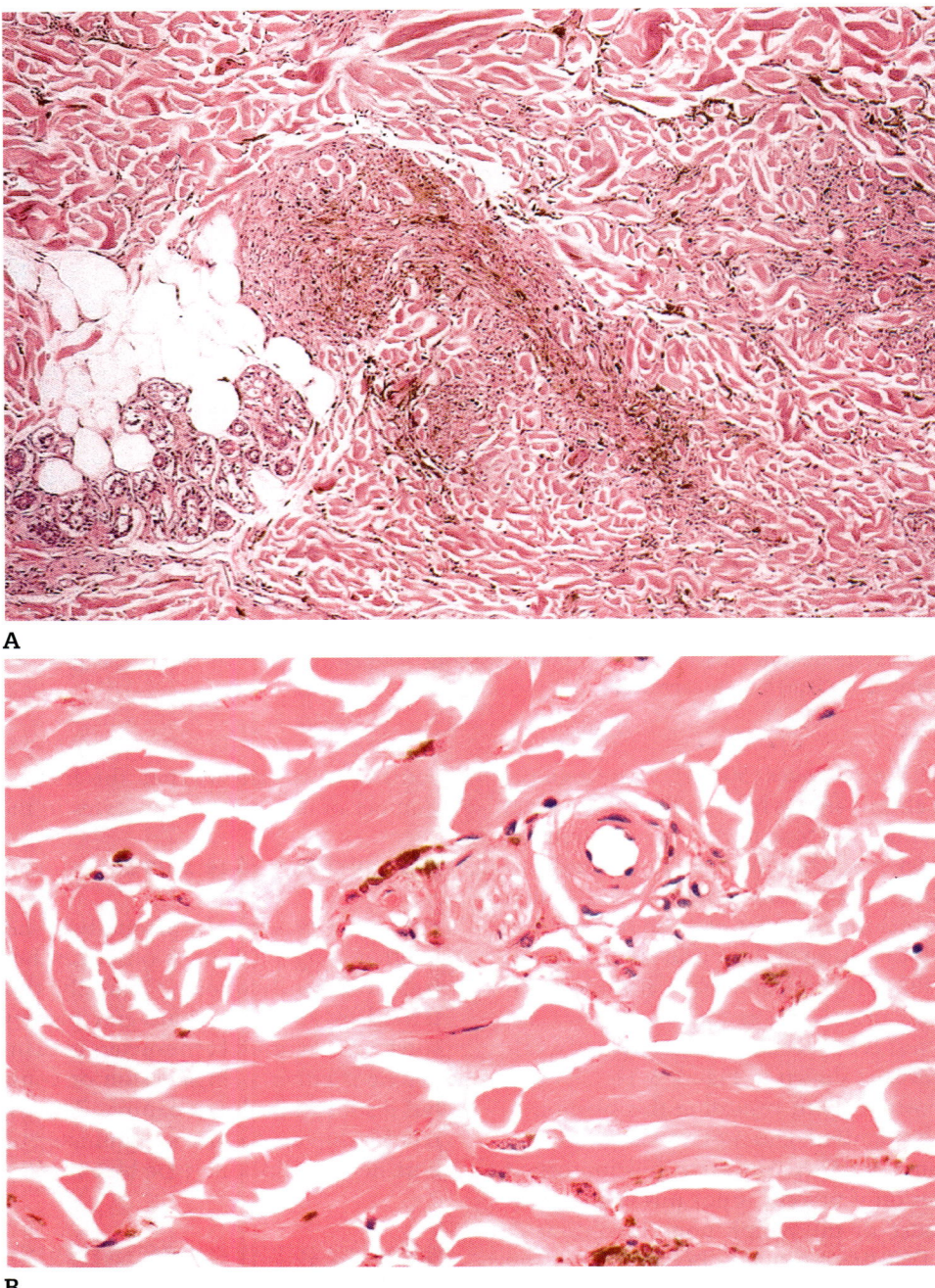

FIGURE 8-12 Plaque-type blue nevus. **A,** Periappendageal aggregates of pigmented melanocytes are seen. **B,** There are intervening Mongolian-spot-like areas of solitary melanocytes and macrophages separated by fibrous tissue.

Histopathological Features The histologic features are similar to ordinary blue nevi, but large lesions often show some heterogeneity of melanocytes, including slender dendritic cells, fascicles of spindle cells, aggregates of epithelioid melanocytes, and occasionally clear cell melanocytes. In plaque-type blue nevi, melanocytes in the dermis are often predominantly arranged in a periappendageal distribution. They also tend to be associated with blood vessels and nerve trunks. Foci of hypercellularity, similar in appearance to CBN, may be present, and it is important not to confuse these foci with malignant melanoma (60) (Fig. 8-12).

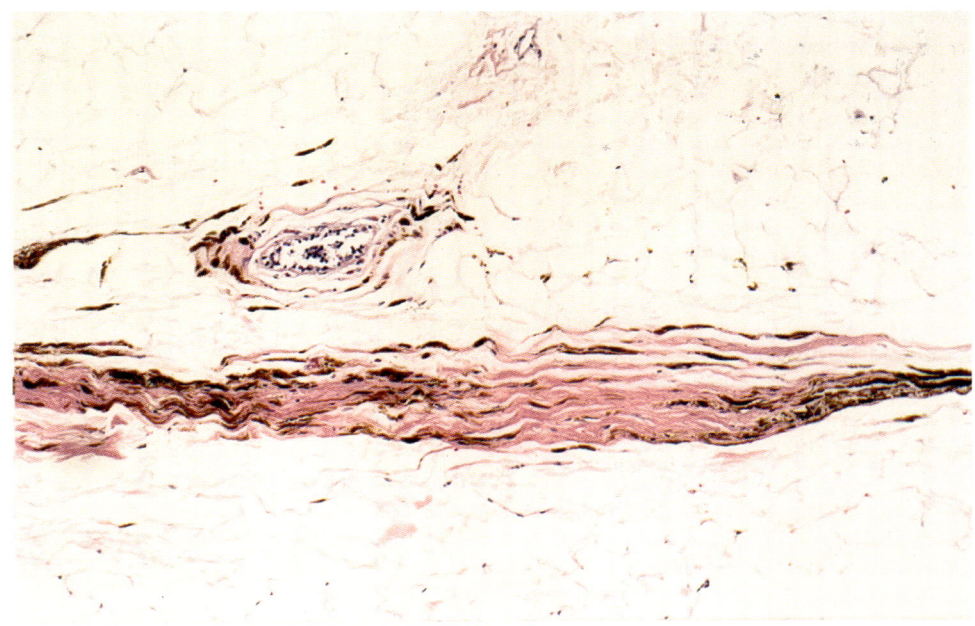

C

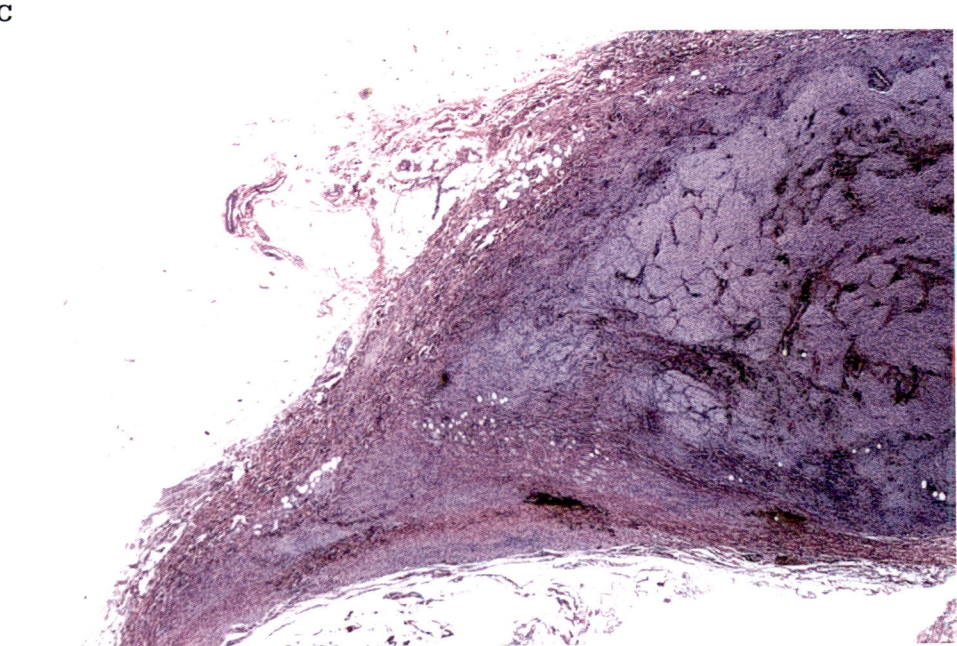

D

FIGURE 8-12 *Continued.* **C,** Melanocytes are seen within and around a peripheral nerve and at the periphery of a small blood vessel. **D,** A cellular melanocytic nodule is seen in the subcutis.

Neurocristic Hamartoma

Clinical Features The term *neurocristic hamartoma* has been suggested for a subset of pigmented spindle cell lesions, whose features were thought to reflect combined melanocytic and schwannian differentiation (60–63). A variant thereof, so-called pilar neurocristic hamartoma, is a lesion that is clinically characterized by multiple perifollicular papules occupying an area of skin measuring several centimeters in diameter (60). The clinical features of subsequently reported neurocristic hamartomas resemble patchlike or plaque-type blue nevi.

Histopathological Features Histologically, the lesions of pilar neurocristic hamartoma resembled perifollicular blue nevi. Subsequent reports described neurocristic hamartomas as mixtures of melanocytes, Schwann cells, and neuromesenchyme. However, neurocristic hamartoma is not a widely accepted entity among pathologists, and there is obvious histologic overlap between neurocristic hamartoma and patchlike nevi and plaque-type blue nevi. Because melanocytes show considerable phenotypic placticity and heterogeneity, it has been argued that neurocristic hamartomas are not composite tumors of Schwann cells and melanocytes but rather melanocytic nevi with prominent schwannian differentiation.

Target Blue Nevus

Target blue nevus is an uncommon type of blue nevus that is important to recognize because of its possible clinical confusion with melanoma (64) (Table 8-7).

Clinical Features The two cases reported to date have occurred on the dorsal aspect of the foot of young adult males (64). The lesions were about 1 cm in greatest diameter, were dome shaped, and showed a target appearance. Each lesion was characterized by a central dark blue nodule surrounded by a flesh-colored annulus and more peripheral blue-black macular annulus. Both patients reported that their lesions had changed in color during the previous year.

Histopathological Features On scanning magnification, one can detect a zonal alteration in the number of pigment-containing cells corresponding to the target-like clinical appearance (64). The dark central nodule has the features of a typical blue nevus—a fibrotic tumor containing pigmented dendritic cells and fusiform cells. The flesh-colored annulus, although exhibiting dermal sclerosis, is remarkable for significantly reduced numbers of pigment-containing cells. However, the most peripheral zone of the lesion has, in contrast, significant numbers of the pigmented dendritic cells.

Differential Diagnosis The variation in numbers of pigmented dendritic cells in the target blue nevus might suggest an atypical lesion. However, careful inspection will disclose an overall orderly arrangement of the cellular population and fibrosis. In addition, cytologic atypia is generally minimal or absent.

Mucosal or Visceral Blue Nevi

Blue nevi have been reported at various mucosal and internal sites (65–70). Common blue nevi are usually an incidental finding and readily recognized as such, if a biopsy is performed. Their occurrence at internal sites is thought to be related to aberrant neural crest migration. Mucosal and internal cellular blue nevi may be difficult to recognize as such on a partial biopsy and confusion may arise with metastatic melanoma or a melanotic nerve sheath tumor.

REFERENCES

1. Levene A. On the natural history and comparative pathology of the blue naevus. Ann Rep Coll Surg Engl 1980;62:327–34.
2. Lovas GL, Wysocki GP, Daley TD. The oral blue nevus: histogenetic implications of its ultrastructural features. Oral Surg 1983;55:145–50.
3. Nakai T, Rappaport H. A study of the histogenesis of experimental melanotic tumors resembling cellular blue nevi: the evidence in support of their neurogenic origin. Am J Pathol 1963;43:175–99.
4. Misago N. The relationship between melanocytes and peripheral nerve sheath cells (part II): blue nevus with peripheral nerve sheath differentiation. Am J Dermatopathol 2000;22:230–6.
5. Mandybur TI. Melanotic nerve sheath tumors. J Neurosurg 1974;41:187–92.
6. Carney JA. Psammomatous melanotic schwannoma. Am J Surg Pathol 1990;14:206–22.
7. Sun J, Morton TH, Gown AM. Antibody HMB-45 identifies the cells of blue nevi. Am J Surg Pathol 1990;14:748–51.
8. Busam KJ, Barnhill RL. The immunophenotype of blue nevi. J Cutan Pathol 1996;23:67.
9. Busam KJ, Chen YT, Old LJ, et al. Expression of Melan-A (MART-1) in benign melanocytic nevi and primary malignant melanoma. Am J Surg Pathol 1998;22:1067–72.

TABLE 8-7 Target blue nevus.

Clinical features
    Young adults
    Approximately 1 cm
    Location dorsal aspect of foot (two cases)
    Dome-shaped nodule
    Central gray-black to blue-black area surrounded by flesh-colored annulus and more peripheral macular blue-black annulus
    History of recent change, usual
Histopathological features
    Central nodule contains pigmented dendritic cells, fibrosis, and possibly spindle cells in dermis
    Flesh-colored annulus shows fibrosis and reduced number of pigmented dendritic cells
    Outer pigmented annulus shows some pigmented dendritic cells
Differential diagnosis
    Melanoma with regression

10. El Bahrawy A. Ueber den mongolenfleck bei Europaern. Arch Dermatol Syphil 1922;141:171–92.
11. Larsen NP, Godfrey LS. Sacral pigment spots. Am J Phys Anthropol 1927;10:253–74.
12. Pratt G. Birthmarks in infants. Arch Dermatol 1953;67;302–5.
13. Ota M, Tanino H. Nevus fusco-caeruleus ophthalmo-maxillaris and melanosis bulbi. Tokyo Shinshi 1939; 63(3133):1243–5.
14. Hirayama T, Suzuki T. A new classification of Ota's nevus based on histopathological features. Dermatologica 1991; 183:169–72.
15. Nödl F, Krüger R. Maligner blauer nävus bei nävus Ota. Hautarzt 1984;35:421–4.
16. Sun C-C, Lu Y-C, Lee EF, Nakagawa H. Naevus fusco-caeruleus zygomaticus. Br J Dermatol 1987;117:545–53.
17. Hidano A, Kaneko K. Acquired dermal melanocytosis of the face and extremities. Br J Dermatol 1991;124:96–9.
18. Ito M. Nevus fusco-caeruleus acromino-deltoideus. Tokohu Exp Med 1954;60:10.
19. van Krieken JH, Boom BW, Scheffer E. Malignant transformation in a naevus of Ito. A case report. Histopathology 1988;12:100–2.
20. Burkhart CG, Gohara A. Dermal melanocytic hamartoma. Arch Dermatol 1981;117:102–4.
21. Degos R. Dermatologie. Paris: Editions Medicales Flammarion, 1953.
22. Tièche M. Ueber benigne melanome ("chromatophorome") der haut "blaue naevi". Virchows Arch Pathol Anat 1906; 186:212–29.
23. Montgomery H. The blue nevus (Jadassohn-Tieche): Its distinction from ordinary moles and malignant melanomas. Am J Cancer 1939;36:527–39.
24. Dorsey CS, Montgomery H. Blue nevus and its distinction from Mongolian spot and the nevus of Ota. J Invest Dermatol 1954;22:225–36.
25. Leopold JG, Richards DB. The interrelationship of blue and common naevi. J Path Bact 1968;95:37–46.
26. Radentz WA, Vogel P. Congenital common blue nevus. Arch Dermatol 1990;126:124-5.
27. Rodriguez HA, Ackerman LV. Cellular blue nevus. Clinicopathologic study of forty-five cases. Cancer 1968;21:393–405.
28. Modly C, Wood C, Horn T. Metastatic malignant melanoma arising from a common blue nevus in a patient with subacute cutaneous lupus erythematosus. Dermatologica 1989;178:171–5.
29. Shenfield HT, Maize JC. Multiple and agminated blue nevi. J Dermatol Surg Oncol 1980;6:725–8.
30. Busam KJ. Metastatic melanoma to the skin simulating blue nevus. Am J Surg Pathol 1999;23:276–82.
31. Bhawan J, Cao SL. Amelanotic blue nevus: a variant of blue nevus. Am J Dermatopathol 1999;21:225–8.
32. Carney JA, Stratakis CA. Epithelioid blue nevus and psammomatous melanotic schwannoma: the unusual pigmented skin tumors of the Carney complex. Semin Diagn Pathol 1998;15:216–24.
33. O'Grady TC, Barr RJ, Billman G, Cunningham BB. Epithelioid blue nevus occurring in children with no evidence of Carney complex. Am J Dermatopathol 1999;21:483–6.
34. Groben PA, Harvell JD, White WL. Epithelioid blue nevus: neoplasm sui generis or variation on a theme? Am J Dermatopathol 2000;22:473–88.
35. Seab JA Jr, Graham JH, Helwig EB. Deep penetrating nevus. Am J Surg Pathol 1989;13:39–44.
36. Mehregan DA, Mehregan AH. Deep penetrating nevus. Arch Dermatol 1993;129:328–31.
37. Ball NJ, Golitz LA. Melanocytic nevi with focal epithelioid cell components: a review of seventy-three cases. J Am Acad Dermatol 1994;30:724–9.
38. Kamino H, Tam ST. Compound blue nevus: a variant of blue nevus with an additional junctional dendritic component. A clinical, histopathologic, and immunohistochemical study of six cases. Arch Dermatol 1990;126:1330–3.
39. Ferrara G, Argenziano G, Zgavec B, et al. "Compound blue nevus": a re-appraisal of "superficial blue nevus with prominent intraepidermal dendritic melanocytes": with emphasis on dermoscopic and histopathologic features. J Am Acad Dermatol 2002;46:85–9.
40. Allen AC. A reorientation on the histogenesis and clinical significance of cutaneous nevi and melanomas. Cancer 1949;2:28–56.
41. Gartmann VH. Neuronaevus blue Masson—cellular blue nevus Allen. Archiv Klin Exper Dermatol 1965;221:109–21.
42. Leopold JG, Richards DB. Cellular blue nevi. J Pathol Bacteriol 1967;94:247–5.
43. Avidor I, Kessler E. "Atypical" blue nevus—a benign variant of cellular blue nevus. Dermatologica 1977;154:39–44.
44. Tran TA, Carlson JA, Basaca PC, Mihm MC. Cellular blue nevus with atypia (atypical cellular blue nevus): a clinicopathologic study of nine cases. J Cutan Pathol 1998;25: 252–8.
45. Connelly J, Smith JL Jr. Malignant blue nevus. Cancer 1991;67:2653–7.
46. Goldenhersch MA, Savin RC, Barnhill RL, Stenn KS. Malignant cellular blue nevus. Case report and literature review. J Am Acad Dermatol 1988;19:712–22.
47. Temple-Camp CRE, Saxe N, King H. Benign and malignant cellular blue nevus. A clinicopathological study of 30 cases. Am J Dermatopathol 1988;10:289–96.
48. Granter SR, McKee PH, Calonje E, et al. Melanoma associated with blue nevus and melanoma mimicking cellular blue nevus: a clinicopathologic study of 10 cases on the spectrum of so-called "malignant blue nevus." Am J Surg Pathol 2001;25:316–23.
49. Antonescu CR, Tschernyavsky SJ, Woodruff JM, et al. Molecular diagnosis of clear cell sarcoma: detatcion of EWS-

ATF1 and MITF-M transcripts and histopathological and ultrastructural analysis. J Mol Deiagn 2002;4:44–52.
50. Epstein JI, Erlandson RA, Rosen PP. Nodal blue nevi. A study of three cases. Am J Surg Pathol 1984;8:907–15.
51. Sterchi JM, Muss HB, Weidner N. Cellular blue nevus simulating metastatic melanoma: report of an unusually large lesion associated with nevus-cell aggregates in regional lymph nodes. J Surg Oncol 1987;36:71–5.
52. Lamovec J. Blue nevus of the lymph node capsule. Report of a new case with review of the literature. Am J Clin Pathol 1984;81:367–72.
53. Pariser H, Beerman H. Extensive blue patchlike pigmentation. A morphologic variant of blue nevus? Persistent extrasacral Mongolian blue spot? Diffuse mesodermal pigmentation? Arch Dermatol Syphil 1949;59:396–404.
54. Upshaw BY, Ghormley RK, Montgomery H. Extensive blue nevus of Jadassohn-Tièche. Report of case. Surgery 1947;22:761–5.
55. Pittman JL, Fisher BK. Plaque-type blue nevus. Arch Dermatol 1976;112:1127–8.
56. Hendricks WM. Eruptive blue nevi. J Am Acad Dermatol 1981;4:50–3.
57. Tsoitis G, Kanitakis C, Kapetis E. Naevus bleu multinodulaire en plaque, superficiel et neuroide. Ann Dermatol Venereol 1983;110:231–5.
58. Pfaltz M, Schnyder UW. Verlauf und Ultrastruktur beim plaqueartigen Naevus bleu. Hautarzt 1989;40:355–7.
59. Heymann WR, Yablonsky TM. Congenital appearance of plaque-type blue nevus. Arch Dermatol. 1991;127:587.
60. Busam KJ, Woodruff JM, Erlandson RA, Brady MS. Large plaque-type blue nevus with subcutaneous cellular nodules. Am J Surg Pathol 2000;24:92–9.
61. Tuthill RJ, Clark WH Jr, Levene A. Pilar neurocristic hamartoma. Its relationship to blue nevus and equine melanotic disease. Arch Dermatol 1982;118:592–6.
62. Pearson JP, Weiss SW, Headington JT. Cutaneous malignant melanotic neurocristic tumors arising in neurocristic hamartomas. A melanocytic tumor morphologically and biologically distinct from common melanoma. Am J Surg Pathol 1996;20: 665–77.
63. Mezebish D, Smith K, Williams J, et al. Neurocristic cutaneous hamartoma: a distinctive dermal melanocytosis with an unknown malignant potential. Mod Pathol 1998;11:573–8.
64. Bondi EE, Elder D, Guerry D IV, Clark WH Jr. Target blue nevus. Arch Dermatol 1983;119:919–20.
65. Bogomoletz W. Blue nevus of oral mucosa. Br J Dermatol 1968;80:611–3.
66. Jao W, Fretzin DF, Christ ML, Prinz LM. Blue nevus of the prostate gland. Arch Pathol 1971;91:187–91.
67. Tobon H, Murphy AI. Benign blue nevus of the vagina. Cancer 1977;40:3174–6.
68. Kjaerheim A, Martinez MG, Montes LF. Blue nevus of the oral cavity. Oral Surg 1970;29:718–28.
69. Lach B, Russell N, Benoit B, Atack D. Cellular blue nevus ("melanocytoma") of the spinal meninges: electron microscopic and immunohistochemical features. Neurosurgery 1988;22:773–80.
70. Lam KY, Law S, Chan GS. Esophageal blue nevus: an isolated endoscopic finding. Head Neck 2001;23:506–9.

CHAPTER 9

Melanocytic Nevi with Phenotypic Heterogeneity

Raymond L. Barnhill

As previously discussed, the developmental biology of melanocytic nevi is poorly understood and thus explanations for the variance in cell type, melanin content, stroma, and other characteristics currently do not exist. To better characterize the wide range of cellular and stromal variations that may occur in melanocytic lesions, we have coined the overarching term *melanocytic nevus* (or tumor) *with phenotypic heterogeneity* (MNPH). Accordingly, the goal of this chapter is to describe the salient features of the most common melanocytic lesions with phenotypic heterogeneity the pathologist is likely to encounter. A number of closely related processes reported in the literature as "combined" nevus, deep penetrating nevus, plexiform spindle cell nevus, inverted type A nevus, and melanocytic nevus with focal dermal epithelioid cell components or dermal nodules are emphasized because of their unusual histologic features. As outlined in Table 9-1, a number of these lesions tend to show rather similar attributes, and these morphologic similarities and differences are discussed in the chapter.

PHENOTYPIC HETEROGENEITY AND NOMENCLATURE

The nevi described below are related because of depth, architecture, and the presence of pigmented cells (which may be oval, elongate, epithelioid, spindle, or dendritic). Discriminating features that might be of aid are listed in Table 9-1 and include superficial or deep disposition, configuration (i.e., wedge shaped, plexiform, bulbous), cell type (pigmented spindle cell, epithelioid cell, dendritic cell), and two or more populations of cells (1–25).

Also as noted in Table 9-1, deep penetrating nevus and plexiform spindle cell nevus (and MNPH showing components of the latter two nevi) share attributes with Spitz nevi and blue nevi. For example, occasional Spitz nevi may extend deeply into the reticular dermis in a wedge-shaped pattern, and some may even involve subcutaneous fat (see Chapter 7). Such nevi also may be characterized by bulbous lobular aggregates of cells that protrude into the deep dermis or the subcutis. In some instances, one may have difficulty deciding whether such a nevus is a variant of Spitz nevus, pigmented spindle cell nevus, deep penetrating nevus, plexiform nevus, or blue nevus. Thus a distinction among these various nevi might simply be based on depth of involvement by the nevus and perhaps nuances of cell type and architecture.

Generally speaking, the designation of a lesion as blue nevus has been based on a constellation of clinical and histologic features. A major criterion is the presence of a bluish color, accompanied by localization to certain anatomic sites such as the dorsal aspects of the hands and feet, buttocks, and sacrococcygeal area and a certain spectrum of histologic features. If one applies the clinical criterion of blue color for diagnosis of nevi, the resulting spectrum of lesions would be rather large and would include ordinary and cellular blue nevi and bluish nevi with varying proportions of pigmented spindle cells, epithelioid cells, and intermediate cells. The latter nevi would probably include plexiform spindle cell nevus, deep penetrating nevus, and any number of MNPH.

In regard to histologic features, the limits of blue nevus have not been clearly delineated. The most prototypic blue nevi contain aggregates of heavily melanized dendritic melanocytes, circumscribed fibrosis, and melanophages. Cellular blue nevi encompass dermal lesions containing not only dendritic melanocytes but also less heavily melanized spindle cells. Blue nevi rigorously characterized by bundles of dendritic melanocytes containing heavy melanin granules may exhibit a wedge configuration, plexiform architecture, and deep extension

TABLE 9-1 Comparison of histologic features in certain melanocytic nevi and those demonstrating phenotypic heterogeneity.

Characteristic	Blue color	Depth		Architecture				Cellular characteristics					
		Superficial	Deep	Inverted wedge	Plexiform	Bulbous contour	Sclerosis	Epithelioid cells	Pigmented epithelioid cells	Spindle cells	Pigmented spindle cells	Dendritic cells	Conventional nevus cells
MNPH	±	++	+	±	+	++	±	±	±	±	±	±	—
Spitz nevus	—	++	+	++	±	+	+	++	+	++	+	—	—
Pigmented spindle cell nevus	—	++	—	—	—	—	—	—	+	—	++	—	—
Blue nevus	++	++	++	++	++	++	++	—	—	—	+	++	+
Cellular blue nevus	++	+	++	+	++	++	++	+	+	++	+	+	+
Epithelioid blue nevus	+	++	++	+	+	+	±	+	+++	+	+	+	—
Deep penetrating nevus	++	+	++	++	++	++	+	±	+	+	++	±	—
Plexiform spindle cell nevus	++	+	++	++	++	+	±	±	+	+	++	±	—
Inverted type A nevus (melanocytic nevus with focal dermal epithelioid cell component; nevus with pigmented dermal nodules)	+	+	+	+	±	+	±	+	++	±	+	—	++

into the reticular dermis. Thus even unequivocal blue nevi may show overlap with deep penetrating nevus, plexiform nevus, and Spitz nevi. One may encounter melanocytic nevi with varying admixtures of pigmented spindle cells, epithelioid cells, and dendritic melanocytes. Such nevi are considered nevi with phenotypic heterogeneity, blue nevus, and so on, depending on the components present, the architecture, and the stringency of one's criteria. For similar nevi without dendritic melanocytes one confronts similar problems of nosology.

In general, we propose that such nevi are designated as MNPH with specification as to the components present. It is possible that one might define such lesions as either blue nevi, using rather broad criteria (such as blue color and the presence of heavily melanized spindle cells and/or epithelioid cells and any of the following features: wedge-shaped configuration, plexiform morphology, and deep extension); spindle and epithelioid cell nevi (because of the presence of both spindled and epithelioid cells); deep penetrating nevi; or plexiform pigmented spindle cell nevi. Thus categorization of such lesions may be quite arbitrary.

Classification of Melanocytic Lesions with Phenotypic Overlap

Because of overlapping morphologic features, reproducible diagnosis of some of the lesions described in this chapter may not be possible. A reasonable approach is a descriptive diagnosis of such lesions as MNPH according to the guidelines in Table 9-1. For example, a lesion involving the deep reticular dermis might be characterized as a superficial and deep pigmented spindle cell nevus (or melanocytic proliferation or tumor) or a superficial and deep plexiform nevus (or melanocytic proliferation or tumor) composed of pigmented dendritic cells and spindle cells. With this approach, one would be able to avoid forcing a lesion not easily classified into one particular category or another. Certain lesions fulfilling sufficient criteria for diagnosis may be classified under standardized terminology for example, Spitz nevus and blue nevus. The use of the term *MNPH* is acceptable for nevi with two or more distinct cell types. However, we advise that the particular cell types should be specified in the diagnosis or an appended note.

MELANOCYTIC NEVUS WITH PHENOTYPIC HETEROGENEITY

The recognition of two or more fairly distinct populations of melanocytes in melanocytic nevi dates back to the turn of the last century (1,2) (Table 9-2). The term *combined nevus* was used initially to describe the combination of ordinary nevus and blue nevus elements (1–5). However, we subsequently extended the spectrum of combined nevus to *melanocytic nevus with phenotypic heterogeneity* to include components of any type of nevus, including blue nevus (ordinary, cellular, congenital, epithelioid, etc.), congenital

TABLE 9-2 Summary of published accounts of combined nevus (MNPH).

Author	Year	Number of cases	Observations
Tèiche	1906	—	Concept of combined nevus; ordinary plus blue nevus
Dubreuilh and Petges	1912	1	Ordinary and blue nevus
Allen and Spitz	1953	2	Ordinary and blue nevus
Evans	1956	5	Ordinary and blue nevus
Leopold and Richards	1968	20	Ordinary nevus plus common blue or cellular blue nevus
Gartmann and Müller	1977	97	Combinations of ordinary nevus, common blue nevus, cellular blue nevus, and Spitz nevus
Weedon and Little	1977	32	Combination of Spitz nevus and other nevus cell component, not further specified by authors
Fletcher and Sagebiel	1981	50	Combinations of ordinary nevus, common blue nevus, cellular blue nevus, and Spitz nevus
Rogers et al.	1985	22	Combinations of Spitz nevus, ordinary nevus, and blue nevus
Pulitzer et al.	1991	95	Combinations of ordinary common blue, cellular blue, Spitz, and pigmented spindle cell nevus

nevus, Spitz nevus, pigmented spindle cell nevus (deep penetrating nevus and plexiform pigmented spindle cell nevus), nevi with pigmented dermal components that have been characterized under a number of terms including inverted type A nevus, nevus with focal dermal epithelioid component, and nevi with dermal nodules (6–12).

Clinical Features

The characteristics of the MNPH (combined nevus) are probably related to the predominant cellular population present, for example, whether blue nevus, Spitz nevus, or other (1–10) (Table 9-3). Most patients were relatively young with a mean age of 30.3 years in one large series (10). A predominance of women has been consistently reported in several studies. Most of these nevi measure < 5 mm in greatest diameter (8,10).

In nevi with a significant component of blue nevus, the most common sites of involvement are the face, back, and shoulder (8). Such nevi are often diagnosed as blue nevi because of the predominant dark color. Some of these nevi may also demonstrate a small, well-circumscribed blue or blue-black focus—often 1–3 mm in diameter, within an otherwise ordinary flesh-colored, tan, or brown nevus (see below) (8,12,13).

Nevi with prominent components of Spitz nevus occur commonly on the extremities as do conventional Spitz nevi (9). Such nevi are often diagnosed as an unusual nevus, Spitz nevus, dermatofibroma, or possibly melanoma.

Histopathological Features

As discussed above, nevi designated as MNPH may potentially encompass the entire phenotypic repertoire of melanocytic nevi (1–10) (Table 9-3). It should also be kept in mind that the lesions reported in various studies as combined nevi are most likely a skewed sampling of nevi selected for unusual, atypical, or poorly characterized features (8–10). Furthermore, some of the morphologic combinations reported are based on subjective interpretations that may not necessarily be reproduced by other observers. With these caveats in mind, the common presentations of MNPH will be described.

One of the most common patterns of MNPH is that of an ordinary nevus and blue nevus (Figs. 9-1 and 9-2). In our experience, the ordinary nevus component, as with all MNPH, may be compound or dermal, often overlies or is adjacent to the blue nevus component, and commonly has a congenital pattern (Fig. 9-1). The blue nevus elements most often consist of heavily pigmented dendritic melanocytes, melanophages, and variable fibrosis. Less commonly, the fusiform cells typical of cellular blue nevus may also be present with or without dendritic cells. The component of blue nevus may extend deeply into the reticular dermis as nests or fascicles, often in a plexiform configuration (Fig. 9-2). Despite the two or more components, such nevi are usually symmetric, well-circumscribed, orderly, and display little or no cellular atypia.

Another common pattern of MNPH, which probably includes inverted type A nevus and melanocytic nevus with dermal epithelioid cell components or dermal nodules, is that of an ordinary nevus in combination with discreet foci of pigmented spindle cells and/or pigmented epithelioid cells (11,12) (Fig. 9-3). The latter cells are often enlarged, contain abundant granular melanin, and are disposed in nests or fascicles in the deep portions of or beneath the ordinary nevus, sometimes or commonly in plexiform arrangements. The sizes of the nests or fascicles may vary from being minuscule to large lobular or digitate aggregates. The nuclei are usually slightly enlarged round, oval, or elongate and uniform but on occasion show slight to moderate atypia. Melanophages are also frequently associated with these pigmented foci. It should be pointed out

TABLE 9-3 Melanocytic nevus with phenotypic heterogeneity.

Clinical features
  Any age (3–74 years), but usually < 40 years
  Women > men
  Head and neck (especially for blue nevus variants), upper trunk, proximal extremities
  Often component of blue, blue-black
  May have small (1–5 mm) blue, blue-black focus in ordinary nevus
  Size < 6–7 mm, in most instances

Histopathological features
  Symmetrical
  Well circumscribed
  Orderly arrangements of cells
  Two or more of the following:
    Ordinary nevus component
    Pigmented dendritic melanocytes
    Pigmented spindle/epithelioid cells
    Amelanotic spindle cells
    Spitz nevus cells
  Ordinary nevus component often overlies or is adjacent to other component
  Congenital pattern often
  Deep involvement occurs
  Variable component of melanophages
  Plexiform configuration on occasion
  Sclerosis of collagen

Differential diagnosis
  Congenital nevus
  Cellular blue nevus
  Deep penetrating nevus
  Plexiform spindle cell nevus
  Spitz nevus
  Melanoma

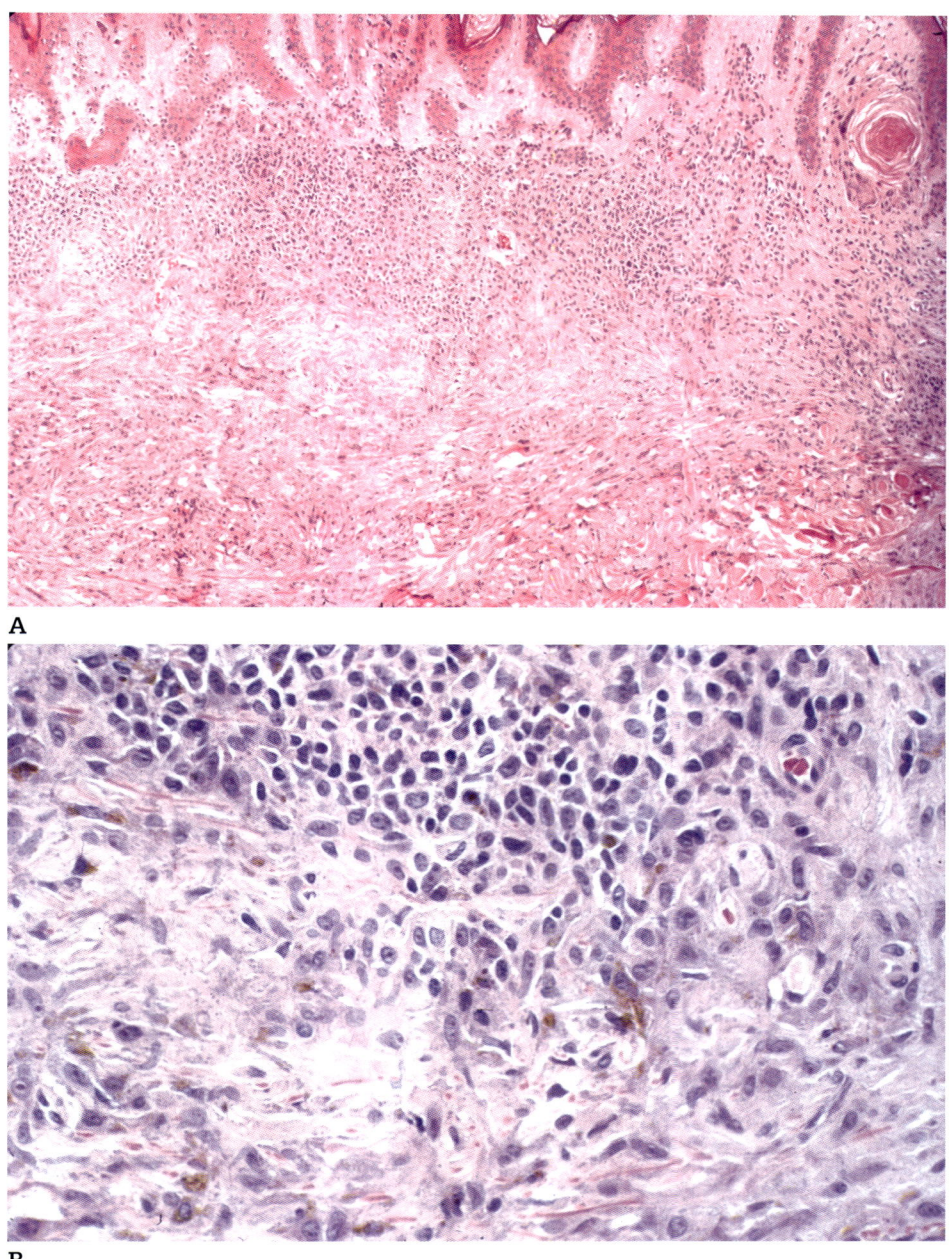

FIGURE 9-1 MNPH, composed of ordinary compound nevus overlying blue nevus. **A,** Note the well-defined zone of small nevus cells in the superficial dermal overlying the blue nevus. **B,** A sheet of small type B nevus cells collides with blue nevus cells. There is slight fibrosis associated with the blue nevus cells.

that this pattern of MNPH is also probably morphologically identical to that of deep-penetrating nevus and plexiform pigmented spindle cell nevus (13–16).

Spitz nevi uncommonly are observed in association with ordinary nevus elements (Fig. 9-4) (9). The topographic relationships of these two components include the Spitz nevus component being adjacent to, beneath, or admixed with the common nevus elements.

Besides the above relatively well recognized forms of MNPH, almost any combination of cell types is possible

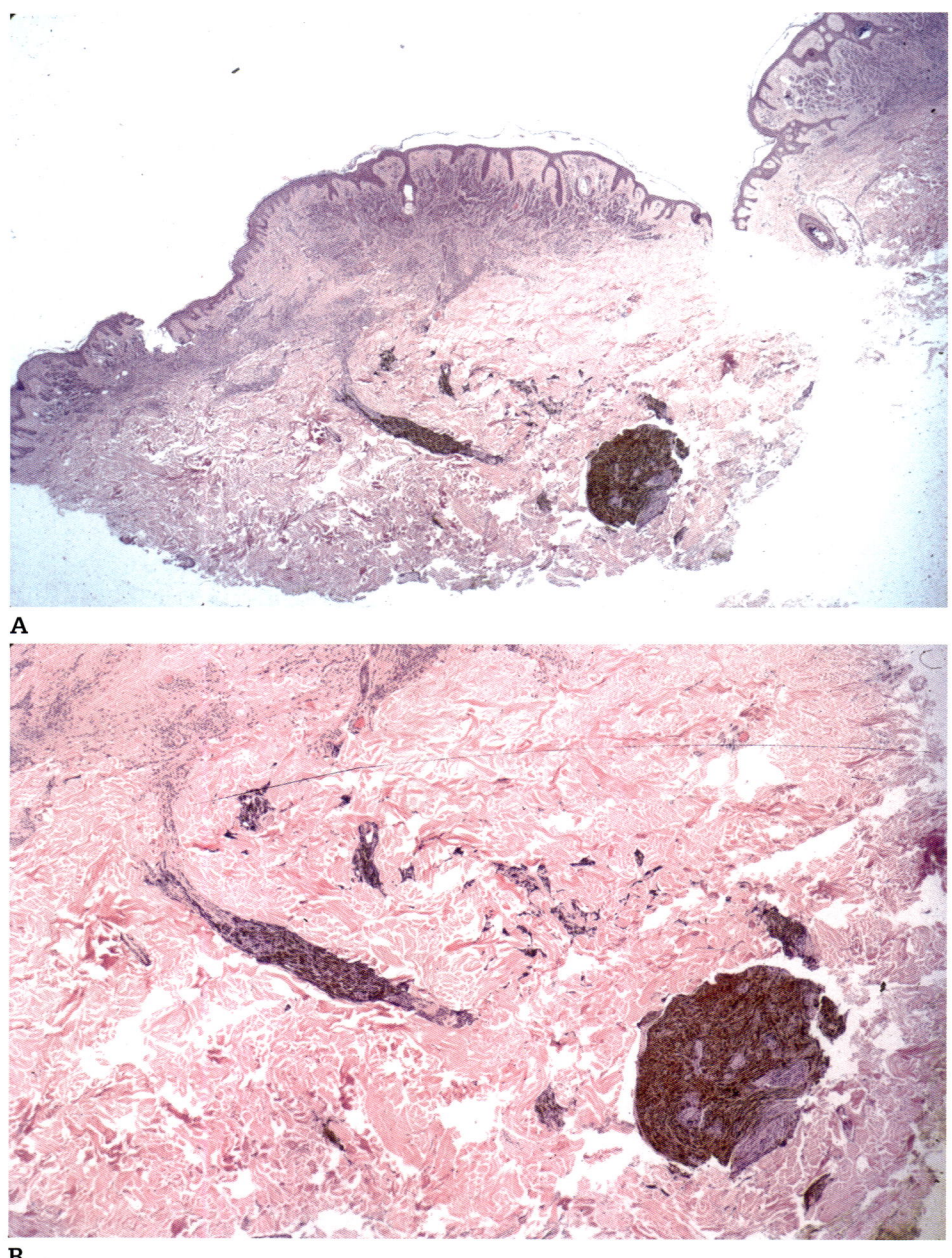

FIGURE 9-2 MNPH composed of dermal nevus overlying the blue nevus in the deep dermis. **A,** Note the clear separation of the two components. **B,** The blue nevus has a plexiform configuration in the deep reticular dermis. The heavily pigmented elements are associated with neurovascular structures.

but rare. Thus one may encounter nevi containing various admixtures of ordinary nevus cells, dendritic melanocytes, Spitz nevus cells, and perhaps other transitional cell types. Atypical features may also be observed such as melanocytic disordered patterns and cytologic atypia of the intraepidermal component (6–10).

INVERTED TYPE-A NEVUS

The morphologic pattern invoked by inverted type-A nevus is one probably also encompassed by MNPH and melanocytic nevus with focal dermal epithelioid cell components or dermal nodules (11–13). The term describes

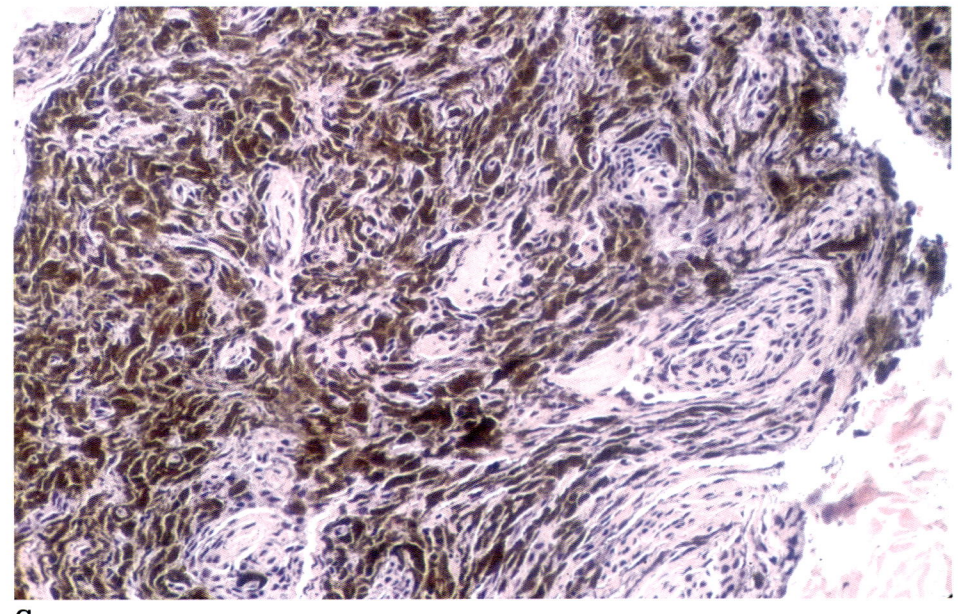

FIGURE 9-2 *Continued.* **C,** A compact nest of pigmented dendritic melanocytes and melanophages associated with cutaneous nerves.

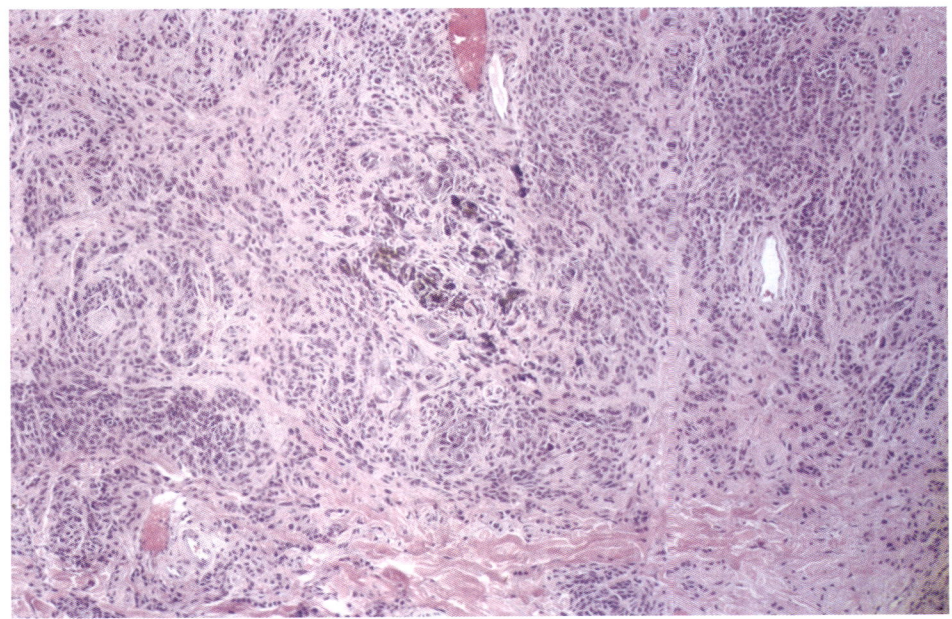

FIGURE 9-3 MNPH with a focal aggregate of pigmented epithelioid cells. **A,** Most of the field shows nests and cords of small-type B nevus cells. However, there is a small circumscribed aggregate of pigment-containing cells in the center of the field.

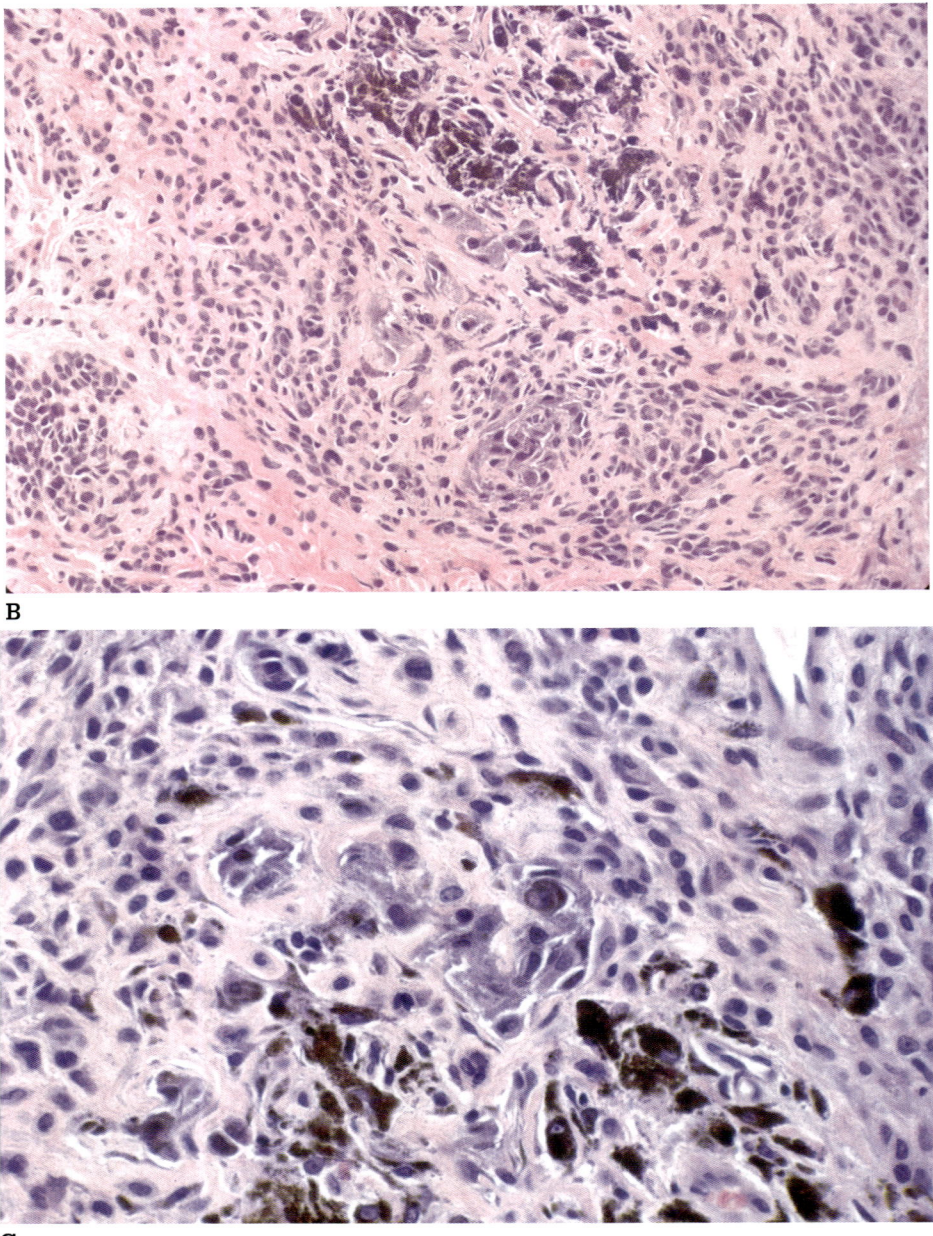

FIGURE 9-3 *Continued*. **B,** The cells within this aggregate are epithelioid cells and melanophages. These findings also fit the morphologic pattern of inverted-type A or melanocytic nevus with focal dermal epithelioid cell component. **C,** The epithelioid cells are enlarged with abundant cytoplasm containing melanin. The surrounding stroma is slightly sclerotic.

the presence of discrete nests of epithelioid cells, usually pigmented, within the dermal component of an ordinary nevus (Fig. 9-3). These nests are often deep and may be multifocal. In general, the term has not been accepted into general usage and may not offer any advantages over other terms.

MELANOCYTIC NEVUS WITH FOCAL DERMAL EPITHELIOID CELL COMPONENTS OR DERMAL NODULES

As mentioned above, the presence of a focal distinct epithelioid cell component in an ordinary nevus is charac-

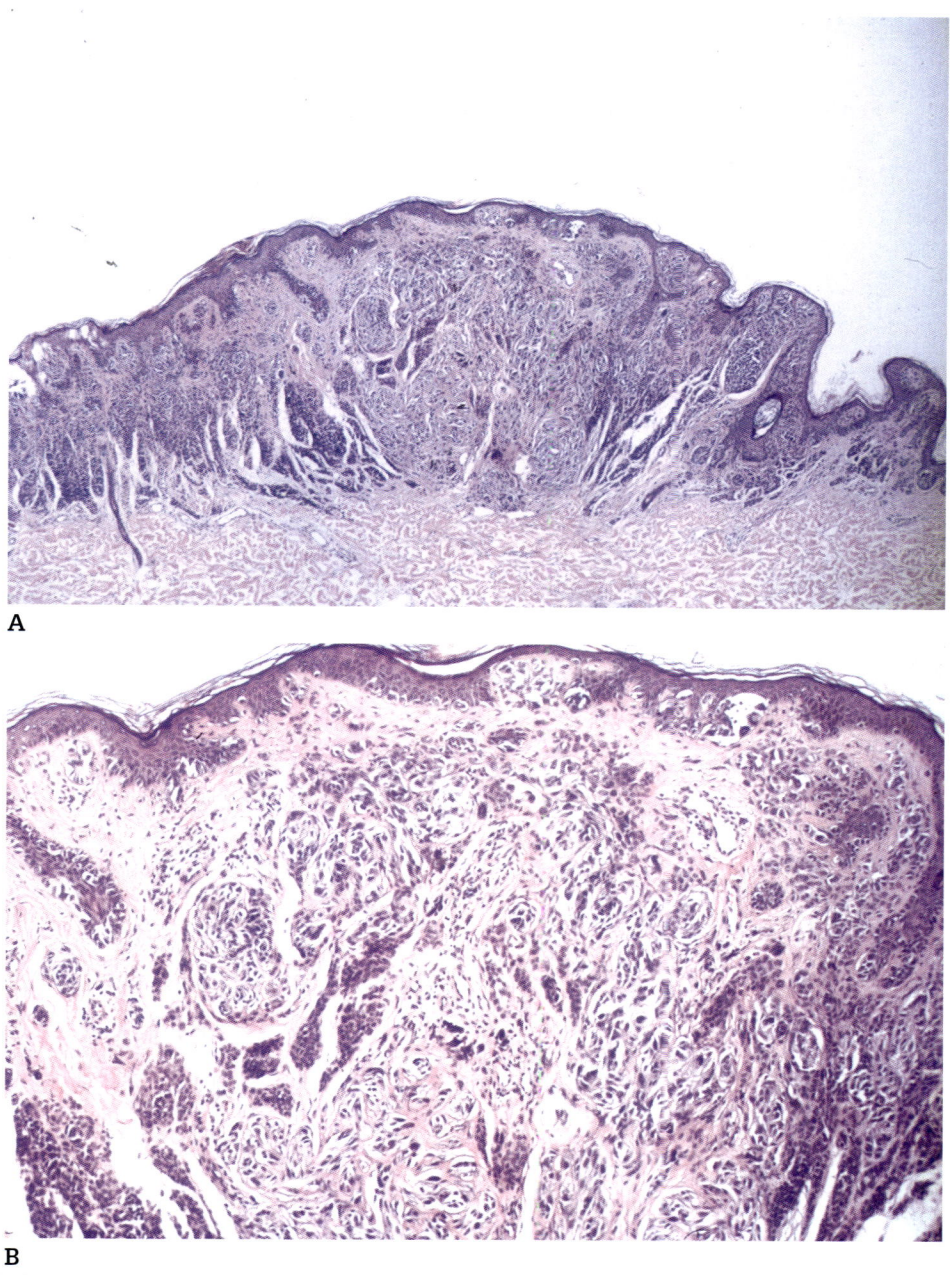

FIGURE 9-4 MNPH composed of ordinary compound nevus and Spitz nevus. **A,** The dome-shaped lesion with a central component of spindle and epithelioid cells is surrounded by ordinary compound nevus. **B,** The central portion of the lesion contains spindle and epithelioid cell elements in small nests and fascicles.

teristic of one pattern of MNPH (Fig. 9-3). This same morphologic description has recently been termed melanocytic nevus with focal dermal epithelioid cell components (MNFDECC) or dermal nodules (Table 9-4) (12). In their study of 73 cases, Ball and Golitz (12) reported that MNFDECC were characterized by the recent appearance of a 1- to 5-mm black macule or papule in a preexisting nevus and a corresponding histologic focus of atypical epithelioid cells. These authors stressed the importance of distinguishing such a newly developed focus from melanoma. In regard to the pathogenesis of MNFDECC, the authors postulated the development of an abnormal clone of cells, perhaps with a growth advantage over the surrounding ordinary nevus cells. As ev-

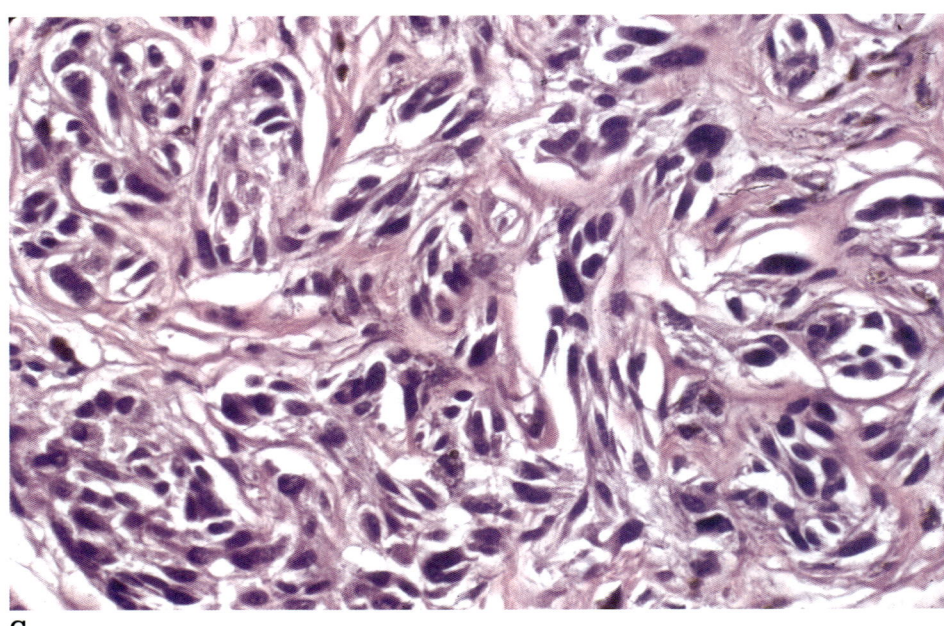

FIGURE 9-4 *Continued.* **C,** Higher magnification of panel B showing bundles of spindled cells and some epithelioid cells. The stroma is slightly fibrotic, and the compartmentalization of the cellular bundles has the appearance of schwannian differentiation.

idence for their hypothesis, they showed p53 expression in some of the foci compared to no expression in the background nevus. This hypothesis has merit and suggests that focal tumor progression might account for some varieties of MNPH in which the emergence of a new, altered, or aberrant population of cells has occurred, but it requires further study.

TABLE 9-4 Melanocytic nevus with focal dermal pigmented epithelioid cell component.
Clinical features
Mean 31.3 years (1 month to 78 years)
Women = men
Head and neck, trunk
6.2 mm mean, with central 1–5 mm dark brown or black macule or papule of recent onset
Histopathological features
Ordinary nevus
Congenital pattern may be present
Central focus or foci containing large epithelioid melanocytes in variably sized nodular aggregates
Heavily pigmented
Cytologically bland or atypical
Occupying 5–80% of nevus
Associated melanophages
Often transition of surrounding nevus
Differential diagnosis
Melanoma

Differential Diagnosis

The differential diagnosis of MNPH depends, of course, on the particular cellular populations present. However, the histologic change often of most concern to pathologists is an aberrant focus of cytologically altered/atypical cells in an otherwise ordinary nevus. Such a finding is of concern for early transformation to melanoma or even fully evolved melanoma (Table 9-5). The latter histologic alteration as already mentioned is present most commonly in the dermis. However, as discussed in Chapter 10, the development of melanoma in the dermal component of a nevus is highly unusual. Therefore, such a diagnosis must be carefully weighed and based on sufficient criteria of atypicality, mitotic activity, and nodular (confluent) proliferation.

Although MNPH are heterogenous, they tend to be present in fairly young individuals (< 40 years), measure < 5–6 mm, and exhibit an overall symmetry and regular appearance. As previously mentioned, the presence of a focal aggregate of pigment-laden epithelioid/spindle cells is usually the feature of concern. Although occasional aggregates of epithelioid cells are large, many are small and well circumscribed. Cytologic atypia is usually low grade or insignificant compared to melanoma. The surrounding nevus, which is usually of ordinary type, is generally unremarkable with reference to atypicality. An occasional mitosis may be observed in such a focus without

TABLE 9-5 Comparison of MNPH[a] and melanoma.

Characteristic	MNPH	Melanoma
Symmetry	Frequent	Uncommon
Size	< 6 mm, often	> 1 cm, often
Lateral borders	Sharply defined	Poorly defined
Focus, foci of altered cells	Present, well demarcated	Variable
Cytologic atypia	Usually absent or low grade	High grade
Mitotic activity	Absent or minimal	Frequent
Mononuclear cell infiltrates	Uncommon	Frequent

[a]Focus of epithelioid/spindle cells in ordinary nevus (as also observed in inverted type-A and clonal nevi).

undue concern; however, the presence of two or more mitoses per high power field should prompt careful inspection for melanoma.

DEEP PENETRATING NEVUS

The term *deep penetrating nevus (DPN)* was introduced in 1989 with the report of 70 unusual nevi with disturbing morphologic features (14). The authors alleged that although DPN was related to blue nevus, cellular blue nevus, and Spitz nevus, it seemed to occupy a reasonably well defined niche among the latter entities. One particular point emphasized by the authors was the frequent confusion of DPN with melanoma (14). DPN also shows features in common with plexiform spindle cell nevus (15,16) (see below).

Clinical Features
In the single report of DPN, most patients ranged in age from 10 to 30 years (14) (Table 9-6). The most common sites of DPN included the face, upper trunk, and proximal extremities. Most lesions measured < 1 cm in greatest diameter and were clinically diagnosed as blue nevus or cellular blue nevus. On follow-up, ranging from 1 to 23 years (mean, 7 years), none of the lesions had recurred or metastasized (14).

Histopathologic Features
Scanning magnification discloses in most instances a symmetric, well-circumscribed lesion with involvement of the deep reticular dermis and possibly subcutis (14) (Table 9-6). The overall architecture is usually that of an inverted wedge extending into the deep dermis (Fig. 9-5). The superficial dermal portion is characterized by a diffuse proliferation of pigmented spindle cells that show progressive organization as discreet fascicles or nests with descent into the deep dermis. Junctional nests are noted in some lesions. The fascicles of spindle cells tend to be associated with neurovascular and adnexal structures of the lower reticular dermis. These cellular aggregates often exhibit bulbous contours and may bulge into the subcutis, as do cellular blue nevi (Fig. 9-5A). Melanophages are usually intimately associated with the spindle cells. Some nevi may show cytologic atypia.

PLEXIFORM SPINDLE CELL NEVUS

Plexiform spindle cell nevi are notable for a plexiform arrangement of pigmented spindle cells, often involving the deep reticular dermis (15–17). The recognition of this unusual nevus is important so that it is distinguished from melanoma. A close relationship to superficial pigmented spindle cell nevus, Spitz nevus, blue nevus, and DPN has been emphasized (16).

TABLE 9-6 Deep-penetrating nevus.[a]

Clinical features
- 10–30 years
- Face, upper trunk, proximal extremities
- < 1 cm
- Raised lesions with bluish color

Histopathological features
- Symmetric
- Well circumscribed
- Inverted wedge configuration
- Extension of cellular fascicles into deep dermis or subcutis
- Pigmented spindle cells in fascicles associated with neurovascular bundles
- Junctional nests, occasionally
- Diffuse involvement of superficial dermis
- Cytologic atypia, occasionally

Differential diagnosis
- Spindle and epithelioid cell nevus
- Cellular blue nevus
- Other variants of MNPH
- Melanoma

[a]Plexiform spindle cell nevus is similar to DPN but shows a striking plexiform configuration not always present in DPN. Neither does the plexiform nevus always extend as deeply as DPN.

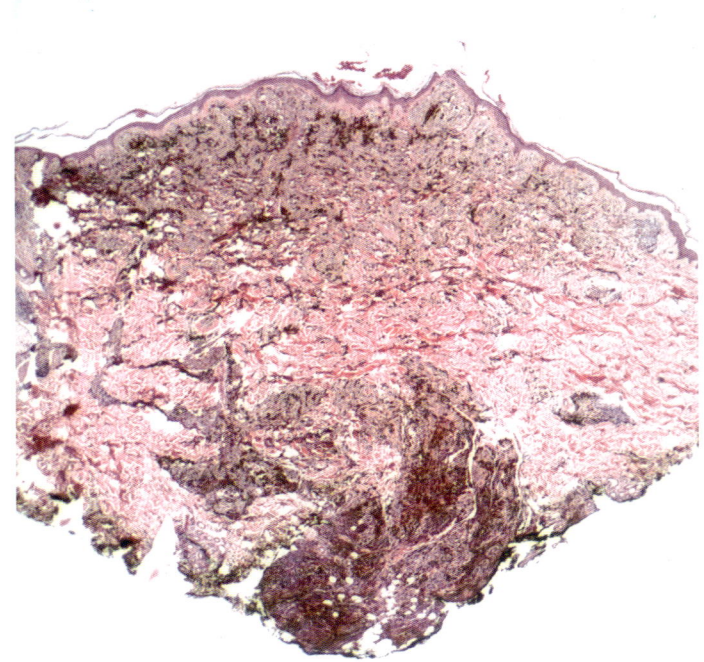

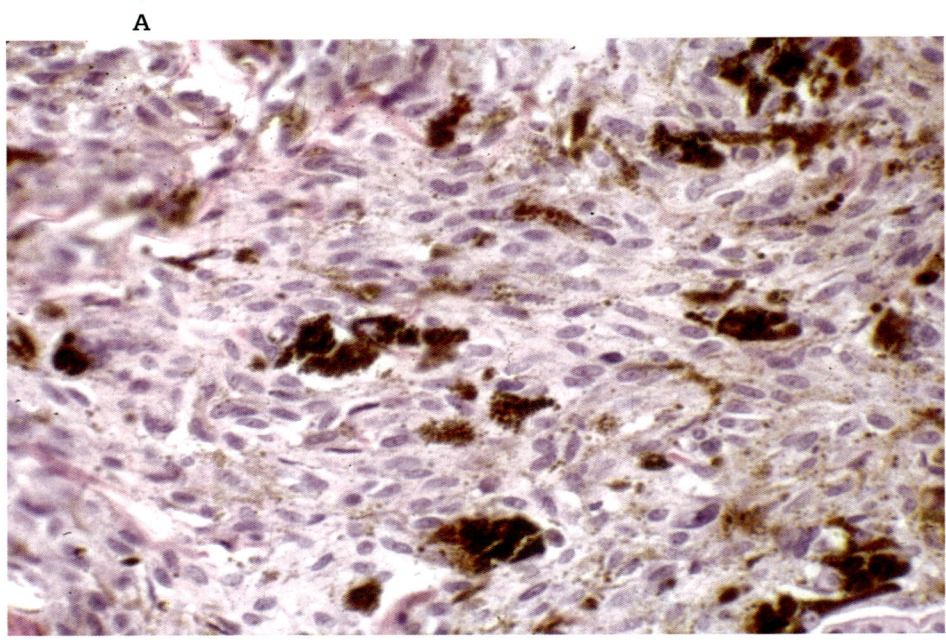

FIGURE 9-5 Deep penetrating nevus. **A,** Note the wedge-shaped configuration and deep extension of the rounded bundles of the pigmented spindle cells. **B,** Tightly packed fascicles of fusiform cells and scattered melanophages. The nuclei within the fusiform cells have dispersed chromatin patterns.

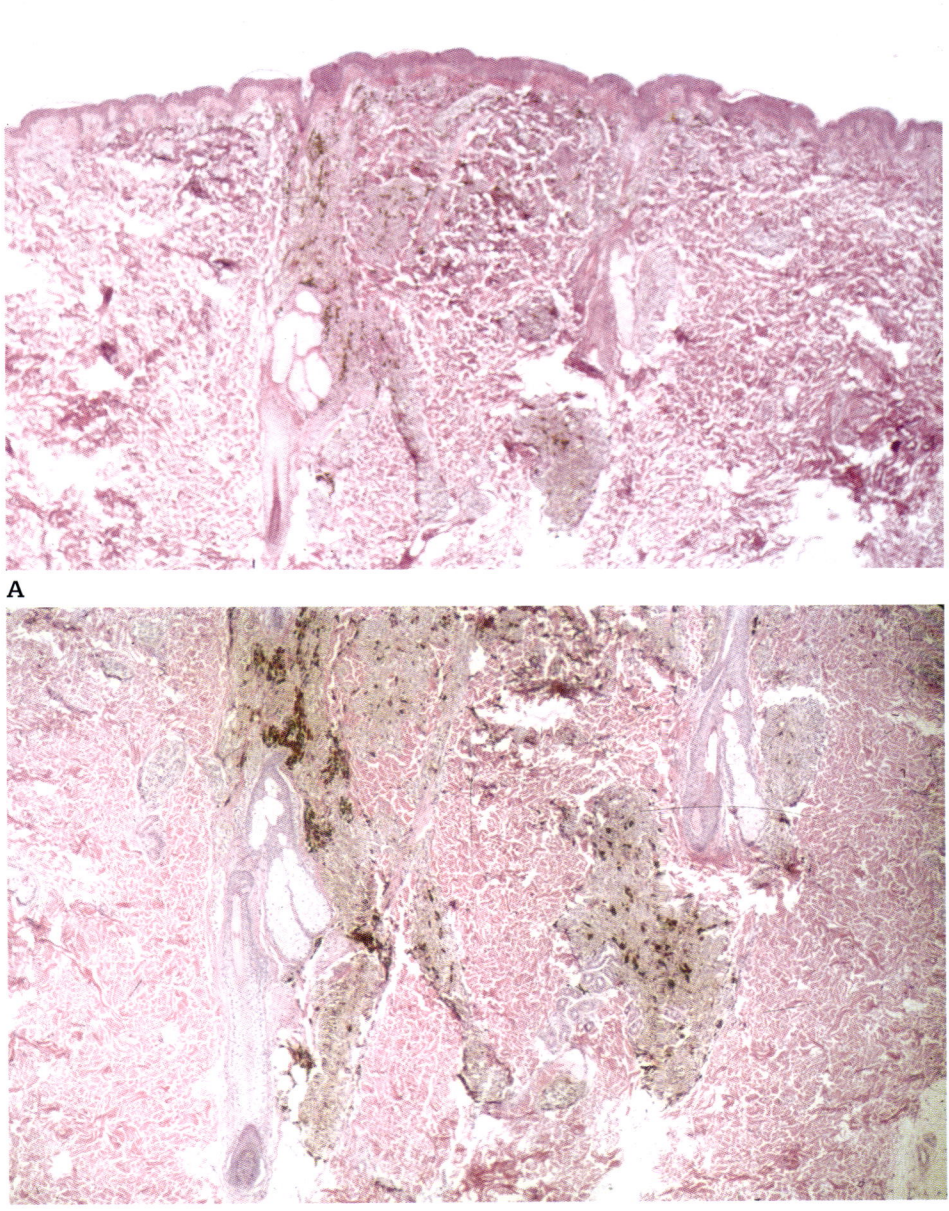

FIGURE 9-6 Plexiform pigmented spindle cell nevus. **A,** Characteristic appearance on scanning magnification of the fascicles of the pigmented spindle cells in plexiform arrangement. **B,** The fascicles are associated with appendages, blood vessels, and nerves. There is normal collagen separating these cellular aggregates.

Clinical Features

The lesions thus far reported occurred in young adults (mean age, 22.5 years) and involved the shoulders and back primarily (15). Clinically, the lesions were described as raised, bluish or black, suggesting blue nevus, an atypical nevus, or melanoma.

Histopathological Features

Most lesions are slightly raised, symmetric, and exhibit a wedge-shaped configuration in the reticular dermis (15–17). The most striking feature is the plexiform arrangement of fascicles of pigmented spindle cells that track along adnexal structures and neurovascular bundles (Fig. 9-6).

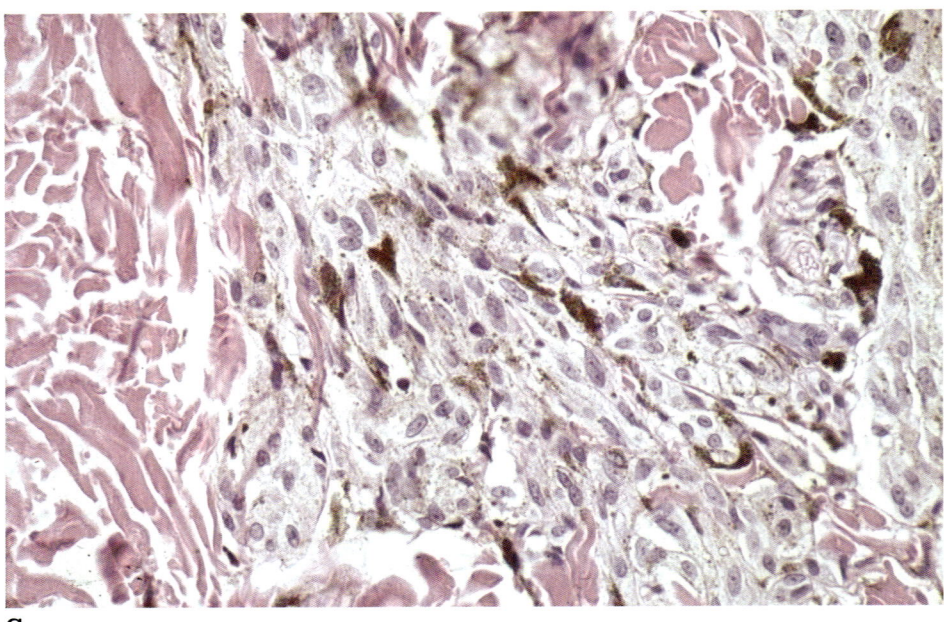

FIGURE 9-6 *Continued.* **C,** This field shows uniform-appearing fusiform cells. The cells contain fine granular melanin and monotonous nuclei with dispersed chromatin. There is a striking resemblance to the spindle cells of superficial pigmented spindle cell nevus.

Other common features include junctional nests, diffuse involvement of the superficial dermis, and infiltration of cutaneous nerves and arrector pili muscles. The spindle cells contain abundant granular melanin and oval or elongate nuclei with delicate chromatin patterns and inconspicuous nuclei (Fig. 9-6C). Occasional low-grade cytologic and rare mitotic figures are observed. Melanophages are often present in association with the spindle cell elements.

Differential Diagnosis

Because of the presence of pigmented spindle cells and frequent deep involvement, plexiform spindle cell nevi are closely related to DPN. However, they are discriminated from DPN by their striking plexiform configuration (often lacking in DPN) and frequent absence of bulbous cellular aggregates and deep involvement.

Because of the unusual nature of nevi described as deep penetrating or plexiform, the immediate concern is to discriminate such lesions from melanoma, whether primary or metastatic (Table 9-7). The most worrisome features include the depth of involvement, the presence of fascicles of pigmented spindle cells, perineurial infiltration, the plexiform or lobular configuration of such lesions, and especially cytologic atypia and mitoses, if present. Particular features helping in this differential diagnosis include the usual size < 6–7 mm (almost always < 1 cm), overall symmetry, nondisruptive growth patterns, lack of high-grade atypia, and lack of significant mitotic activity in such nevi. Nonetheless, some of these

TABLE 9-7 Comparison of deep penetrating nevus, plexiform spindle cell nevus, and melanoma.

Characteristic	Deep penetrating nevus	Plexiform spindle cell nevus	Melanoma
Symmetry	Frequent	Frequent	Uncommon
Size	< 1 cm, often	< 1 cm, often	> 1 cm, often
Lateral borders	Sharply defined	Sharply defined	Often ill-defined
Dermal configuration	Inverted wedge, lobular	Inverted wedge, plexiform	Variable, irregular
Deep extension	Present, often into subcutis	Variable, occasionally into subcutis	Variable
Rounded lobular aggregates in dermis	Frequent	Variable	Uncommon
Cytologic atypia	Absent to low grade	Absent to low grade	High grade
Mitotic activity	Absent or minimal	Absent or minimal	Frequent

nevi are quite challenging because of their large size, the confluent masses of cells without evidence of maturation, and the cytologic atypia. As a result, the biologic potential of a small minority of such lesions may be difficult to predict. Rare instances of lymph node metastases have been observed (10). The most appropriate management of these lesions is to communicate to the clinician the uncertain but possibly aggressive potential of such tumors and to ensure that they are excised with uninvolved surgical margins. The patient should also have careful periodic examinations for possible recurrence or metastasis. If sufficient criteria for unequivocal melanoma are lacking, our policy is to avoid labeling a patient with that diagnosis.

As discussed above, these nevi show overlap with other variants of MNPH, cellular blue nevus, and atypical variants of Spitz nevus.

REFERENCES

1. Tèiche M. Über benigne melanome ("chromatophorome") der hart-blaue naevi. Virchows Arch A 1906;186:212–29.
2. Dubreuilh W, Petges G. Le naevus bléu. Ann Dermatol 1912;2:552–62.
3. Allen AC, Spitz S. Malignant melanoma: a clinicopathologic analysis of the criteria for diagnosis and prognosis. Cancer 1953;6:1–45.
4. Evans RW. Histologic appearance of tumors. Med J Edinb Lond 1956;1:230–50.
5. Leopold JG, Richards DB. The interrelationship of blue and common naevi. J Pathol Bacteriol 1968;95:37–46.
6. Gartmann H, Müller H. Über das gemeinsame vorkommen von blauem naevus und naevuszell-naevus in ein und derselben geschwulst ("combined nevus"). Z Hautkr 1977;52:389–98.
7. Weedon D, Little JA. Spindle and epithelioid cell nevi in children and adults. Cancer 1977;40:217–25.
8. Fletcher V, Sagebiel RW. The combined nevus: Mixed patterns of benign melanocytic lesions must be differentiated from malignant melanomas. In: Ackerman AB, ed. Pathology of Malignant Melanoma. New York: Masson, 1981: 273–83.
9. Rogers GS, Advani H, Ackerman AB. A combined variant of Spitz's nevi. Am J Dermatopathol 1985;7:61–78.
10. Pulitzer DR, Martin PC, Cohen AP, Reed, RJ. Histologic classification of the combined nevus. Analysis of the variable expression of melanocytic nevi. Am J Surg Pathol 1991;15:1111–22.
11. Mihm MC Jr, Googe PB. Problematic Pigmented Lesions. Philadelphia, Lea & Febiger, 1990.
12. Ball NJ, Golitz LE. Melanocytic nevi with focal atypical epithelioid cell components: a review of seventy-three cases. J Am Acad Dermatol 1994;30:724–9.
13. Collina G, Deen S, Cliff S, et al. Atypical dermal nodules in benign melanocytic naevi. Histopathology 1997;31:77–101.
14. Seab JA Jr, Graham JH, Helwig EB. Deep penetrating nevus. Am J Surg Pathol 1989;13:39–44.
15. Barnhill RL, Barnhill MA, Berwick M, Mihm MC Jr. The histologic spectrum of pigmented spindle cell nevus: a review of 120 cases with emphasis on atypical variants. Hum Pathol 1991 22:52–8.
16. Barnhill RL, Mihm MC Jr, Magro CM. Plexiform spindle cell naevus: a distinctive variant of plexiform melanocytic naevus. Histopathology 1991;18:243–7.
17. Cooper PH. Deep penetrating (plexiform spindle cell) nevus. A frequent participant in combined nevus. J Cutan Pathol 1992;19:172–80.
18. Smith KJ, Barrett TL, Skelton HG III, Lupton GP, Graham JH. Spindle cell and epithelioid cell nevi with atypia and metastasis (malignant Spitz nevus). Am J Surg Pathol 1989;13:931–9.
19. McGovern VJ. Spitz nevus. In: Blaustein A, ed. Melanoma: Histological Diagnosis and Prognosis. New York: Raven Press, 1982;37–44.
20. Rodriguez HA, Ackerman LV. Cellular blue nevus. Clinicopathologic study of forty-five cases. Cancer 1968;21:393–405.
21. Carney JA, Stratakis CA. Epithelioid Blue Nevus and Psammomatous Melanocytic Schwannoma: The Unusual Pigmented Skin Tumors of the Carney Complex. Seminars in Diagnostic Pathology, 1998;15(3):216–224.
22. Groben PA, Harvell JD, White WL. Epithelioid blue nevus: neoplasm sui generis or variation on a theme? Am Jour Dermatopathol 2000;22(6):473–488.
23. Moreno C, Requena L, Kutzner H, de la Cruz A, Jaqueti G, Yus ES. Epithelioid blue nevus: a rare variant of blue nevus not always associated with the Carney complex. J Cutan Pathol 2000;27:218–223.
24. O'Grady TC, Barr R, Billman G, Cunningham BB. Epithelioid Blue Nevus occurring in children with no evidence of Carney complex. Am J Dermatopathol 1999;21(5):483–486.
25. Carney JA, Ferreiro JA. The Epithelioid Blue Nevus: A multicentric familial tumor with important associations, including cardiac myxoma and psammomatous melanotic schannoma. Am J Surg Pathol 1996;20(3):259–272.

CHAPTER 10

Malignant Melanoma

Raymond L. Barnhill

The purpose of this chapter is to provide a highly practical approach to the histopathologic diagnosis of melanoma of the skin and its differential diagnosis. Emphasis is placed not only on the major forms of conventional melanoma but also on unusual and rare variants that are difficult to recognize. (1–342)

DESCRIPTIVE EPIDEMIOLOGY

Over the past several decades, there has been a significant increase in the incidence of and mortality from cutaneous melanoma among white populations worldwide (1) (Table 10-1). From the 1960s through the mid-1980s the incidence of melanoma among white populations has consistently risen, with increases averaging between 3 and 7% per annum. The highest incidence rates worldwide have been observed in Queensland, Australia; for example, during the period from 1979/1980 to 1987, the incidence of melanoma among men doubled to a rate of 55.8/100,000 and rose to 42.9/100,000 in women. In contrast, darkly pigmented peoples, including Africans, Asians, Native Americans, and Hispanics have much lower and fairly stable incidences of melanoma. Recent studies have indicated that the rates of increase in incidence and mortality among whites are diminishing (i.e., they are not rising as rapidly) in many Western countries; and, in fact, incidence rates in some subgroups (younger women in the United States) have actually declined (2–6). Most of the increase in incidence in recent years reflects increasingly a high proportion of thin (< 1.0 mm) pagetoid (or superficial spreading) melanomas developing in intermittently sun-exposed skin. During the same period, the incidence of thick (> 4.0 mm) melanomas in some countries remained stable (2,3).

Mortality rates in countries with the highest incidences have begun to slow their rate of increase, plateau, or even diminish in some subgroups (again, in younger women). However, some Western countries with previously lower incidences of melanoma are now experiencing recent increases in the incidence and mortality of melanoma. It is prudent to keep in mind that the quality of data collected has changed drastically over the last century, and this alone may greatly influence the time trends of cancer incidence and mortality (2). In addition, all data concerning melanoma should be adjusted for age, sex, body site, and Breslow thickness to be meaningful.

Cutaneous melanoma affects fairly young individuals, with a mean age at diagnosis of ~50 years. However melanoma is rare before puberty and accounts for only 0.3% of melanomas occurring in individuals < 14 years of age in the United States (7). In general, melanoma seems to have an equal incidence in men and women although a sex ratio favoring women has been reported from some European countries. In recent years, older men (> 55 years) have been noted to have a substantially greater incidence of melanoma (and also significantly thicker melanomas) than women of comparable age (2). The latter incidence rates continue to rise with age. Melanomas may occur at any cutaneous or mucosal site. However, melanomas developing in whites most commonly involve the backs of men and the legs of women and less often affect other exposed sites. The preferred sites for Africans, Asians, and other dark-skinned peoples include plantar skin, other acral sites, the subungual areas, and mucosal sites.

Risk Factors

Risk factors for the development of melanoma include both endogenous and environmental factors and their

TABLE 10-1 Descriptive epidemiology of malignant melanoma of skin.
Melanoma represents 4.2% of all cancers by incidence (excluding nonmelanoma skin cancers)
Incidence is latitude dependent; 1990 crude incidence rates for whites (per 100,000 population per year):   Northern United States (Connecticut), 12.4   Southern United States (Arizona), 26
Total new cancer cases estimated in the United States for 2000:   Malignant melanoma, 53,600   Primary brain tumor, 17,000   Thyroid, 20,700   Multiple myeloma, 14,600   Larynx, 8,900   Hodgkin's disease, 7,000
Incidence of melanoma is increasing: Connecticut registry data (per 100,000 population per year):   1935–1940, 1.1   1946–1949, 2.4   1956–1960, 3.3   1966–1970, 5.2   1976–1980, 8.5   1986–1990, 12.4   1995–1999, 20.0 (SEER)[a]
Overall deaths in the United States for 2000: 7,400; melanoma represents 1.3% of all cancer deaths
Overall 10-year survival (clinical stage I): 71%
10-year survival based on Clark's anatomic levels of invasion (clinical stage I):   II (into papillary dermis), 95%   III (filing papillary dermis), 75%   IV (into reticular dermis), 70%   V (into subcutaneous fat), 45%
10-year survival of clinical stage I tumors based on primary tumor thickness (mm):   < 0.76, 95%   0.76–1.49, 84%   1.50–2.49, 69%   2.50–3.99, 58%   4–7.99, 69%   > 8.0, 30%
Most frequent sites in whites: Male: back, anterior torso, upper extremity, head and neck   Female: back, lower leg, upper extremity, head and neck
Most frequent sites in blacks and Asians: soles, mucous membranes, palms, nail beds
Frequency of melanoma by type of tumor   Conventional melanomas   Pagetoid melanoma (intermittently sun-exposed skin, usual), 67%   Nodular melanoma (without appreciable adjacent intraepidermal component), 10%   Solar melanoma (continuously sun-exposed skin), 5–10%   Acral melanoma (glabrous skin, including nail apparatus), 2–5%   Rare and unusual forms of melanoma, 5–10%   Desmoplastic–neurotropic melanoma, 1%

[a]SEER, Surveillance, Epidemiology, End Results.

complex interactions (1). The most significant factors are numbers of nevi (both typical and atypical), cutaneous and pigmentary phenotypic characteristics (such as eye color, hair color, skin color, and freckling), skin phototype (propensity to tan and burn), family and personal history of melanoma and nonmelanoma skin cancer, significant sun exposure, and probably nonsolar UV radiation exposure. The role of sunlight in the cause of melanoma has been suspected for many years, particularly exposure in childhood, and also the effects of intermittent, or recreational, sun exposure in adults. It is has been suggested that at least 65% of melanomas worldwide may be related to sun exposure. Nevertheless, the complex relationship between solar irradiation and melanoma remains elusive. Between 5 and 12% of melanomas arise in individuals having one or more first-degree relatives with melanoma (8).

The easy accessibility of the skin to examination coupled with the fact that the detection of melanoma in an early stage is potentially curable (in stark contrast to the lack of effective treatment for metastatic melanoma) has prompted campaigns for the screening and early detection of melanoma. However it is unclear if such efforts will have any effect on reducing the incidence of thick and potentially lethal melanomas (1–3).

CRITERIA FOR DIAGNOSIS AND CLASSIFICATION OF MELANOMA

Puisque ces mystères me dépassent, feignons d'en être l'organisateur.
—JEAN COCTEAU

The overwhelming majority of melanomas begin as intraepidermal or intraepithelial proliferations, which may or may not have some relationship to a melanocytic nevus (9–37) (Fig. 10-1A,B). Estimates of the frequency of melanomas developing in continuity with a nevus of any kind vary widely; approximately a third of melanomas have nevus remnants (38–40). The duration of this intraepidermal phase ranges from months to many years, during which these proliferative lesions show progressive degrees of architectural and cytologic atypicality (41).

Increasing cytologic atypia of melanocytes accompanies the aberrant architectural appearance. The melanocytes vary in degree of atypia and the proportion of cells with nuclear atypia. Atypical melanocytes usually have enlarged nuclei that exhibit variation in nuclear shapes and chromatin patterns and may have large nucleoli. Thickening of nuclear membranes and irregular nuclear contours are also characteristic. The cyto-

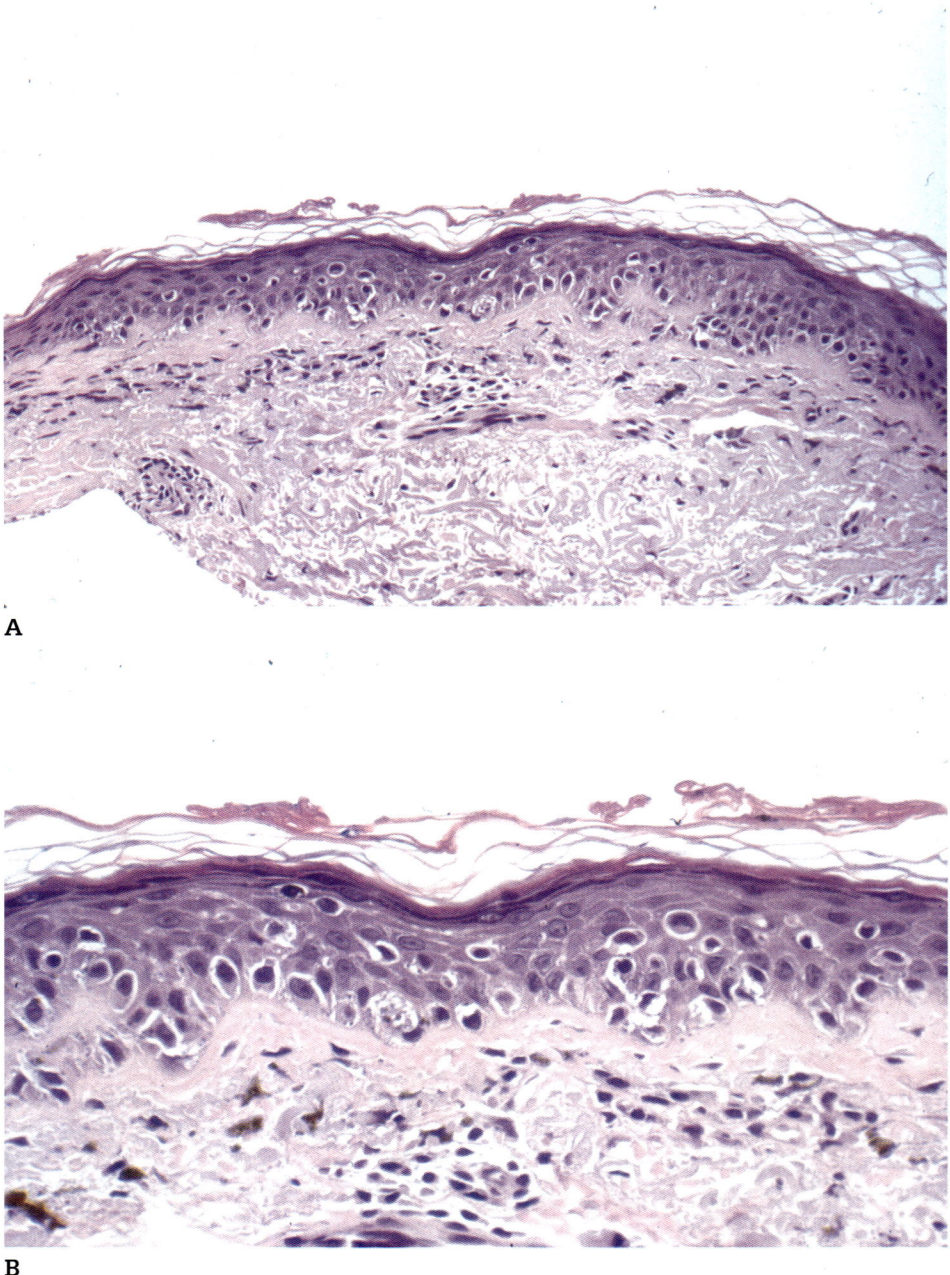

FIGURE 10-1 Melanoma in situ. The lesion has developed de novo within the epidermis. This is the most frequent pathway of melanoma development. Atypical melanocytes are disposed as single cells along the basal layer and in pagetoid array.

plasms of such melanocytes may be abundant with a pink granular quality, may contain granular or finely divided (dusty) melanin (Fig. 10-2), or may show retraction, resulting in a clear space around the nuclei. Melanocytes with scant cytoplasm typically have high nuclear/cytoplasmic ratios.

Approach to Criteria for and Classification of Melanoma

The histopathologic criteria for diagnosis (and attempts at classification) of melanoma are related to the most important properties of such lesions that have resulted in recurrences and metastases in patients with careful longitudinal

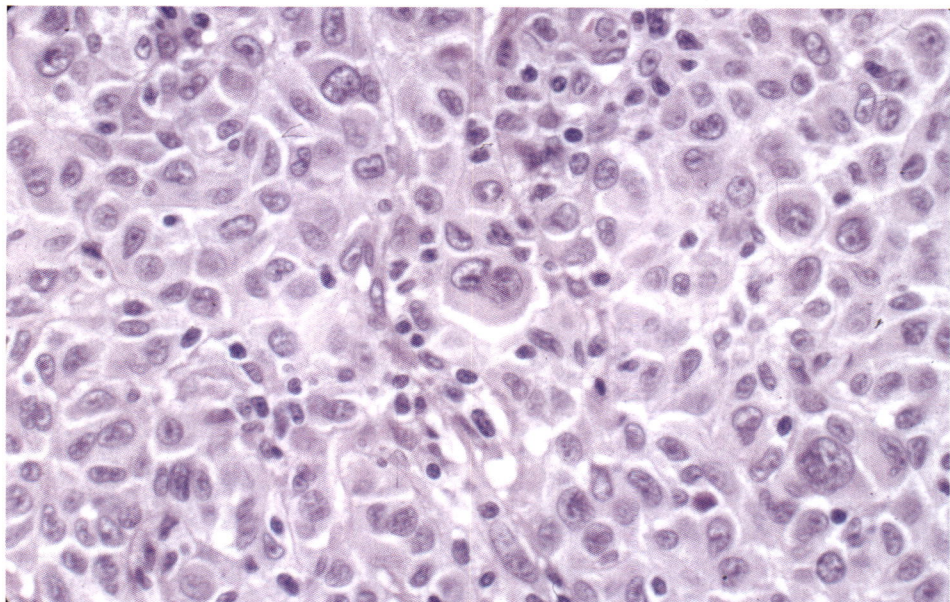

FIGURE 10-2 Epithelioid melanoma cells in a sheet-like pattern in the dermis, the most common cellular phenotype of melanoma. Such a field might be observed in any type of melanoma. The cells have a monomorphous appearance and are characterized by abundant eosinophilic cytoplasm.

follow-up (9–37). These various criteria are assessed along with clinical information, such as age, and clinical criteria, referred to below. Since no criterion is absolute for the diagnosis of melanoma, all such information must be systematically assembled in arriving at a diagnostic interpretation. The histopathologic criteria for diagnosis of melanoma are related to the location of melanocytes in the skin or mucosa, the organizational patterns of melanocytes, their cytologic properties, other morphologic characteristics (tissue, stromal and host response), the anatomic site of the lesion, and other attributes (Table 10-2). At present, histopathologic diagnosis remains subjective but is fairly reproducible for the vast majority of conventional melanomas on review by pathologists who are experienced with melanocytic lesions. There has been no analytic weighting of the most important criteria. Nonetheless, some of the more objective and organizational criteria—such as size, asymmetry, pagetoid spread, confluent nesting of melanocytes, and dermal mitoses—seem to be more reproducible than other more subjective criteria—such as cytologic atypia (with the exception of pronounced cytologic atypia).

Based on the parameters listed in Table 10-2 we will systematically discuss the histopathologic criteria for diagnosis and a simple approach to nomenclature and classification of melanoma. As has been discussed in the literature, attempts at classification of melanoma have often been illogical since they have commonly employed clinical, topographic, histomorphologic, cytologic, and other terms in the same classification scheme (16,41). In general, we accept that classifications are often flawed and artificial because much biologic information is lacking.

Granted the limitations of classification, we propose the following practical approach (Table 10-3) to the classification of melanoma.

- **Conventional melanoma** with no attempt at subclassification other than recording descriptively the organizational pattern(s) of the overlying and/or adjacent intraepithelial component as pagetoid, lentiginous, and/or nested and the anatomic site. Nonetheless, we believe that some recognition should be given to the **solar melanomas** and their precursor atypical melanocytic proliferations (lentigo maligna, Hutchinson melanotic freckle, or *la melanose circonstrite precancereuse de Dubreuilh*) because of their apparent direct relationship to cumulative sun exposure and their historical importance and to the **acral melanomas** (including melanomas involving both glabrous, nearby nonglabrous skin, and the nail apparatus) because of their importance in peoples of color and potential causal differences.
- **Other unusual morphologic or cytologic variants** based on distinctive features and management issues: desmoplastic melanoma, neurotropic melanoma, melanomas resembling melanocytic nevi ("nevoid" melanoma), melanomas arising in congenital nevi;

TABLE 10-2 Classification of melanoma.

Location in the skin
   Intraepidermal
   Dermal
   Subcutaneous
   Soft tissue
Organizational patterns of melanocytes
   Intraepidermal component
      Pagetoid
      Lentiginous
      Nested
      Two or more patterns
   Dermal component
      Single cell infiltration
      Nests of cells
      Aggregative (nodule formation)
      Two or more patterns
Specific morphologic features:
   Epidermal surface configuration
      Verrucous
      Papillomatous
      Polypoid
   Stromal alterations
      Desmoplasia
      Myxoid alteration
   Other alterations
      Neurotropism
      Neural differentiation (neurogenic, neural transforming)
      Angiotropism
      Alveolar/glandular
Cell type
   Epithelioid
   Spindle
   Dendritic
   Nevus-like
   Small
   Balloon
   Clear
   Anaplastic giant
   Rhabdoid
   Signet ring
Anatomic site of lesion
   Intermittently and completely sun-protected sites
   Continously sun-exposed sites (solar)
   Acral (nonglabrous and nearby glabrous skin), including
      the nail apparatus
   Mucosal sites
Origin from precursor lesion
   Nevus of any kind
   Other precursor

and other rare cytologic and morphologic variants that are important to recognize because of differential diagnosis (e.g., small cell melanoma, balloon cell melanoma, melanoma, myxoid melanoma).

We make reference to the historical classification of melanoma, because it is still used by many and some of its aspects are useful.

Historical Perspectives: The Radial and Vertical Growth Phases As a Basis for the Classification of Melanoma

Recognizing that the vast majority of melanomas develop through a progressive proliferation of melanocytes within the squamous epithelium, often over years, Clark and co-workers (9,10) proposed a classification of melanoma. This classification culminated from data in the literature and the authors' observations and was based on the concept of the so-called radial, or horizontal, growth phase (RGP) of melanoma. The latter term described the progressive centrifugal (and thus radial) growth or enlargement of melanoma over time. Several years later, the RGP was employed not only for the horizontally expanding intraepithelial proliferation but also for the vertical microinvasion of melanoma into the papillary dermis (9,10,17,22,23,29,30) (Fig. 10-3A,B). At some point in this evolution of melanoma within the squamous epithelium (and/or within the papillary dermis), the tumor was conjectured to acquire additional neoplastic properties, which resulted in an inexorable tumoral proliferation within the dermis. This latter phase of tumor progression was designated the vertical growth phase (VGP) and was thought to supervene on a RGP in about 90% of melanomas (9,10,22,29,30) (Fig. 10-3C,D; Table 10-3). It has been theorized that the proposed VGP develops de novo, or from rapid progression of the intraepidermal component, in 10–15% of tumors (see below). Hypothetically, the genesis of the VGP as described above does not rule out an origin from the dermis or the adnexa (eccrine sweat ducts or hair follicles).

The proponents of the VGP suggest that the VGP signals a qualitative change in the biology of a melanoma (9,10,22,29,30) and, in particular, the onset of the metastatic phenotype because of its purported histomorphologic resemblance to metastatic melanoma. Such tumoral foci are have been described as a single cellular nodule or plaque composed of smaller cohesive nests (29,30) (Table 10-3). The constituent cells within the latter configurations are tightly packed, are frequently monomorphous with marked cytologic atypia, and commonly display mitotic activity and individual cell necrosis (Figs. 10-3C,D and 10-4).

Experimental work has suggested differential properties between the latter two phases of tumor progression. Cell surface antigen phenotype, cytogenetics, growth of isolated cells in soft agar and in cell culture are some of the experimental characteristics suggesting differences between the RGP and VGP as well as with melanocytic nevi (28). Although the concepts of RVP and VGP are of interest, they have not yet been fully validated by biologic data. For example, approximately two thirds of melanoma proposed to be VGP do not metastasize, while rare cases

TABLE 10-3 Practical classification of malignant melanoma.

Conventional melanomas
    Intraepithelial component categorized as pagetoid, lentiginous, nested, or two or more patterns
        Intraepithelial melanoma (melanoma in situ)
        Intraepithelial melanoma with invasion of dermis, subcutis, etc.
    Absence of intraepidermal component
Conventional melanomas subclassified because of etiological and anatomic site differences
    Solar melanomas
    Acral melanomas
    Mucosal
Unusual or rare variants of melanoma
    Desmoplastic–neurotropic
    Neurotropic
    Melanomas resembling melanocytic nevi (nevoid melanoma; Spitzoid melanoma)
    Melanomas arising in or resembling a blue nevus (malignant blue nevus)
    Melanomas arising in a dermal nevus
    Melanomas arising in a congenital nevus
    Melanomas resembling experimentally induced and spontaneous melanomas in animals
    Verrucous
    Pleomorphic (sarcomatoid)
    Small cell
    Balloon cell
    Signet ring cell
    Rhaboid
    Myxoid
    Clear-cell sarcoma (malignant melanoma of soft parts)

of melanomas with features of only RGP result in metastases (29). Alternative hypotheses suggest that the undoubted tumor progression of melanoma is (a) either continual rather than a discreet event and thus corresponds fairly well with Breslow thickness and/or (b) that the switch to the metastatic phenotype has no precise relationship to such morphologic constructs as the proposed RGP and VGP (Fig. 10-4).

Clark's classification was thus based on clinical features and intraepithelial patterns of melanocytes in the RGP versus invasive melanomas lacking an RGP (so-called pure vertical growth phase). The rationale for classifying melanomas according to presence and type or absence of the radial growth phase has been ascribed to distinctive clinical and histopathologic features and potential differences in cause and prognosis.

Although clinical, epidemiologic, histopathologic, and other experimental differences exist among the conventional melanomas subclassified as superficial spreading, lentigo maligna, and acral lentiginous (20,26,27,35), some proportion of melanomas (10–20% or more) demonstrate such morphologic and cytologic heterogeneity that they commonly prove difficult to subcategorize (16,24). *In fact, differences in morphologic features of melanomas are generally related to anatomic site, age, degree of sun-exposure, and other poorly understood factors* (16). Often there are no consistent differences other than the clues provided by site that allow for the reliable subclassification of melanoma.

When considering the complexity of biologic and neoplastic systems, we question the rationale of using such nomenclature without more scientific data. For example, the term *superficial spreading melanoma* has no clear biologic basis as a unique subtype of melanoma since the initial intraepidermal proliferation of all melanomas is "superficial" and "spreads" horizontally; thus the latter term applies to any type of conventional intraepithelial melanoma. The term *nodular melanoma* is also artificial, since any melanoma may result in a bulky invasive component after some period of intraepidermal proliferation, possibly of limited or sometimes lengthy duration (18). To categorize a tumor as nodular based on the limitation of the intraepidermal component to less than three epidermal rete ridges beyond the invasive tumor is clearly arbitrary (9,10).

The case can still be made for differences in tumorigenesis among melanomas arising on the most sun-exposed surfaces, intermittently sun-exposed skin, and sun-protected sites, such as acral skin. However, much more research is needed at the basic science level to establish these potential differences in tumor biology. In a study of head and neck melanomas the parallel increasing incidences of the proposed subtypes of superficial spreading, lentigo maligna, and nodular melanoma are evidence ar-

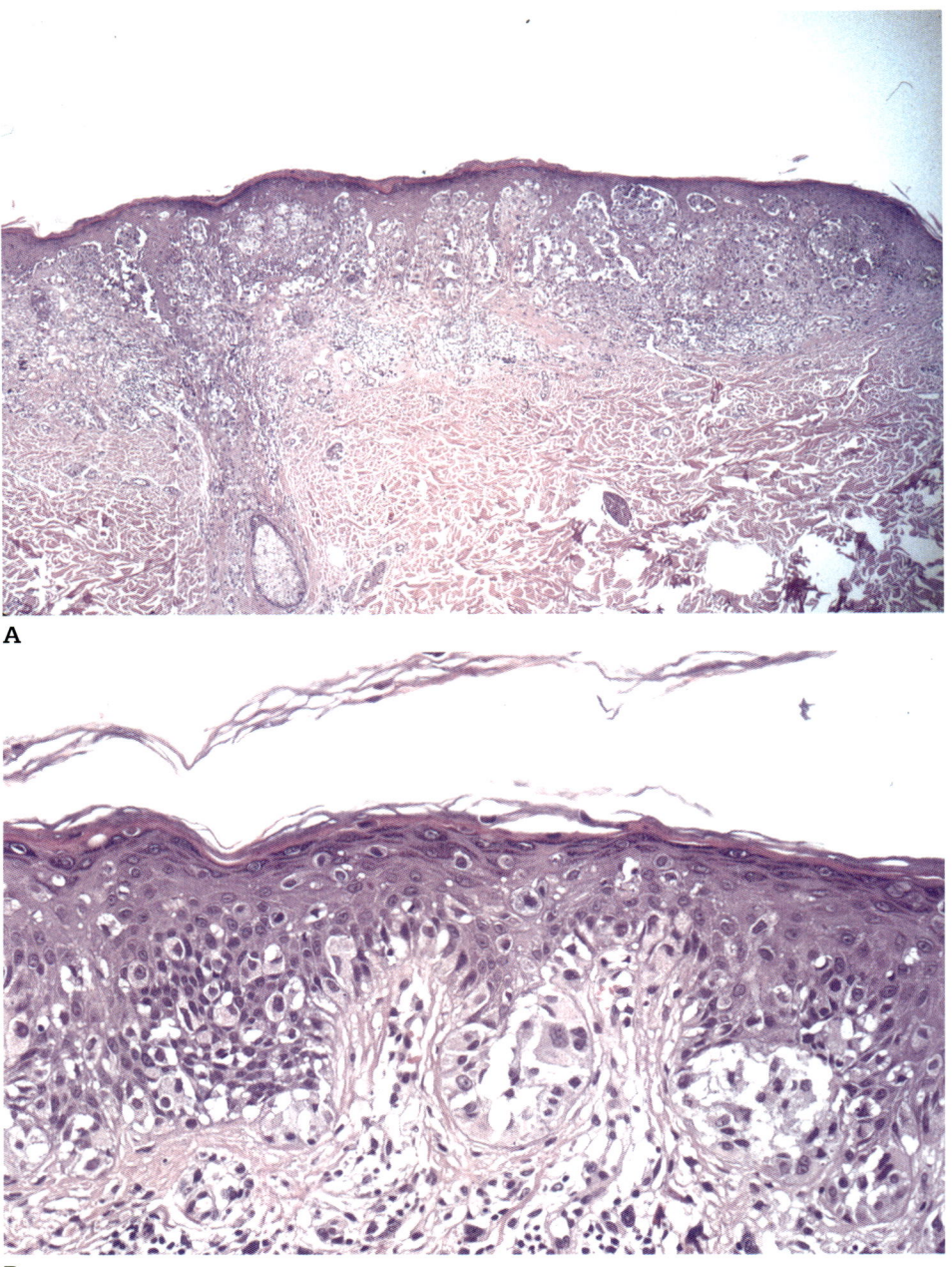

FIGURE 10-3 Melanoma. **A,** Note the microinvasive (level II) component in the papillary dermis. **B,** Higher magnification shows pagetoid infiltration (melanocytosis) of the epidermis by melanoma cells and small nests of melanoma cells in the papillary dermis. This has been described by some as the RGP and level II invasion.

guing against a unique relationship of the putative variant lentigo maligna with cumulative sun exposure (42). In regard to prognostic factors, it has been well established that after adjusting for tumor thickness, conventional melanomas do not show differences in overall survival among the proposed subtypes.

CONVENTIONAL MELANOMAS

Clinical Features

Particular Reference to Melanomas Involving Intermittently Sun-Exposed Skin The following discussion

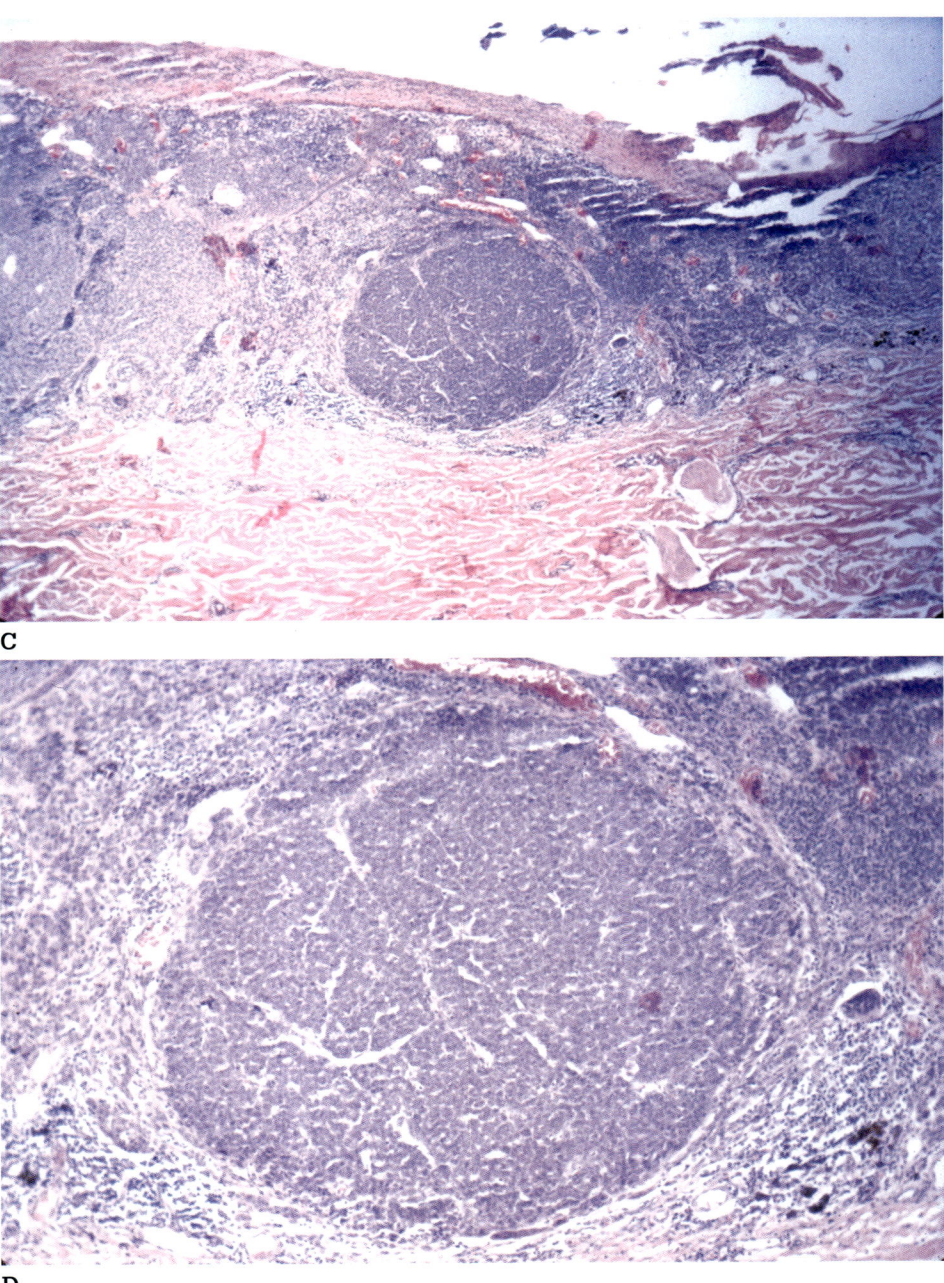

FIGURE 10-3 *Continued.* **C,D,** Malignant melanoma with cohesive aggregate of melanoma cells in the papillary dermis and level III invasion. The invasive component of melanomas exhibiting the latter morphologic attribute has been termed by some as the VGP.

applies to cutaneous melanoma viewed as a single disease entity, although we realize that there are some melanomas occurring at particular sites that have rather distinctive features suggesting causal differences that require further study (43,44) (Tables 10-4–10-6). As already mentioned, cutaneous melanoma is a disease of white adults. Patients are most commonly diagnosed with melanoma in the 4th through 7th decades. Men and women are equally affected.

The majority of melanomas (perhaps in the range of 70%) developing in whites are generally localized to intermittently sun-exposed skin (i.e., glabrous cutaneous surfaces), which is often covered and thus not continuously exposed to sunlight and usually does not demon-

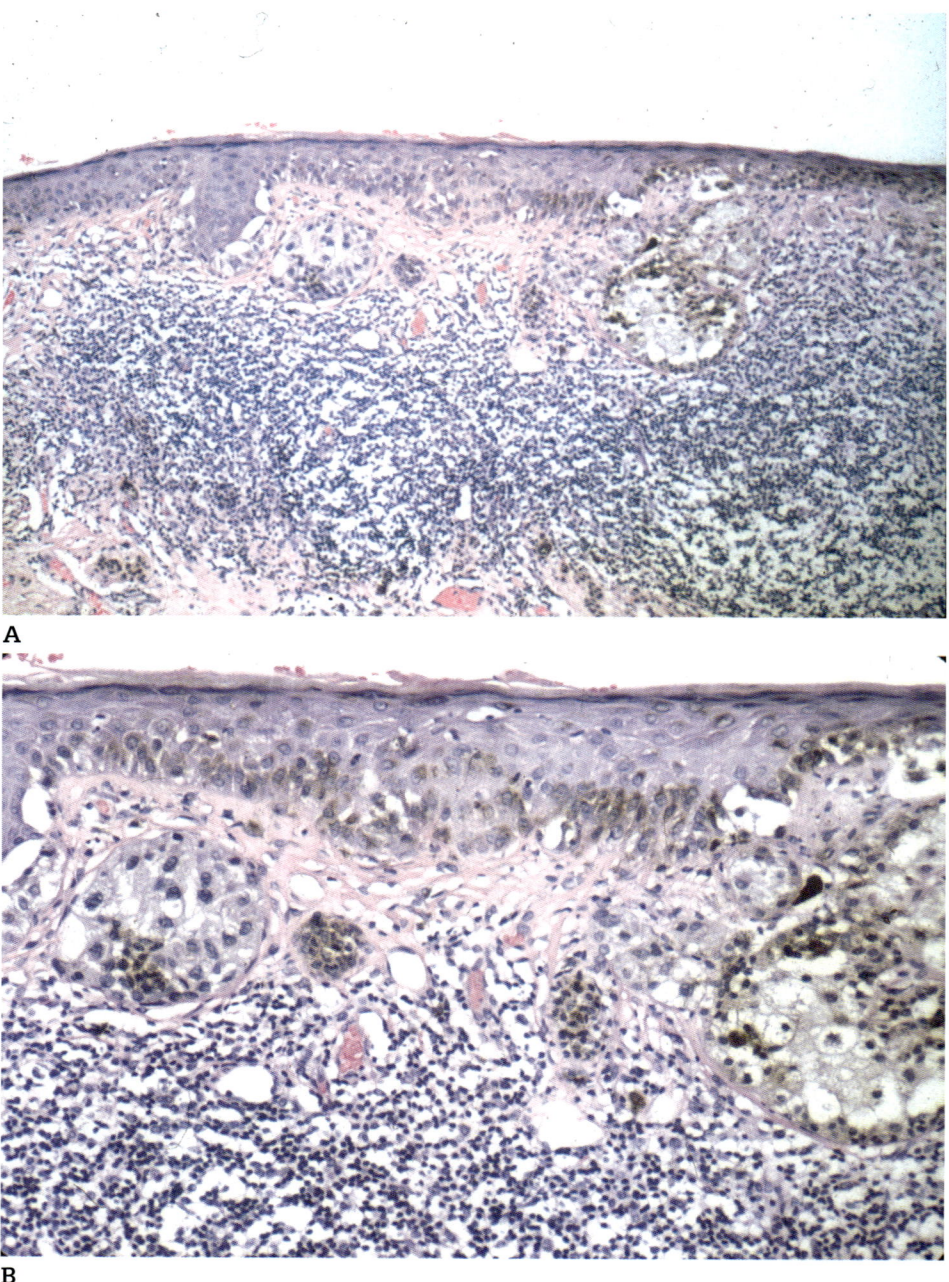

FIGURE 10-4 Melanoma, superficially invasive (level II). **A,** The lesion shows asymmetry, effacement (loss of the epidermal rete pattern), and thinning of the epidermis. Note the cohesive nests of epithelioid melanoma cells in the papillary dermis. Such epidermal alterations strongly suggest melanoma, in addition to the highly abnormal arrangement and cytologic atypia of the melanocytes. A dense mononuclear cell infiltrate expands the papillary dermis. **B,** Higher magnification showing cohesive nests of melanoma cells in the papillary dermis. Some authors label this early VGP melanoma and consider it a marker for increased metastatic risk.

strate significant solar elastosis histologically (such melanomas have been commonly termed by many as pagetoid or superficial spreading melanoma based on clinical, histopathologic, and other findings). The most common sites include the trunk (back) followed by the lower extremities and head and neck for white men and the lower extremities followed by the back, upper extremities, and head and neck for white women. However, melanomas

TABLE 10-4 Clinical features of conventional melanomas of the skin.

Type	Median age (years)	Location	Size (cm)	Duration of intrapidermal and/or microinvasive growth	Topography	Color
Pagetoid (intermittently sun-exposed skin)	44	All sites, often on trunk of men, legs of women	0.5–15	1–7 years	Palpable	Various shades of brown, black, gray, red
Mainly nodular	53	All sites	0.3–5	Months to 2 years[a]	Palpable	Bluish, black; pink (amelanotic)
Solar (continuously sun-exposed skin)	65	Sun-exposed sites, usually head and neck	0.2–20	5–15 years	Flat initially	Various shades of tan, brown, black with frequent hypopigmentation
Acral	65	Palms, soles, nailbeds	0.5–15	1–10 years	Flat initially, palpable	Various shades of tan, brown, black

[a]Period of evolution (short-lived or absent intraepithelial growth phase).

with a prominent pagetoid pattern may involve any anatomic site.

These pagetoid forms of melanoma are often present anywhere from 1 to 7 years before diagnosis and may develop in association with an atypical (dysplastic) nevus or demonstrate an ordinary nevus remnant. There seems to be an association with multiple primary melanomas, familial melanoma, and an atypical (dysplastic) nevus phenotype. The early lesions may be essentially flat with slight elevation of borders and often increase in size as an asymmetrical plaque with irregularity or notching of borders. With progression, one may observe a papular or nodular component superimposed on the surrounding plaque. Patients often notice change in size and color and with more advanced lesions itching, ulceration, and bleeding. The mean diameters range from 0.8 to 1.2 cm but may be as small as 0.3 cm or as large as 4.0 cm or more. The latter group of melanomas demonstrate vary-

TABLE 10-5 Salient histologic features of conventional melanomas.

Characteristic	Pagetoid	Mainly nodular	Solar	Acral
Pattern of intraepidermal growth	Pagetoid, nested	—	Lentiginous, nested, pagetoid	Lentiginous, nested, pagetoid
Epidermis	Hyperplastic	—	Atrophic	Marked hyperplasia
Usual cell type	Epithelioid	—	Spindle, epithelioid	Spindle, epithelioid
Papillary dermis	Inflamed, thickened	—	Variably inflamed	Inflamed, thickened
Frequency of regression	Common	Uncommon	Common	Common
Solar elastosis of dermis	Slight	Slight or Variable	Marked	None
Usual cell type of invasive component	Epithelioid	Epithelioid	Spindle	Spindle, highly pleomorphic cell
Desmoplasia	Uncommon	Uncommon	Common	Common
Neurotropism	Uncommon	Uncommon	Common	Common
Precursor nevus	Common (20–33%)	Less common (8%)	Uncommon (3%)	Uncommon

TABLE 10-6 Melanomas of intermittently sun-exposed skin

Clinical features
  In general onset after puberty, but all ages affected
  Most frequent 30–70 years
  Whites >> Africans, Asians
  Women ≥ men
  Most common sites, lower extremities and trunk of women and trunk (back) of men
  Pain, pruritus
  Often > 1 cm (range 2 mm to > 15 cm)
  Inially macular, later stages may be papular and nodular
  Asymmetry
  Irregular and often notched borders
  Complexity and variation in color often with admixtures of tan, brown, black, blue, gray, white, red
  May be entirely skin colored (amelanotic) or black
  Ulceration and bleeding may be present
Histopathologic features
Architecture
  Asymmetry
  Heterogeneity of lesion
  Large size (> 6 mm), but many exceptions
  Poor circumscription of proliferation
  Melanin not uniformly distributed
Organizational abnormalities of intraepidermal component
  Pagetoid spread
    Upward migration of melanocytes in random pattern, single cells predominate over nests
    Cells often reach granular and cornified layers
  Lentiginous melanocytic proliferation
    Melanocytes reach confluence
    Nesting of melanocytes (sun-damaged skin)
    Melanocytes not equidistant
    Proliferation of melanocytes along adnexal epithelium
  Nesting pattern
    Variation in size, shape, and placement of nests
    Nests replace large portions of squamous epithelium
    Diminished cohesiveness of cells in nests
    Confluence of nests
  Loss of epidermal rete pattern (effacement)
  Mononuclear cell infiltrates, often bandlike
  Fibroplasia of papillary dermis
  Regression frequently present
Cytology
  Nuclear changes
    Majority of melanocytes uniformly atypical
    Nuclear enlargement
    Nuclear pleomorphism (variation in sizes and shapes)
    Nuclear hyperchromasia with coarse chromatin
    One or more prominent nucleoli
  Cytoplasmic changes
    Abundant granular eosinophilic cytoplasm in epithelioid cells
    Finely divided (dusty) melanin
    Variation in size of melanin granules
    High nuclear to cytoplasmic ratios in spindle cells
    Retraction of cytoplasm
  Mitoses (in dermal component)
  Atypical mitoses
  Necrotic cells
Invasive component usually in dermis
  Architecture
    Tumefactive cellular aggregates
    Pushing, expanding pattern without regard for stroma
    Hypercellularity
    Less host response
  Cytology
    As above
    Increased nuclear to cytoplasmic ratios
    Mitoses in dermal component
    Atypical mitoses
    Necrotic cells
Differential diagnosis
  Melanocytic tumors
    Atypical (dysplastic) melanocytic nevus
    Halo nevus with atypia
    Spitz nevus/tumor
    Pigmented spindle cell nevus
    Recurrent melanocytic nevus
    Other melanocytic nevi with prominent pagetoid spread
  Nonmelanocytic tumors
    Squamous cell carcinoma
    Paget's disease, mammary or extramammary
    Sebaceous carcinoma
    Cutaneous T cell lymphoma
    Epidermotropic eccrine carcinoma
    Metastatic carcinoma, other
    Angiosarcoma
    Kaposi sarcoma
    Leiomyosarcoma
    Atypical fibroxanthoma
    Malignant fibrous histiocytoma

ing shades of brown admixed with complex hues of red, pink, blue, gray, white, and black. Foci of regression may result in considerable heterogeneity of the gross morphologic features and are represented by areas of white (depigmentation), gray, blues, and pink (see below).

Solar Melanomas Both the solar and acral melanomas develop in somewhat older individuals with an average age of 60–65 years. (22) The solar melanomas arise in the sites of greatest sun exposure (e.g., the head and neck, with the cheek being the single most common site followed by the nose and forehead).

Acral Melanomas Acral melanoma, although accounting for 5% or less of melanomas among whites, is the most frequent form of melanoma among Asians, Africans, and other people of color (22,32–34). However, approximately the same incidence of acral melanoma occurs in all ethnic groups. Acral melanomas may involve glabrous skin and nearby nonglabrous skin of the palms, soles, digits, and also the nail apparatus. The sole is the single most common site for melanoma developing in nonwhite populations. Subungual melanoma (SUM) is a distinctive variant of acral melanoma that most often involves the nailbed of the great toe or thumb where it commonly presents as an ulcerated tumor (22,32–34).

Melanoma with Nodular Component Any melanoma may show progression to a papule or nodule, often dusky blue, blue-black, or pink in color (43,44), superimposed on a macular, macular and papular, or plaque-like "surround" component. However, such a surround component may be completely absent; historically, such melanomas have been termed nodular. Often such papular or nodular lesions are ulcerated and may demonstrate hemorrhagic crust.

Other Miscellaneous Features Melanomas lacking pigment (amelanotic melanoma) and those resembling keratoses are particularly difficult to diagnose without a high index of suspicion. The phenomenon of regression that may be present in up to 50% of melanomas may introduce considerable complexity to the gross morphologic features of melanoma (45). These features correlate with the degree of destruction of melanoma focally, multifocally, or universally (complete regression). The resulting alterations include blue, blue-gray, gray, and whiteish coloration that corresponds to variable melanin accumulation or absence of pigment in the skin. Highly irregular and complex patterns may ensue clinically. Melanomas may rarely resemble halo nevi or may undergo complete regression, resulting in circumscribed depigmentation (43–45).

Histopathologic Features

Melanoma In Situ and Intraepithelial Melanoma The fundamental problem surrounding the histopathologic diagnosis of melanoma in general is the lack of a single criterion that is specific for melanoma and this is especially true for melanoma in situ. The reason for this is obvious: *melanoma in situ is a misnomer*—that is, it is theoretically cured with complete removal, and there is no definitive biologic parameter, such as metastasis, that may be correlated with histopathologic criteria. Melanoma experts have thus formulated criteria based on the assessment of the intraepidermal component of invasive melanomas that have metastasized (15,41). However, in some respects, this is a straw man; with tumor progression, the characteristics of intraepithelial melanoma evolve and thus may be different from true in situ lesions. In fact, some proportion of invasive melanomas have limited or absent intraepithelial components, rendering the intraepithelial component "nondiagnostic" (46,47). It has been shown that there is a negative correlation between pagetoid spread and Breslow thickness (46). Therefore, the criteria for the diagnosis of melanoma in situ are theoretical, since (a) true in situ lesions currently lack a biologic marker and (b) criteria based on invasive lesions are not entirely representative (15). As a result, the diagnosis has become highly subjective, and often a question of threshold and the experience of the observer. Accordingly, the atypical nevus for one pathologist is the melanoma in situ for another and the converse. Criteria are easily written in articles and textbooks but are often difficult to apply at the microscope. Experience and common sense must reign when interpreting borderline lesions, and the pathologist must resist the compulsion to force a lesion into one category or another without thoughtful deliberation (48,49).

We believe that lesions currently diagnosed as melanoma in situ include a virtual wastebasket of (a) atypical intraepidermal melanocytic proliferations or atypical nevi; (b) lesions with reactive changes that are not neoplastic, as from acute UV radiation exposure or external trauma; (c) atypical intraepidermal melanocytic proliferations that are biologically indeterminate, (d) invasive melanomas due to sampling error (50), and (e) true melanomas in situ (48,49). It is likely that in the future one will be able to evaluate such lesions more objectively, for example, with techniques such as fluorescence in-situ hybridization (FISH), for markers such as fairly specific cytogenetic alterations. Until objective examination is possible, we recommend that all such lesions potentially diagnosed as melanoma in situ be adequately sampled for an invasive component and that clinical information is thoughtfully weighed for factors potentially influencing the histologic characteristics.

The diagnostic evaluation involves the progressive use of multiple criteria, both architectural and cytologic (listed in Table 10-7). This exercise must begin at scanning magnification with a low-power image analysis (tumor silhouette). Often assessment (the Gestalt) at this level is all that is needed for the diagnosis and, at the very least, provides crucial information about the nature of the lesion (Table 10-7). Examination at high magnification allows one to assess cytologic details and to confirm one's impression from low power.

Size

First of all the diameter of the lesion in millimeters is an important factor—that is, the larger the lesion, the more suspicious or confident one can be about the diagnosis of melanoma. There is no absolute threshold for diagnosis and thus melanomas may be as small as 2–3 mm, the so-called small-diameter melanoma (51,52); however,

TABLE 10-7 Histopathologic and clinical criteria for melanoma versus a benign melanocytic lesion.

Factor	Melanoma	Benign Lesion
Size	≥ 6 mm, often ≥ 10 mm < 6 mm small-diameter melanoma, metastatic melanoma	< 5–6 mm, often
Symmetry	Asymmetrical with respect to epidermal thickness, melanocytic elements, melanin distribution, host response, usually	Symmetrical, usually
Circumscription	Poorly circumscribed at peripheries with single-cell intraepithelial patterns, often	Well circumscribed with well-defined nests at periphery, often
Heterogeneity	Heterogenous with two or more cellular phenotypes or variable cellular populations, often	Often homogeneous cellular populations
Intraepidermal patterns	Loss of rete-oriented pattern; cells scattered in pagetoid patterns above level of dermal papillae; single cells reaching confluence along dermal epidermal junction; irregular and haphazard nesting; discohesive and large nests	Single cells on elongated rete ridges; little or no pagetoid spread; regular, uniform nesting; cohesive, relatively small nests
Dermal patterns	Confluence of cells with little or no maturation (sheetlike patterns of cells)	Regular spacing and maturation with depth
Cellularity, cellular density	High cellular density, crowding of cells	Lower cellular density
Melanin synthesis	Variable or no loss of synthesis with depth	Loss of synthesis with depth
Epidermal reaction	Hyperplasia, thinning, ulceration; variable epidermal thickness; stratum corneum shows alteration (hyperkeratosis, parakeratosis, scale crust)	Uniform thickness of epidermis, often; stratum corneum basketweave or unaffected
Maturation (differentiation)	Melanoma cells fail to exhibit diminished cellular and nuclear sizes and overall cellular density with depth in dermis	Melanocytes exhibit diminished cellular and nuclear sizes and overall cellular density with depth in dermis; progression from polygonal cells to lymphocyte-like cells to schwannian cells (neurotization) with depth
Mitosis	Likelihood of melanoma increases with absolute number in dermis and depth of mitoses; atypical mitoses	Not present in dermal component, usually
Necrosis	Single cells or confluent necrosis	Not present, usually
Host response	Often bandlike and asymmetrical infiltrates with superficially invasive melanoma; diminished inflammation with increasing tumor thickness	Little or no inflammation; perivascular infiltrates; bandlike infiltrates in halo nevi
Regression	Often all stages (early, intermediate, late); multifocal common in thin melanoma; often asymmetrical	Uncommon, often symmetrical
Cytological features	Uniform atypia • *Epithelioid cells:* Abundant pink granular or dusty cytoplasm; nuclear enlargement; nuclear pleomorphism; dispersed chromatin with prominent nucleoli; hyperchromatism • *Spindle or cuboidal cells:* often retraction of cytoplasm and high nuclear to cytoplasmic ratios; nuclear enlargement; pleomorphism; hyperchromatism • *Small cells:* often uniformity of cell type; pleomorphism; hyperchromatism	Little or no, or variable; atypia
Age	Melanoma rare before age 10 years or puberty; increases with age, particularly men > 55 years	Benign lesions likely to be present in younger individuals statistically
Gender	Men more likely to have melanomas on back vs. distal legs of women	Spitz nevi and related lesions common on thighs, arms in women > men
Anatomic site	Men more likely to have melanomas on back and trunk vs. distal legs followed by trunk of women	Benign lesions more likely on sun-protected sites and areas such as the thighs, buttocks, arms
Clinical characteristics	Melanomas often > 6 mm and generally > 10 mm, up to 20 cm; asymmetry, irregular and notched borders; complex coloration with tan, brown, black, gray, blue, white; pruritus, pain, bleeding, ulceration; history of changing or new lesion	Often < 6 mm; symmetry, regular and well-defined borders; uniform color, tan, brown; present for long period of time without change (exception: early "nodular" melanomas)

one must have other convincing criteria to ensure the diagnosis. Most melanomas are thus > 5–6 mm and many are > 10 mm in diameter.

Complexity, Symmetry, Homogeneity, and Circumscription

Another important feature at scanning magnification is the overall complexity of a lesion. In other words, to what extent or how does the lesion deviate from the idealized profile of a benign nevus? Is the lesion asymmetrical, heterogenous, and poorly defined? In general, benign lesions show a mirror-image symmetry if the lesion is bisected. On the other hand, melanomas tend to demonstrate increasing degrees of asymmetry, and such asymmetry may involve not only the melanocytic component but also the epidermis, melanin distribution, and host response (Fig. 10-4). Likewise, benign lesions commonly show a homogeneity of cellular elements—the melanocytes are fairly uniform and their architectural arrangements fairly similar throughout the lesion. Conversely, melanomas progressively show variation in cytologic features and architectural arrangements as one assesses a lesion throughout and compares one half of the lesion to the other half. Melanomas often have poorly defined peripheries: The intraepidermal melanocytic proliferative component gradually diminishes peripherally so that it is difficult to observe where the lesion ends, as compared to well-demarcated junctional or dermal nesting that ends abruptly in benign nevi. Exceptions to the latter criteria clearly occur, and consequently one may encounter nodular and so-called nevoid melanomas (see below) that are symmetrical, well circumscribed, and may have fairly homogenous melanocytic populations.

Cellular Density

The overall cellularity or cellular density of the lesion is a useful criterion. That is to say, is the epidermis being replaced by large numbers of melanocytes; are the melanocytes reaching confluence along and replacing the dermoepidermal junction; are large numbers of melano-cytes scattered throughout the epidermis in pagetoid patterns; are large nests of melanocytes replacing the epidermis? Increasing cellular density (cellular crowding) is an important attribute, suggesting melanoma in the epidermis and the invasive component; there are lesser degrees of cellularity in a benign lesion. There are exceptions to this criterion as evidenced by sparsely cellular melanomas developing in markedly sun-exposed skin.

Squamous Epithelial Alterations

Of particular importance is the state of the squamous epithelium and stratum corneum in a melanocytic lesion. Benign melanocytic lesions usually demonstrate a uniform or symmetrical appearance of the squamous epithelium—the epidermis shows the same thickness throughout the lesion, irrespective of whether there is epidermal hyperplasia, elongated rete, or no alteration in thickness. Similarly, the stratum corneum is often unaffected and basketweave in benign lesions. On the other hand, melanomas often disrupt epidermal homeostasis by stimulating epidermal proliferation and as a result hyperplasia and/or thinning and atrophy (Fig. 10-4). Often, asymmetry of the epidermis is present along with variation in epidermal thickness, melanin synthesis, and in the properties of the cornified layer. Characteristic features of the epidermis commonly observed with melanoma include effacement or loss of the epidermal rete pattern, dermoepidermal separation, and a "scalloping" of the dermoepidermal junction that usually accompanies confluence of melanoma cells at the junction. Epidermal atrophy, erosion, ulceration, and/or epidermal hyperplasia may be present, and replacement of the epidermis by aggregates of melanoma cells may be seen. Certain morphologic alterations of the epidermis are often associated with particular patterns of melanoma, for example, melanomas from intermittently sun-exposed skin demonstrate pagetoid spread and those from acral skin commonly show epidermal hyperplasia. On the other hand, solar melanomas often are typified by epidermal atrophy. Melanin is usually distributed in a regular and uniform pattern along the basilar and suprabasilar portions of the epidermis in benign lesions. In addition, there is often greater melaninization of the lower-most poles of the epidermal rete; in contrast, melanoma results in irregular and disorderly patterns of pigment distribution in the epidermis. In general, all melanomas provoke alterations of the stratum corneum, with the common occurrence of hyperkeratosis and parakeratosis.

Organizational Patterns within the Squamous Epithelium

The organizational pattern of melanocytes in the squamous epithelium is one of the most important criterion used to assess a lesion for melanoma. The three patterns are pagetoid spread, single-cell or lentiginous proliferation along the basilar portion of the epithelium, and nested arrangements of melanocytes. Since melanomas are often heterogeneous, commonly more than one pattern is present in any given lesion.

Pagetoid Pattern
- Melanomas with pagetoid intraepidermal component (Superficial spreading melanoma)

Pagetoid spread, scatter, or melancytosis is one of the most important and often the single most important feature used to establish a diagnosis of melanoma (Fig. 10-5).

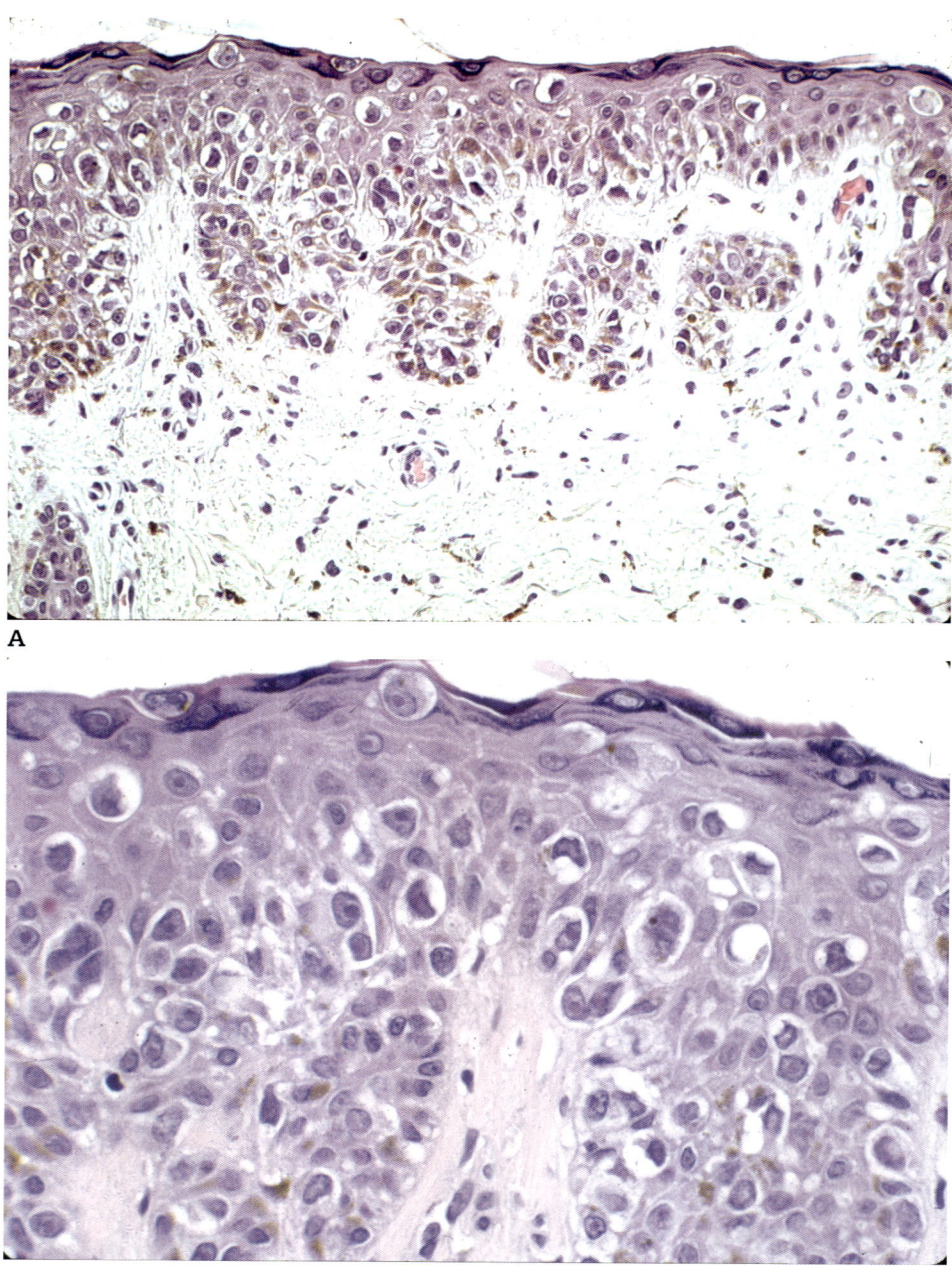

FIGURE 10-5 Melanoma in situ with pagetoid pattern is the most frequent histomorphologic pattern of intraepidermal melanoma. **A,** Pagetoid spread of epithelioid cells throughout epidermis. The presence of single and small nests of melanoma cells in the superficial malpighian layer of the epidermis (i.e., an imaginary horizontal line linking the most superficial limits of the dermal papillae) provides compelling evidence for melanoma. **B,** Significant cytologic atypia of melanocytes provides confirmatory evidence for melanoma.

This pattern is observed in a large proportion of melanomas (ranging from 32.1 to 76% of melanomas in various studies) (46,48) and has been proposed as the major histopathologic criterion for pagetoid or superficial spreading melanoma. The latter variant of melanoma has been said to account for as many as two thirds of all melanomas in white populations. However, pagetoid spread was absent in 44.4% of melanomas in one series (46).

The term *pagetoid spread,* or scatter, originated from the resemblance of intraepidermal melanoma to Paget's disease of the breast; the pattern is defined by a scattering of single and small nests of melanoma cells through

TABLE 10-8 Prevalence of pagetoid melanocytosis in various melanocytic lesions.

Lesion	Percent	Number of cases
Melanoma	76	103
Spitz tumors	38	47
Nevi of palms and soles	61	18
Pigmented spindle cell nevi	20	10
Recurrent nevi	60	10
Vulvar nevi	80	5
Nevi of infancy and childhood	100	3[a]
Ordinary acquired nevi	0	100

Source: Adapted from Stern and Haupt (1998) (49).
[a] Cases preselected for pagetoid melanocytosis.

all levels of the squamous epithelium (46,48). The biologic basis of this phenomenon is not understood (47), and it may represent a transepidermal elimination process. Because this finding may be observed in benign conditions (Table 10-8), one must be careful when pagetoid spread is encountered and carefully assess the context of the lesion (48,49,53,54).

In an attempt to precisely define this phenomenon, the term *pagetoid melanocytosis* was invoked to describe the upward discontinuous extension of melanocytes into the superficial dermis without reference to cytologic features (48,49). The following criteria have been proposed: (a) the cells in the superficial epidermis must be recognized as melanocytes, (b) the latter melanocytes are discontinuous from and are clearly not a direct extension of junctional melanocytes or nests of melanocytes, and (c) the pagetoid melanocytes must occupy the superficial epidermis above the most superficial dermal papilla. Confounding factors include direct extension of epidermal basal-layer junctional nests of melanocytes and tangential sections that falsely suggest pagetoid spread. Although precise (quantifiable) criteria are lacking, additional features (not always present) favor melanoma versus a benign process: (a) the pagetoid spread should involve a large front of the squamous epithelium (i.e., it should be diffuse) and involve, at the very least, a single 400× HPF; (b) it should demonstrate sufficient cellular density (greater cellular density favors melanoma but is not an absolute criterion); (c) the melanocytes should be clearly atypical (Fig. 10-6); and (d) pagetoid melanocytes should be noted in the superficial epidermis without underlying basilar melanocytes or nests, either centrally or lateral to the main portion of the lesion (termed by some "free-floating" pagetoid melanocytosis) (Fig. 10-6). Although there are no quantitative data avail-

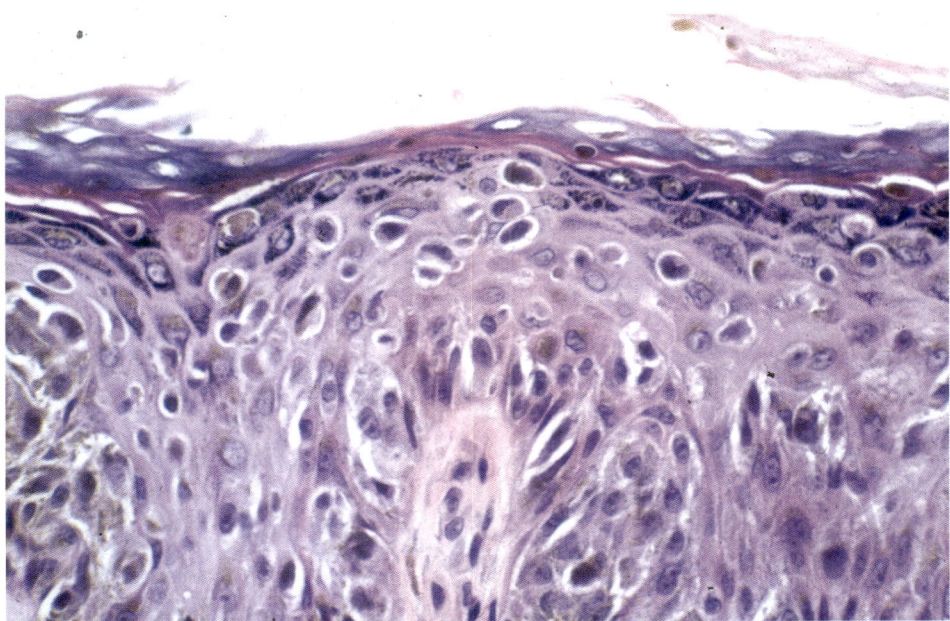

FIGURE 10-6 Pagetoid pattern of melanoma in situ. Note the high cellular density and cytologic atypia of melanoma cells scattered throughout superficial epidermis.

able on the density of pagetoid spread needed to diagnose intraepidemal (or in situ) melanoma, this criterion, as with all others, depends on context and the extent to which other important criteria are present.

Epithelioid melanoma cells containing abundant granular eosinophilic or dusty finely divided (pigment-laden) cytoplasm are probably most commonly encountered in the setting of pagetoid scatter. The nuclei of the latter cells usually have dispersed chromatin patterns and prominent eosinophilic nucleoli. However, one may observe considerable heterogeneity of cell type, including relatively small round or cuboidal cells with scant cytoplasm and nuclei that are hyperchromatic and irregular.

Lentiginous Pattern
- Melanomas with intraepidermal lentiginous component
    - Solar melanomas with lentiginous intraepidermal component ("Lentigo maligna" melanoma)
    - Acral melanomas with lentiginous intraepidermal component ("Acral lentiginous" melanoma)
    - Mucosal melanomas with lentiginous intraepithelial component

A large number of melanomas demonstrate predominately single-cell or lentiginous patterns of melanocytes along the basal layer. The pattern is especially common in melanomas involving chronically sun-exposed skin (9–11,42,55–79), acral skin (80–102), and mucosal sites (84). For melanoma in situ the melanocytes must achieve a sufficient frequency and degree of cytologic atypia over a sufficient front of the squamous epithelium to be diagnostic. In general, the melanocytes should be contiguous, replacing basal-layer keratinocytes or approaching this frequency (Fig. 10-7). Of particular importance for the diagnosis if epidermal rete ridges are present is the loss of a rete-oriented pattern of melanocytic proliferation. Thus the melanocytes are contiguous along the basal layer instead of being concentrated along the lower-most aspects of the elongated rete ridges. The latter feature signifies a loss of growth control.

Solar melanomas—that is, melanomas developing on the most sun-damaged surfaces, such as the central face, and histologically exhibiting clear-cut solar elastosis—most commonly, but not exclusively, demonstrate lentiginous proliferation of melanocytes, hence the terminology *lentigo maligna* and related lesions (Fig. 10-7). As discussed below, solar melanomas may also show predominatedly pagetoid and/or nested patterns of melanoma in situ and thus also seem to be directly related to cumulative sun exposure.

The predominately lentiginous melanocytic lesions constitute a histopathologic continuum from solar lentigo to frank melanoma in situ (termed here *solar intraepidermal melanocytic proliferation*), as discussed in Chapter 4). The rather ambiguous term *lentigo maligna* has been applied indiscriminately to this continuum of lentiginous melanocytic proliferation (LMP), often without precise definition. In our view, the latter term has been used in the following ways:

- As a synonym for melanoma in situ to apply to all such lentiginous lesions of sun-exposed skin, without strict criteria.
- To describe all intraepidermal melanocytic proliferations of sun-damaged skin, ranging from those with increased numbers of basilar melanocytes and no atypia to those with pronounced melanocytic atypia that qualify as melanoma in situ.
- To describe the RGP of lentigo maligna melanoma, without any more precise definition.

We appreciate that *lentigo maligna* is firmly entrenched in the lexicon of cutaneous melanoma and that its useage will not disappear soon. Nonetheless, to foster more precise communication and clarity, we recommend that LMP of sun-damaged skin should be more specifically defined as to degree of cytologic atypia or as melanoma in situ, based on histologic criteria (Table 10-9; see also below).

One must observe sufficiently atypical melanocytes replacing the basal layer of the epidermis as the minimal essential criterion for melanoma in situ. Other important features include effacement or loss of the epidermal rete ridges (Fig. 10-7), clustering or nesting of atypical melanocytes (in general not associated with epidermal rete ridges, as in a lentiginous junctional nevus) as they progressively show greater frequency along the basal layer, the involvement of skin adnexal structures by the atypical melanocytic proliferation, and usually the beginnings of pagetoid spread.

The threshold for diagnosis of melanoma in situ in this context is one of the most difficult problems in all of melanoma pathology (74,76). We contend that these intraepidermal proliferations of sun-exposed skin constitute a spectrum of lesions (solar intraepidermal melanocytic proliferation), ranging from proliferations with relatively low cellular frequency and slight cytologic atypia to clear-cut melanoma in situ (Table 10-9); a characterisitic feature of the latter group of lesions is their highly heterogeneous nature, necessitating adequate sampling in all instances. Probably a proportion or many of these lesions originate from solar lentigines and lentigious junctional nevi and show progressive melanocytic frequency and atypia. The distinction of many of these

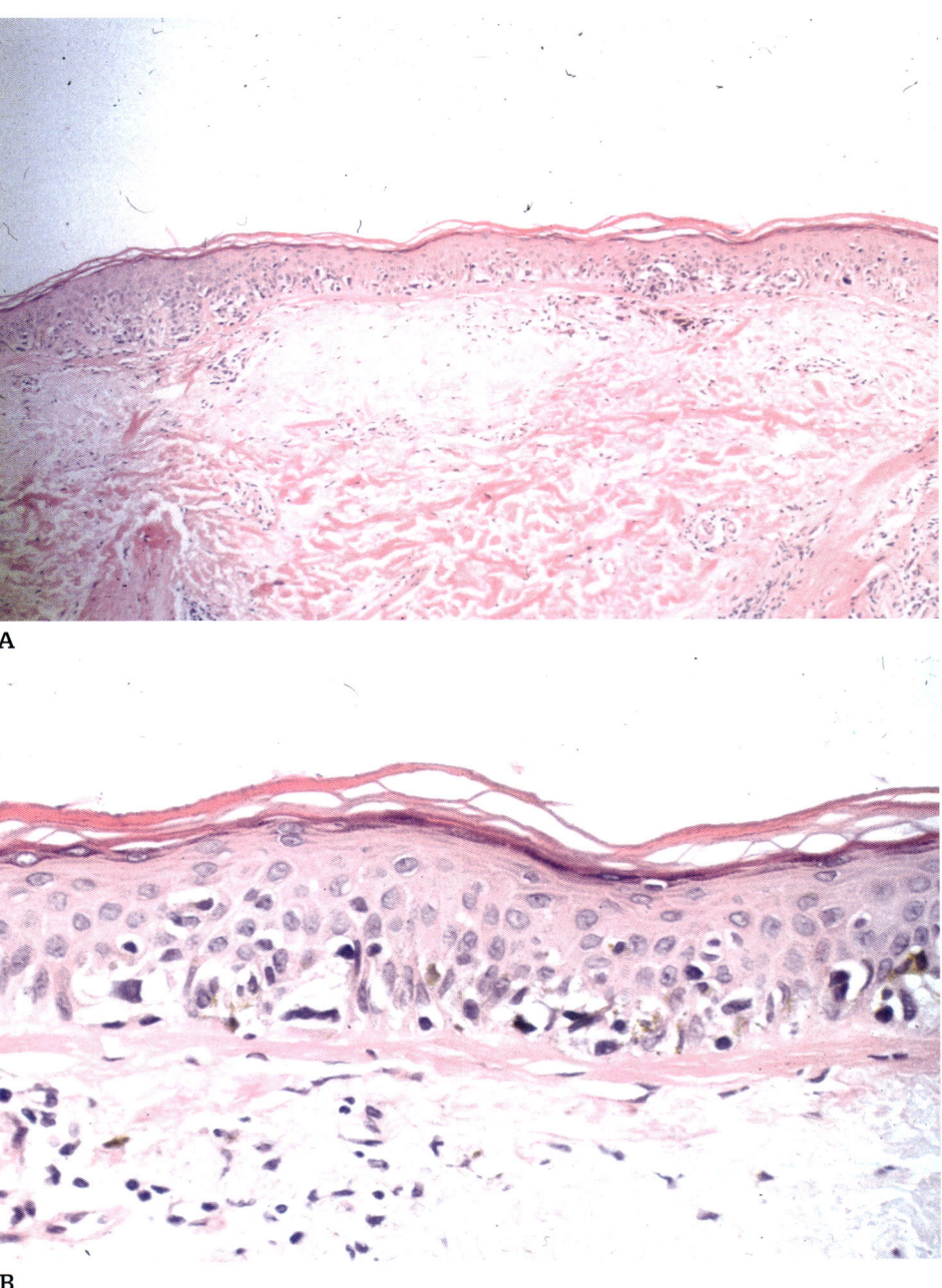

FIGURE 10-7 Lentiginous pattern of (solar) melanoma in situ **A,** The key features include effacement of epidermis (not always present), contiguous single-cell (lentiginous) proliferation of atypical melanocytes along the basal layer, and prominent solar elastosis. This lesion also demonstrates intraepidermal nesting of melanoma cells, which is also a criterion for solar melanoma in situ, and thus it would also be designated lentigo maligna (or melanoma in situ, lentigo maligna type) by many authors. **B,** Higher magnification of panel A showing the location of atypical melanocytes in the basilar portion of the epidermis.

early subtle proliferations from the background changes of sun-exposed skin is difficult or impossible in many instances and requires clinical information and common sense for their interpretation (Table 10-9).

The threshold at which point these atypical proliferations become biologically significant and require appropriate surgical excision is controversial and has not been adequately studied. Our general criteria (Table 10-9) include

TABLE 10-9 Comparison of features of solar intraepidermal melanocytic lesions.

Feature	SMH[a]	SL[a]	SLN[a]	SIMP[a] with atypia	SMIS[a] (formerly lentigo maligna)
Epidermal rete	Unchanged	Elongated or unchanged	Usually elongated	Variable; elongated or effaced	Often effaced
Lentiginous melanocytic proliferation	Variable, usually slight	Slight or none	Present	Present	Present
Frequency of melanocytes	Slightly increased	Normal or slightly increased	Increased	Increased	Increased; contiguous or near contiguous
Nesting of melanocytes	Usually absent	Absent	Present; usually cohesive	Usually absent	Usually present; often discohesive
Proliferation of melanocytes along adnexae	Usually absent	Usually absent	Usually absent	Usually absent	Usually present and extensive
Pagetoid spread	Absent	Absent	Usually absent	Usually absent	Often present
Cytologic atypia	Often absent or slight; pleomorphism	Usually absent	Present or absent	Variable; usually slight to moderate	Often uniform; moderate to severe

[a]SMH, solar melanocytic hyperplasia, chronic photoactivation; SL, solar lentigo; SLN, solar lentiginous nevus; SIMP, solar intraepidermal melanocytic pro-

contiguous or near contiguous proliferation of basilar melanocytes with nuclei that are larger than nearby keratinocytic nuclei (Fig. 10-7). We believe that all such lesions with features of solar intraepidermal melanocytic proliferation (SIMP) should be either adequately sampled or completely removed for full histopathologic examination to exclude melanoma in situ or invasive melanoma. Melanoma in situ may ensue as one begins to observe clustering or intraepidermal nesting of atypical melanocytes, proliferation along adnexal epithelium, and some pagetoid spread. The melanocytes commonly show retraction of cytoplasm and somewhat angulated or slightly spindled nuclei that are pleomorphic and often hyperchromatic. With somewhat greater atypicality the melanocytes exhibit nuclei with prominent pink nucleoli; the cells may at this point have an epithelioid appearance with abundant cytoplasm.

As with atypical intraepidermal melanocytic proliferations of sun-damaged skin, the threshold for diagnosis of melanoma in situ of acral skin is especially subjective and requires much better definition (Fig. 10-8). The criterion of contiguous or near contiguous proliferation of atypical melanocytes, particularly exending between epidermal rete ridges mentioned above, supports melanoma in situ at these sites. It must be kept in mind that the initial lesions may show relatively limited or variable cytologic atypia. More developed lesions demonstrate intraepidermal nesting and pagetoid spread. The melanocytes may be heavily pigmented with prominent dendrites, and some may show striking retraction of cytoplasm (Fig. 10-8). In contrast to solar melanomas, melanomas involving acral skin often exhibit epidermal hyperplasia.

Nested Pattern

Nested intraepidermal melanocytic proliferation occurs commonly in melanoma but almost always accompanies pagetoid and/or lentiginous patterns (Figs. 10-9 and 10-10). However, intraepidermal melanoma may be almost entirely nested (uncommon) and can be extremely difficult to distinguish from a melanocytic nevus. Histopathologic criteria include asymmetry; poorly circumscribed peripheries; intraepidermal aggregates of melanocytes that are usually large, often replacing (or obliterating) large portions of the squamous epithelium; nests that vary considerably in size, shape, degree of cellular cohesion, and placement or spacing; significant cytologic atypia of melanocytes, although sometimes subtle; and prominent disturbance to the epidermis, including hyperkeratosis, parakeratosis, epidermal thinning and atrophy, hyperplasia, and dermoepidermal separation (some or all present).

CONVENTIONAL MICROINVASIVE MELANOMA

After a period of intraepidermal proliferation, some proportion of, perhaps most, in situ melanomas invade the papillary dermis (9–34), often inially as single cells, as small aggregates of cells, or both, constituting level II invasion (Figs. 10-3 and 10-10; Table 10-10). In contrast, the more advanced level III involvement (see below) is defined by tumor cell aggregates *filling and expanding* the papillary dermis but not clearly involving the reticular dermis (Fig. 10-11).

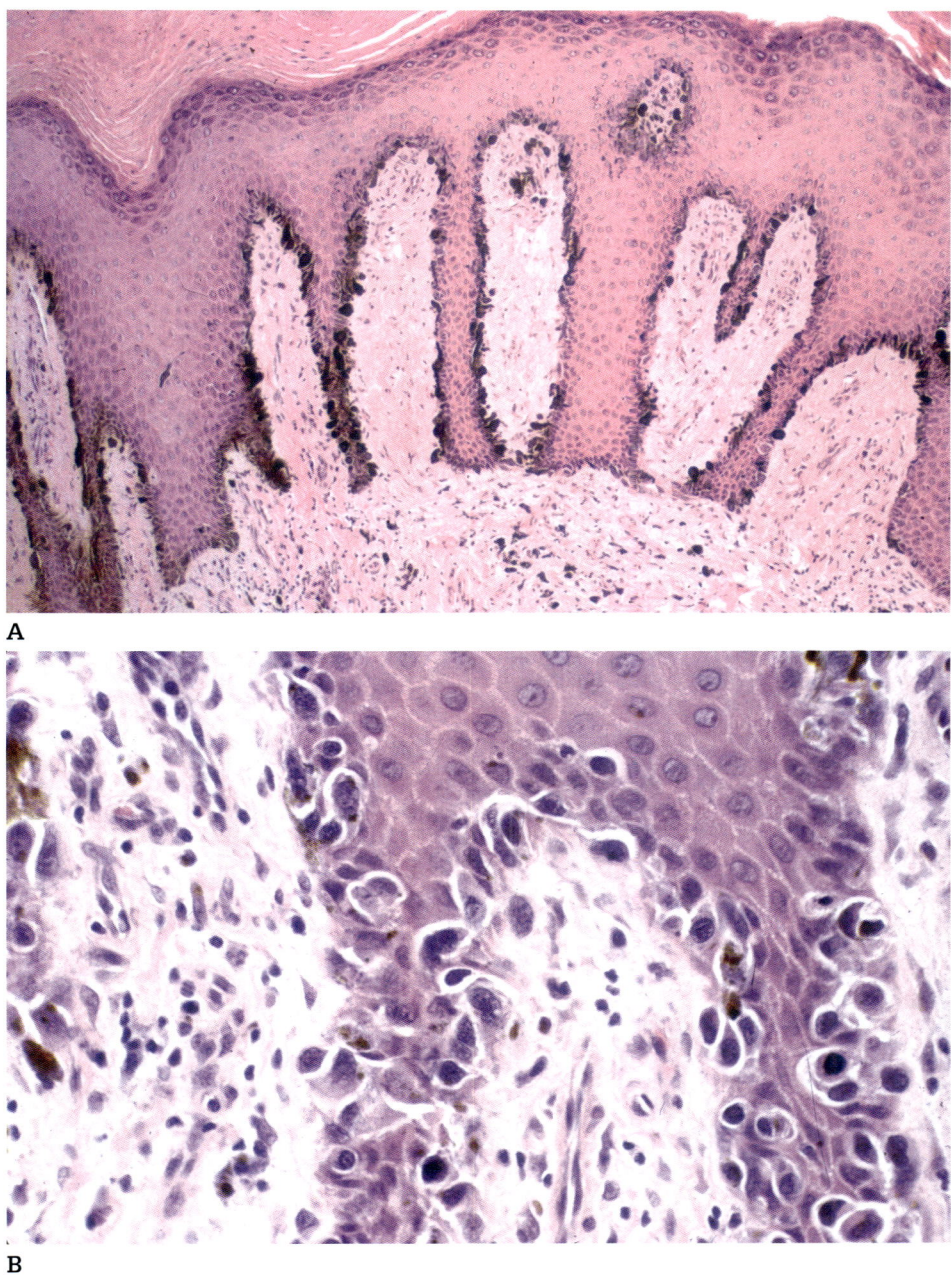

FIGURE 10-8 Lentiginous pattern of acral melanoma in situ. **A,** Increased number of atypical basilar melanocytes. Note the pronounced hyperpigmentation of the basal layer of the epidermis and striking nuclear pleomorphism and hyperchromatism of melanocytes. The epidermis is hyperplastic. **B,** The basilar melanocytes are contiguous and demonstrate high nuclear/cytoplasmic ratios, highly significant nuclear enlargement, pleomorphism, and hyperchromatism.

The criteria for diagnosis include identifying melanoma cells with histologic characteristics similar to the intraepidermal cells that, at the same time, have no connection to the intraepidermal component and skin appendages and are clearly distinguishable from a dermal nevus remnant, if present, and other cells types, such as macrophages and endothelial cells (Table 10-6). The recognition of papillary dermal invasion is facilitated by observing tumor cells generally beneath the plane of the epidermal rete or basal layer of the epidermis, searching

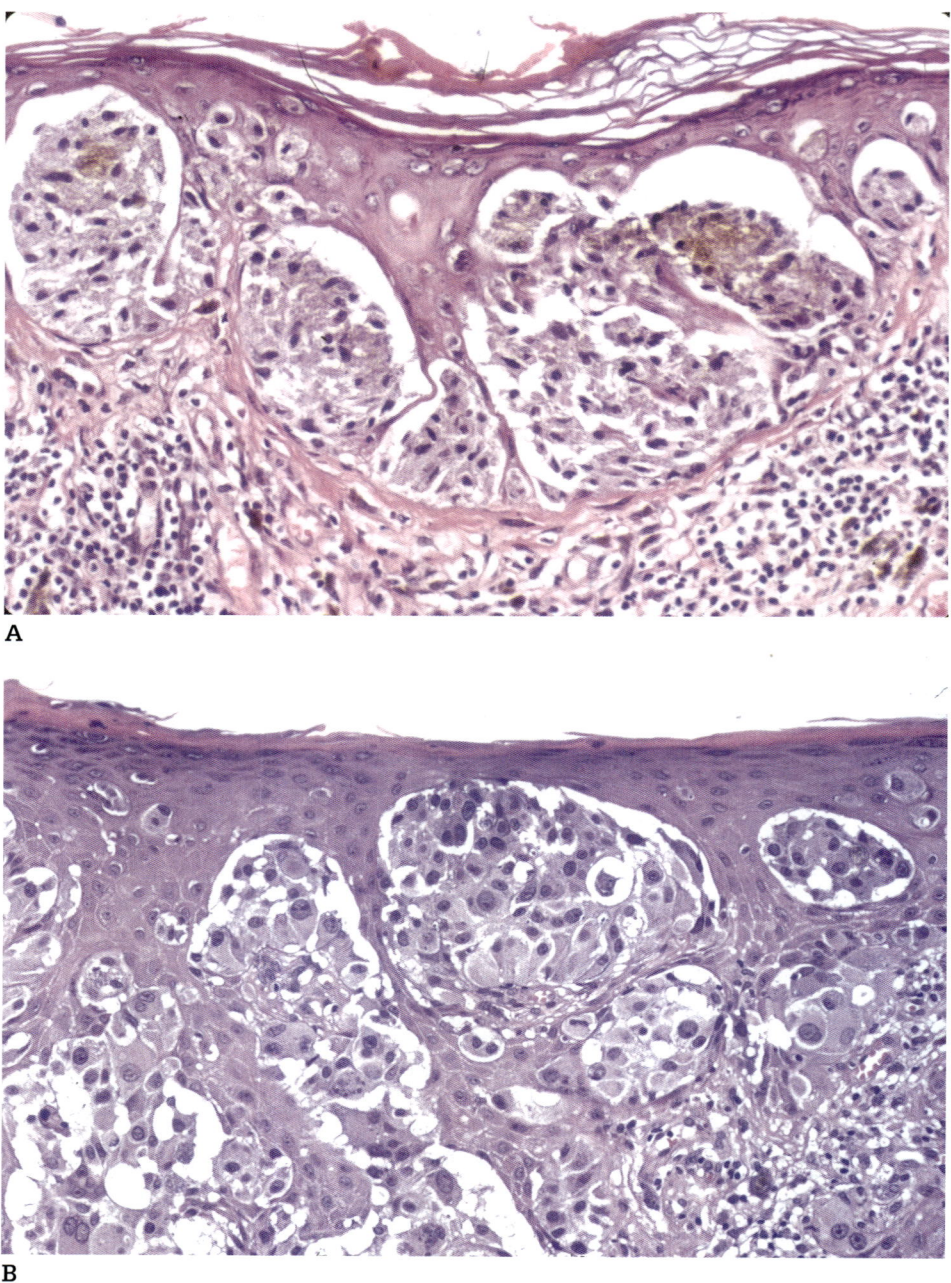

FIGURE 10-9 Nested pattern of melanoma in situ. **A, B,** Large irregular and discohesive nests of melanoma cells replacing and distorting the epidermis are the predominant features. The overall asymmetry of nesting; the large size, irregular shapes, irregular placement, and discohesion of the nests; the marked confluence of the melanocytes; and significant cytologic atypia of the melanocytes provide the criteria for melanoma in situ.

for multifocal invasion, examining of serial sections to confirm multifocal invasion and the absence of epidermal connection, and potentially conducting immunohistochemisty studies with markers for melanocytic lineage such as Mart-1 (Fig. 10-3). Although melanoma cells may track downward along the epithelium of hair follicles and eccrine ducts, this does not constitute true dermal invasion. Serial sections again may be necessary to determine if suspicious tumor foci in the dermis are connected to adnexal structures or are truly independent and thus in-

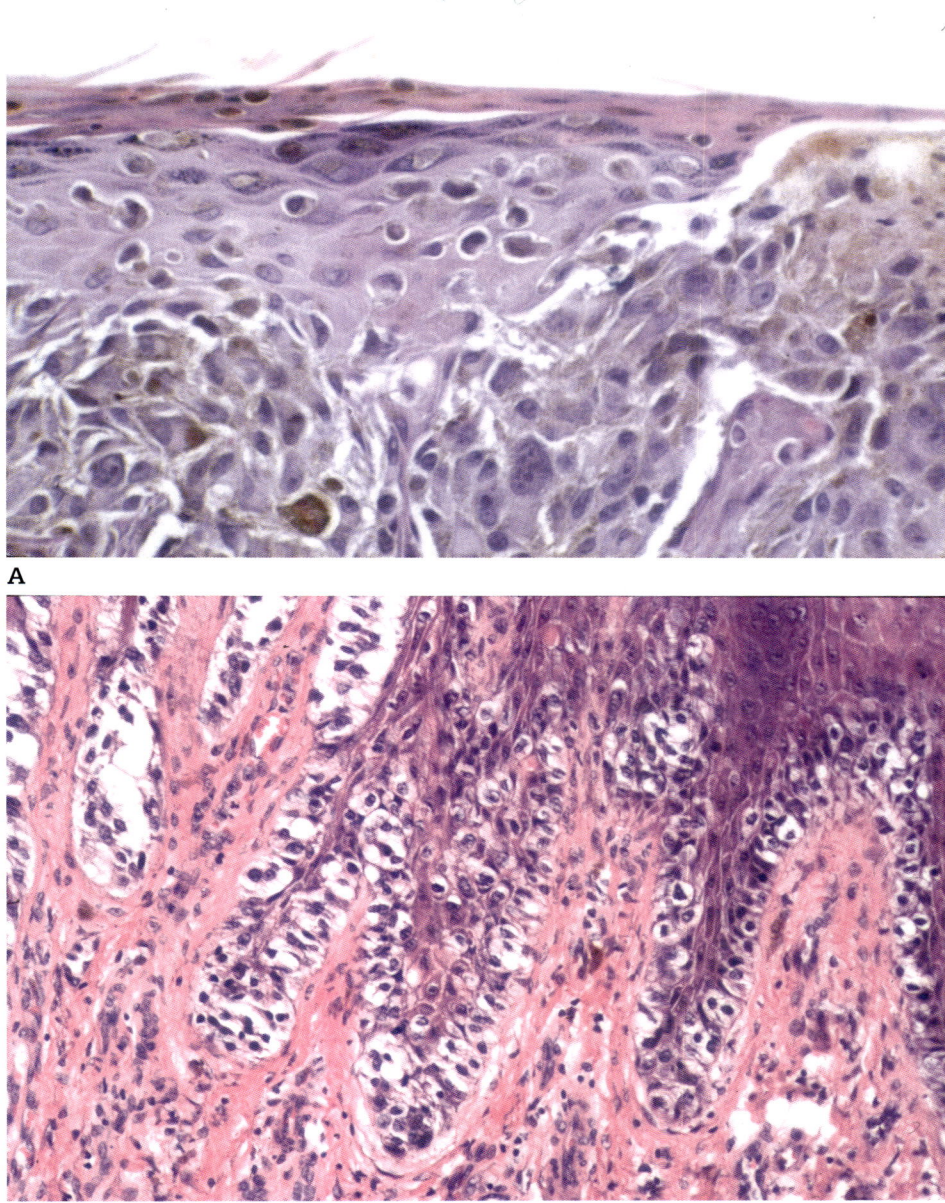

FIGURE 10-10 Melanoma with more than one intraepidermal pattern. **A,** In many (perhaps most) melanomas both pagetoid and nested arrangements of intraepidermal melanoma cells are present. **B,** Acral melanoma in situ with both lentiginous and nested patterns of melanocytes. Pagetoid infiltration is frequently present in well-developed acral melanomas.

vasive. In rare instances, melanoma may show invasion from the adnexae rather than the epidermis. Accordingly, the determination of Breslow thickness must be made from the point of invasion from the adnexal structure, in some instances horizontally rather than vertically, from the overlying epidermal granular layer.

The melanoma cells may be of any type, including epithelioid cells, polygonal cells, spindle cells, and relatively small cuboidal cells with minimal cytoplasm. At this stage, the invading melanocytic cells seem to lack proliferative attributes and the capacity for cohesive nodular growth (10,22,29). Thus mitotic figures are rarely observed. Mi-

TABLE 10-10	Anatomic levels of invasion.
Level	Description
I	Entirely intraepidermal; melanoma in situ
II	Microinvasive into papillary dermis
III	Expansion of papillary dermis by cohesive cellular nodule or plaque (but confined to papillary dermis)
IV	Invasion of reticular dermis
V	Invasion of subcutaneous fat

CONVENTIONAL INVASIVE MELANOMA

With expansion of the papillary dermis (level III) and invasion of the reticular dermis (level IV) and subcutaneous fat (level V) the vast majority of melanomas are characterized by the propensity of the melanoma cells to aggregate into progressively larger and more cohesive nests and plaques, as more poorly defined collections of tumor cells, or (rarely) to invade as single cells or files of cells (9,10,22,32).

Histomorphologic criteria at this stage include asymmetry; ulceration of the epidermis; high cellular density (crowding) of melanocytes in the dermal component with confluent or sheet-like patterns (Fig. 10-11); little or no maturation with depth, as is observed in nevi and Spitz tumors (i.e., the same degree of melanoma cell density and often pigment synthesis are present throughout the invasive component); heterogeneity of melanoma cells often present (i.e., admixture of epithelioid cells, spindle cells, and pigmented and nonpigmented cells); dermal mitoses, including atypical forms; single-cell necrosis or necrosis en masse; substantial cytologic atypia; and lymphocytic infiltrates, often beneath or infiltrating the invasive front of the tumor (see below) (Table 10-6).

Any melanoma cell type or combination or cell types may be present; however, the most common melanoma cell observed in the conventional forms of melanoma is a relatively large epithelioid or polygonal cell that is char-

croinvasive melanomas often show a striking host response in the papillary dermis, typically a dense cellular infiltrate of lymphocytes and monocyte/macrophages in a perivascular or bandlike pattern (Fig. 10-4). Melanin-containing macrophages and vascular proliferation often accompany the mononuclear cell infiltrates. The phenomenon of regression, often focal or multifocal, may be present in up to 50% of microinvasive melanomas (see below) (45,103). Regression is defined by clear-cut obliteration of melanoma in circumscribed or more expanded zones of the epidermis and dermis or possibly the dermis alone (described as dermal regression), accompanied by particular alterations of the papillary dermis. The latter findings generally include some combination or all of the following: lymphocytic infiltrates, which constitute the initial host response; accumulation of melanophages; prominent vascularity; and progressive fibroplasia (scarring) as the end stage of the process (104).

FIGURE 10-11 Malignant melanoma with level III invasion.

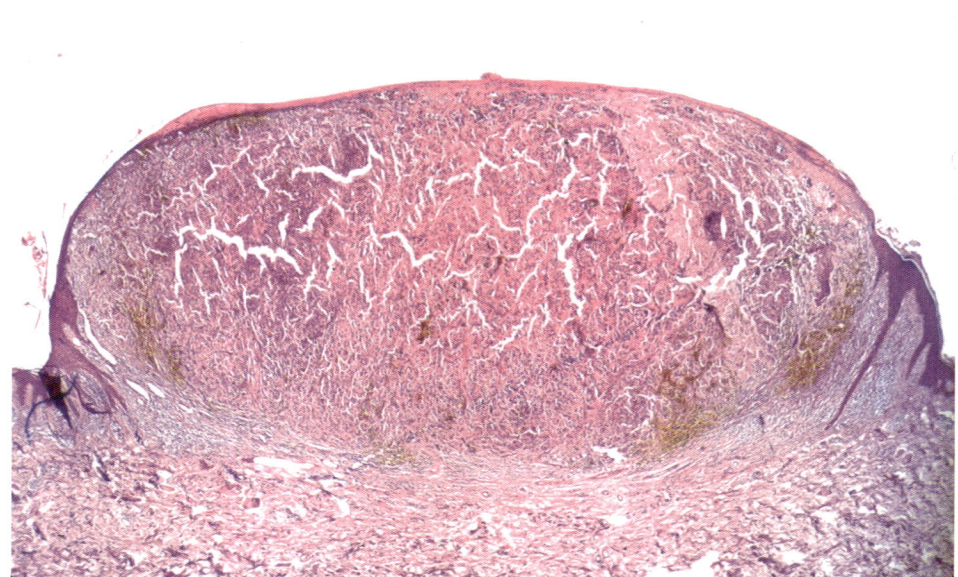

acterized by abundant cytoplasm exhibiting finely granular or dusty melanin or granular eosinophilic cytoplasm (9,10,21,22,32). The melanin granules commonly vary considerably in size and shape. The nuclei are enlarged, are pleomorphic, have dispersed chromatin or are hyperchromatic, have irregular and thickened nuclear membranes, and often have prominent pink or amphophilic nucleoli. Less frequently, spindle cells, small cuboidal cells, or large bizarre mononuclear or multinucleate cells may predominate or are admixed with the other cell types. As mentioned above, many melanomas are notable for considerable heterogeneity of cell type, so that the cells vary in nuclear size and shape and amount of cytoplasm from one focus to another.

Some melanomas invade the reticular dermis as files or small groups of tumor cells infiltrating collagen bundles. In some instances, the tumor cells may show a tropism for, or a propensity to track along, hair follicles, eccrine ducts, cutaneous nerves, or blood and lymphatic vessels. As referred to above, this tropism for cutaneous appendages is thought to be contiguous tumor extension from the intraepidermal component. However, although neurotropism and angiotropism are both poorly understood, they seem to represent the affinity of *invasive* tumor cells for the latter structures and thus connote a mechanism of direct tumor extension along these structures and migratory metastasis.

The host response in invasive melanomas is highly complex and heterogeneous. In general with increasing tumor thickness one observes an overall diminution in the lymphocytic infiltrates present. Therefore, melanomas generally measuring < 1–2 mm in thickness usually demonstrate the most substantial lymphocytic infiltrates, which are often disposed in dense perivascular or band-like patterns in the papillary dermis. The latter infiltrates may permeate or simply be situated beneath the invading tumor cell aggregates, or both. The former phenomenon has been termed tumor-infiltrating lymphocytes (TILs) and specifically refers to the juxtaposition of lymphocytes to tumor cells (satellitosis) and displacement of invasive tumor (29). Such infiltrates are often asymmetrical and may be focal or diffuse; they may be accompanied by other host response changes, including melanophages, fibroplasia, and increased dermal vasculariy or vascular ectasia.

The presence of melanin-containing macrophages in melanoma may simply indicate significant melanin content in the lesion or may be a marker of tumor destruction (regression). As mentioned above, histologic regression is very closely related to and often accompanies host response in early melanomas (see later in this chapter). Strictly defined, regression connotes the obliteration of tumor by host (immunologic) response. In particular regression may result in highly complex focal, multifocal, or diffuse alterations in a tumor, including lymphocytic infiltrates, accumulation of melanophages, fibroplasia, and vascular ectasia in any combination and accompanied by variable intraepidermal and dermal obliteration of tumor.

Any invasive melanoma may exhibit discrete foci of tumor in the reticular dermis and/or subcutaneous fat clearly removed from the main invasive part of the melanoma. The latter foci have been termed *microscopic satellites* and were defined as at least 0.05 mm in diameter (105). The latter size threshold is clearly arbitrary, and it is certain that this phenomenon requires further study for clarification of its biologic nature. Seemingly discontinuous or continuous extensions of the main tumor and local microscopic metastases probably account for most such satellite foci. Angiotropic and neurotropic tumor aggregates and both lymphatic and vascular intraluminal deposits account for some or many microscopic satellites (106) (Fig. 10-12).

Approximately one third of conventional melanomas are associated with a contiguous melanocytic nevus (38–40), such as a junctional or compound nevus (occasionally atypical) or most commonly a dermal nevus remnant. There has been controversy as to whether atypical intraepidermal components identified as atypical nevi are truly precursor lesions or simply the peripheral, less atypical portion of the melanoma (40). Such distinctions are often difficult and subjective.

Differential Diagnosis of Conventional Melanomas with Intraepithelial Component

Pagetoid Pattern The differential diagnosis of melanoma with a predominately pagetoid intraepidermal component includes first of all various other melanocytic proliferations (Table 10-6). One must often consider multiple features in aggregate and exclude benign or reactive conditions that may exhibit pagetoid spread, in particular, nevi in children and adolescents, acral nevi, nevi activated by sunlight exposure and other factors, recurrent/persistent melanocytic nevi, congenital nevi particularly in early life, atypical (so-called dysplastic) nevi, Spitz tumors (pagetoid Spitz tumor) (48,49,54), and pigmented spindle cell nevi (36,37,53). The latter entities often show a general symmetry and the Gestalt at scanning magnification is one of an orderly and usually uniform process, only limited pagetoid spread, sparse melanocytes (commonly) that are often limited to the lower half of the squamous epithelium (and thus do not satisfy the definition of pagetoid melanocytosis referred to above), generally nests with greater frequency than single melanocytes, melanocytes with little or no cytologic

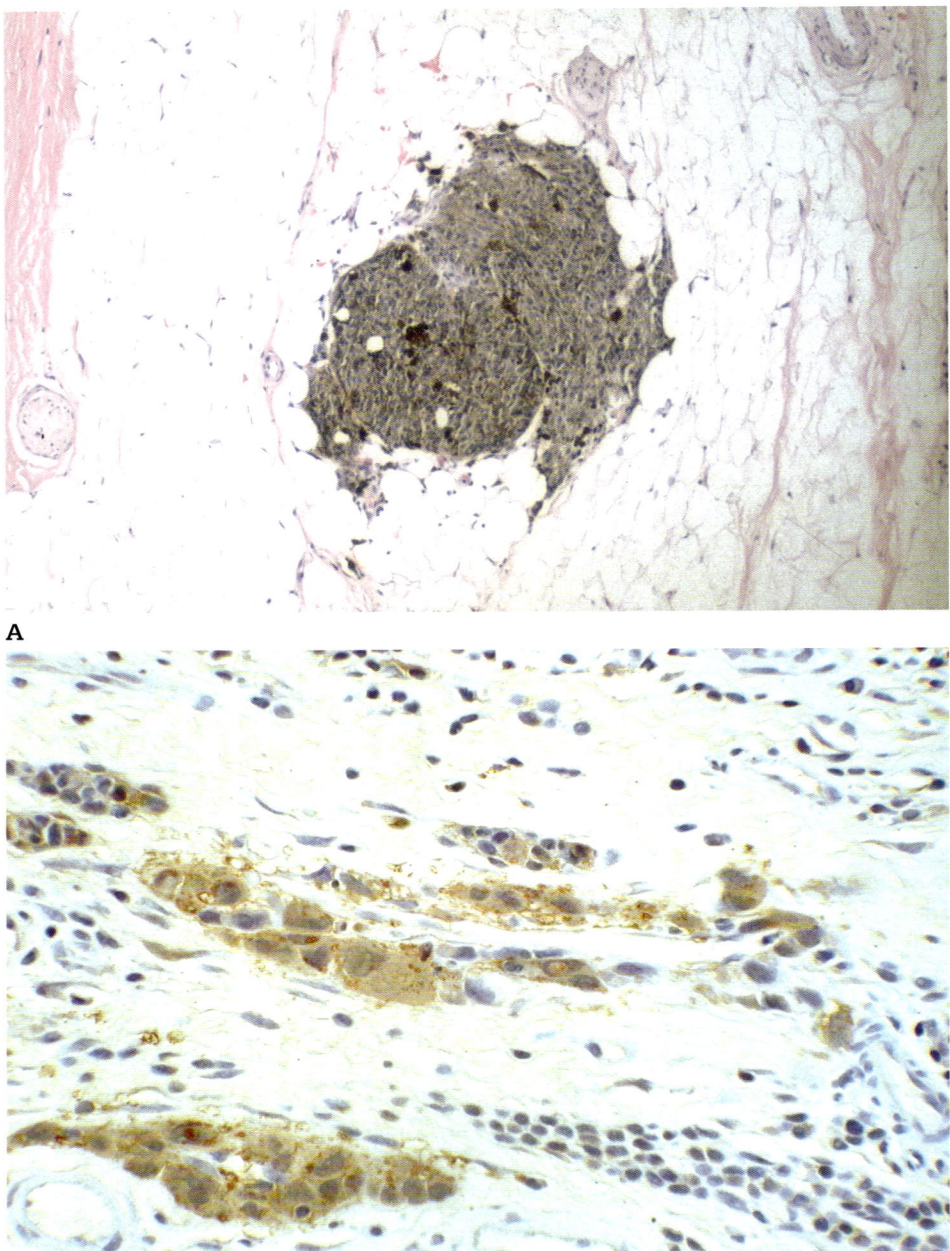

FIGURE 10-12 Melanoma. **A,** A microscopic satellite of a melanoma in subcutaneous fat, there is a small cohesive aggregate of melanoma cells clearly separate from the main portion of the primary melanoma. **B,** Angiotropic melanoma. The melanoma cells cuff microvessels at the base of a primary melanoma and are clearly identified by S-100 protein immunostaining.

atypia, and—of critical importance—lack of other features of melanoma. The misdiagnosis of melanocytic nevi, including Spitz tumors, pigmented spindle cell nevi, congenital nevi, recurrent melanocytic nevi, and nevi in children as melanoma, is primarily related to overreaction to focal or limited pagetoid spread.

Intraepidermal Epithelioid Cell Melanocytic Proliferations

A particular problem encountered with some frequency is that of intraepidermal proliferations of epithelioid melanocytes suggesting melanoma in situ. In general the proliferations include pagetoid variants of Spitz

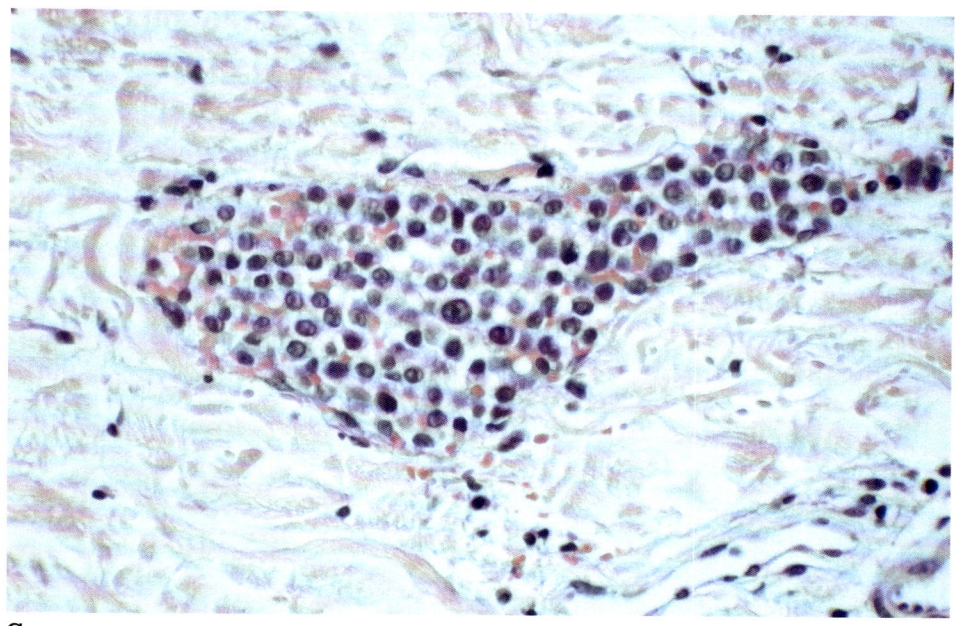

FIGURE 10-12 Continued. **C,** Vascular invasion by melanoma cells in a primary melanoma. Melanoma cells pack the lumen of the vascular channel. The latter phenomenon is exceptionally rare in our experience.

nevus/tumor, intraepidermal melanoma, and proliferations that are biologically indeterminate (36,37,54). Such proliferations commonly involve the thighs of women. Features arguing in favor of a pagetoid variant of Spitz nevus/tumor in addition to clinical parameters include small size (e.g., < 5–6mm), overall symmetry, sharp circumscription, pagetoid spread generally limited to the lower half of the epidermis and characterized by relatively low cellular frequency, junctional nesting typical of a Spitz tumor, and melanocytes with cytologic features of a Spitz tumor (i.e., polyangular contours, ground glass eosinophilic cytoplasm, and nuclei with dispersed or uniform chromatin). Spitz tumors also display in general a characteristic maturation of cells with infiltration into the dermis. The cells are remarkable for a diminution in cellular and nuclear sizes and also a diminution in size of aggregates of cells descending into the dermis. The cells also typically infiltrate the stroma in an orderly and regular pattern. Nonetheless, there is a subset of this general category of proliferations that defy categorization as clearly being Spitz in origin or melanoma or evolving melanoma.

Intraepidermal Pigmented Spindle Cell
Melanocytic Proliferations
Closely related to the problem of distinguishing pagetoid Spitz tumors from melanoma is the dilemma of differentiating pigmented spindle cell nevi (PSCN) and atypical variants from intraepidermal melanoma (37,53). PSCN may exhibit two patterns, not mutually exclusive, that may be confused with intraepidermal melanoma: pagetoid spread (Fig. 10-13) and large intraepidermal nesting with irregularity and discohesion. To distinguish such lesions from melanoma, one must evaluate the lesion in the context of all the other features present. Thus such lesions often occur in children, are small in diameter (e.g., 2–4 mm), are well demarcated, and exhibit rather uniform cytologic features of melanocytes.

An especially difficult problem is the separation of PSCN from a predominantly intraepidermal pigmented spindle cell form of solar melanoma developing in markedly sun-damaged skin but also occasionally at other sites. Such melanomas usually exhibit greater asymmetry, larger intraepidermal nests with greater cellularity, and greater cytologic atypia of spindled melanocytes as compared to PSCN.

Atypical (Dysplastic) Nevi
In general, pagetoid spread is an uncommon or rare finding in atypical (dysplastic) melanocytic nevi (AMN) (see Chapter 5) (39,40). However, on occasion, AMN with pronounced atypia may be misdiagnosed as pagetoid melanoma because of appearances suggesting early pagetoid spread, confluence of cellular aggregates along the dermoepidermal junction, prominent variation in nesting pattern, significant cytologic atypia, entrapment

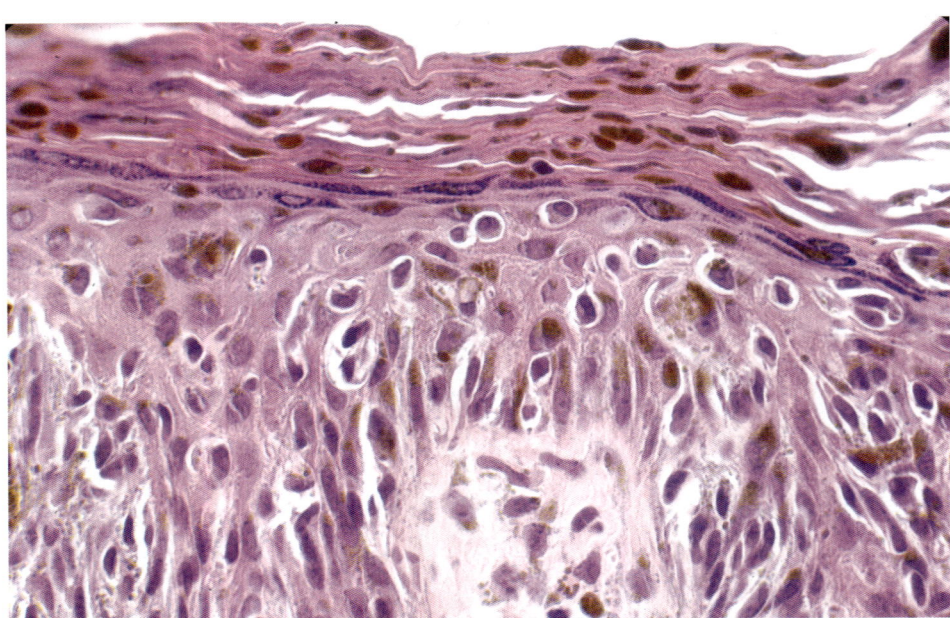

FIGURE 10-13 Pigmented spindle cell nevus with pagetoid spread showing individual melanocytes scattered throughout the superficial epidermis in tissue from a child. The lesion was small, symmetrical, and well circumscribed and had an orderly arrangement of intraepidermal nests of melanocytes. The pagetoid cells lack the cytologic atypia of melanoma in situ (see Figs. 10-5 and 10-6).

of nests of dermal nevus cells in the papillary dermis, and dense mononuclear cell infiltrates. On occasion, the distinction of AMN from melanoma is exceedingly difficult. Nonetheless, discrimination of pagetoid melanoma from AMN is usually possible because of the greater asymmetry and disorder encountered in melanoma. Usually, AMN will maintain an overall symmetry, a fairly uniform appearance throughout the lesion, a nevic organization as exemplified by fairly organized junctional nesting, and a basilar proliferation of melanocytes that is still concentrated along the epidermal rete and with greater density toward the lower poles of the rete. Thus the intervening epidermis between rete will contain a lesser density of melanocytes than that on the epidermal rete. If pagetoid spread is present, this architectural pattern is often more prominent about the epidermal rete and *confined to the lower-most epidermis*. Occasional AMN exhibit effacement of the epidermal rete pattern and confluence of melanocytic cells along the dermoepidermal junction in this zone. The latter changes are commonly associated with dense mononuclear cell infiltrates. The latter changes may strongly suggest melanoma, and the findings must be carefully interpreted in the overall context of the lesion. AMN are generally characterized by variable or discontinuous cytologic atypia—that is, the degree of nuclear enlargement, pleomorphism, and hyperchromatism varies from cell to cell (39,40). This cytologic feature is very helpful in discriminating AMN from the more uniform or contiguous cytologic atypia of melanoma.

A finding that raises the possibility of melanoma is entrapment of atypical nevus cells in a fibrotic papillary dermis of AMN. Such findings may even suggest partial regression of melanoma. A distinction from melanoma should be based on a systematic evalualtion of all the cytologic and architectural characteristics of the lesion. It is important that the dermal nevus cells in question usually lack the marked and uniform cytologic atypia especially manifested as pleomorphism, hyperchromasia, and prominent nucleoli of melanoma cells.

In general, halo nevi have dense mononuclear cell infiltrates, histologic regression in some instances, and varying degrees of architectural and cytologic atypia that may suggest pagetoid melanoma. The typical halo nevus of children and adolescents is characterized by overall symmetry, orderly appearance, and little or no cytologic atypia. The lymphoid cells that permeate the dermal nevus have a uniform density and well-defined inferior horizontal margin. The nevus cells of halo nevi may demonstrate cellular enlargement with prominent eosinophilic cytoplasm, but their nuclear details are usually little altered. In contrast, there is a variant of halo nevus that has prominent pattern and cellular atypia and is perhaps best categorized as an AMN. The discussion of AMN (above) is relevant to this form of (atypical) halo nevus.

Melanomas with pagetoid patterns often show considerable overlap with lentiginous melanomas, since the latter melanomas may display junctional nesting, pagetoid spread, and the presence of epithelioid cells in either the intraepidermal or dermal components (32). The presence of pagetoid melanocytosis may signify tumor progression of some solar melanomas to a higher-grade tumor equivalent to pagetoid melanoma (21). The application of strict criteria may allow distinction of pagetoid melanoma from solar melanoma. Thus, in the case of solar melanoma, one usually observes prominent solar elastosis, epidermal atrophy and effacement, prominent involvement of adnexal units by the melanocytic proliferation, and strikingly pleomorphic melanoma cells with scant cytoplasm, in at least some portion of the lesion (32).

On occasion, nonmelanocytic lesions are considered in the differential diagnosis of pagetoid melanoma (Table 10-6). The principal conditions include Paget's disease, either mammary or extramammary; squamous cell carcinoma in situ; sebaceous carcinoma, epidermotropic eccrine carcinoma; cutaneous T cell lymphoma; and other epidermotropic carcinomas, such as Merkel cell (neuroendocrine) carcinoma (107,108). In most instances, the dilemma can be resolved simply by careful attention to histologic details in routinely stained sections (107).

After observing pagetoid spread in a given lesion, it is important to study the lesion at scanning magnification and ask these questions: Does the lesion have other attributes that support a diagnosis of melanoma? Is the clinical context consistent with melanoma? For example, the absence of melanin (with exceptions), the presence of mucin-containing cells in Paget's disease, and the presence of cells with intercellular bridges and dyskeratotic cells in squamous cell carcinoma in situ argue against melanoma. In some instances, adjunctive studies, such as mucin and melanin stains or immunohistochemistry (107) (Table 10-11), may provide additional help or may be critical for diagnosis. For example, the antibodies against S-100 protein, (109,110,) HMB-45 (111), Mart-1 (112), mift (113), and tyrosinase (114) are fairly specific for melanoma, whereas the CAM 5.2 and 21N antibodies are specific for Paget's disease. CAM 5.2 is a monoclonal antibody directed against cytokeratins with molecular weights of 8, 18, 19, 39, 43, and 52 kDa, which are expressed in glandular epithelium (115). The polyclonal antibody 21N reacts with the c-erb B2 protein, which is found in many adenocarcinomas (116). Guidelines for the further delineation of proliferations with a pagetoid pattern are outlined in Table 10.11 (see also Chapter 2).

Lentiginous Pattern In general, the lentiginous melanomas must be distinguished from lentigines demonstating some atypia, lentiginous nevi, atypical nevi, and pigmented spindle cell nevi of sun-damaged and acral sites, respectively (see below).

Nested Pattern Predominately nested forms of melanoma must be distinguished from melanocytic nevi with prominent intraepidermal nesting such as pigmented spindle cell nevi and congenital and other atypical nevi. The latter differential diagnosis is especially problematic when the lesion has nesting at its peripheries and is composed of relatively small nevus-like melanocytes that have a general uniformity. Histopathologic features that we

TABLE 10-11 Histochemical and immunohistochemic evaluation of pagetoid involvement of the epidermis.

Marker[a]	Pagetoid melanoma	Paget's disease	Squamous cell carcinoma in situ	Cutaneous T cell lymphoma	Sebaceous carcinoma
PAS+D	−	±	−	−	−
Alcian blue	−	±	−	−	−
Fontana-masson (melanin)	+	±	±	−	−
S-100 protein	+	−	−	−	−
HMB-45	+	−	−	−	−
Keratin	−	±	+	−	±
21N	−	+	−	−	−
EMA	±	+	+	−	+
CEA	−	±	−	−	−
GCDFP-15	−	+	−	−	−
LCA	−	−	−	+	−
CD$_3$ (panT)	−	−	−	+	−

[a]PAS+D, periodic acid-Schiff plus diastase for neutral glycosaminoglycans; Alcian blue, for acidic glycosaminoglycans (nonsulfated); CAM 5.2, monoclonal antibody against several cytokeratins; 21N, polyclonal antibody against c-erb B2 protein; EMA, epithelial membrane antigen; CEA, carcinoembryonic antigen; GCDFP-15, gross cystic disease fluid protein 15; LCA, leukocyte common antigen; CD$_3$ (pan T), surface markers common to all T lymphocytes; −, generally negative; +, generally positive; ±, uncommonly positive.

have found useful in attempting to resolve this problem include size of the lesion (lesions with large diameters argue in favor of melanoma); asymmetry; considerable variation in the size, shape, and tendency to confluence of nests (in particular the large size of intraepidermal nests replacing the epidermis); significant discohesion of junctional nests (Fig. 10-7); significant thinning and scalloping of epidermis with dermoepidermal separation; significant atypia of melanocytes within nests (e.g., nuclear pleomorphism, hyperchromatism, irregular and thickened nuclear membranes, and prominent nucleoli); and other important attributes such as subtle but definite pagetoid spread. In some instances, after assessing all such features, one may not be able to arrive at a definite diagnosis of melanoma. In this situation, the lesion should be described as biologically indeterminate and managed with complete excision and careful monitoring of the patient.

CONVENTIONAL INVASIVE MELANOMAS WITH LITTLE OR NO ADJACENT INTRAEPIDERMAL COMPONENT

Melanomas characterized by a bulky invasive component and limited or absent adjacent intraepidermal component that have been previously termed nodular melanoma may account for 10–15% of melanomas in white individuals (9–11,18,21,22,32) (Table 10-12). In all likelihood, this group of melanomas includes an assortment of melanomas either originating from the rapid clonal progression of a limited or short-lived intraepidermal component no longer recognizable or originating from the de novo development of an invasive component of intraepithelial, adnexal, or dermal origin.

Clinical Features

This group of melanomas may develop on any anatomic site; however, as with the general group of conventional melanomas, the most common site is the trunk. The tumor usually presents as a protuberant or polypoid blue-black papule or nodule associated with obliteration of skin markings and frequent ulceration and crust (43,44). A subset lack pigment and present as pink (amelanotic) tumors. A high index of suspicion is needed to diagnose amelanotic tumors.

Histopathologic Features

Scanning magnification discloses a raised, dome-shaped, or polypoid tumor, often but not always exhibiting some asymmetry (9–11,18,21,22,32,34) (Figs. 10-11 and 10-14; Table 10-12). The epidermis over the tumor is usually thin, is effaced, and may be ulcerated. Variable upward

TABLE 10-12 Conventional melanoma with little or no adjacent intraepidermal component (nodular melanoma).

Clinical features
  30–70 years (often 40–50, but any age)
  Men = women
  Any site, especially trunk dorsal surfaces of hands
  0.3–5 cm
  Rapid evolution, often (4 months to 2 years)
  Papule or nodule, pigmented or amelanotic (advanced)
    Often protuberant, polypoid
    Black, blue-black, pink
  Ulceration, bleeding
  Asymmetry but symmetry may be present often
  Well-defined borders, often
Histopathologic features
  Dome-shaped polypoid or sessile tumor often
  May be pedunculated
  Asymmetry (often symmetrical)
  Epidermis commonly thinned, effaced, ulcerated
  Overlying intraepidermal component may or may not be present and usually does not extend peripherally beyond dermal invasive tumor
  Pagetoid spread, lentiginous melanocytic proliferation, intraepithelial nesting may be present
  Cohesive aggregate or aggregates of tumor cells fill subjacent dermis, subcutis
  No maturation, usually
  Host response at base and/or tumor-infiltrating lymphocytes, common
  Epithelioid cells often make up invasive component, but spindle cells, small cuboidal cells common; heterogeneity, often
  Partial regression, relatively uncommon
  Precursor nevus (~ 6% of cases)
Differential diagnosis
  Spitz tumor
  Pigmented spindle cell nevus
  Atypical halo-like nevus
  Metastatic melanoma
  Cellular blue nevus with atypia
  Squamous cell carcinoma
  Adnexal carcinomas
  Atypical fibroxanthoma
  Fibrous histiocytoma
  Adult xanthogranuloma
  Lymphoma, particulary large cell anaplastic variants
  Cellular neurothekeoma
  Malignant peripheral nerve sheath tumor
  Capillary hemangioma
  Malignant glomus tumor or with atypia
  Angiosarcoma
  Kaposi sarcoma
  Leiomyosarcoma

migration of melanoma cells in the epidermis may be present, but intraepidermal spread often does not extend beyond the margins of the invasive tumor.

The dermal component is typified by a cohesive nodule or smaller nests of tumor cells that have a pushing or expansile pattern of growth (Figs. 10-11 and 10-14). The tumor cells most frequently are epithelioid (Fig. 10-7), but other cell types—including spindle cells, small epithelioid cells resembling nevus cells, and giant mononuclear or multinucleate ("monstrocellular" forms) (Fig. 10-14D)—may predominate or be admixed with other cell types. The cell population usually appears monomorphous, but closer examination reveals frequent cellular enlargement, nuclear enlargement, variation in nuclear size and shape, hyperchromatism and prominent nucleoli. High nuclear-cytoplasmic ratios are often noted. The cytoplasm of epithelioid cells has eosinophilic granular qualities or contains melanin granules that may vary in size. Epithelioid cells often contain finely divided dusty melanin granules, but melanin may be absent. The surrounding stroma may demonstrate variable mononuclear cell infiltrates, fibroplasia, telangiectasia, and melanophages.

Differential Diagnosis

Such melanomas may be confused with metastatic melanoma, Spitz tumors with varying degrees of atypia, atypical halo nevi, cellular blue nevi with of without atypia, squamous cell carcinoma, atypical fibroxanthoma, fibrous histiocytoma, leiomyosarcoma, myoid fibroma, lymphoma (particularly large cell anaplastic lymphoma), cellular capillary hemangioma, and Kaposi sarcoma (Table 10-12). Epidermotropic metastatic melanoma involving the papillary dermis may prove difficult to distinguish from nodular melanoma (117). Metastatic melanoma is often fairly monomorphous and often shows less epidermal involvement and little stromal response, whereas nodular melanoma is often polymorphous and exhibits greater stromal response. However, distinction may be impossible in certain cases, and discrimination must rely on clinical information and clinical course.

Certain Spitz tumors, particularly those with atypia, enter into the differential diagnosis of nodular melanoma (see Chapter 7). Clinical information is pertinent to the diagnosis, since melanoma is uncommon in the young, whereas atypical lesions are more suspicious for melanoma in adults.

SOLAR MELANOMA

Solar melanoma is also called by many lentigo maligna melanoma, melanoma associated with Hutchinson's melanotic freckle, and lentigo malin des vieillards of Dubreuilh. Originally described by Sir Jonathan Hutchinson, this variant of melanoma is appropriately termed *solar melanoma* (SM) because its development is directly related to cumulative sunlight exposure (9–11,32,34,55–79) (Table 10-13). SM are defined by their localization to continuously/chronically sun-exposed skin and the presence of significant solar elastosis histologically. They are also distinctive lesions because of their gross morphologic appearance, characteristic slow evolution, development in elderly individuals, and often distinctive histopathologic appearance. Approximately 4–15% of melanomas occurring in whites are of the solar subtype (22). There some evidence that they are increasing in frequency. They generally affect older individuals with a median age at diagnosis of 65 years for invasive SM. However, they may be observed in younger individuals living in geographic areas with high insolation. There is a predilection for the head and neck, with the cheek being the single most commonly affected site followed by the nose and forehead. Uncommonly they may develop at other sites of chronic sun exposure such as the dorsal surfaces of the hands or lower legs. Often the solar melanomas develop after an indolent period of growth (20–30 years and even up to 50 years) as an atypical intraepidermal melanocytic proliferation (lentigo maligna, Hutchinson melanotic freckle, SIMP) before in situ and invasive melanoma ensues (Table 10-9; see below).

As previously discussed, it is likely that there is continuum of lesions that constitute the solar melanocytic neoplastic system (Table 10-9). This system probably includes the exceedingly common lesions of solar lentigo and solar lentiginous nevi as the initial lesions. The occurrence of such lesions in the same distribution and with overlapping clinical features suggest some relationship of the latter two lesions with solar intraepidermal melanocytic neoplasia (lentigo maligna). The likelihood of progression of such lesions, particularly solar lentigo is poorly defined and almost certainly is remote. However, the ensuing steps of progression after solar lentigo, the lentiginous melanocytic proliferations with slight, moderate, and severe atypia are observed and generally provoke controversy as to the their appropriate terminology and biologic significance (Table 10-9). We thus propose that there is in fact a continuum of such atypical lesions and that with each progressive step of atypia the risk of disease progression rises. The basis for such a system is supported by analgous lentiginous lesions associated with photochemotherapy (PUVA) and xeroderma pigmentosum (XP) (118). Closely related melanomas are the most common form of melanoma occurring in patients with XP, a rare genetic disease associated with defective DNA repair. Thus the solar melanomas are likely to have some defect in DNA repair (118,119).

The risk of progression of lentigo maligna (SIMP) to invasive melanoma is not well defined but nonetheless has been estimated to range between 2.2 and 30%, depending on the age of the patient and other factors (120). We

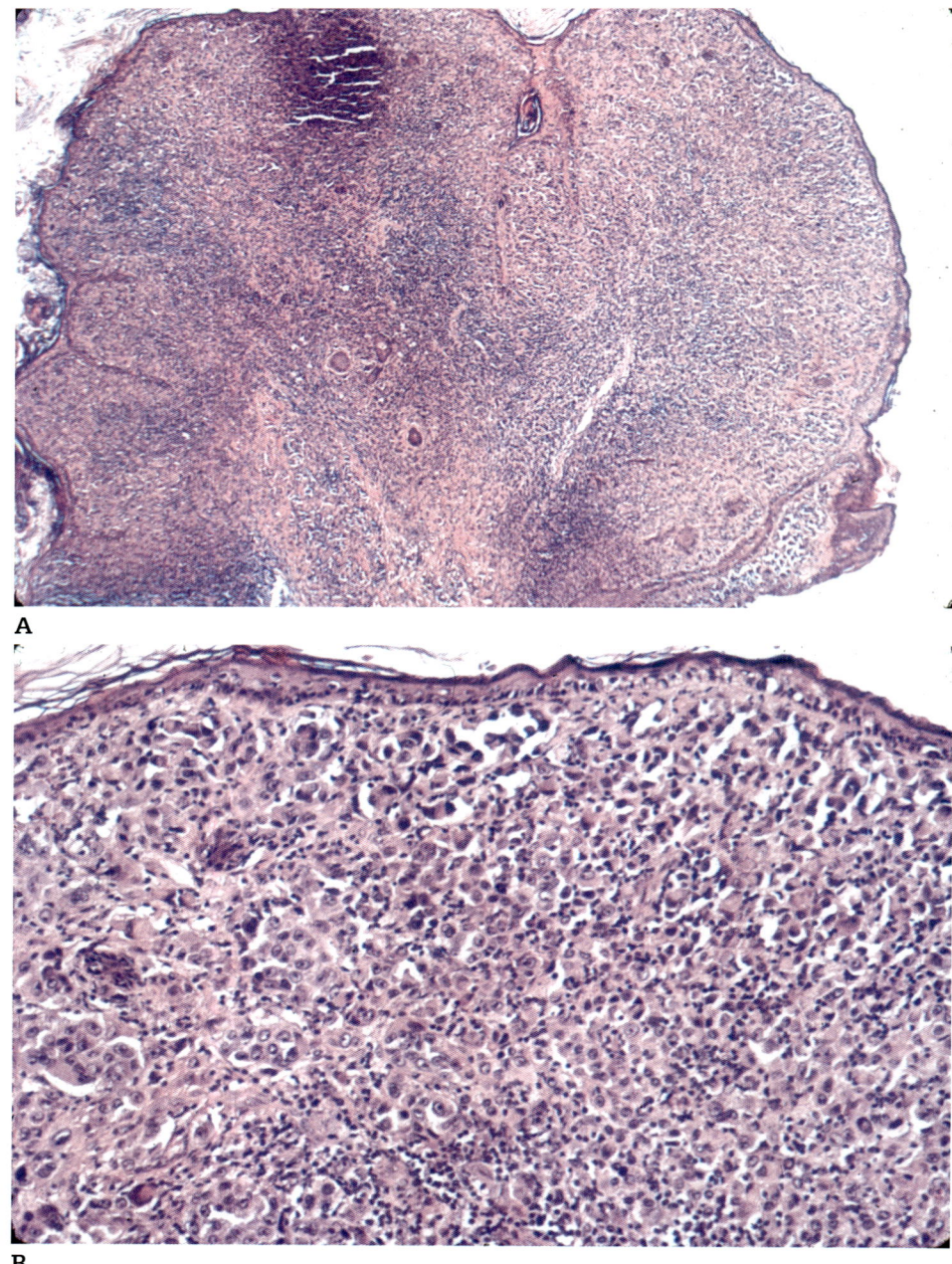

FIGURE 10-14 Predominately nodular form of melanoma. **A,** This tumor has a polypoid configuration with virtually all of the tumor above the horizontal plane of the epidermis. **B,** Note the effacement and general sparing of epidermis. Such melanomas must be distinguished from metastases.

believe that this risk is almost certainly related to the degree of atypicality of the SIMP lesion present and whether unequivocal melanoma in situ is present. The presence of the melanoma in situ would presumably increase the risk for the development of invasive melanoma. Rapid progression to invasive melanoma from lesions designated as lentigo maligna has been documented to occur in a matter of months (121,122).

Clinical Features

The solar melanomas are primarily defined by their clinical attributes (Table 10-13). The clinical lesion often be-

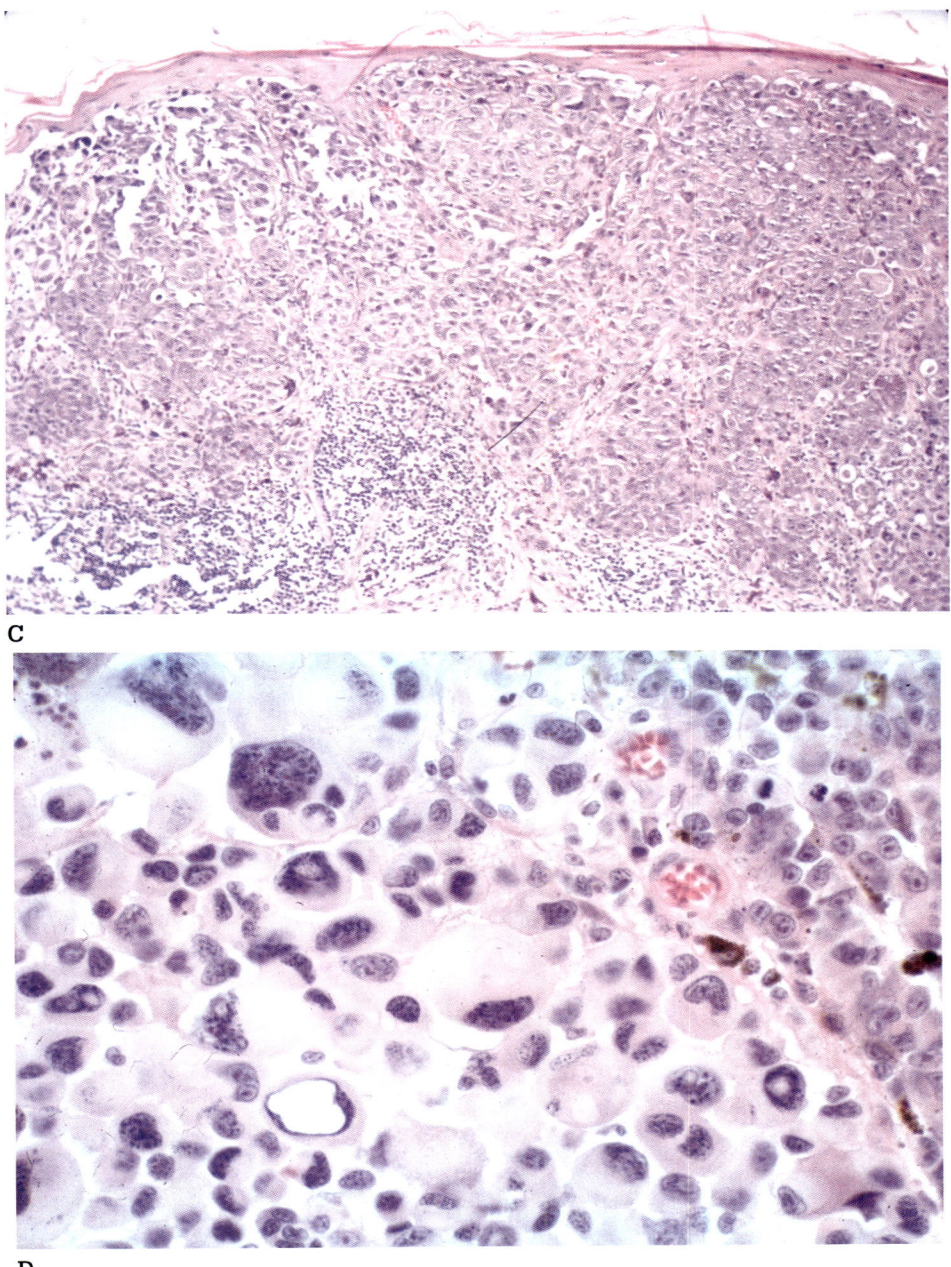

FIGURE 10-14 *Continued.* **C,** Typical nests of epithelioid cells in the dermis. **D,** Anaplastic melanoma cells present.

gins as a tan macule, as small as 2 mm but sometimes attaining diameters of 3 cm or more, while remaining noninvasive (43,44,66). One generally observes the progressive development of shades of brown, flecks of black, and a uniform black color superimposed on the tan background. The latter color changes are generally accompanied by increasing asymmetry, diameter of the lesion, irregularity of borders and often at the same time regression of another portion of the lesion (63). Increasing complexity of color with shades of blue, gray, and white often ensue and indicate pigment incontinence in the dermis and regression. The development of palpable foci usually connote invasion. Uncommon lesions may exhibit little or no pigmentation and hence are amelanotic; a high index of suspicion is clearly needed to diagnose melanoma in the latter circum-

TABLE 10-13 Solar melanoma.

Clinical features
- 60–70 years
- Men = women
- Sun-exposed surfaces: cheek (most common), nose, forehead, ears, neck, dorsal surfaces of hands
- 0.2–20 cm
- Initial tan macule, suggesting a varnish-like stain
- Tan, brown, black macule or patch (black flecks characterisitic) (early lesions)
- Pink, gray, white with progression and areas of regression
- Papule or nodule, pigmented or amelanotic (advanced, often but not always)
- Ulceration, bleeding
- Asymmetry
- Irregular, notched borders

Histopathologic features
- Effacement and thinning of epidermis, common
- Prominent solar elastosis
- Solar intraepidermal melanocytic proliferation (lentigo maligna)
    - Solar intraepidermal melanocytic proliferation (insufficient for melanoma in situ)
        - Lentiginous melanocytic proliferation
        - Pleomorphic melanocytes (variable cytological atypia)
        - Occasional extension of melanocytic proliferation downward along appendages
        - Absence of nesting and pagetoid spread, usually
    - Melanoma in situ
        - Contiguous or near contiguous lentiginous melanocytic proliferation
        - Intraepidermal nesting of melanocytes
        - Pagetoid spread
        - Promient extension of melanocytic proliferation downward along appendages, often with nesting
        - Significant cytologic atypia
        - Melanocytes somewhat spindled to increasingly epithelioid
- Pigmented spindle cell variant (often on ears)
    - Prominent intraepidermal discohesive nesting of atypical spindle cells
    - Spindle cells often comprise invasive component but polygonal, small cells common
- Appendage-associated nesting of atypical melanocytes suggests invasion and may be florid (not true invasion)
- Partial regression relatively common
- Precursor nevus present (~ 3% of cases)
- Desmoplasia, neurotropism, angiotropism common

Differential diagnosis
- Solar lentigo
- Solar melanocytic hyperplasia (photoactivation)
    - De novo
    - Occurrence with nevi, fibrous papule, basal cell carcinoma, actinic keratosis, etc.
- Atypical intraepidermal melanocytic proliferation, not otherwise specified
- Solar lentiginous junctional or compound melanocytic nevi with or without atypia (may overlap atypical nevi)
- Pigmented spindle cell nevus
- Pigmented actinic keratosis
- Squamous cell carcinoma, spindle cell type
- Atypical fibroxanthoma
- Cellular neurothekeoma
- Malignant peripheral nerve sheath tumor
- Angiosarcoma
- Kaposi sarcoma
- Leiomyosarcoma

stance. Although precise data are lacking, an invasive component may develop in approximately 5–30% of solar melanomas (120) and is often a black, raised focus or pink (amelanotic) tumor.

Histopathologic Features

The solar melanomas are first of all defined by their occurrence on the most sun-exposed surfaces and by the histologic presence in almost all cases of prominent solar elastosis (Table 10-13). They present histologically in two patterns: (a) most commonly as a lentiginous melanocytic proliferation, historically termed lentigo maligna (Figs. 10-15 and 10-16), and (b) much less commonly as a intraepidermal nested proliferation of pigmented spindled melanocytes, resembling pigmented spindle nevus (Fig. 10-17). The nature of lentigo maligna, as previously discussed, has been controversial since many consider it to be a spectrum of melanocytic lesions, including a precursor to melanoma and melanoma in situ; on the other hand, others believe that all such lesions are melanoma in situ. One particular reason for this is that the concept of melanoma in situ is a recent development, whereas the clinicopathologic entities of Hutchinson's melanotic freckle and lentigo malins des viellards (later la melanose circonstrite precancereuse de Dubreuilh) were described long before before the modern-day attempts to define criteria for in situ melanoma. Thus, until recently, authors have generally made no effort to define the threshold criteria for lentigo maligna versus a solar lentigo or melanoma in situ in this context versus lentiginous melanocytic proliferations with atypia. We clearly hold the former position that lentigo maligna constitutes a spectrum of lesions (Table 10-9).

Lentiginous Melanocytic Proliferations with Some Degree of Atypicality That Fall Short of Melanoma In Situ This spectrum of the SIMPs includes the the following features: (a) an increased number of basilar melanocytes that are either cytologically normal or pleomorphic (see detailed discussion above) (66) (Fig. 10-9C; Table 10-9), (b) solar elastosis, (c) atrophy and effacement of the epidermis (Fig. 10-9A), (d) extension down appendageal structures by the melanocytic proliferation (9,10,66,74) (Fig. 10-9C,D), (e) a variably atypical population of melanocytes (the atypia can be graded, if present, as slight, moderate, or severe), and (f) absence of intraepidermal nesting and appreciable pagetoid spread.

Melanoma In Situ In addition to criteria b, c, and d listed above, melanoma in situ includes one or more of the following g, h, i, and j: (g) contiguous lentiginous melanocytic proliferation, (h) nesting of melanocytes, (i) pagetoid spread of individual or nests of melanocytes, and (j) more significant and uniformly appearing cytologic atypia of melanocytes compared to the first group of lesions. The latter features involving at least a single high-power field ($\times 400$) constitute the minimal essential criteria for a diagnosis of solar melanoma in situ (Figs. 10-1, 10-7, and 10-15).

Other features that are useful in recognizing this coterie of lesions are irregular distribution of pigment in the epidermis, multinucleate melanocytic giant cells, and lymphocytic infiltrates in the dermis. The multinucleate giant cells with peripherally arranged nuclei in a wreathlike pattern have been termed "starburst" cells; they are commonly observed but are not unique to solar melanomas and their precursor lesions (71,72).

The evolution of such lesions is typified by increasing frequency of basilar melanocytes and the development of nests of cells with diminished cohesion (Figs. 10-1, 10-7, and 10-15). There may be extensive involvement of appendageal epithelium in some cases, with large cellular nests (Fig. 10-15D,E). Recognition of prominent appendageal involvement by SM, or any melanoma, is of critical importance so that the lesion is not misdiagnosed as invasive melanoma rather than simply as an intraepithelial or in situ component. One of the most difficult problems associated with SM is undoubtedly the distinction of invasive tumor from both intraepidermal and appendageal intraepithelial nests of melanoma cells. Serial sections may aid in resolving this dilemma. With progression of LM (SIMP) to true melanoma in situ, there is a tendency for upward migration of cells and eventually to microinvasion of the papillary dermis (Fig. 10-15). The cell type present in this spectrum of lesions is heterogenous. One commonly observes a melanocyte with retracted cytoplasm; and often elongate, stellate, or spindled configuration (32,34); and a high nuclear/cytoplasmic ratio (Fig. 10-7). The nuclei are commonly pleomorphic and hyperchromatic (Fig. 10.9E,F). With progression, the cells become more epithelioid in and exhibit nuclear enlargement and prominent nucleoli. Epidermal hyperplasia may also be encountered in the latter context.

Pigmented Spindle Cell Variant of Solar Melanoma

A characteristic and uncommon variant of SM already mentioned is composed of confluent fascicles of pigmented spindle cells along the dermoepidermal junction and involves appendages (Fig. 10-17) (37). The lesions may be fairly well circumscribed but often show some asymmetry, limited pagetoid spread, and cytologic atypia.

Extension of SM into the dermis may be difficult to recognize because of the sometimes subtle nature of the

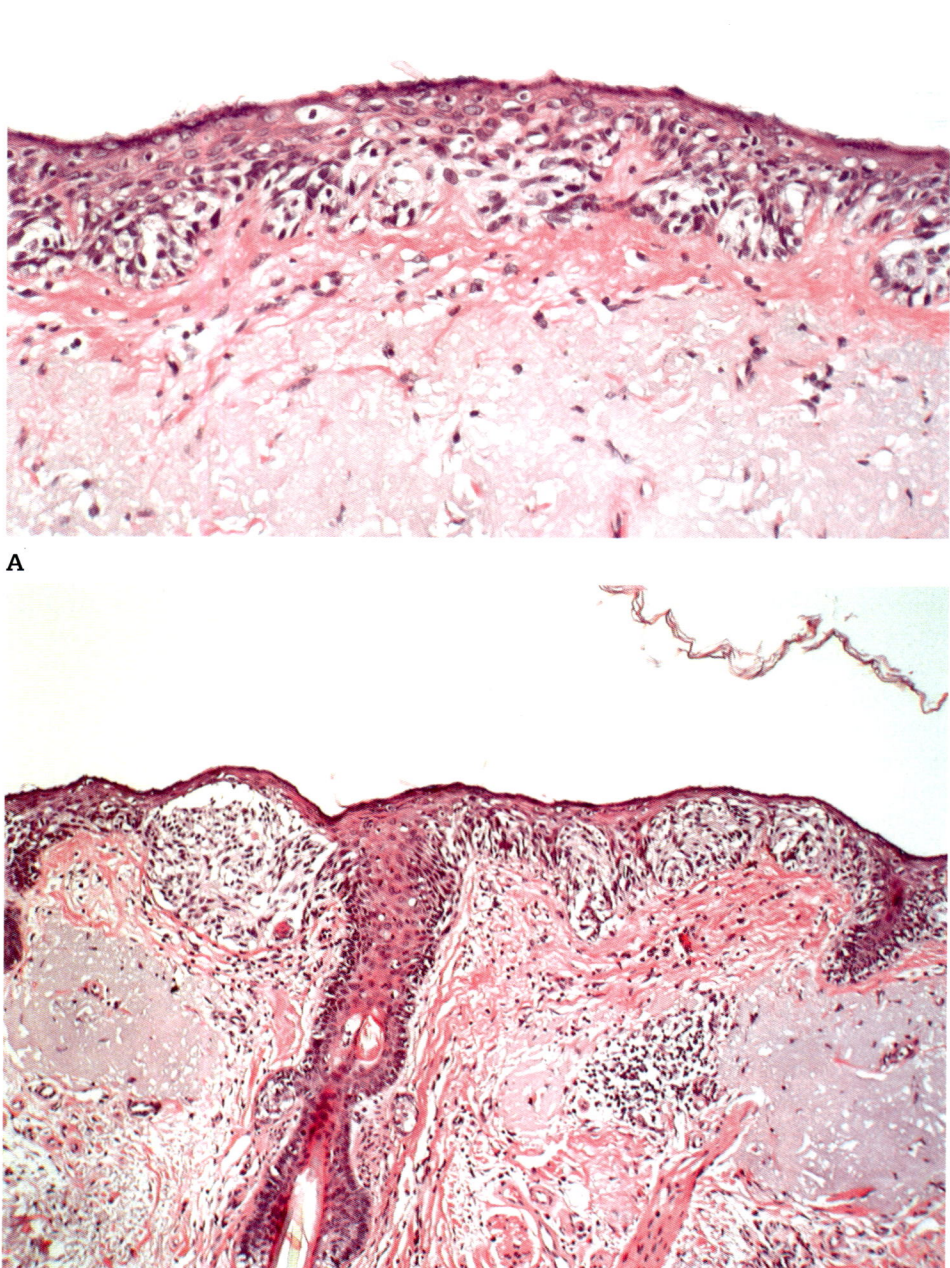

FIGURE 10-15 Solar melanoma. **A,** Advanced solar melanoma in situ showing epidermis effacement and confluent nesting of atypical melanocytes along the basilar portion of the epidermis. **B,** Note the large nests of melanocytes replacing the epidermis in this advanced melanoma in situ.

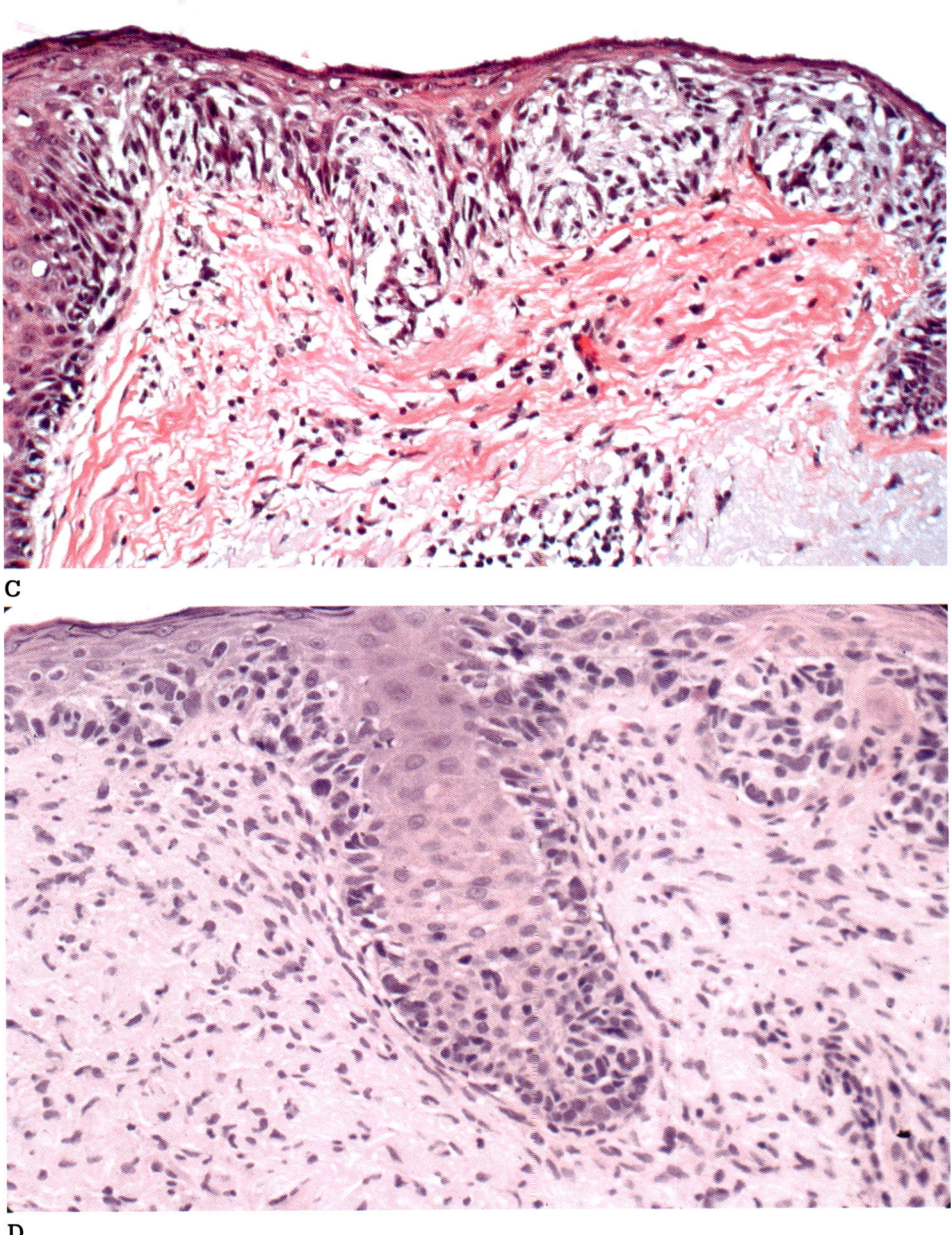

FIGURE 10-15 *Continued.* **C,** Note the large nests of melanocytes replacing the epidermis in this advanced melanoma in situ. **D,** There is a striking basilar proliferation of variably atypical melanocytes in both the epidermis and the follicular epithelium.

cytologic atypia of invasive melanocytes, prominent cellularity of the stroma, and activation of mesenchymal cells (Fig. 10-15F,G). The invasive dermal component of SM is frequently composed of spindle cells, either occurring singly or in bundles (Fig. 10-16) (66), with varying stromal desmoplasia and invasion of nerve twigs (see desmoplastic melanoma). Invasion of the dermis may originate from appendageal-associated melanoma cells or nests. In the latter instances, depth of invasion (Breslow thickness) should not be measured from the granular layer of the epidermis, since this value would overestimate tumor depth. The measurement of tumor thickness instead should ideally be taken from the granular layer of the hair follicle or sweat gland. The stromal response usually in-

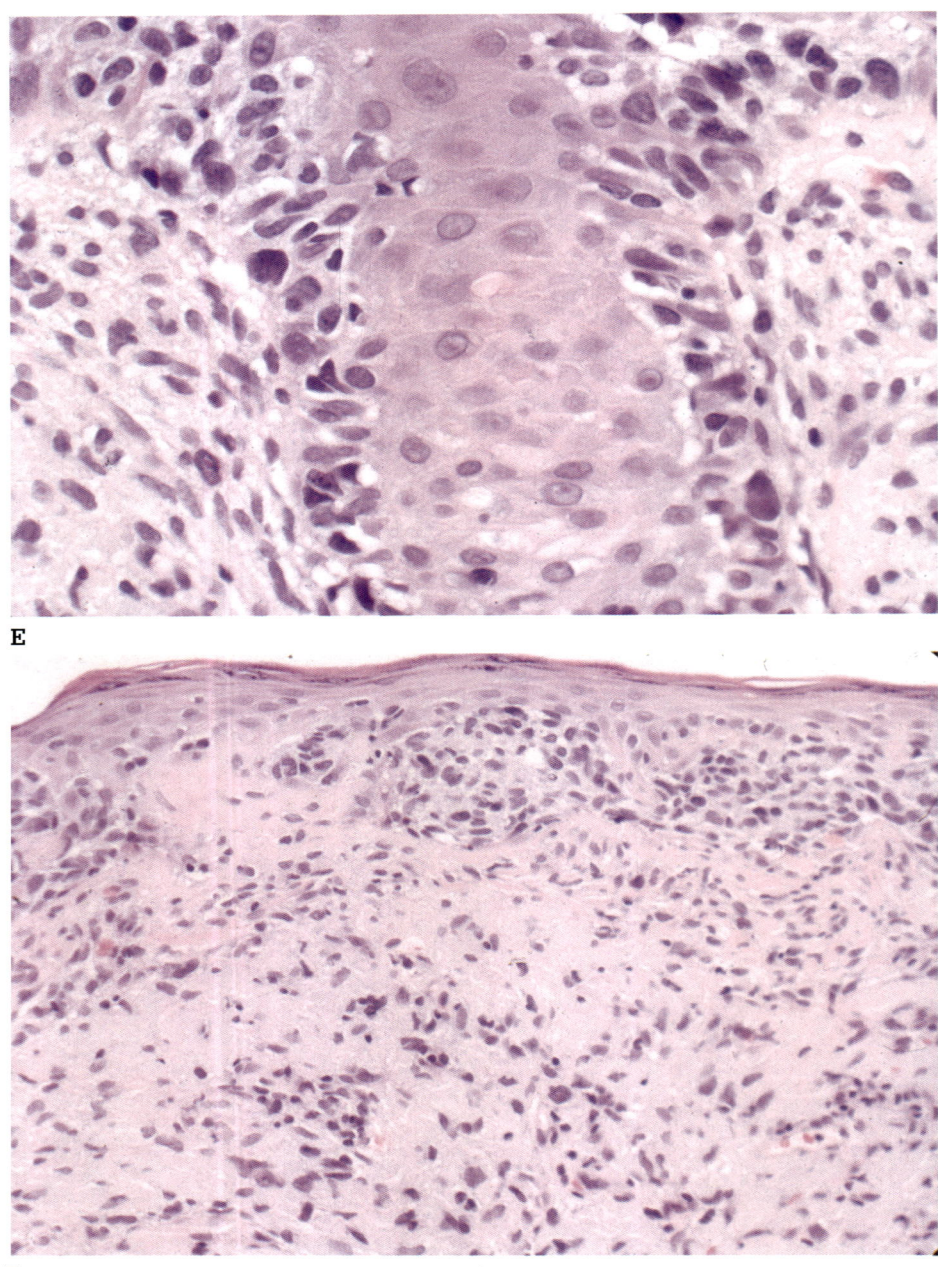

FIGURE 10-15 *Continued.* **E,** Higher magnification of panel D showing prominent involvement of a hair follicle by the atypical proliferation of melanocytes. Note the highly pleomorphic and hyperchromatic character of the nuclei. **F,** Confluent nesting of melanoma cells along the dermoepidermal junction. Invasive melanoma cells are also present throughout the papillary dermis.

cludes lymphocytic infiltrates, prominent vascularity, and melanin-containing macrophages.

The invasive component SM may also be comprised of any cell type including epithelioid cells and small nevuslike cells.

Differential Diagnosis

Lentigo maligna (SIMP) and solar melanoma must be distinguished from solar lentigo (SL), lentiginous nevi of sun-damaged skin, pigmented seborrheic keratosis, melanoacanthoma, atypical (dysplastic) nevus, pig-

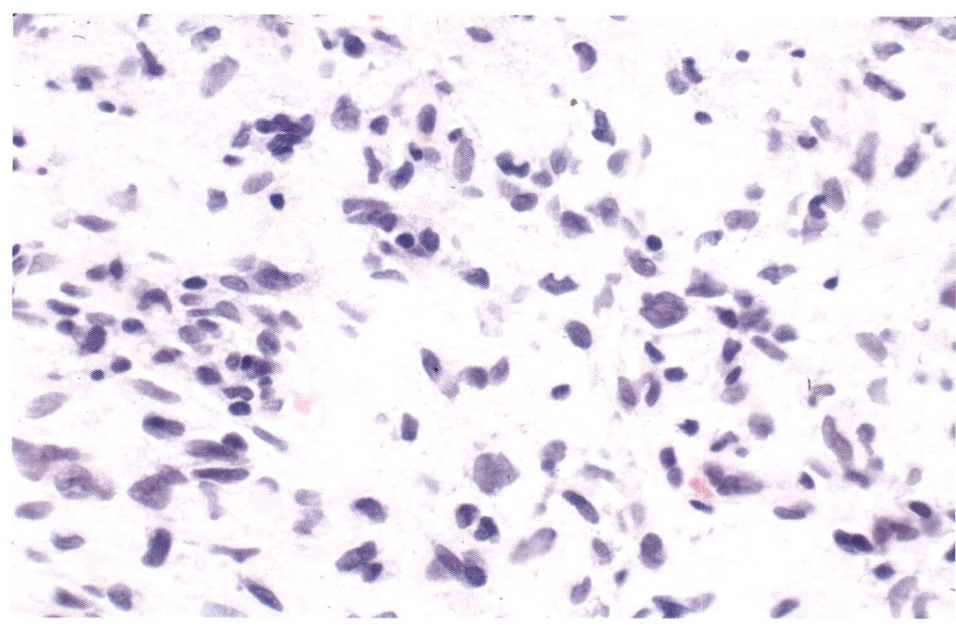

FIGURE 10-15 *Continued.* **G,** Higher magnification of panel F showing invasive melanoma cells dispersed somewhat haphazardly in the solar elastosis. The tumor cells display high nuclear to cytoplasmic ratios and prominent nuclear pleomorphism.

mented spindle cell nevus, and the melanocytic hyperplasia (or melanocytosis) occurring in chronically sun-damaged skin either alone or associated with melanocytic nevi or other neoplasms, such as pigmented actinic keratoisi, basal cell carcinoma or angiofibroma, and other forms of melanoma (Tables 10-9 and 10-13). Finally, one must keep in mind the rare occurrence of concomitant atypical melanocytic proliferation and SM and other tumors, such as actinic keratosis, squamous cell carcinoma, and basal cell carcinoma.

Solar Lentigo and Lentiginous Melanocytic Nevi

Lentigo maligna (SIMP) may in fact develop from some varieties of solar lentigines and solar lentiginous melanocytic nevi. Solar lentigines are usually characterized by small size (often < 3–4 mm), elongated peglike epidermal rete but not always, a uniform pattern of melanin pigmentation of the epidermis, the lack of or possibly an increased frequency of basilar melanocytes (but not as great as that seen in SIMP), the lack of extension of melanocytes down adnexal structures, generally no junctional nesting of melanocytes, and little or no cytologic atypia. On the other hand, atypical lentiginous proliferations of melanocytes in sun-damaged skin, including fully-developed SM, are often larger than SL (but not necessarily so), often show effacement of the epidermal rete (thus lack elongated epidermal rete, but there are exceptions), show uneven patterns of epidermal pigmentation, often demonstrate proliferation of melanocytes along the adnexal structures, commonly have nesting of melanocytes in proliferations consonant with melanoma in situ, show a consistently increased frequency of basilar melanocytes (often > 15 melanocytes/0.5 mm), have some degree of pagetoid spread, and display cytologic atypia of melanocytes.

It is clear with experience that there are some lesions that are difficult to place in one category or the other. The latter group of lesions is most likely made up of SL that are indeterminate or incipient neoplasias. Such lesions should be adequately sampled, since they may show heterogeneity and therefore one should not miss areas with more advanced atypia. Because of frequent heterogeneity there should be clear communication with clinicians about the level of concern for an individual lesion. Complete removal may be prudent, so that such difficult lesions are sufficiently sampled.

Solar lentiginous melanocytic nevi may likewise enter into the differential diagnosis and much of the same discussion applies to this group of lesions as for SL. Both junctional and compound variants are observed. Commonly, these lesions are also characterized by elongated epidermal rete with lentiginous melanocytic hyperplasia and junctional nests localized to the lower-most poles of the rete. The junctional nests in these nevi are usually well

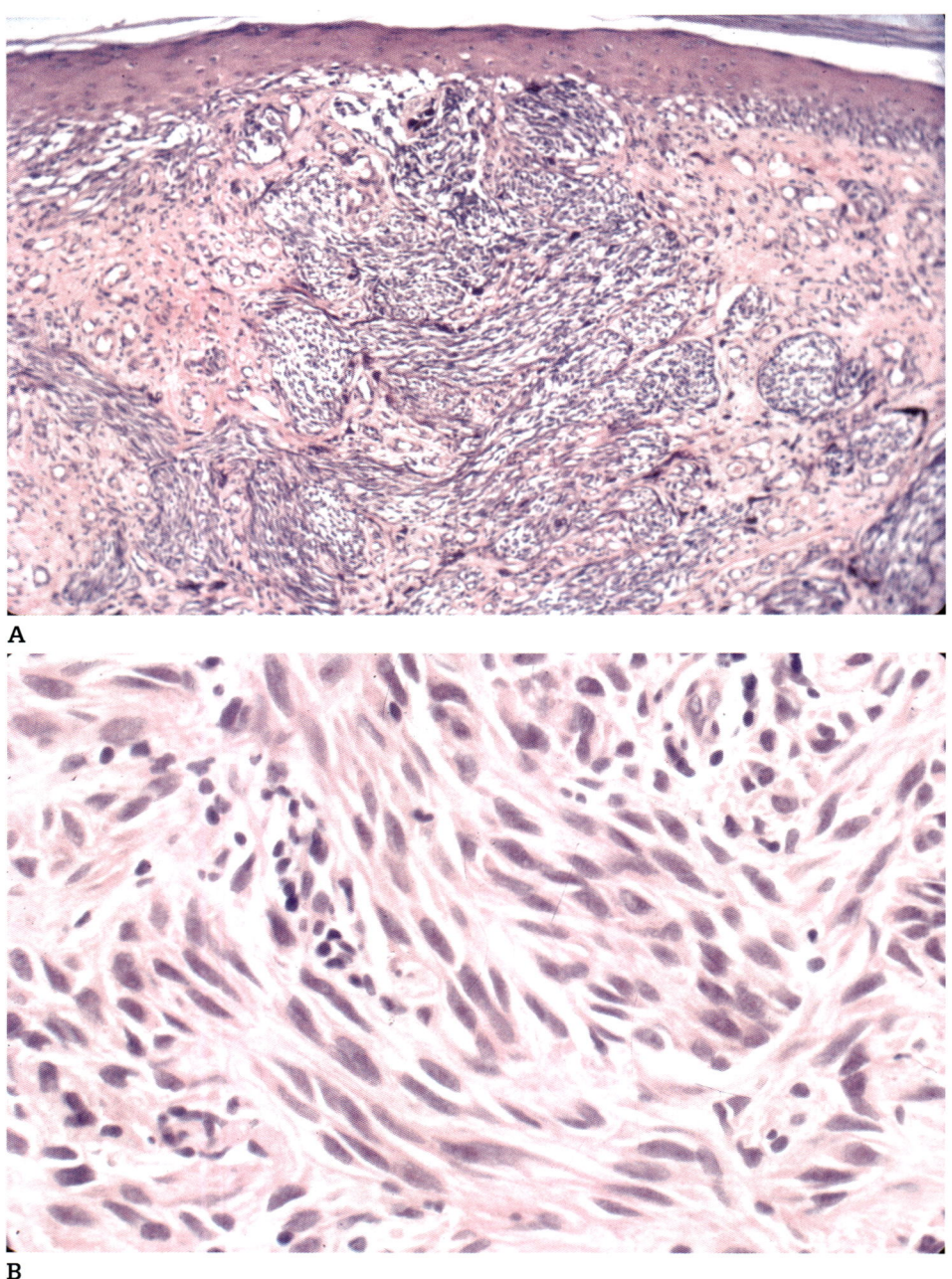

FIGURE 10-16 The invasive component of solar melanoma commonly consists of bundles of monomorphous spindle cells, as noted in these fields.

defined, equidistant, and usually of fairly similar size and shape, versus the more irregular and haphazard nesting observed in SM. The other features mentioned above for SL usually allow for distinction from SM. Nonetheless, as mentioned for SL, there are a minority of lesions that occupy a gray area and must be managed with caution and carefully sampled for more significant atypicality; the patients must be followed.

Pigmented Spindle Cell Nevus Well-differentiated forms of solar melanoma with spindle cells may cause confusion with PSCN. Typical PSCN usually involves covered skin and commonly occurs in children and young adults (37,53); whereas SM invariably develops in sun-exposed skin and usually in older persons. An effaced epidermis, cellular nests with diminished cohesion, and a prominent basilar single cell proliferation of markedly atypical spin-

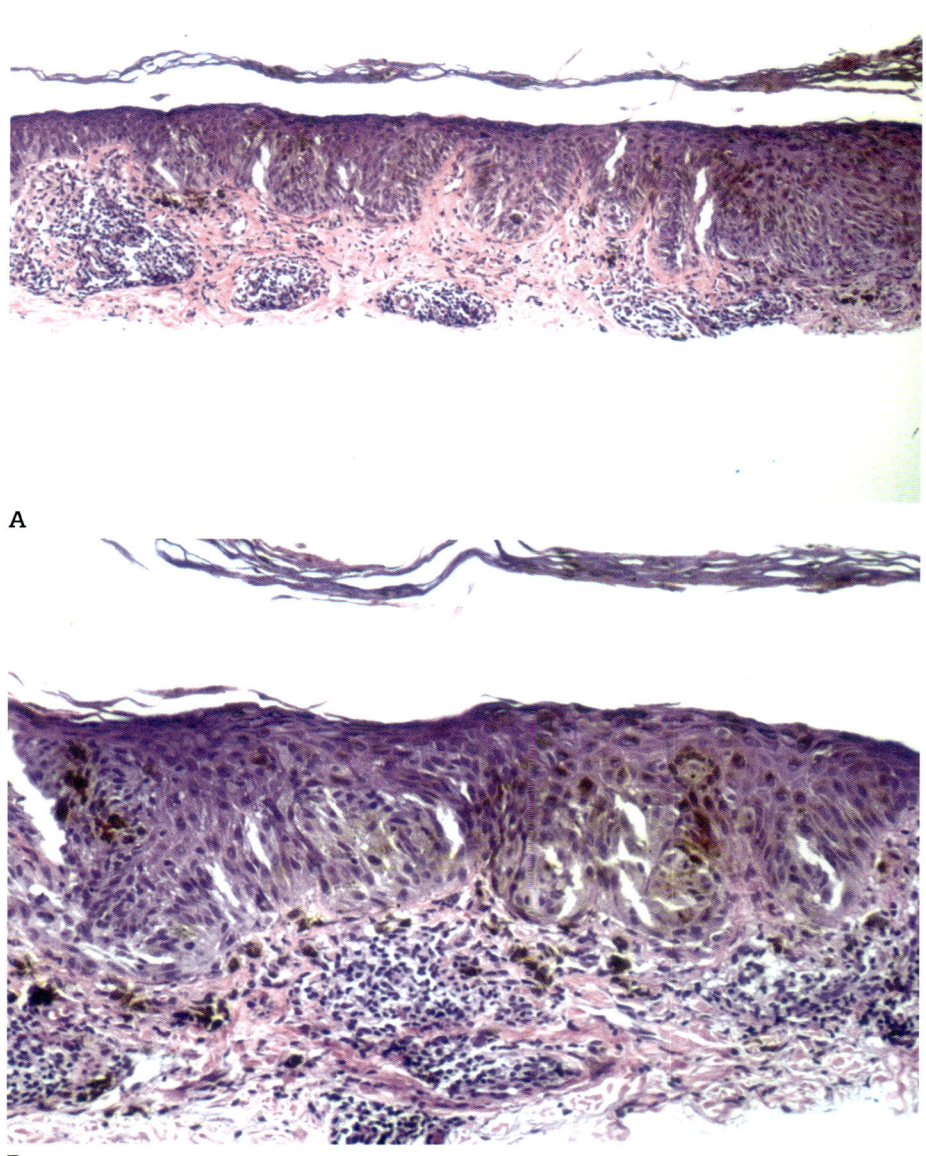

FIGURE 10-17 Solar melanoma, pigmented spindle cell variant. **A,** Intraepidermal proliferation of pigmented spindle cells in nests mimicking PSCN. **B,** Although the lesion is composed of pigmented spindle cells, the pattern of intraepidermal nesting is more asymmetrical and irregular versus a conventional PSCN.

dle cells argue in favor of SM. PSCN are usually well circumscribed with well-formed, orderly, and regular fascicles of pigmented spindle cells. Epidermal hyperplasia usually encountered in PSCN contrasts with the atrophy of SM. Cytologically, PSCN is usually composed of monotonous fusiform cells with nuclei containing delicate chromatin. Nonetheless, atypical varieties of PSCN may show considerable overlap with SM.

Solar melanoma may exhibit epithelioid cells with some upward migration through the epidermis, suggesting pagetoid melanoma. Careful evaluation of such tumors will usually disclose a predominance of basilar melanocytic

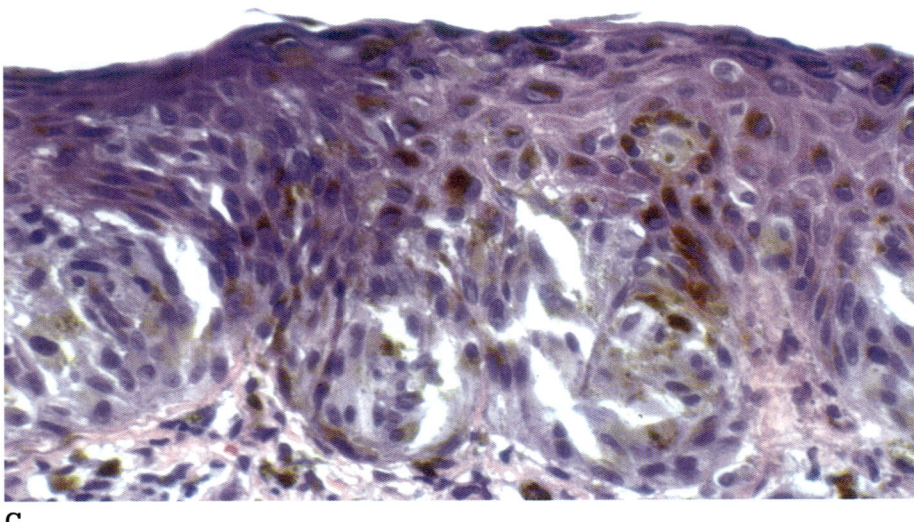

FIGURE 10-17 *Continued.* **C,** Both melanomas of this type and PSCN may exhibit pagetoid spread.

cells, effacement of the epidermis, marked solar elastosis, and prominent involvement of skin appendages.

Solar Melanocytic Hyperplasia; Melanocytic Hyperplasia of Chronically Sun-Exposed Skin; Melanocytosis of Chronically Sun-Exposed Skin; Chronic Sun Damage The distinction of melanocytic hyperplasia of chronically sun-damaged skin—termed here solar melanocytic hyperplasia (SMH)—from true solar intraepidermal melanocytic neoplasias encompassing lentiginous melanocytic proliferations with varying degress of atypia and melanoma in situ (formerly lentigo maligna) and solar melanoma is one of the most challenging problems in all of melanoma pathology. Before proceeding further, SMH is defined as an increase in the number of single basilar melanocytes, nuclear enlargement and pleomorphism of melanocytes is commonly present, solar elastosis, and a pigmented lesion that may or may not be present clinically (74,77,123,124). It has been established that the number of basilar melanocytes is directly related to cumulative sun exposure and that chronically sun-exposed skin has an approximate twofold increase in the number of basilar melanocytes (123).

The practical problem of SMH is principally encountered in the following situations: the distinction of SMH from SIMP in general and in the special circumstance of assessing the peripheral margins of SIMP and the distinction of SMH from SIMP occurring in association with melanocytic nevi, angiofibromas (125), and other neoplasia (such as basal cell carcinoma). When approaching the problem of SMH versus solar intraepidermal melanocytic neoplasia, one must realize that both are related to cumulative sun exposure, probably have some relationship, and are almost certainly part of a continuum. For example, in studies of SIMP (lentigo maligna) it is clear that one may encounter lentiginous melanocytic proliferations (LMP) with little or no cytological atypia along side LMP with atypia (66). Thus in some circumstances SMH and SIMP may be histologically indistinguishable, and one must have information about the clinical lesion to differentiate the two processes. However, there is still the problem that SMH may rarely be a precursor to SIMP. Therefore, it must be acknowledged that not all such melanocytic proliferations can be easily categorized as SMH or as SIMP (see below).

Based on the definition of SMH mentioned above, it is clear that one needs criteria beyond that of lentiginous melanocytic hyperplasia and low-grade cytologic atypia of melanocytes to recognize SIMP reliably. The following criteria, particularly when observed with increasing frequency correlate with SIMP (74): (a) nests of (clusters of three or more) melanocytes in a solar intraepidermal melanocytic proliferation almost always indicate melanoma in situ, (b) pagetoid spread generally indicates melanoma in situ, (c) significantly increased numbers of (> 15 and especially > 25 melanocytes/0.5 mm of basal layer) and contiguous basilar melanocytes have a high correlation with SIMP, (d) significant cytologic atypia (nuclear enlargement, pleomorphism, variation in chromatin patterns, and prominent nucleoli) clearly correlates with SIMP and uniform atypia of increasingly epithelioid melanocytes with melanoma in situ, (e) melanocytes extending down adnexal structures generally correlate with SIMP, (f) irregular distribution of melanin is seen in the epidermis, (g) often a high nuclear to cytoplasic ratio of melanocytes suggests SIMP (125), and (h) prominent dendrites of melanocytes (reaching the upper third of the malpighian layer) are rare but fairly specific for SIMP (74). Clinical criteria must also be closely considered as well, especially size and abnormal gross morphologic features. Other methodologies—including nuclear morphometry (77) and immunostaining with markers such as HMB-45 and Ki-67 (for proliferation rate)—provide additional information but are of little practical value in this situation (74). No single criterion when viewed alone can be construed as entirely specific for SIMP; however, with the accumulation of the latter features one can confidently diagnose SIMP. After a comprehensive assessment of all information available, the pathologist should be able to place a lesion into one of three categories: SMH, SIMP/SM, or intraepidermal melanocytic proliferation or lesion possibly with atypia, not otherwise specified. We reserve the third category for lesions defying unequivocable classification until more information becomes available.

The interpretation of surgical margins for SIMP continues to be a major challenge to the histopathologist. Although the latter discourse on SMH vs. SIMP also applies just as much to this subject, there are a few additional considerations that are relevant to this specific context. It is well established that the peripheries of SIMP may be poorly defined and may extend as far as 3–10 cm beyond the clinically defined margins of the lesion (74,77). However, additional confounders entering into this assessment of surgical margins besides that of SMH include a potential "field effect" from melanoma itself and a reactive intraepidermal melanocytic hyperplasia from a previous surgical procedure. The biologic nature and significance of a so-called field effect from melanoma has never been adequately explained. However, studies examining the peripheral intraepidermal component of acral melanoma with fluorescence in situ hybridization (FISH) suggest that the field effect could be neoplastic (126). Furthermore, since some portions of well-documented SIMP (LM) may demonstate LMP with little or no melanocytic atypia, such peripheral LMP associated with SIMP must be considered potentially neoplastic until proved otherwise (66). The melanocytic hyperplasia associated with a previous surgical procedure is usually (but not always) confined to the area above a scar and usually is limited in nature.

The other major factors to consider when interpreting surgical margins are that diagnostic features of SIMP may not be present at the peripheries of the lesion, and often one has only limited tissue to examine. Thus, for example, intraepidermal nesting of melanocytes is often absent at the peripheries of SIMP. In this instance, the most helpful features include significantly increased numbers of melanocytes (e.g., > 25 melanocytes/0.5 mm), any pagetoid spread, and significant cytologic atypia of melanocytes for interpreting a margin as positive (74). Probably the most significant criterion for a negative margin is a rapid decline in numbers of melanocytes as one approaches the margin.

Particular lesions of chronically sun-exposed skin may exhibit atypical intraepidermal melanocytic proliferation that may closely mimic if not be identical to SIMP (74,77). We believe this type of proliferation to be closely related to if not the same as SMH. However, these proliferations differ from conventional SMH, since they develop in association with compound or dermal nevi, fibrous papules, basal cell carcinomas, actinic keratoses, and other tumors. Thus there may be other factors operative in the pathogenesis of these atypical hyperplasias in addition to sunlight. Especially in the case of nevi, other external insults such as physical or chemical trauma may result in reactive hyperplasias analgous to that observed in the recurrent/persistent melanocytic nevus.

The histologic findings generally include lentiginous melanocytic hyperplasia possibly contiguous and variable cytologic atypia of melanocytes; however, other features (such as nesting of melanocytes, involvement of adnexal structures, and some pagetoid spread) may strongly suggest SIMP. The latter constellation of findings commonly overlies an otherwise conventional dermal nevus or fibrous papule of the central face, generally removed without significant clinical concern. The frequency of these changes have not been clearly established, except in the case of fibrous papules. Among 150 fibrous papules 7% demonstrated these atypical findings (125). Helpful distinguishing features are that these proliferations are clearly associated with another distinct lesion and they are almost always confined to the epidermis overlying the lesion and, therefore, are well circumstribed and of small diameter, particularly in the case of dermal nevi and fibrous papules; in contrast SIMP is usually more extensive and poorly defined. Other features favoring an atypical SMH over SIMP are lower cellular density and variable cytologic atypia of melanocytes, lower nuclear to cytoplasmic ratios, and occasional large melanocytes that are Spitz like and sometimes multinucleate (125). One must keep in mind the possibility of SIMP being present as an independent process or "collision" tumor. It is not possible to categorize all such atypical proliferations as reactive or neoplastic; thus the term intraepidermal melanocytic proliferation or lesion, not otherwise specified, with or without atypia is appropriate.

It is important to ensure that all such proliferations are fully examined and sampled histopathologically and all relevant clinical information compiled.

ACRAL MELANOMA (PALMAR-PLANTAR MELANOMA, VOLAR-SUBUNGUAL MELANOMA)

Acral melanoma (AM) may be strictly defined as any melanoma arising on glabrous or volar (non-hair-bearing) skin of the soles, palms, and digits and also from the nail apparatus (22,32,34,81–102). Although the latter anatomic domains are indeed unique, the latter definition is difficult to adhere to since glabrous and nonglabrous skin merge imperceptibly; therefore, some proportion of acral melanomas will involve both glabrous and nonglabrous skin; in addition, some authors have included melanomas of the dorsal skin of the hands and feet as AM. Nonetheless, as discussed here, acral melanomas are strictly defined as involving only glabrous skin or the nail apparatus of the distal extremities. 85% of AM involve volar (palms, soles, and digits) surfaces versus 15% arising from the nail apparatus (subungual areas). Among AM, almost 90% occur on the foot with the following distibution: soles, 68–71%; toes, 11%; subungual areas of the feet, 9–10%; palms, 4%–10%; fingers, 2%; and subungual areas of the hands, 5.6–10% (86). In addition to these topographic considerations, patients with AM are generally older (e.g., commonly 60–70 years of age), have particular histopathologic findings, and may have a different biologic basis compared to other melanomas. There seem to be no clear differences in frequency between men and women. Although rare among white populations (range 1–13.5%), AM is the most frequent form of melanoma among Asians (29–46%), Africans (60–70%), and other ethnic groups of color (22,32) (Table 10-14). However, it should be emphasized that AM has approximately the same incidence in all ethnic groups (92). Reed and co-workers (83,84) first recognized that melanomas involving glabrous skin of the soles may feature a rather characteristic pattern of lentiginous intraepidermal melanocytic proliferation. However, pagetoid and nested intraepidermal patterns of melanocytes are also frequently present (94,101).

The cause of AM is poorly understood among the various subtypes of melanoma, as sunlight would not seem to be a risk factor. The role of precursor lesions in the cause of AM has received considerable attention but requires further study because of the rarity of these melanomas and the lack of longitudinal studies (89,104,127,128). Melanocytic nevi may possibly account for a small numberof AM (104), since a nevus remnant is observed in 10–13% of AM, compared to about 30% in conventional melanomas from all other sites (22). The description of pigmented macules on the sole (including some termed atypical melanosis) raises the possibility of another perhaps more frequent precursor lesion to AM (127,128). Lewis and Johnson (127) suggested that plantar melanomas in Africans may have some association with the rather common lentiginous lesions occurring on the soles in these populations. Lentiginous macular lesions on volar surfaces vary with respect to size and gross morphologic features. In addition to simple lentigines and nevi, such lesions may show considerable latitude in the features present with alterations ranging from slight lentiginous or intraepidermal melanocytic proliferation with little or no atypia, to lesions with clearly increased lentiginous or intraepidermal melanocytic proliferation and variable nesting and atypia of melanocytes, and finally to lesions with all of the latter alterations but also including well-developed pagetoid spread, nesting, and significant cytological atypia. The fact that the intraepidermal component of AM early on or at it peripheries may show minimal or variable atypia suggests a relationship to or origin from such lentiginous macular lesions. Suffice it to say careful, longitudinal studies are needed on the matter of precursors to AM.

The association of AM with weight-bearing areas of the foot: the heels, metatarsal areas, and toes (a much higher incidence) compared to the palms has long suggested that trauma may be a factor in the cause of AM (86). Whereas the justification for distinguishing AM from other conventional melanomas has been questioned, recent studies examining chromosomal aberrations in AM with comparative genetic hybridization and FISH suggest that this subgroup may possess distinctive properties (126). In particular, a group of 15 AM had significantly greater numbers of gene amplifications compared to a similar number of pagetoid (superficial spreading) melanomas. It is also of interest that such amplifications were present in AM in situ and in melanocytes up to 3 mm distant from the clinical lesion, suggesting the early development of such genetic alterations in AM. Viruses and chemical carcinogens have also been suggested as possible causal agents for AM.

Clinical Features

Acral melanoma usually evolves through an intraepidermal macular phase, characterized by increasing size, irregularity of borders, and variegation of color (22,44, 84–86) (Table 10-14). The macular phase often has a predominant dark brown to jet black color but may be lighter brown or even tan in some instances. The latter growth phase is often less variable compared to conventional melanomas at other sites. One may also observe depigmented and gray areas indicative of regression. The borders may be highly irregular with notching. The greatest

TABLE 10-14 Acral melanoma.

Clinical features
  60–70 years
  Men = women
  Equal incidence in all racial groups
  Most prevalent form of melanoma in Africans, Asians, Native Americans, other peoples of color
  Glabrous (volar) skin and nail unit
    Palms, soles, digits (85%)
    Nail unit (15%)
  Feet (90% of cases)
    Soles (68–71%)
    Toes (11%)
    Nail units (16–20%)
    Palms (4–10%)
    Fingers (2%)
  0.3–15 cm
    ≥ 0.7 cm, often
    < 0.7 cm with irregular borders, color, or "parallel ridge" pattern on epiluminescence microscopy
  Often jet-black macule early, but also tan, brown, gray, blue, pink, white
  Pigmented or amelanotic papule or nodule (advanced) with ulceration, bleeding, eschar
  Irregular borders, notching

Histopathologic features
  Prominent acanthosis with elongated epidermal rete common
  Thickened stratum corneum
  Contiguous or near contiguous lentiginous melanocytic proliferation in almost all lesions
  Intraepidermal melanocytes appear to lie in lacunae (clear spaces)
  Variable cytologic atypia with minimal atypia in early lesions
  Pagetoid spread (particularly in more advanced lesions)
  Intraepidermal nesting (particularly in more advanced lesions)
  Proliferation of melanocytes downward along eccrine ducts (even into deep dermis and subcutis)
  Pronounced pagetoid spread, large intraepidermal nests, significant numbers of melanocytes in stratum corneum in advanced lesions
  Polygonal to spindled melanocytes often with prominent dendrites
  Nuclear enlargement, hyperchromatism, pleomorphism prominent
  Invasive component
    Cohesive nests, sheets of cells, or loosely aggregated files of cells
    Spindle cells common, but also polygonal, small, and highly pleomorphic cells are noted
    Nevoid and sarcomatoid variants occur
  Desmoplasia, neurotropism, angiotropism common

Differential diagnosis
  Melanotic macule
  Lentigo
  Atypical intraepidermal melanocytic proliferation, not otherwise specified
  Acral melanocytic nevus with or without atypia (may overlap atypical [dysplastic] nevus)
  Pigmented spindle cell nevus
  Squamous cell carcinoma, spindle cell type
  Atypical fibroxanthoma
  Cellular neurothekeoma
  Malignant peripheral nerve sheath tumor
  Angiosarcoma
  Kaposi sarcoma
  Leiomyosarcoma

diameter of the lesion may range from 0.3 to 15.0 cm or greater. Any pigmented lesion on the sole (and perhaps other acral sites) measuring > 7 mm and lesions ≤ 7 mm with irregular borders, color, or both or having a so-called parallel ridge patten on epiluminescence microscopy are suspicious for melanoma and should be biopsied (102). With tumor progression, a focal elevated portion that is often dusky blue, black, or amelanotic may develop. With time, one may observe nodule formation; this is commonly accompanied by ulceration, hemorrage, and crusting. Some AM present as a frankly nodular melanoma with little or no adjacent macular component. In some proportion or all such cases, the macular component has presumably been obliterated by the rapid progression to an advanced tumor. AM are often diagnosed at an advanced stage because of neglect and failure to seek medical attention or misdiagnosis as traumatic injury or a banal process such as verruca.

Histopathologic Features

The attributes of glabrous skin seem to account for some but not all of the histopathologic features of AM (22,32,34,86–86,94) (Table 10-14). The minimal essential criteria for diagnosis of intraepidermal acral melanoma (as at all other sites) remain controversial, since one is dealing with a continuum of atypicality in macular lesions, the interpretations are highly subjective, and there is currently no consensus about criteria. Therefore, the threshold for diagnosis will vary from one pathologist to another based on the accumulation of abnormal features considered important and his or her experience.

Our operational criteria are (a) contiguous or near contiguous lentiginous (basilar single-cell) melanocytic proliferation, which is the common denominator in almost all lesions and almost exclusively presents in early lesions or at the peripheries of more advanced lesions; (b) variable cytologic atypia of melancytes, including minimal atypia in early lesions or at the peripheries; (c) prominent acanthosis of the epidermis with elongated rete ridges; (d) thickened stratum corneum; (e) pagetoid spread common particularly with more advanced lesions; (f) intraepidermal nesting, especially with more advanced lesions; and (g) proliferation of melanocytes downward along eccrine ducts (Figs. 10-8, 10-10B, and 10-18). In well-developed AM, the intraepidermal component shows pronounced pagetoid spread, large nests of melanocytes, and significant numbers of melanocytes in the stratum corneum in addition to lentiginous melanocytic proliferation (94). Uncommonly, there may be tracking of the intraepidermal tumor downward along eccrine ducts into the deep dermis and subcutaneous fat. The intraepidermal melanocytes commonly appear to lie within lacunae, to have polygonal to spindled morphologies, and may display prominent dendrites that extend throughout the epidermis (83–86) (Figs. 10-10B and 10-18B). The nuclei are enlarged, hyperchromatic, and often highly pleomorphic (Fig. 10-11B). Some melanocytes are commonly bizarre, and frankly anaplastic giant cells may be observed. A proportion of, but not all, AM contain melanocytes with prominent dendritic processes. With tumor progression, there is a tendency for upward migration and dermal invasion. Variable degrees of melanization are present.

FIGURE 10-18 Acral melanoma. **A,** There is a disorderly proliferation of atypical basilar melanocytes that show confluence, dyscohesive nesting, and some pagetoid spread. The epidermal is hyperplastic.

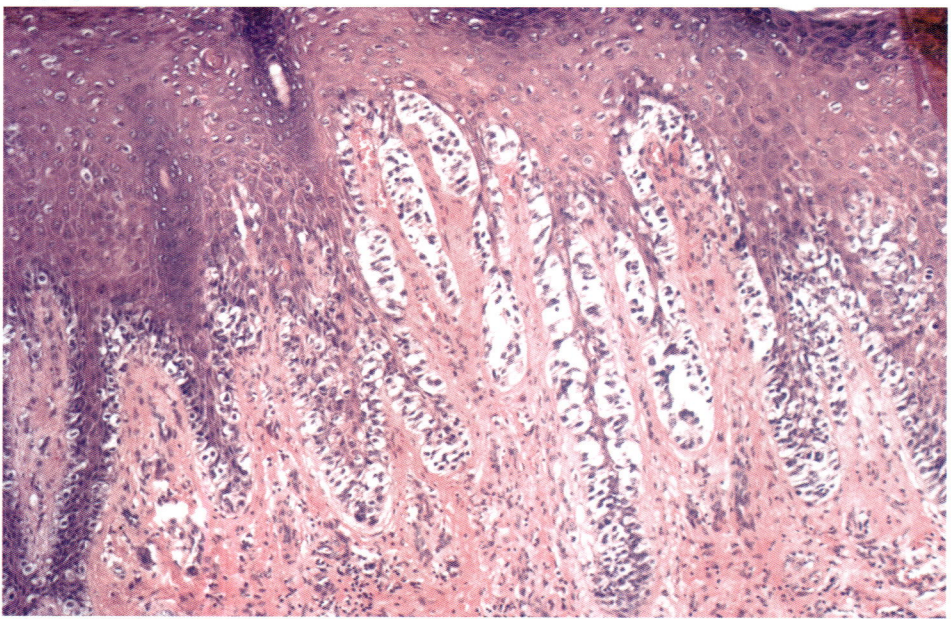

A

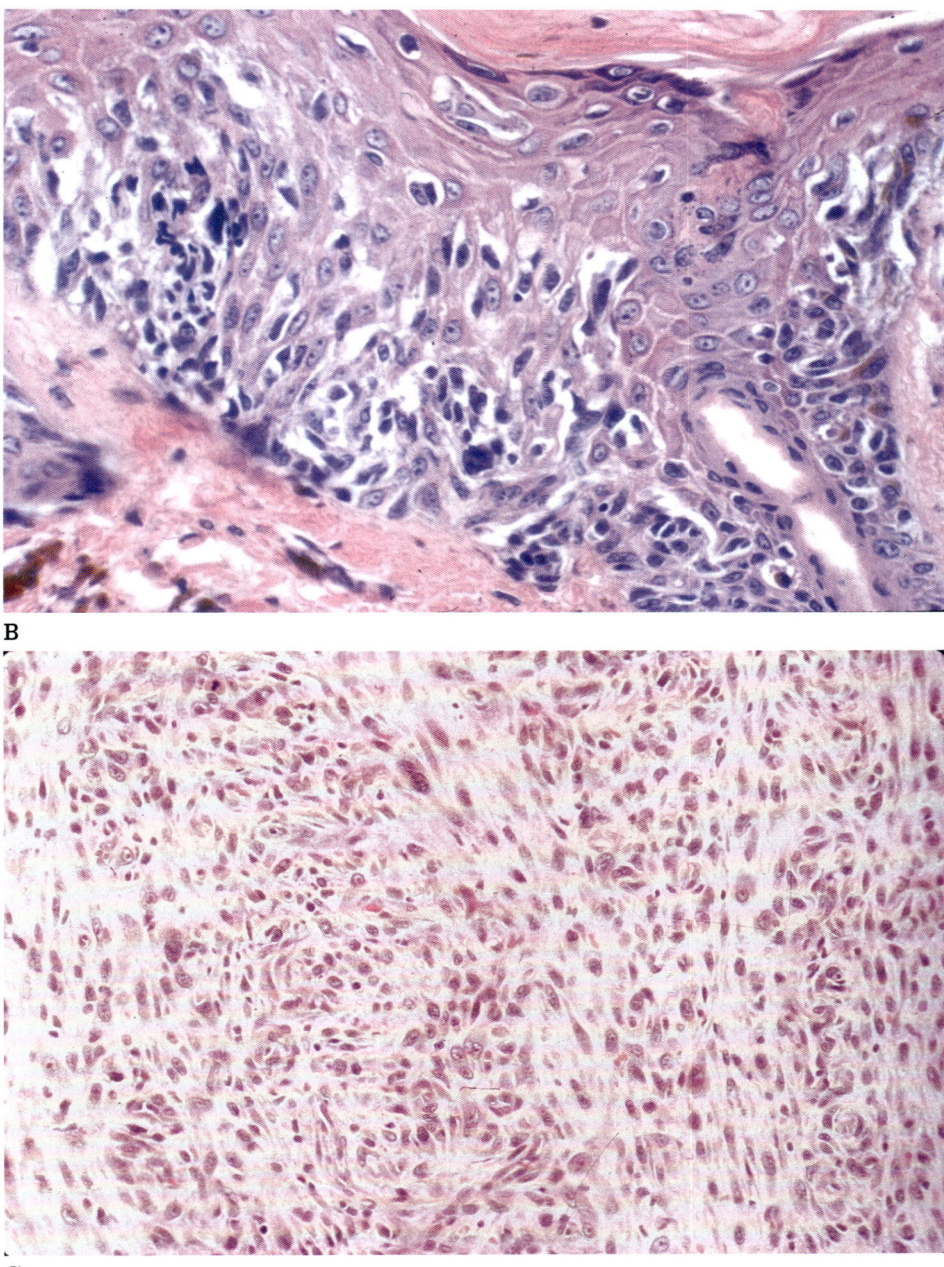

FIGURE 10-18 Continued. **B,** There is prominent upward migration of cells throughout epidermis. **C,** Fascicles of plump spindle cells are distributed throughout the dermis.

From the center of the lesion toward the periphery, there is commonly a diminution in both the frequency and atypia of intraepidermal melanocytes so that the diagnosis of melanoma may legitimately be in doubt (this point holds for all melanomas with a peripheral intraepidermal component).

As described above, the intraepidermal or microinvasive phase is usually typified by relatively dense mononuclear cell infiltrates in a thickened, fibrotic papillary dermis that often contains foci of regression (22,32,34, 86–86). Many of these tumors are advanced at the time of diagnosis, with central polypoid or fungating tumors that are often ulcerated and frequently extend deeply into the dermis. (Table 10-14).

The dermal component is most often composed of spindle cells (Figs. 10-18C), but epithelioid cells, small cells, and highly pleomorphic cells resembling a sarcoma are occasionally noted (22,32,34,83–86). The invasive component may be composed of cohesive nests, sheets, or more loosely aggregated files of melanocytes or individually invasive melanocytes. One particular variant is a nested arrangement of small cuboidal melanocytes that may closely mimic a nevus (84). A proportion of AM exhibit desmoplasia, neurotropism, angiotropism, or any combination of these features (see below). In the latter group of tumors, spindle cells or less commonly small nevuslike cells or epithelioid cells are loosely aggregated in a collagenized dermis.

SUBUNGUAL MELANOMA (MELANOMA OF THE NAIL APPARATUS)

Subungual melanoma (SUM) is a distinctive variant of AM originating from melanocytes in the nail matrix, nailbed epithelium, or the periungual epidermis (i.e., the nail apparatus) (129–138). Some have suggested that the term *subungual melanoma* may not accurately reflect the origin of melanomas from this site and thus prefer *melanoma of the nail apparatus* (129). In their advanced stages, SUM have generally destroyed or disrupted the nailplate and nailbed and thus are subungual. These lesions are commonly diagnosed at an advanced stage because they are rare, often resemble rather banal conditions such fungal infections of the nail, and so frequently lack pigmentation, which is a major clue to the diagnosis of melanoma. Thus SUM are often associated with a poor prognosis with 5-year survival rates ranging from 16 to 72%. This unusual form of melanoma was first reported in 1834 by Alexis Boyer, surgeon to Napoleon, who described a 57-year-old man with a pigmented band involving the left fifth finger that progressed to an inflamed painful nodule after many years (138). Sir Jonathan Hutchinson applied the term *melanotic whitlow* to the latter entity because of its striking resemblance to common fungal infection or a "whitlow," which he attributed to a "melanocytic sarcoma"; he is also credited with the observation that hyperpigmentation extending onto periungual skin, Hutchinson's sign, often indicates subungual melanoma (130). Subungual melanomas account for 1–3% of all melanomas in most series. However they may make up 15–20% of melanomas among African-Americans, 10–31% among Asians, and 33% among Native Americans (131–138). As referred to above, there is generally an equal distribution between the hands and feet. The median age of patients with subungual melanoma is approximately 64 years, with a range of 20–95 years (131–138).

As with other AM, local traumatic injury may be an causal factor in the development of SUM, as originally proposed by Hutchinson, but is nonetheless difficult to substantiate (138). Since many SUM diagnosed early are associated with pigmented nail bands present for some period of time, it is likely that some proportion of SUM develop from melanocytic hyperplasias that probably evolve through an atypical intraepidermal melanocytic proliferation to melanoma (137,139,140). In a similar fashion, junctional nevi involving the nail unit may give rise to melanoma, since they occur with some frequency in Africans, Asians, and Native Americans (140,141). Such nevi also have a predilection for the thumb and index finger, as do SUM, and are asymptomatic and inapparent for long periods of time. The role of precursor lesions remains conjectural at this time without more definitive evidence.

Clinical Features

These tumors in 70–90% of cases involve the nailbed of the great toe or thumb, followed in frequency by the index finger and other digits (137,139,140) (Table 10-15). The dominant hand is more commonly affected than the nondominant one. The initial manifestation of early SUM most commonly (in three quarters of cases) is a solitary longitudinal pigmented band of the nail plate (melanonychia striata longitudinalis) (frequently > 3 mm in width) without nail deformity (133,137,140) (Table 10-16). The color is usually brown or black. In general, all such pigmented bands increase in breadth (> 6 mm is highly suspicious for melanoma), show increased complexity of color with shades of brown and black, have irregular or blurred borders, may show some roughening of the nail surface, and commonly demonstrate brown to black macular pigmentation extending onto the proximal or lateral periungual skin (Hutchinson's sign) or the free edge of the nail plate (142). Saida and Ohshima (133) reported the duration of such bands before diagnosis to range from 3–10 years. The presence of multiple pigmented bands in adults, particularly in African-Americans, almost always indicates a benign process (139). In adults the most common cause of a pigmented band is a melanotic macule and in children a junctional nevus (143). Patients may also present with complete pigmentation of the nail, which may vary from tan to black. The rapid progression of longitudinal melanonychia especially to complete pigmentation of the nail is particularly worrisome for SUM (144). The occurrence of this phenomenon in young children should be approached with caution, since such lesions may be benign and regress completely hence the term *regressing nevoid nail melanosis* (145,146). There also may be progressive nail deformity with thickening, split-

TABLE 10-15 Subungual melanoma.

Clinical features
   60–70 years (range, 20–95 years)
   Men = women
   Equal incidence in all racial groups
   Prevalent in Africans, Asians, Native Americans, other peoples of color
   Hands = feet
      Great toe or thumb (70 to 90% of cases) followed by index finger, other digits
      Dominant hand > nondominant hand
   0.3–6 cm
   Solitary longitudinal pigmented band involving nail in 75% of cases
      Frequently ≥ 3 mm in width (> 6 mm highly suspicious for melanoma)
      Brown color initially
   Complexity of color with brown, black
   Irregular or blurred borders
   Roughening or dystrophy of nail surface
   15–65% amelanotic
   Hutchinson's sign: brown or black pigmentation extending onto proximal or lateral periungual skin or the free edge of the nail plate
   Advanced lesions
      Loss of nail
      Mass under nail
      Pain
      Bleeding
      Ulcerated pigmented or amelanotic nodule
   Clinical diagnosis often a banal condition such as fungal infection

Histopathological features
   Thickening of nail matrical or nailbed epithelium
   Lentiginous melanocytic proliferation in almost all lesions
   Variable cytologic atypia with minimal atypia in early lesions
   Pagetoid spread (particularly in more advanced lesions)
   Intraepidermal nesting (particularly in more advanced lesions)
   Proliferation of melanocytes downward along eccrine ducts (even into deep dermis and subcutis)
   Pronounced pagetoid spread, large intraepidermal nests, significant numbers of melanocytes in stratum corneum in advanced lesions
   Polygonal to spindled melanocytes often with prominent dendrites
   Nuclear enlargement, hyperchromatism, pleomorphism prominent
   Invasive component
      Cohesive nests, sheets of cells, or loosely aggregated files of cells
         Spindle cells common, but also polygonal, small, and highly pleomorphic cells are noted
      Nevoid and sarcomatoid variants occur
   Desmoplasia, neurotropism, angiotropism, common

Differential diagnosis
   Longitudinal melanonychia
   Melanotic macule
   Lentigo
   Regressing nevoid nail melanosis
   Atypical intraepidermal melanocytic proliferation, not otherwise specified
   Nailbed melanocytic nevus with or without atypia
   Squamous cell carcinoma, spindle cell type
   Cellular neurothekeoma
   Malignant peripheral nerve sheath tumor
   Angiosarcoma
   Kaposi sarcoma
   Leiomyosarcoma

TABLE 10-16 Causes and simulators of longitudinal melanonychia.

Single band		Multiple bands
Nonneoplastic	Neoplastic	Nonneoplastic

Carpal tunnel syndrome
Foreign body (subungual)
Hematoma (longitudinal)
Irradiation (local)
Postinflammatory hyperpigmentation
Trauma (acute)
Trauma (chronic)
	Melanocytic
	  Acquired melanocytic nevus
	  Congenital melanocytic nevus
	  Proliferation of normal melanocytes
	  Proliferation of atypical melanocytes
	  Postoperative recurrent/persistent melanocytosis
	  Melanoma in situ
	  Metastatic melanoma
	  Subungual melanoma
	Nonmelanocytic
	  Basal cell carcinoma
	  Bowen's disease
	  Mucous cyst
	  Subungual fibrous histiocytoma
	  Verruca vulgaris
	  Breast carcinoma
		Dermatologic disorders
		  Laugier-Hunziker symdrome
		  Lichen planus
		  Lichen striatus
		Drugs and ingestants
		  Antimalarials, arsenic, bleomycin, busulfan, cyclophosphamide, diquat, daunorubicin, doxorubicin, fluoride, 5-fluorouracil, gold therapy, hydroxyurea, ketoconazole, melphalan, mepacrine, mercury, methotrexate, minocycline, nitrogen mustard, nitrosourea, phenothiazine, phenytoid, psoralen, sulfonamide, tetracycline, timolol, zidovudine
		Microbial
		  AIDS
		  Acrothecium nigrum
		  Alternaria grisea tenius
		  Bacteria co-existing with onychomycosis
		  Blastomycetes
		  Candida
		  Fusarium oxysporum
		  Hendersonula toruloidea
		  Homodendrum elatum
		  Pinta
		  Proteus mirabilis
		  Secondary syphilis
		  Trichophyton soudanense
		Exogenous/nonmicrobial
		  Irradiation (systemic)
		Racial variation
		  African-American
		  Hispanic, Native American, and other dark-skinned peoples
		  Japanese
		Systemic diseases and states
		  Addison's disease
		  Adrenalectomy for Cushing's disease
		  Hemosiderosis
		  Hyperbilirubinemia
		  Hyperthyroidism
		  Malnutrition
		  Peutz-Jeghers syndrome
		  Porphyria
		  Pregnancy
		  Vitamin B_{12} deficiency

ting or destruction of the nail. The possibility of an amelanotic SUM must always be kept in mind, since a significant proportion (15–65%) lack pigment (138).

More advanced lesions are typified by a mass under the nail, loss of the nail, pain, bleeding, and ulceration (131). Lesions presenting late may have the appearance of an ulcerated black or amelanotic nodule with hemorrhagic crusting and granulation tissue. Mean diameter ranges from 0.3 to 6.0 cm. SUM are commonly not recognized and often initially treated as a fungal infection (onychomycosis), chronic paronychia, pyogenic granuloma, bacterial infections, granulation tissue, verruca, subungual hematoma, squamous cell carcinoma, etc. (131,136).

Histopathologic Features

Early lesions are characterized by slightly increased numbers of atypical melanocytes in the nail matrix or nailbed (133) (Table 10-15). A lentiginous pattern is predominant but pagetoid spread and some nesting also may be observed (133). Pleomorphic polygonal melanocytes are most commonly present, often with some component of dendritic melanocytes. As with acral melanomas at other sites, the squamous epithelium is often thickened and one observes increasing density of basilar intraepidermal melanocytes, increasing pagetoid spread and nesting with more advanced lesions (Fig. 10-19). Polygonal melanocytes generally are noted more commonly than spindle cells, but the two forms may occur together.

Approximately 50% of invasive SUM exhibit an adjacent intraepidermal component that is predominantly lentiginous, as described above; however, as mentioned above, for all AM the intraepidermal component often features significant pagetoid spread and nesting of melanocytes as well (131,134,135) (Fig. 10-13). Because SUM are often diagnosed at an advanced stage, anywhere from 15 to 38% of cases may have no demonstrable adjacent intraepidermal component. Many such tumors as a result are fungating and ulcerated.

The invasive component, as with other forms of AM, is usually composed of polygonal cells and/or spindle cells, but small cells and highly pleomorphic cells are also occasionally noted (Fig. 10-19C). Some tumors may exhibit deep extension with invasion of bone, a number are desmoplastic–neurotropic and possibly angiotropic, and some may exhibit a prominent fibrovascular stromal alteration (131). The pattern of dermal invasion may include cohesive aggregates of cells, distinct nests and bundles of cells, sheets of spindle cells suggesting a sarcoma, or more widely spaced fascicles of cells or individual cells. A significant proportion is amelanotic.

Differential Diagnosis

The differential diagnosis for AM (including SUM in general) primarily includes melanotic or pigmented macules, atypical clinical lesions described as atypical melanosis, lentigines, and melanocytic nevi of acral skin (Tables 10-14 and 10-15). Melanotic macules and lentigines of acral skin are closely related and are distinguished only by increased numbers of melanocytes in lentigines since both may exhibit basal layer hyperpigmentation. Lentigines usually do not exhibit the frequency of melanocytic proliferation or cytologic atypia that is typical of AM (84,131). Nonetheless, lentigines are likely to belong to a continuum with early AM in situ and thus a subset of atypical lesions may be difficult to categorize as clearly lentigo or AM in situ. The latter group of lesions is best described as an intraepidermal melanocytic proliferation with atypia and indeterminate biologic potential until more information becomes available.

A small number of lesions involving the soles of Japanese individuals have been reported as mimics of AM under the term *atypical melanosis,* owing to their atypical clinical features of large, irregular borders, and color variegation (128). However, histologically they demonstrate only slightly increased numbers of intraepidermal melanocytes without cytologic atypia.

Occasional acral nevi may have alarming features, such as upward migration of cells throughout the epidermis, prominent lentiginous melanocytic proliferation, and varying degrees of cytologic atypia. Although upward migration may be noted in acral nevi, particularly in children, the constituent cells seldom reveal more than low-grade cytologic atypia, and the pattern of pagetoid spread is usually orderly and confined to the lowermost epidermis. Other characteristics of acral nevi include fairly small diameter, a general symmetry, regular size, spacing, and cohesive qualities of the junctional nesting. As with all melanocytic nevi, atypical variants involve acral skin, constituting a continuum of abnormality from normal to AM. There has been considerable discussion in other sections about this general topic and the need to assess multiple clinical and histopathologic parameters when interpreting any given lesion. Therefore, a size of ≥ 7 mm, asymmetry, poor circumscription of the lesion, effacement of the epidermis, loss of the epidermal rete-oriented pattern of melanocytic nesting and proliferation, increasing cellular density, prominent density of pagetoid spread, large confluent intraepidermal nests, significant atypia of melanocytes (i.e., nuclei at least twice the size of keratinocytic nuclei with pleomorphism), hyperchromatism, and finally large nucleoli are all features supporting intraepidermal melanoma (91,102). As we already discussed for other entites, a small percentage of lesions cannot be confidently diagnosed as nevus or AM. As noted above, we recommend that such lesions be designated as an atypical melanocytic proliferation that is biologically indeterminate. One particular note of caution is that well-differentiated AM may exhibit dermal components with little or no inflammatory response. In such cases, careful evaluation for cytologic atypia, necrotic cells, and mitotic activity are helpful in recognizing melanoma.

The differential diagnosis for AM includes nonmelanocytic lesions, such as tinea nigra, intracorneal, and hemorrage (talon noir), verruca, pyogenic granuloma, eccrine poroma, and squamous cell carcinoma (84–86).

The differential diagnosis for SUM includes some of the entities above, including fungal infection of the nail, traumatic injury with dystrophy of the nail, paronychia, pyogenic granuloma, subungual hematoma, verruca, bacterial and viral infections, and squamous cell carcinoma (131,136,138).

LONGITUDINAL MELANONYCHIA (MELANONYCHIA STRIATA)

Longitudinal melanonychia (LM) is directly related to a focal increase in the number or function of melanocytes

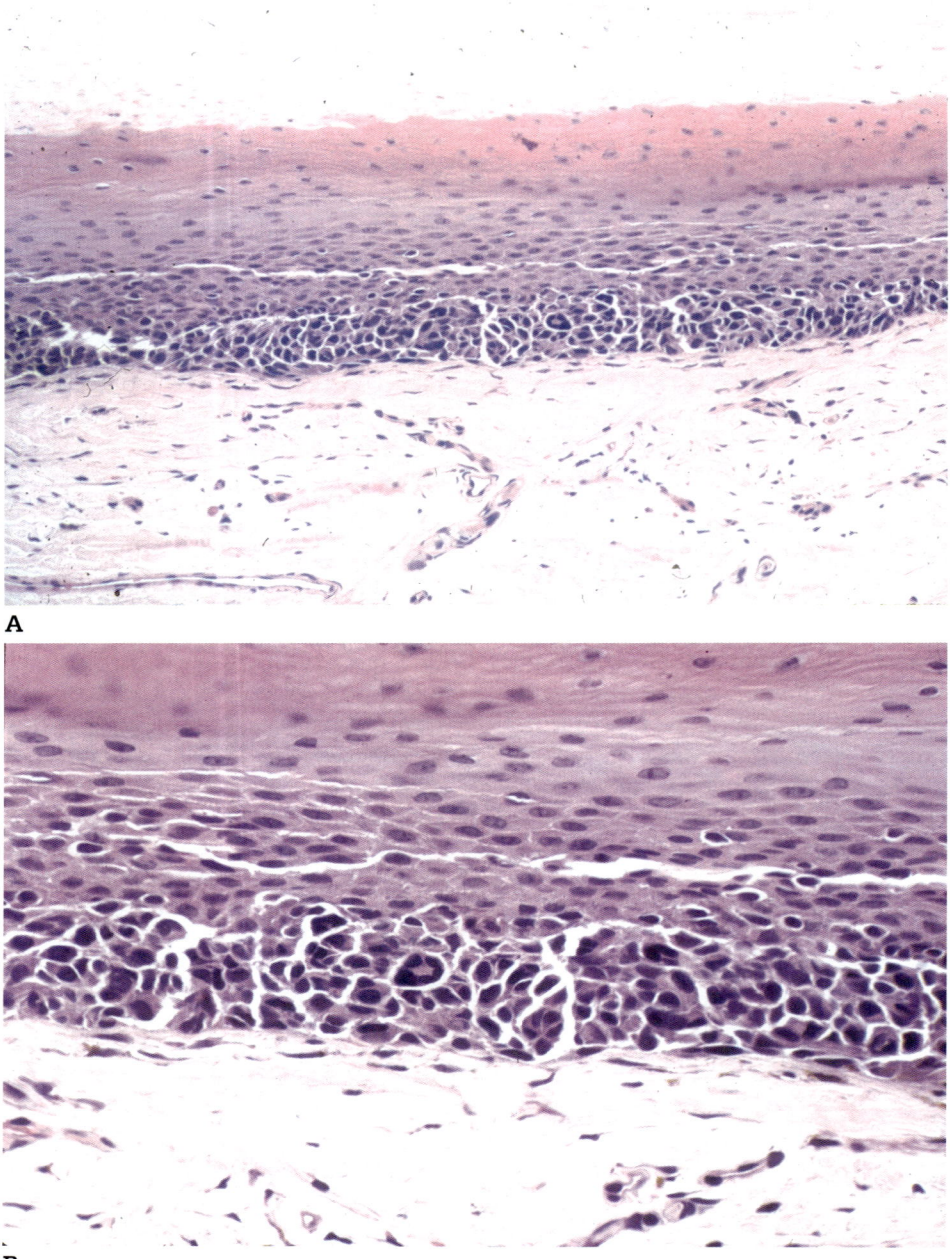

FIGURE 10-19 Subungual melanoma in situ. **A,B,** The basilar portion of the squamous epithelium is replaced by confluent nests of atypical melanocytes.

in the nail matrix, or both, resulting in melanin deposition in the nail plate (139–141) (Table 10-16). In addition to melanin, blood and other chromagins produce pigmented bands that may be indistinguishable from true LM by both clinical history and clinical observation. The cause may be from a melanocytic process or from a variety of nonneoplastic causes, including trauma, fungal infection, drug ingestion, and Addison's disease (141).

Melanocytic lesions resulting in MS are melanotic macules (hyperactive melanocytes), increased numbers of normal melanocytes (including lentigines), atypical melanocytic proliferations, junctional nevi, and melanoma in situ or invasive melanoma. In general, a nailbed biopsy is needed for definitive diagnosis unless clinical factors provide convincing evidence to the contrary (139). Age and race must be considered in the evaluation of LM. In general, a soli-

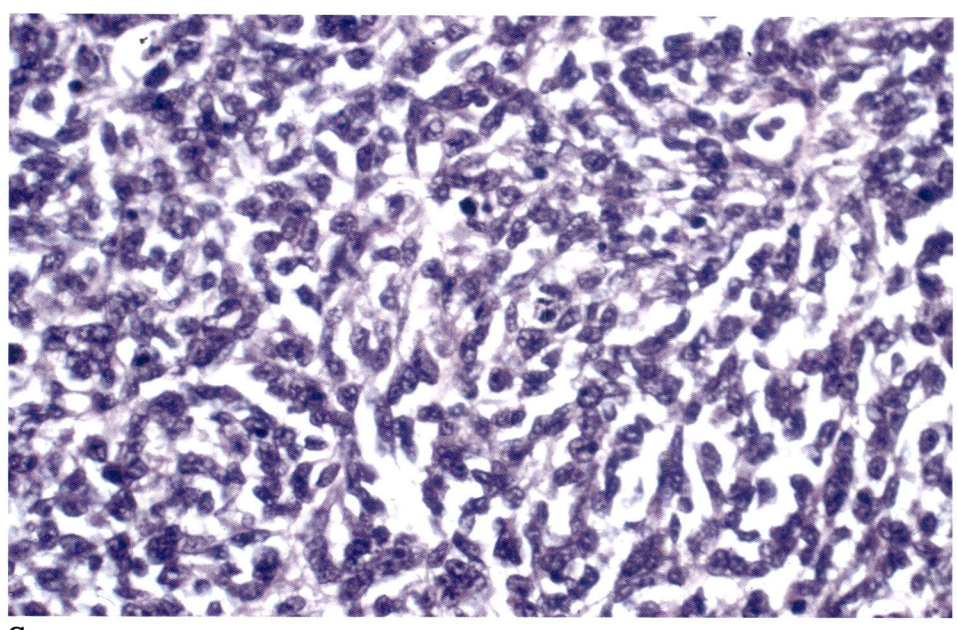

FIGURE 10-19 *Continued.* **C,** Small cell invasive component of subungual melanoma.

tary LM developing in whites must be assessed by nailbed biopsy to exclude melanoma. LM are much more prevalent in non-white groups, with 77% of blacks over the age of 20 years and almost 100% over the age 50 having them. They are also common in Asians, Hispanics, and other populations of color. They may be followed using the guidelines referred to above—that is, an adult patient, especially elderly, with any of the following features particularly in combination: a pigmented band > 6 mm, variegated brown or homogenous black color, irregular or blurred borders, rapid onset or a rapidly changing pigmented band, and periungual pigmentation would necessitate nailbed biopsy (139,140).

OTHER MORPHOLOGICAL AND CYTOLOGICAL VARIANTS OF MELANOMA

Malignant Neuroectodermal Tumor (Desmoplastic Melanoma, Desmoplastic–Neurotropic Melanoma, Neurotropic Melanoma)

Desmoplastic melanomas (DM) and their closely related variants pose one of the most significant challenges to pathologists for correct diagnosis before such lesions reach an advanced and inoperable stage. Why are they so difficult to recognize? It is simply a question of unsuspecting clinicians and pathologists encountering a rare and unfamiliar lesion that, on the one hand, often has a deceptively bland appearance and, on the other, commonly lacks features typical of a conventional melanoma and of a melanocytic lesion itself. The clinical impression is often that of a banal nonmelanocytic lesion, in general more than half of DM and its variants are amelanotic, many lack or have an inconspicuous intraepidermal melanocytic component, and they often appear innocuous histologically, commonly suggesting a benign scar-like fibrous process. Initial diagnoses often rendered include a scar, fibromatosis, dermatofibroma, a benign peripheral nerve sheath tumor, or blue nevus. As a result, they often escape detection until they are advanced and multiple recurrences or metastases have developed.

First described in 1971 by Conley et al. (147), DM is defined by the distinctive histomorphologic features of spindled melanocytes disposed in a collagenized stroma (147–169) (Table 10-17). Reed and Leonard (170) subsequently drew attention to a subset of desmoplastic melanomas with striking neural differentiation resembling a neuroma and/or invasion of cutaneous nerves by tumor cells and coined the term neurotropic melanoma (171). Since the 1970s, several hundred cases of these various tumors have been reported, and it is increasingly apparent that desmoplastic melanoma and its closely related variants constitute a continuum of neuroectodermal tumors expressing the various neurocristic phenotypic (158–160,163,165,170) options of the melanocyte. The

TABLE 10-17 Desmoplastic melanoma and desmoplastic neurotropic melanoma.

Clinical features
  60–65 years
  Men ≥ women (1.75–2:1)
  Sun-exposed skin, head and neck, but also extremities, acral, mucosal sites
  Firm nodule or indurated depressed lesion
  Flesh-colored or with pigmented lesion (29–43%)
  1–5 cm
  Dysesthesias, nerve palsies, intractable pain, occasionally

Histopathologic features
  Intraepidermal melanocytic proliferation in 85%
    Solar intraepidermal melanocytic proliferation with atypia (lentigo maligna) to melanoma in situ, most common
  Fibrous nodule in dermis and possibly subcutis
  Absence of pigment, often
  Short to long curvilinear fascicles of spindle cells
  Storiform appearance
  Spindle cells with serpiginous often tapered nuclei
  Nuclear atypia varies from subtle pleomorphism to frank anaplasia
  Neurotropism, common
    Perineurial and/or endoneurial invasion
    Schwannian, perineurial differentiation
  Angiotropism common
  Aggregates of lymphocytes within tumor common
  Variable myxoid stroma
  Occasional mitoses in dermis, often 1–4/mm^2

Differential diagnosis
  Scar
  Sclerosing blue nevi including variants with hypercellularity
  Desmoplastic (sclerosing) Spitz nevus/tumor
  Neuroma
  Neurofibroma
  Neurothekeoma, particularly cellular variants
  Malignant peripheral nerve sheath tumor
  Myxoma
  Dermatofibroma
  Dermatofibrosarcoma protuberans
  Atypical fibroxanthoma
  Malignant fibrous histiocytoma
  Fibromatosis
  Spindle cell squamous cell carcinoma
  Leiomyosarcoma

histomorphologic phenotype of this group of tumors may include any one or more of the following characteristics:

- Desmoplasia, which is the most common phenotype.
- Neurotropism (see below), which is defined by perineurial and/or endoneurial invasion of cutaneous nerves by tumor cells or neural differentiation (also known as neural or neurosarcomatous transformation) as characterized by formation of nerve-like structures recapitulating perineurium and endoneurium or delicate sheets of spindle cells reminiscent of neurofibromas, neuromas, and in some instances indistinguishable from malignant peripheral nerve sheath tumors.
- Less commonly, myofibroblastic, neuroendocrine, and other forms of mesenchymal differentiation, usually accompanying desmoplasia and neutrotropism (163,165).

In the following discussion, *DM* is defined as a desmoplastic melanoma without neurotropism, *desmoplastic–neurotropic melanoma* (DNM) demonstrates both desmoplasia and neurotropism (i.e., perineurial or endoneurial invasion or both, or neural differentiation, or both); and *neurotropic melanoma* (NM) exhibits neurotropism but no desmoplasia. Since the initial report of DM and its variants, several hundred cases have appeared in the literature and information concerning the natural history and biologic potential of this group of tumors is beginning to emerge. The incidence of DM and its variants is difficult to establish, since the vast majority of cases are diagnosed at tertiary care centers. Nonetheless, from our population-based study from the Connecticut Tumor Registry, only 1% of 650 melanomas demonstrated any desmoplasia and/or neurotropism, substantiating the rarity of this group of melanomas (172).

Desmoplastic Melanoma and Desmoplastic–Neurotropic Melanoma

Clinical Features Desmoplastic melanoma and desmoplastic–neurotropic melanoma (DM/DMN) most frequently arise in association with the solar lentiginous melanomas; because of this linkage, the mean and median patient ages are about 60 years and the chronically sun-exposed skin of the head and neck the most common site (Table 10-17). As with solar melanoma, there is a predilection for the cheek, nose, and scalp. The next most common sites are the extremeties, followed by the trunk. However, these melanomas may develop at any site, including acral and mucosal locations. In virtually all series, men are more commonly affected than women with a male/female ratio of 1.75:2.1 (22,147–171) (Table 10-17). As already mentioned, in the majority of cases DM and DMN often present as a painless, rather inconspicuous, firm or indurated flesh-colored lesions that may be papular, nodular, or occasionally depressed (55–74). Thus most commonly melanoma is not even considered in the clinical differential diagnosis. DM and DMN are frequently first diagnosed as recurrent lesions. Firm nodules recurring at the site of previous surgery are a common first manifestation. Initial clinical diagnoses are, therefore, unsuspecting and vague, such as lump or nodule, not otherwise specified, sclerosing basal cell carcinoma, and cyst. If pigmented, the gross morphologic features may vary considerably from a subtle ill-defined tan to brown macule suggesting a solar lentigo to the complex appearance of any type of melanoma. Often the features of a solar melanoma are observed with variegated macular pigmentation and irregular borders (see above). The size ranges from < 1 cm to > 2 cm in greatest diameter. For pigmented lesions, clinical diagnoses are often more focused and often include lentigo, dermatofibroma, pigmented mass, not otherwise specified, and melanoma. The difficulty in recognizing DM and DMN clinically and histologically usually causes a significant delay in intervention and appropriate surgery.

Histopathologic Features Desmoplastic melanoma and desmoplastic–neurotropic melanoma (DM/DMN) must be suspected for any scar-like spindle cell proliferation arising in chronically sun-exposed of elderly individuals. The minimal essential histopathologic criteria include a spindle cell proliferation with varying degrees of atypia embedded in a fibrous stroma and confirmation of the melanocytic/neuroectodermal lineage of spindle cells by observing an atypical intraepidermal melanocytic proliferation and/or by positive immunohistochemisty with S-100 protein or with other equivalent markers, such as p75 neurotrophin receptor (173,174), or with other less-specific antibodies, such as neuron-specific enolase and NKI/C3 in concert with vimentin (163,166). Other corroboratory features are the presence of melanin, aggregates of lymphocytes throughout the tumor, and neurotropism (Table 10-17).

Scanning magnification usually discloses a fibrous nodule displacing the normal dermal collagen or lamina propria and often extending into subcutaneous fat (160,163) (Fig. 10-20A). An intraepidermal melanocytic proliferation of some kind is usually observed in approximately 86% of DM and DMN reported in the literature (163). In a series of 28 cases, 48% of DM had an intraepidermal component of SIMP (lentigo maligna) compared to 15% in the literature (163). An additional 33% of the latter cases and 56% from the literature showed a component best described as an atypical lentiginous melanocytic proliferation rather than solar melanoma in situ (72). About 4% of the cases exhibited a predominately pagetoid intraepidermal pattern. DM and DMN may also be associated with lentiginous melanomas of acral and mucosal sites; however, a recent Australian study reported only three DM and DMN cases among 280 that could be classified as acral lentiginous (169). It must be pointed out that a small percentage of cases may in fact show intraepidermal melanocytic proliferation that is possibly reactive rather than being neoplastic; however this requires further study.

Approximately 15% of the DM and DMN in one study did not show any evidence of an intraepidermal melanocytic component, and this has been similarly observed in 13% of cases reported from the literature. Such lesions are often referred to as de novo in the literature. With increasing depth of DM, there is a tendency for the intraepidermal component to become disassociated from the dermal component or completely lost (163). Nonetheless, recurrent tumors more commonly lack an intraepidermal component. It is also possible that a small percentage of DM and DMN may have some developmental relationship with appendageal melanocytes or from pluripotential neuroectodermal cells in the dermis, perhaps associated with cutaneous nerves. In sum, some type of atypical intraepidermal melanocytic proliferation, whether lentiginous or not and whether sufficiently developed for melanoma in situ or not, is often present in DM and DMN, particularly in sun-exposed skin (Fig. 10-7). Marked solar degeneration of collagen is an almost invariable finding in these sun-exposed sites (163).

As mentioned above, the most common histologic pattern of DM is a predominantly desmoplastic presentation (158–160,163). The immediate invasion of the papillary dermis, whether in early or well-developed lesions, is often composed of vertically oriented spindle cells. With involvement of the reticular dermis, the spindle cells become interspersed among dense collagenous fibers as individual spindle cells, short fascicles of cells, much longer curvilinear bundles of cells, and finally in storiform patterns (Fig. 10-20B). The degree of cellularity may vary enormously, with the majority of lesions being sparsely cellular and having the appearance of a cicatrix or a neuroma; in the most advanced lesions, there is high cellular density present. In some instances, there may be an admixture of other cell types, particularly the epithelioid melanoma cells that typify conventional melanoma.

The nuclei may show considerable latitude in the degrees of atypia present. In some cases, the nuclei are relatively small and demonstrate little or no variation in size and shape, suggesting simply a scar or neurofibroma. Often the nuclei are elongated with wavy and serpiginous nuclear morphologies consistent with schwannian differentiation (Figs. 10-20B–F). However, some nuclei are plump, and occasional bizarre multinucleate giant cell forms are noted. Less commonly, the spindle cells may show myofibroblastic differentiation (163,165). In general, there is recognizable nuclear enlargement, pleomorphism, and hyperchromatism (slight to moderate nuclear atypia) in most DM and DMN; in extreme cases, the spindle cells become frankly anaplastic suggesting a sarcoma.

Most DM and DMN lack pigment; however, pigment incontinence may be observed in the papillary dermis and on occasion accompanied by the alterations of regression.

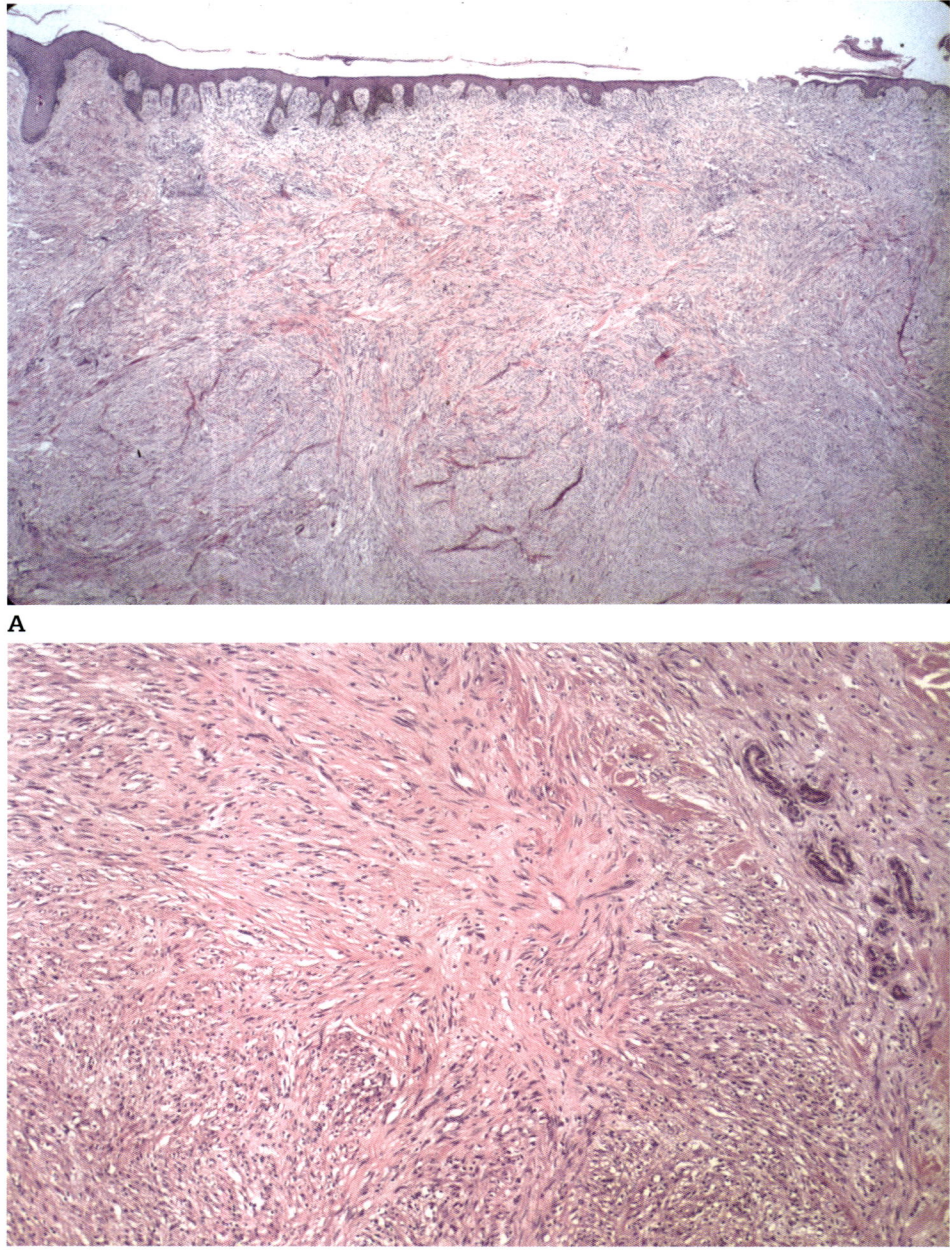

FIGURE 10-20 Desmoplastic neurotropic melanoma. **A,** A fibrotic nodule occupies the dermis. The absence of melanin pigment suggests a nonmelanocytic process, such as a fibroma or scar. **B,** Intersecting fascicles of spindle cells with dense fibrous stroma are seen. One can identify some nuclear pleomorphism of the spindle cells in this lesion.

Occasional spindle cells may contain fine melanin granules within cellular processes, taking on the appearance of a blue nevus (160,163). The tumor stroma is usually fibrous, but myxoid alteration is occasionally encountered and uncommonly may be striking (160,163).

The fascicles of spindle cells may blend with the perineurium of cutaneous nerves so that tumor cells make up the perineurium. Tumor cells may also infiltrate the endoneurium (55,158–160,163). Care must be exercised in assessing neurotropism, as the tumor cells may be arranged in wavy fascicles and resemble neural tissue (160,170,171,175–178) (Fig. 10-15C). Concentric, whorled

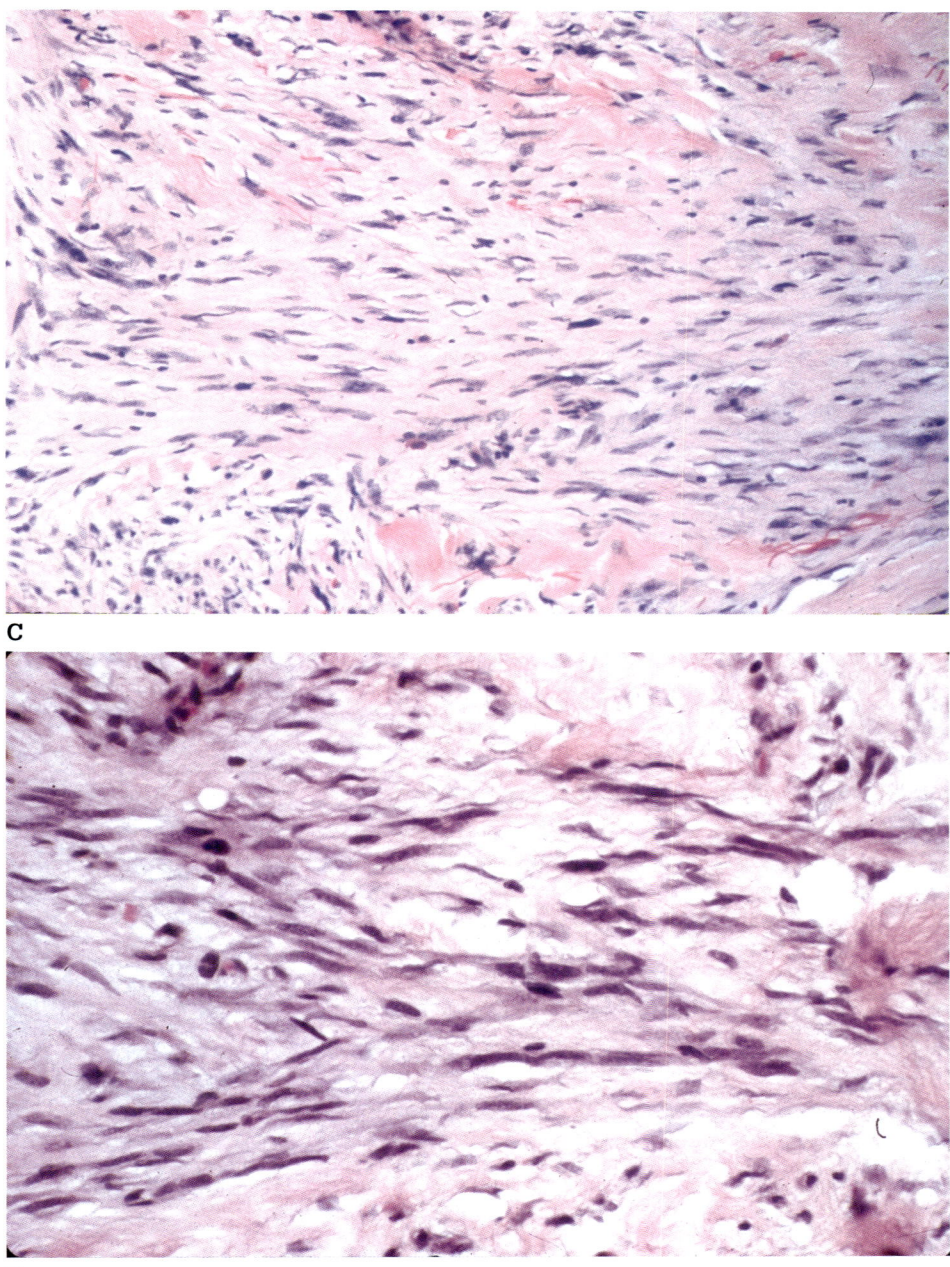

FIGURE 10-20 *Continued.* **C,** Rather widely spaced spindle cells are seen in this field with limited nuclear atypia. **D,** A linear array of spindle cells is disposed in the dense fibrotic matrix.

arrangements of cells may resemble a neuroma. The tumor cells in DM and DMN are also notable for a tropism (angiotropism) or infiltration of the walls of blood or lymphatic vessels. Mitotic figures can usually be found even in the most paucicellular forms of this tumor and commonly number 1–4 mitoses/mm² (160,163,169). A finding typical of DM and DMN mentioned above and useful for recognition of these tumors is the presence of variably dense perivascular lymphocytic infiltrates usually scattered throughout the tumor (160,163,169).

Neurotropic Melanoma

Any form of melanoma may show some degree of desmoplasia, neurotropism, or both (160,163). To be categorized as desmoplastic melanoma, the *predominant pattern* of the invasive dermal component should be desmoplas-

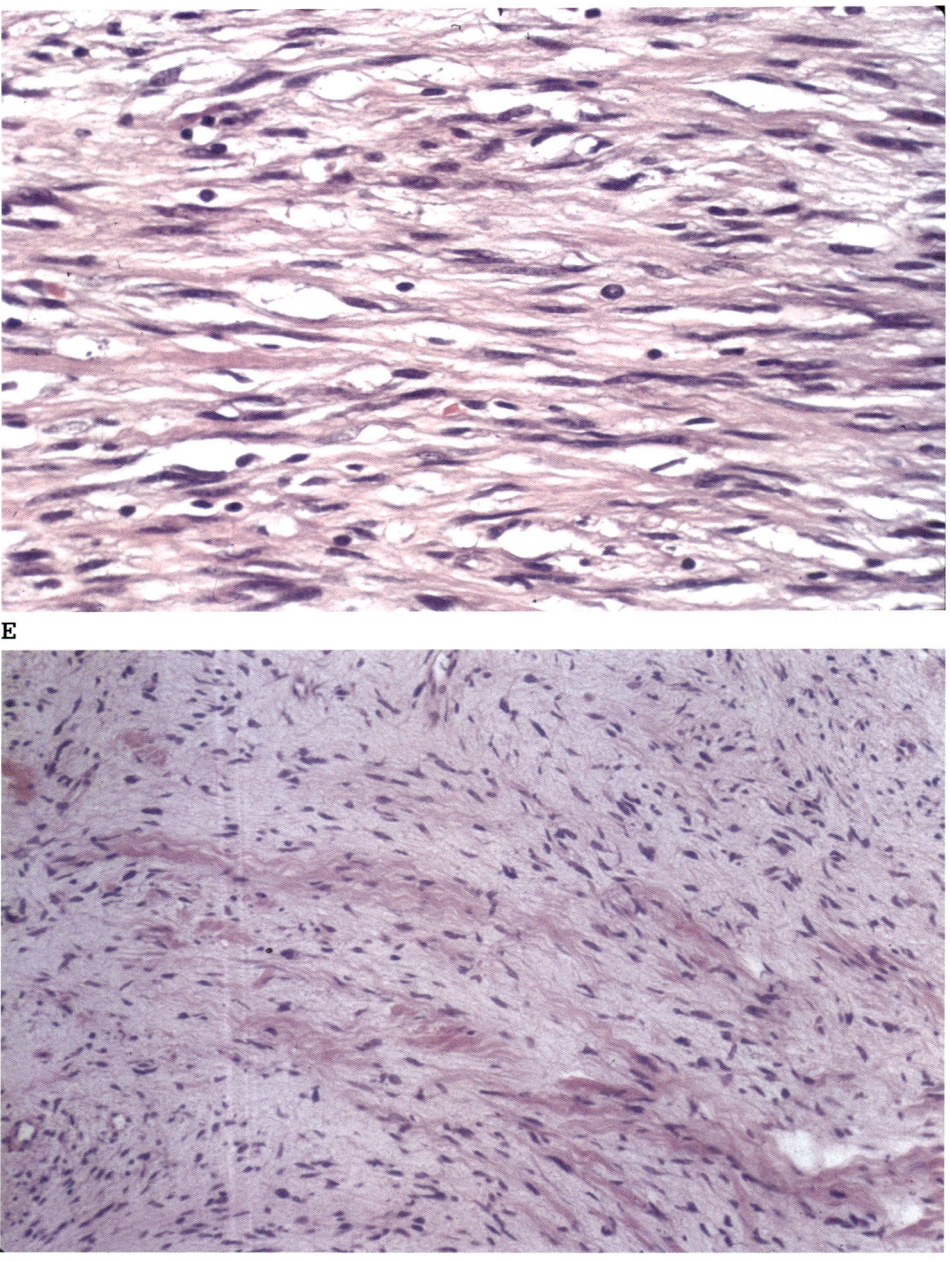

FIGURE 10-20 Continued. **E,** Fascicles of spindle cells contain elongated, wavy pleomorphic and hyperchromatic nuclei. **F,** This field shows nuclei dispersed in delicate matrix resembling a neurofibroma (schwannian differentiation).

tic. The same criterion applies to melanomas designated as neurotropic. Most desmoplastic melanomas have some degree of neurotropism or neuroid differentiation. When prominent desmoplasia and neurotropism are present, the tumor is designated as desmoplastic–neurotropic.

Although Reed and Leonard introduced the term neurotropic melanoma to describe a specific variant of DM that showed infiltration of cutaneous nerves, neural differentiation, or neuroma-like patterns (170), new terms, recently introduced, emphasize different features of tumors in the spectrum of NM (171–178). Jain and Allen (158) described a nerve-centered form of DMN or neurotropic melanoma to depict a principally perineural localization of tumor. The latter tumors are exceedingly rare in our experience. They often present as relatively deep nodular lesions, owing to the macronodular tumoral proliferation about nerves. Smithers et al. (159) designated melanomas with neural differentiation as *neural transforming*. Such tumors have spindle cells with serpiginous morphology dispersed singly or in paucicellular bundles in a delicate, frequently myxoid stroma. We have observed that a large proportion of melanomas demonstrating neurotropism also show the phenomenon of angiotropism, or the propensity of melanoma cells to track along external surfaces of microvessels (106,179).

Clinical Features The clinical presentation of NM closely parallels that of DM and DMN because of their frequent association (160,163,170,171). However, NM without desmoplasia are vanishingly rare, and they may occur in any clinical setting. The most common finding is a firm nodule with features suggesting deep tissue infiltration. Patients with DMN or NM may develop "malignant" neuropathies, and those involving the head and neck may show cranial nerve involvement, particularly the cranial nerves V and VII, with consequent palsies, paraesthesias, and in some cases intractable pain (157,177). Recurrence and extension of tumor into the brain and cerebral metastases are more frequent in neurotropic melanoma than in conventional desmoplastic melanoma (157).

Histopathologic Features Neurotropic melanoma is often associated with atypical lentiginous melanocytic proliferation or lentiginous forms of melanoma within the epidermis and skin appendages (147–169) (Table 10-17). However, some NM may arise with any type of intraepidermal component (e.g., pagetoid involvement) or de novo without an intraepidermal component (180,155). The skin appendages may be the source of some of these tumors.

The term *neurotropism* refers to both the involvement of perineurium and endoneurium of cutaneous nerves by melanoma (spindle) cells and neural differentiation (170) (Fig. 10-21). There may be considerable thickening of the perineurium and expansion of the endoneurial space by the tumor involvement (158–160, 169,170). Extension of tumor along the cutaneous nerves may, however, be extensive and subtle. Histologic clues to nerve involvement include the presence of hyperchromatic spindle cells in the perineurium or endoneurium and mucinous alteration of the nerve. Rarely perineurial accumulation melanophages may be associated with nerve infiltration by melanoma cells and may possibly be a marker of regression in this circumstance. Careful examination of cutaneous nerves at the surgical margins is mandatory to assess adequate excision. Melanoma spindle cells involving cutaneous nerves usually show nuclear enlargement, hyperchromatism, and pleomorphism.

The term *neurotropism* (as originally used by Reed and Leonard) also describes neural or schwannian differentiation in a pattern resembling peripheral nerve sheath tumors, such as neurofibromas or neuromas and the recapitulation of perineurium and endoneurium (170,171,175–178). The tumor cells in such areas are characterized by serpiginous or wavy nuclear configurations and filamentous cytoplasmic processes. The cells are embedded in a variably mucinous and fibrous stroma (Fig. 10-20F). In some instances, the stromal may be so sufficiently myxoid to suggest a myxoma. However, the tumor cells demonstrate loose fascicular arrangements cytologic atypia, and occasional mitotic figures. Some tumors may be indistinguishable from a malignant peripheral nerve sheath tumor without observation of an atypical intraepidermal melanocytic proliferation.

The nerve-centered variant of NM as described by Jain and Allen and in our experience is characterized by a striking predilection of tumor cells to proliferate about, along, and within nerves (158). The end result is the formation of macronodular tumor aggregates that may have plexiform and serpiginous configurations in the dermis, subcutis, and deeper (Fig. 10-21D–F). The spindle cells making up the latter structures generally have some schwannian differentiation; however, they may range from well to poorly differentiated and have the appearance of a high-grade sarcoma (Fig. 10-21F). Other features of DMN or NM may or may not be present, such as an atypical intraepidermal melanocytic component, melaninization, and spindle cell proliferation with desmoplasia and/or neural differentiation in the intervening tissue between nerves.

Immunohistochemistry Immunohistochemistry is needed in almost all DM, DMN, and NM to confirm the diagnosis and to exclude other entities (Table 10-18). Almost 100% of desmoplastic–neurotropic melanomas demonstrate immunoreactivity with antibodies against vimentin, S-100 protein, and p75 neurotrophin receptor (113,163,165,166,173,174,182,183), but uniquely almost all have been reported to be negative for HMB-45 (163,184). If there is positive immunostaining for HMB-45 in DM and DMN, it typically involves nondesmoplastic foci only (i.e., an intraepidermal component), superficial dermal focus of conventional epithelioid melanoma cells, or on occasion the melanoma cells invading nerves (163). Other antibodies used for melanocytic lesions with variable, often infrequent or negative, reactivity with desmoplastic melanoma include Mart-1, MITF (microphthalmia transcription factor), MAGE-1, tyrosinase,

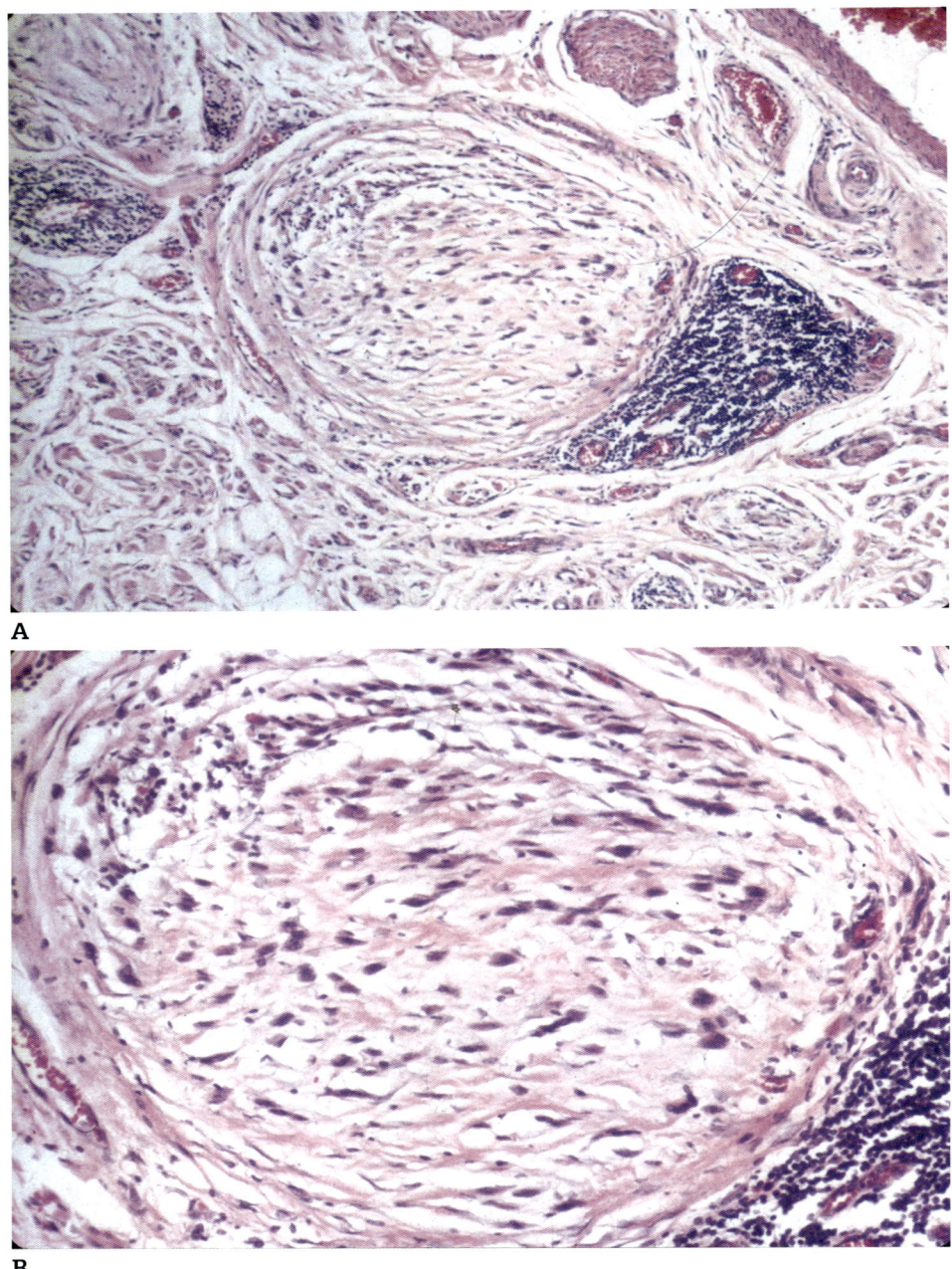

FIGURE 10-21 Neurotropic melanoma. **A,** A cutaneous nerve shows prominent perineurial and endoneurial infiltration by melanoma cells (neurotropism). **B,** Higher magnification of panel A reveals neurotropism by spindle cells with hyperchromatic nuclei.

neuron-specific enolase, NK1/C3, and fibroblast growth factor (113,163,166,182,185,186). Antibodies against keratin, desmin, actin, and Leu-7 (specific for peripheral nerve sheath differentiation but negative in melanocytic tumors), in general, are negative in desmoplastic melanoma. However, the use of refined antigen-retrieval techniques may yield much higher sensitivity with some of the latter antibodies, such as HMB 45 and tyrosinase (114). A battery of markers must always be used to evaluate such tumors. DM and DMN and malignant peripheral nerve sheath tumor (MPNST) may be S-100 protein positive and negative for other markers in some instances. One useful discriminating feature is that the S-100 immunostaining is generally diffuse in melanomas and focal in MPNST.

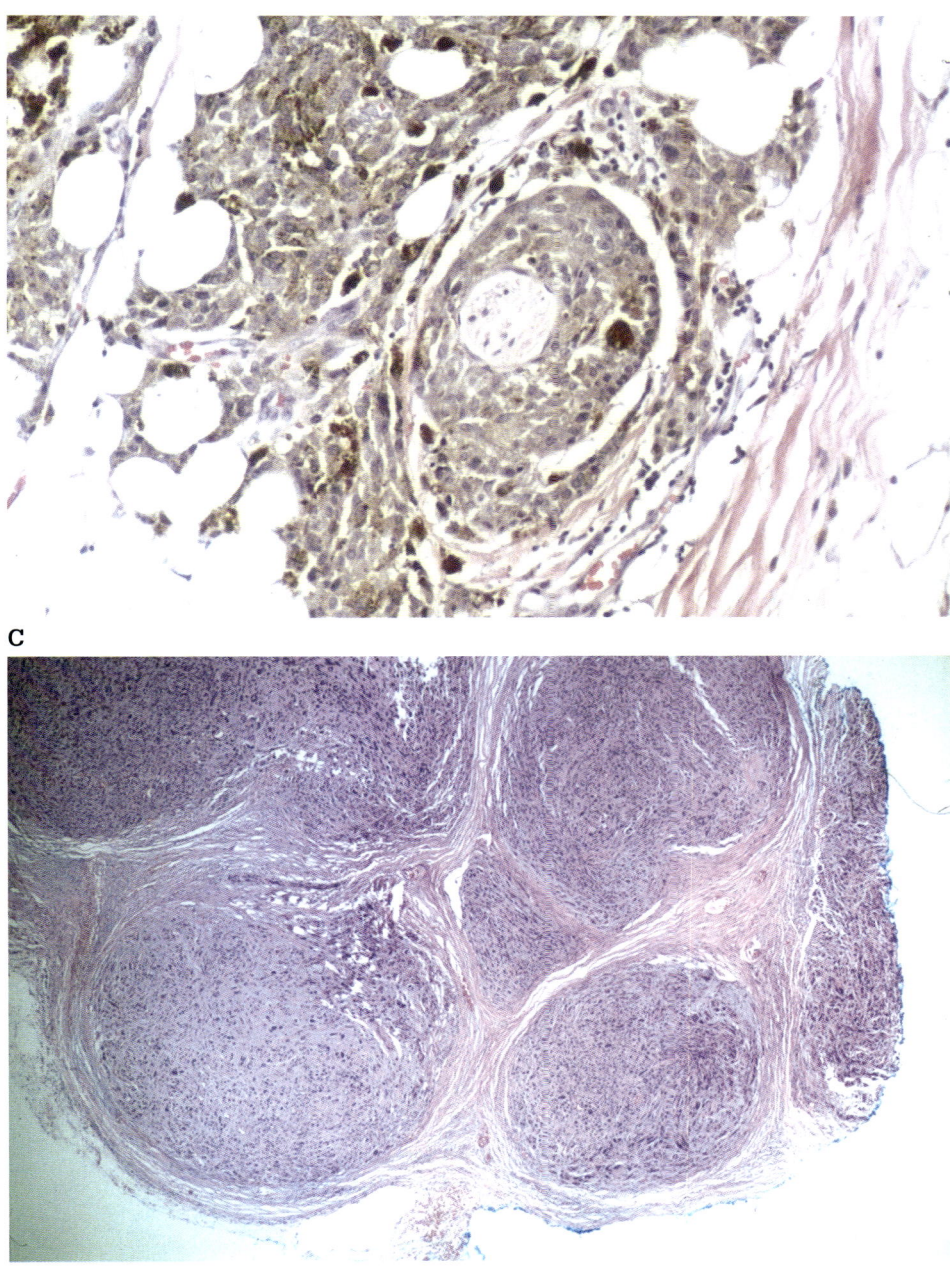

FIGURE 10-21 *Continued.* **C,** Note the perineurial infiltration of a small nerve in the subcutaneous fat. **D,** Nerve-centered (macronodular) variant of neurotropic melanoma showing large nerve bundles infiltrated and cuffed by spindled melanoma cells.

Histogenesis The pathogenesis of desmoplasia and the true nature of the spindle cells in desmoplastic melanoma remain a subject of controversy and debate (147,148,153, 163,165,187,188). Some authors maintain that the fibroplasia results from the induction of collagen synthesis by benign fibroblasts while others believe that melanoma cells function as adaptive fibroblasts to promote collagenization in these tumors (148).

Recent experimental work using human melanoma cell lines injected into nude mice provides new information possibly relevant to the natural history and pathogenesis of DM (187). One particular cell line, UCT-Mel7,

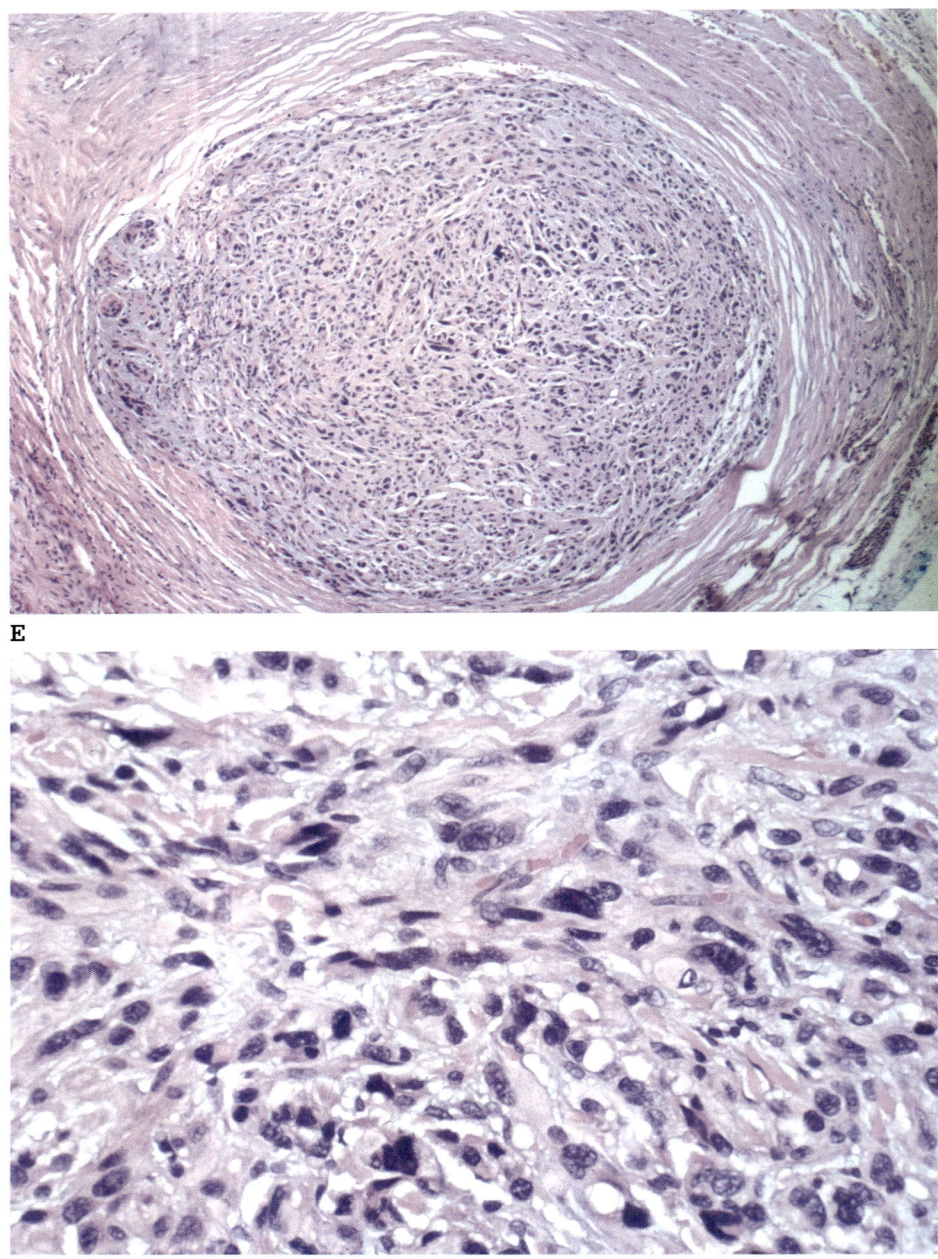

FIGURE 10-21 *Continued.* **E**, Higher magnification of panel D showing the large nerve structure greatly expanded by tumoral infiltration. **F**, The melanoma cells are highly pleomorphic and cytologically suggest a sarcoma.

when injected into nude mice, results in a tumor with many characteristics of DM: desmoplastic stroma and indolent growth in contrast to the inexorable proliferation and dissemination associated with other melanoma cell lines. It is of interest that the desmoplasia elicited by UCT-Mel7 correlated with slow growth (i.e., collagen content of the tumor) was inversely related to cell growth. In additional studies, co-culture of UCT-Mel7 cells with fibroblasts resulted in a twofold increase in collagen synthesis solely by the fibroblast population (188). Increased mRNA expression for collagen was observed in the cultured fibroblasts. These data support the origin of collagen production in DM from fibroblasts rather than melanoma cells.

TABLE 10-18 Results of immunohistochemistry reported for desmoplastic melanoma.

Marker[a]	Carlson et al. (72)[a]	Literature
S-100	100%	94% (165/175)
Vimentin	100%	92% (23/25)
HMB-45	21%	5% (5/92)
Mart-1 (Melan-A)	ND	0–33%
Mift (C5 and D5)	ND	0–35%
MAGE-1	ND	38%
Tyrosinase	ND	0–55%
p75 neurotrophin receptor	ND	100%
NSE	42%	96% (22/23)
EMA	43%	0 (0/1)
FXIIIa	39%	100% (15/15)
Actin, smooth muscle	52%	50% focal
Leu-7	0	0
Keratins AE1.3	0	0 (0/14)
CAM 5.2	0	—

NSE, neuron specific enolase; EMA, epithelial membrane antigen; FXIIIa, Factor XIIIa; ND, not done.

Nevertheless, many authorities counter that the spindle cells in DM are true melanoma cells that have undergone metaplasia to adaptive fibroblasts and thus are themselves capable of collagen synthesis (153). The latter conclusion results from ultrastructural and immunohistochemical studies (148–151,154) and the fact that because of their neural crest origin, melanocytes are capable of collagen production as well as melanin synthesis and schwannian differentiation (160,163,165).

By electron microscopy, the spindle cells of DM and DMN contain premelanosomes and/or melanosomes according to some studies (152,153) (Table 10-19). However, other investigators have not detected evidence of melanin synthesis in the tumor cells of DM (149,151, 157,160,163). From et al. (153) studied desmoplastic melanoma by electron microscopy and noted a progressive transition from large, pleomorphic melanocytes near the dermoepidermal junction to fusiform cells in mid-dermis and to predominantly spindle-shaped cells in a desmoplastic stroma in the deep dermis. All of these cell types contained non-membrane-bound melanosomes and were positive for S-100 protein. Some of the spindle-shaped cells displayed myofibroblastic differentiation (148,163). Valensi (150,151), in ultrastructural studies of desmoplastic melanoma, reported macular desmosomes between the tumor cells and cited this as evidence that the tumor cells were dedifferentiated melanocytic cells with fibroblastic characteristics rather than true fibroblasts.

The idea already mentioned that DM and DMN are malignant neuroectodermal tumors that have a rather close relationship to MPNST is supported by frequent neural differentiation and neurotropism histologically, their immunohistochemical profile (vimentin+, S-100 protein+, most other melanocytic markers generally negative), and their clinical behavior resembling an MPNST. The findings observed in DM and DMN on electron microscopy are often nonspecific; however, the occasional presence of nonbranching, branching, and interweaving cellular processes with focal basal lamina, intermediate junctions, and long-spacing collagen suggest characteristics of perineural cells and schwann cells, and perhaps transitional or primitive forms of the two cell types in these tumors (163). Further support for this thesis includes work showing loss of heterozygosity (LOH) of the neurofibromatosis 1 (NF1) gene and its flanking domains and also the Max-interacting protein 1 (MXI1) in a high proportion of DM and DMN compared to conventional melanoma. The MXI1 is a negative regulator of *Myc* oncoprotein and such LOH has been associated with astrocytomas and glial neoplasia (189).

Natural History and Outcome Desmoplastic melanoma and desmoplastic–neurotropic melanoma is usually diagnosed at an advanced stage, since they are usually at least 4–5 mm in thickness and level IV or V (147–171) (Table

TABLE 10-19 Results of electron microscopy reported for desmoplastic melanoma.

Feature	Carlson et al. (72)	Literature
Intertwining cell processes	100%	45%
Cell junctions	100%	55%
Basal lamina	57%	39%
Lysosomal-like dense bodies	43%	16%
Premelanosomes	0	19%
Melanosomes	0	26%
Long spacing collagen	28%	0
Myo-dense bodies	0	26%

10-10); a mean thickness for all cases reported to date in 1995 was 4.71 mm (163). Because of misdiagnosis, they are commonly first recognized as recurrent or metastatic tumors (190–192). Desmoplastic melanomas frequently recur (range 11–82%) in general owing to inadequate surgical margins (owing to misdiagnosis and the difficulty assessing margins since the tumors are amelanotic, poorly defined, and because of neurotropism (55–61,70). Local recurrences are almost always related to a failure of margin control (resection margins positive, < 1 cm, or unknown), failure to diagnose the tumor correctly (usually inadequate margins), location on the head and neck (often narrower margins), anatomic level V, thickness > 4 mm, and presence of neurotropism (159). Tumors with surgical margins < 1 cm are associated with much higher rates of recurrence compared to those with margins > 2 cm. If one examines lesions with margins 1–2 cm versus those with > 2 cm, there is no difference in rates of recurrence. However there is an odds ratio of 2:1 predicting recurrence. If margins are 2 cm or greater, the recurrence rate is about 5%, which is comparable to that of conventional melanoma. The presence of neurotropism is associated with recurrence rates of 20% compared to 6.8% in DM without neurotropism (169). As with conventional melanoma, local recurrence of DM and DMN is predictive of systemic metastases. DM and DMN seem to recur more rapidly than conventional melanomas, with almost 80% of recurrences appearing within 2 years (169).

In a series of 280 patients with DM and DMN (median thickness, 2.5 mm) reported from Sydney, Australia, the overall 5-year survival rate was 75.2%, and 52% at 10 years; however, when only stage I and II (localized) disease was examined, the 5-year survival rate was 90% (compared to 79% for all melanomas of comparable stage) (169). Factors reported to adversely influence survival for DM and DMN include Breslow thickness, high mitotic rate ($> 4/mm^2$), and in some studies ulceration (193), neurotropism (164), and increased stromal mucin (165). DM with neurotropism are associated with significantly reduced survival compared to DM without neurotropism (164). Attributes affecting time to treatment failure include thickness, high mitotic rate, and surgical margins < 1 cm compared to > 2 cm (169).

DM and DMN result in metastases in just under a third of patients (11–40% in the literature) in most series and seem to behave as a sarcoma (169). These tumors present with regional lymph node involvement much less commonly than conventional melanomas (4 vs. 20%, respectively) (169). Similarly DM and DMN metastasize to regional lymph nodes uncommonly (3–11% of cases) and less often than conventional melanomas. There is an unusually striking predilection for metastasis to the lungs (191) in some series but not in others (169). Systemic metastases are correlated with previous recurrences and tumor thickness (169,191).

Differential Diagnosis The spectrum of tumors potentially confused with desmoplastic and neurotropic melanoma is varied and includes spindle cell proliferations and tumors with a fibrous appearance (147–169,194) (Table 10-17). The principal lesions to be considered include sclerosing blue nevus (70), desmoplastic Spitz nevus/tumor (195), neurothekeoma (nerve sheath myxoma) (196), malignant peripheral nerve sheath tumor, scar, dermatofibroma, atypical fibroxanthoma, malignant fibrous histiocytoma, fibromatosis, dermatofibrosarcoma protuberans, fibrosarcoma, myxoma, spindle cell squamous cell carcinoma, sclerosing basal cell carcinoma, and leiomyosarcoma (70–74,77). The intraepidermal melanocytic proliferation commonly found in desmoplastic melanoma is usually absent in the other conditions.

Sclerosing blue nevus and desmoplastic Spitz nevus/tumor (70,78) are often superficial, small in size, fairly well demarcated, and characterized by an orderly infiltration of the fibrotic stroma by melanocytes and have an overall benign cytologic appearance. In the case of desmoplastic Spitz nevus/tumor, there is a striking zonation of melanocytes in the dermis and progressive maturation or dispersion of individual melanocytes among collagen bundles with depth. The melanocytes are also strikingly epithelioid (and uniform) in appearance in such Spitz tumors and show diminished cellular and nuclear sizes with depth. Mitotic figures, usually encountered in DM and DMN and occasionally in desmoplastic Spitz nevus/tumor, are exceedingly rare or absent in sclerosing blue nevus. Early forms of desmoplastic melanoma may be difficult to distinguish from sclerosing blue nevus (70,71), and it is vital to weigh all clinical and histologic features. For example, desmoplastic melanoma in a young individual on an anatomic site besides the head and neck or acral areas would be highly unusual, and such circumstances would argue against a diagnosis of desmoplastic melanoma. A useful feature for distinguishing DM and DMN from sclerosing blue nevus and desmoplastic Spitz nevus/tumor is often the conspicuous positiviy of the latter tumors with HMB-45 and its negativity in the former group (see below).

The desmoplastic Spitz nevus is characterized by symmetry, an inverted wedge-shaped configuration, and infiltration of the dermis by relatively monotonous epithelioid or spindle cells (78), allowing its distinction from desmoplastic melanoma in most instances. Desmoplastic melanoma may also show a fascicular arrangement of cells that is generally lacking in desmoplastic Spitz nevus.

Relatively cellular variants of neurothekeoma (nerve sheath myxoma) may suggest desmoplastic melanoma

(79). Neurothekeoma commonly arises in the head and neck region, as does desmoplastic melanoma. Neurothekeoma generally occurs in young individuals (average age 20 years), does not demonstrate an intraepidermal melanocytic proliferation, and is typified by a lobular architecture in the dermis (79). Concentric and fascicular arrangements of cells are often noted in neurothekeoma; the constituent cells may be epithelioid or bipolar and stellate, and multinucleate forms are seen. Low-grade nuclear pleomorphism and occasional mitotic figures are occasionally encountered. Distinction from desmoplastic melanoma is based on a regular, organized appearance; orderly infiltration of the dermis; a lesser degree of cytologic atypia; and negative immunoreactivity, particularly with S-100 protein but also with other markers of melanocytic differentiation such as Mart-1, MITF, and tyrosinase (79).

Because of prominent schwannian differentiation, discrimination of desmoplastic–neurotropic melanoma from peripheral nerve sheath tumors may be difficult or impossible. All clinical and histologic characteristics must be considered. Tumors of the head and neck of elderly patients associated with lentiginous melanomas are usually not a diagnostic problem. Tumors in other anatomic sites without an intraepidermal component will cause difficulty, and immunohistochemistry may be of particular value for them (see below) (62,63,80,81).

Lesions demonstrating fibrous or fibrohistiocytic differentiation figure prominently in the differential diagnosis of desmoplastic melanoma and include scars, dermatofibroma (fibrous histiocytoma), juvenile xanthogranuloma, dermatofibrosarcoma protuberans, atypical fibroxanthoma, superficial forms of malignant fibrous histiocytoma, and fibromatosis. These lesions generally lack intraepidermal melanocytic proliferation, melanin pigment, and neurotropism. In general, scars are differentiated from DM and DMN based on the latter features and the presence of horizontally aligned fibrous tissue that is sparsely cellular, vertically-oriented, blood vessels, and absence of adnexal structures. However, in particular situations, such as the distinction of DM and DMN from immature cellular scars, which may exhibit slight nuclear pleomorphism of spindle cells, particularly in re-excision specimens and potentially recurrent lesions, may prove difficult or impossible without resorting to immunohistochemisty. In addition, in some cases there may be relatively few tumor cells admixed with scar tissue. Since S-100 protein marks the tumor cells in almost all DM and DMN, immunohistochemistry would seem to resolve the latter delemma rather easily. However, up to 10% of the cellular population of a scar may be composed of S-100-positive Schwann cells, Langerhans cells, and other cells of uncertain lineage (198). One must then rely on other features, such as cytologic atypia, neurotropism, and lymphocytic infiltrates and the use of additional melanocytic markers, such as tyrosinase (see above).

Atypical fibroxanthoma and malignant fibrous histiocytoma enter the differential diagnosis and often require immunohistochemical evaluation, though they may contain xanthoma cells, not usually seen in desmoplastic melanoma. Fibrohistiohistiocytic tumors as a general rule do not display neurotropism.

Desmoplastic melanomas with extensive mucin may raise problems of differential diagnosis, suggesting, for example, a myxoma. However, myxomas generally lack the cytologic atypia and neurotropism of desmoplastic–neurotropic melanoma and are negative for S-100 protein and other melanocytic markers. The myxomatous variants of desmoplastic melanoma usually have zones of prominent cellularity.

Spindle cell squamous carcinoma and cutaneous leiomyosarcoma may be confused with desmoplastic melanoma, but each lack intraepidermal melanocytic proliferation and melanin synthesis. Squamous cell carcinoma may show keratinization, dyskeratosis, and intercellular bridges. Leiomyosarcoma may exhibit the cytologic characteristics of smooth muscle cells, but immunohistochemistry may be essential to finalize the diagnosis.

Angiotropic Melanoma

The propensity for melanoma to migrate along anatomic structures such as nerves (neurotropism) and skin appendages has been recognized as a common phenomenon for many years. On the other hand, this same capacity of melanoma to migrate along the external surfaces of blood vessels and lymphatics has received almost no attention in the literature (106,179,198–205). The origins of this potential mechanism of tumor dissemination were perhaps first noted in the nineteenth century French medical literature. In his original use of the term *metastasis*, Recamier (198) specifically referred to the spread of tumor cells *along the external* surfaces of vascular channels rather than *within* them (he was inadvertently misquoted by future authors) (199). Subsequently, in his historic paper laying the foundations for surgical margins for melanoma in 1907 W. Sampson Handley (200) referred to Borst who had noted "the tendency of melanotic sarcoma to spread along the perivascular tissues immediately outside the blood-vessels." According to Borst, this attraction of melanoma cells to blood vessels resulted from a "chemiotaxis"—that is, that blood was a necessary food for the production of melanin. Handley explained the phenomenon as anatomic, since lymphatic vessels are in close proximity to arteries and veins, and he believed that melanoma initially disseminated by intralymphatic spread. However, Handley's observations were based on the study of a single lymph node metastasis and the regional spread of tumor from that lymph node, rather than from a primary melanoma.

In more recent years, our group (201–205) proposed for the first time that an important mechanism of melanoma metastasis may be via this phenomenon of migration of tumor cells along the external surfaces of vessels or *extravascular migratory metastasis*. This hypothesized mechanism of tumor spread was based on ultrastuctural and immunopathologic studies; in the latter, melanoma cells are closely apposed to the external surfaces of the endothelial cells of blood vessels. Ultrastructurally, the melanoma cells are linked to the endothelium by an amorphous matrix confined to contain laminin (not organized in a basement membrane) by immunohistochemistry. That morphologic structure was termed the *angio-tumoral complex* (201). According to the proposed mechanism, tumor cells begin the process of local spread by competing with pericytes for the periendothelial position (of pericytes) or pericytic-like location for migration along the external surfaces of vessels.

Our group proposed that the histomorphologic counterpart of the angio-tumoral complex is angiotropic melanoma. Angiotropic melanoma has been referred to and reported anecdotally in the literature, more as a curiosity than as an important biologic phenomenon (206–208). However, we drew attention to the importance of angiotropism as a biologic phenomenon and prognostic factor in localized melanoma and as the likely correlate of extravascular migratory metastasis (106,179). In our experience, angiotropism is observed much more frequently than vascular invasion. For example, in a series of 650 consecutive invasive melanomas, the frequency of vascular invasion was 1.4% (172). In a recently published study of metastasizing melanomas carefully matched with nonmetastasizing melanomas for Breslow thickness, age, gender, and site, the presence of angiotropism strongly correlated with the development of metastases, whereas vascular invasion was not observed in any cases.

Clinical Features and Histopathologic Features There are no gross morphologic features that distinguish angiotropic melanomas from other forms of melamoma at present. Angiotropic melanoma is defined by the cuffing of (the close opposition to) the external surfaces of either blood or lymphatic channels, or both, by aggregates of melanoma cells in at least two or more foci (Fig. 10-12B). By definition, there is no tumor present within vascular lumina (106,179). Angiotropic foci must be located either at the advancing front of the tumor or some distance (usually within 1–2 mm) from the main tumoral mass. Although angiotropism is likely to be present within the mass of an invasive tumor, there is no specific means at present to differentiate simple entrapment of vessels by tumor from angiotropism. Immunohistochemisty with markers such as S-100 protein and Mart-1 may aid in the identification or confirmation of angiotropism (106).

Angiotropism is observed with greater frequency in melanomas that also demonstrate desmoplasia and neurotropism, suggesting closely related mechanisms.

Minimal Deviation Melanoma

In this section we discuss the conceptual basis of minimal deviation melanoma (MDM) without attempting to resolve the controversies of nomenclature, biologic course, or the legitimacy of the entity (211–217). From precedents in other neoplastic systems, the possibility that the biologic behavior of melanomas may correlate with cytomorphology and degree of differentiation seems plausible. To the extent that some melanomas designated as MDM resemble banal compound or dermal nevi, the terms *nevoid melanoma* and *small cell melanoma* might also similarly be applied to such lesions.

The term *MDM* was introduced to embrace the concept that a subset of invasive melanomas is characterized by lesser cytologic atypia and a better prognosis than conventional melanomas of the same thickness (211–217). Thus central to the concept of MDM, is the presence of a cohesive nodule of dermal tumor cells. The growth pattern of such a nodule potentially indicates aggressive properties, such as recurrence or metastasis. Also implicit is the presence of a cell type lacking the characteristics of "fully-evolved" melanoma cells of the invasive component of conventional melanomas. (214–216). Such cells express nuclear and cytoplasmic abnormalities intermediate between a typical basilar melanocyte or nevus cell and a melanoma cell. The cell types presumed to occur in MDM resemble ordinary nevus cells, spindled melanocytes, and epithelioid cells as from Spitz nevi (214–217).

The central problem of MDM is the reliability and significance of recognizing different grades of cytologic atypia and different cell types. At present, there are no specific criteria that clearly distinguish MDM from conventional melanomas or atypical nevi. Neither has the biologic potential of these melanocytic proliferations been sufficiently and objectively correlated with cytologic characteristics—that is, cellular and nuclear morphology (e.g., spindle cell versus epithelioid cell), nuclear area or volume and nuclear pleomorphism. However, a few studies suggest that prognosis may relate to cell type; for example, spindle cell melanomas may be associated with a better outcome than those composed of epithelioid cells (218–220). Measurement of nuclear volume may have prognostic significance in melanoma (221). On the other hand, series of patients with nevoid melanomas and small cell melanomas seem to indicate no better prognosis than that observed with conventional melanoma.

Because of the lack of specific histologic criteria and objective markers, data are not available that confirm or refute MDM as an entity. Therefore, the diagnosis of MDM has probably been applied to a heterogenous collection of lesions, ranging from atypical nevi to conventional melanomas.

Nevoid Melanoma

In a very broad sense, the term *nevoid melanoma* could encompass any form of melanoma having some resemblance to or mimicking any type of melanocytic nevus (222–231). An objection to the use of this term is that a large number of melanomas may more or less resemble banal nevi and that the application of the term may be rather subjective. We clearly acknowledge this problem. A variety of other terms have been employed to describe this general group of melanomas, depending on how stringent one makes the criteria for inclusion—minimal deviation melanoma; verrucous and pseudonevoid melanoma and closely related terms (see below), spitzoid melanoma, small-diameter melanoma, and small cell melanoma (223–226,232–234). It is obvious that some nevoid melanomas might also be characterized as having a small diameter and also being composed of small melanoma cells (i.e., small cell melanoma). However, we employ the term rather restrictively, as have most authors, to describe melanomas that closely resemble ordinary compound or dermal nevi; the latter lesions generally fall into four groups: those with a raised, dome-shaped or polypoid (nodular nonverrucous) configuration that resemble a predominately dermal nevus; those with a distinctly papillomatous or verrucous surface; those resembling a lentiginous melanocytic nevus arising in sun-exposed skin of older individuals; and those with a predominately or exclusively intraepidermal nested appearance mimicking a junctional or compound nevus (222,231).

The importance of this rare group of melanomas cannot be overstated because of the profound diagnostic difficulty they pose to pathologists. The latter conclusion is simply based on the fact that many such lesions are often diagnosed only in retrospect after the development of recurrences or metastases (and unfortunately in some instances only after medicolegal proceedings have begun).

The concept that melanomas may closely resemble melanocytic nevi probably dates back at least to the introduction of the term *minimal deviation melanoma*. Arnold Levene (223) further emphasized this problem when he described "verrucous and pseudonevoid melanomas" in 1980, as variants of melanoma that mimicked warty dermal nevi, both clinically and histologically.

Schmoeckel et al. (222) first coined the term *nevoid melanoma* in their description of 33 melanomas with histologic features suggesting a melanocytic nevus. The latter authors noted that 15 patients developed metastases, and they concluded that nevoid melanoma did not seem to have any better prognosis than conventional melanoma. About 70 additional cases were subsequently reported in the literature (223–231).

Clinical Features From a survey of the literature and our experience, we note that patients of all ages, ranging from children to older individuals (> 80 years of age), may develop NM, with the majority of cases being diagnosed in the 5th decade (222–231) (Table 10-20). Both sexes seem to be equally affected. As with conventional melanomas, NM may occur anywhere on the body surface and most commonly affect the backs of men and the lower extremities of women. Schmoeckel et al. (222) reported that NM had no distinctive clinical features compared to conventional melanomas. However, the clinical findings are probably related to the clinicopathological variant encountered. Verrucous or papillomatous vari-

TABLE 10-20 Nevoid melanoma.

Clinical features
 Women = men
 All ages, commonly 5th decade
 Occurs anywhere, but trunk and lower extremities most common
 No distinctive features but may have verrucous appearance
 Any size, often relatively small diameter but up to 2 cm or more

Histopathologic features
 Striking resemblance to banal compound or dermal nevus at scanning magnification
 Symmetry common
 Well-circumscribed lateral margins
 Pagetoid spread, not common
 Limited intraepidermal component, often
 Relatively small nevuslike cells, monomorphous appearance
 Some maturation may be present but often incomplete or absent
 Single cell infiltration at base
 Cytological atypia
  Nuclear pleomorphism
  Angulated nuclei
  Hyperchromatism
  Prominent nucleoli may be present
 Mitoses in dermal component, particularly deep
 Infiltration of adnexal structures
 Little or no inflammation

Differential diagnosis
 Melanocytic nevus, especially papillomatous dermal nevus
 Metastatic melanoma

ants often suggest a verruca, seborrheic keratosis, or warty melanocytic nevus; whereas the nodular variants are rather more nondescript and commonly suggest a banal nevus, an atypical nevus, or a papule or nodule invoking a wide variety of diagnoses. As with conventional nodular melanomas, particularly amelanotic variants, a high index of suspicion is needed for diagnosis. In many instances, melanoma is not even suspected.

Histopathologic Features The essential histopathologic criteria for diagnosis are as follows: (a) at scanning magnification, the lesion has a striking resemblance to an ordinary compound or dermal nevus (222,229,231) (Fig. 10-18; Table 10-20); (b) the lesion has an overall symmetry (some asymmetry may be present); (c) there is rather sharp circumscription at the peripheries of the lesion; (d) there is an absence of or often only a limited intraepidermal component, commonly with little or no pagetoid spread; (e) a monomorphous population of nevus-like cells in the dermis is usually characterized by a confluent or sheet-like growth pattern in some portion of the lesion (Figs. 10-22 and 10-23), and (f) dermal mitotic figures are seen. Other features that commonly but not invariably present and that may suggest a banal nevus are diameter < 5–6 mm and changes suggesting maturation.

As mentioned above there are four general morphologic variants: (a) the nonverrucous papular or nodular forms that present with only limited or no epidermal hyperplasia (222,227,229,231); (b) the verrucous or papillomatous variants that have a configuration suggesting a common verruca, seborrheic keratosis, or papillomatous nevus (223–226,228,231–235) (Figs. 6-17 and 10-24) (see below); (c) the lentiginous variants arising in sun-exposed skin of older individuals (236,237); and (d) the striking intraepidermal nested variants mimicking a junctional nevus (see above). By definition, these variants usually suggest a banal nevus at scanning magnification, are usually fairly symmetrical, and often are well circumscribed. Ulceration is usually absent. As mentioned, there may be no intraepidermal melanocytic component in a large proportion of cases. The intraepidermal component, if present, may be subtle or limited in nature. One may observe melanocytes arranged as single cells and/or in junctional nests along the dermoepidermal junction (Fig. 10-22B). The latter nesting may result in a confluence of nested aggregates of melanocytes replacing the basilar portion of the epidermis. The epidermis is frequently effaced, thinned, and associated with dermoepidermal separation (Fig. 10-23B). Pagetoid spread may be present in a proportion of cases and is an important finding in confirming a diagnosis of melanoma; however, it is often not a conspicuous feature.

The lentiginous variants originally described by Kossard et al. (236,237) raise an image of a lentiginous junctional or compound nevus at scanning magnification. Features suggesting melanoma include large diameter (up

FIGURE 10-22 Nevoid melanoma. **A,** This lesion resembles a conventional compound nevus at scanning magnification because of its small diameter and the relative small size of the melanocytes; nonetheless, the lesion is slightly asymmetrical.

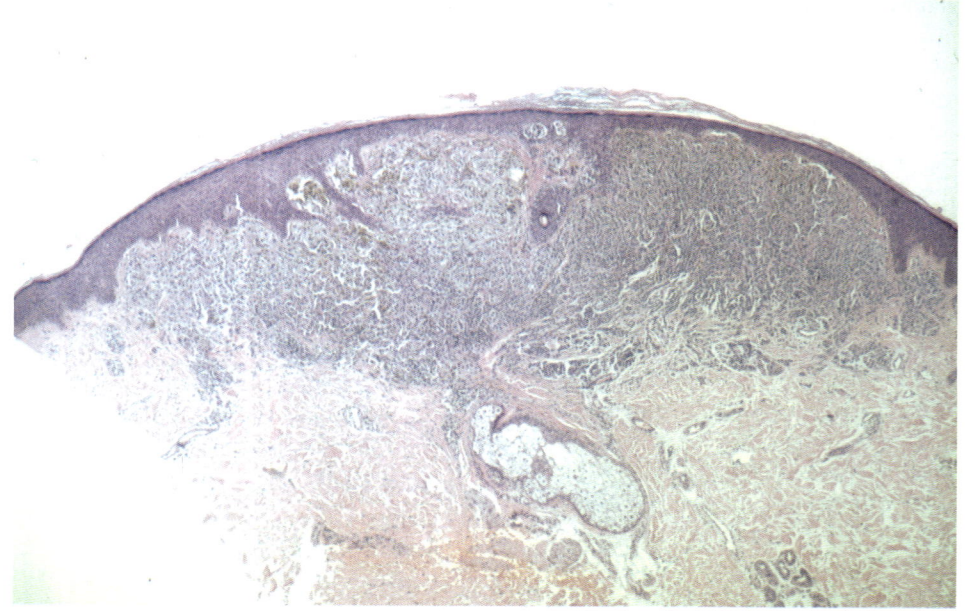

A

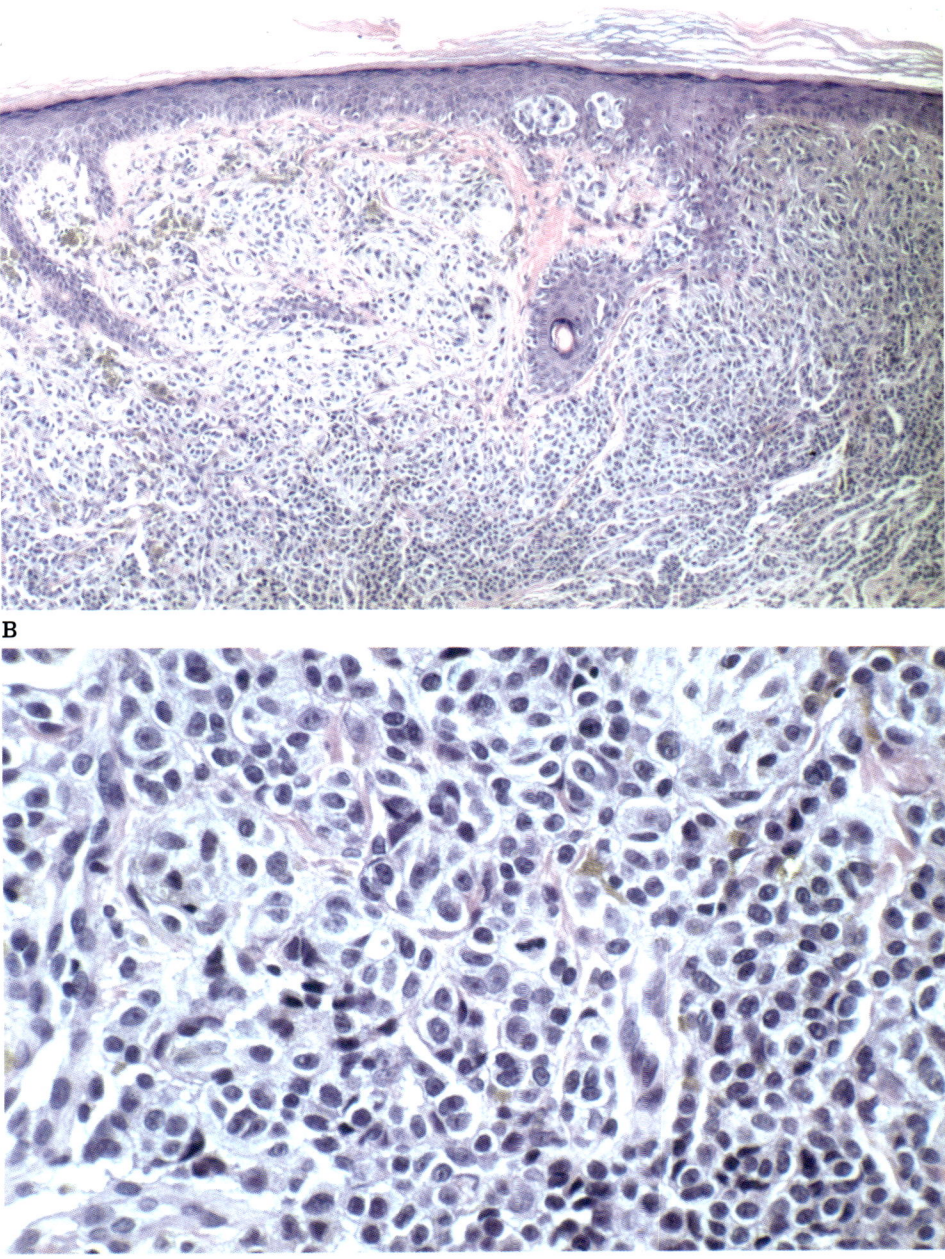

FIGURE 10-22 *Continued.* **B,** There is focal intraepidermal nesting present. The dermis contains nests of fairly small nevuslike cells that are monotypic, show confluence, and lack maturation, all features suggesting melanoma. **C,** Examination at high magnification allows for the recognition of abnormalities essential for diagnosing melanoma: striking nuclear atypia (nuclear enlargement, pleomorphism, and thickening of nuclear membranes). In addition, mitoses are easily found.

to 1 cm or more), asymmetry, poorly defined margins, effacement and atrophy of the epidermis, host response (including partial regression), large junctional and dermal nests of melanocytes that tend to confluence, some pagetoid spread (often subtle), and the lack of maturation.

The principal finding in the dermis includes a sheetlike or confluent arrangement of relatively small cuboidal or polygonal melanocytes closely mimicking nevus cells (Figs. 10-22B and 10-23A). Often, the dermal melanocytic population fills the papillary dermis

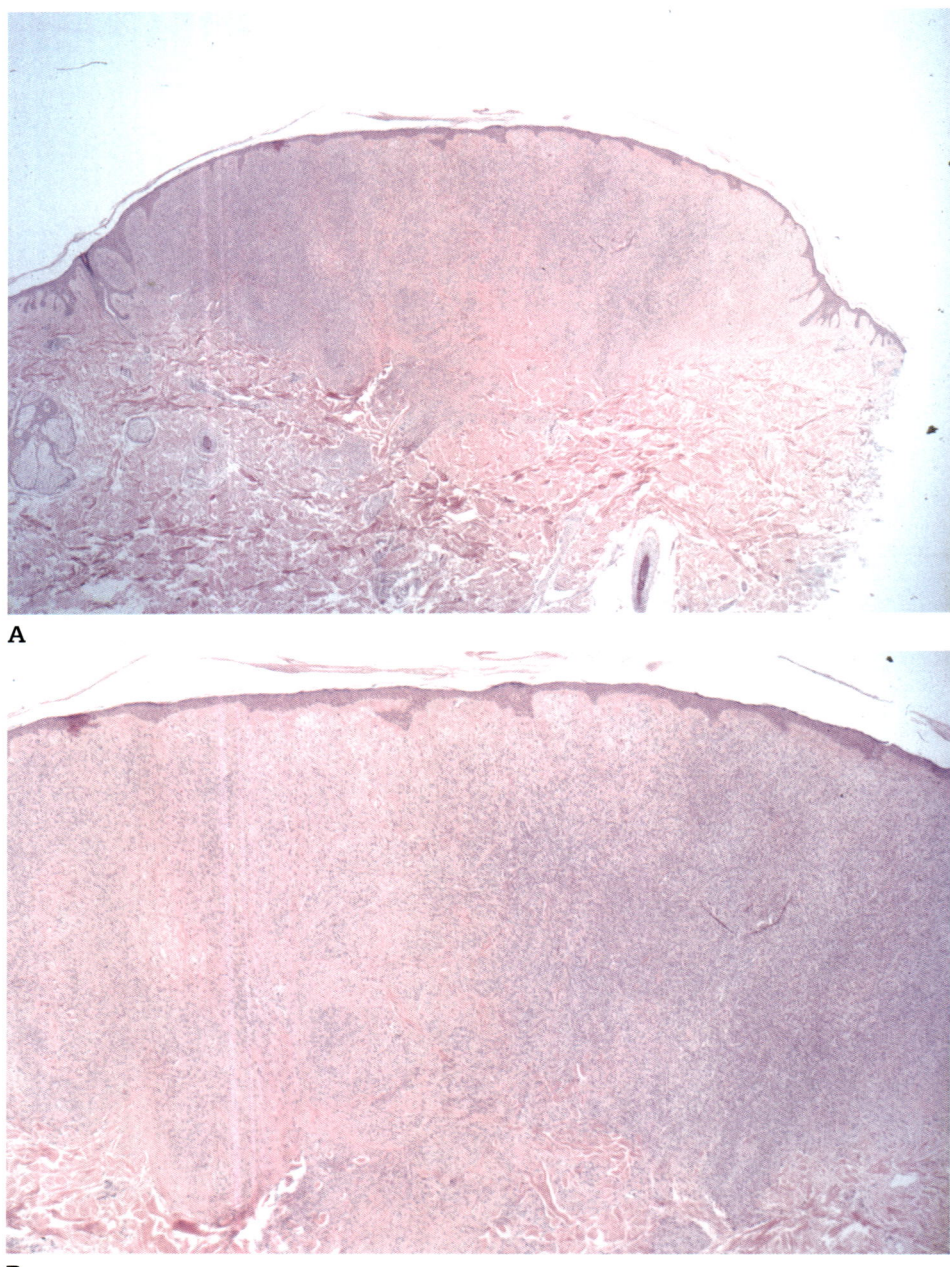

FIGURE 10-23 Nevoid melanoma. **A,** At scanning magnification, this tumor closely mimicks a dermal nevus because of its remarkable symmetry and the general homogeneity and bland cytologic apprearance of the melanocytes. The lesion was diagnosed as an atypical nevus. Regional lymph node metastases developed 7 years after diagnosis. **B,** The epidermis is largely spared. The lesion fails to show maturation, because there is confluence of melanocytes in the dermis.

and is closely opposed to the epidermis, resulting in a strikingly crowded or hypercellular apprearance (Figs. 10-22 and 10-23). In many cases, the melanocytes extend into the reticular dermis with some diminished cellular density and also some reduction in cellular and nuclear sizes, suggesting some maturation. In some lesions, one may observe fairly discreet nesting of melanocytes in some areas, suggesting a nevus; however, other parts of the lesion usually demonstrate the confluence and hypercellulariy that favors melanoma (Figs. 10-22B and

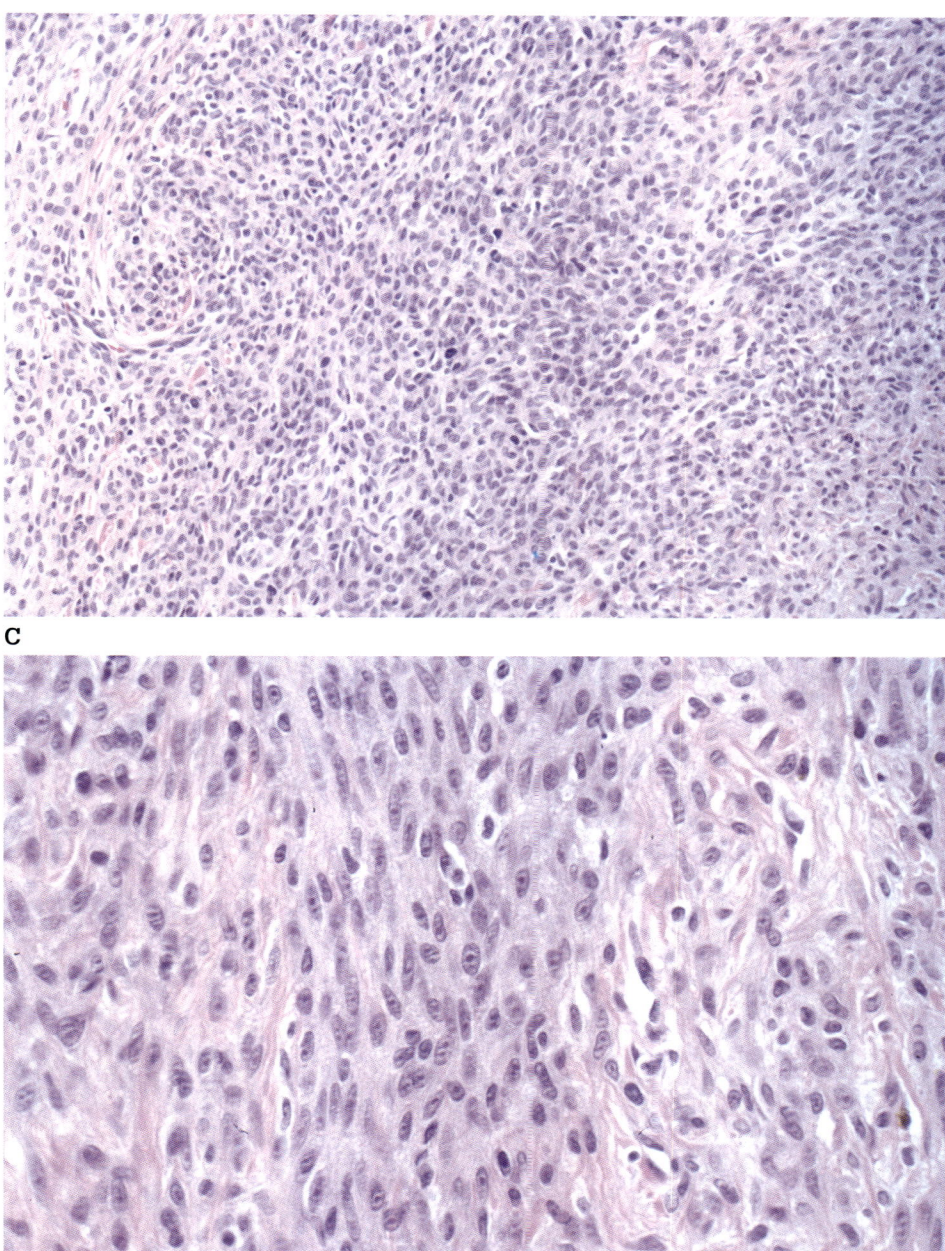

FIGURE 10-23 *Continued.* **C,** Note the prominent cellularity of the melanocytes and the absence of maturation. **D,** High magnification shows confluent spindle cells in the dermis. The nuclei are enlarged with pleomorphism and prominent nucleoli. Uncommon mitoses are present throughout. This lesion underscores the need to examine such borderline tumors at high magnification for additional features that are crucial for histopathologic interpretation.

10-23B). Furthermore, the heterogeneity of the lesion is another feature consonant with melanoma. Although the lateral margins are commonly well demarcated, the base of the melanoma is often poorly defined and characterized by the presence of single cells infiltrating collagen. In most instances, there is no host inflammatory response.

The cytologic features observed merit some discussion. As with all melanomas one encounters a heterogeneity of cell type from lesion to lesion. The melanocytes

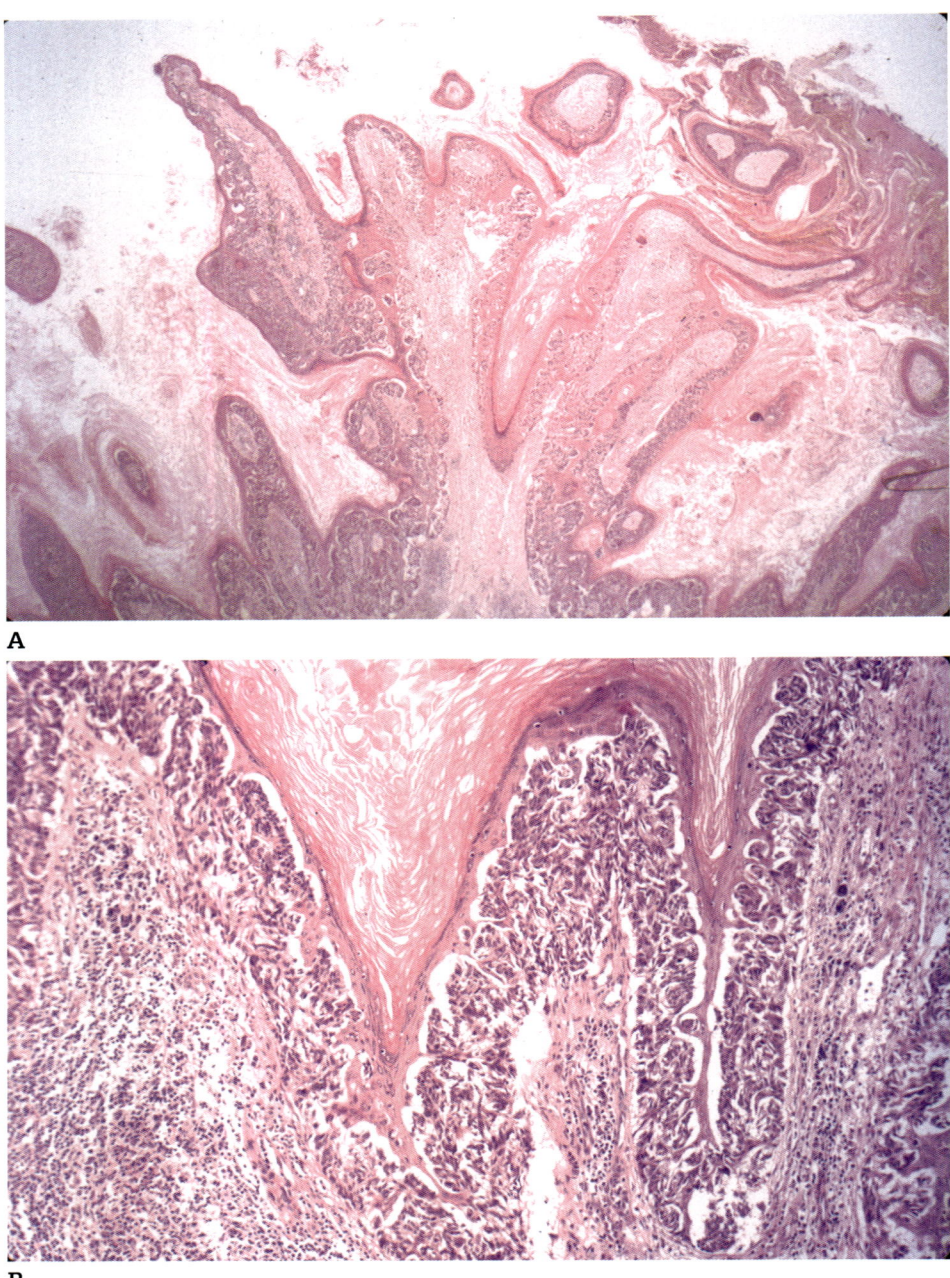

FIGURE 10-24 Verrucous (nevoid) melanoma. **A,** Note the prominent papillomatous configuration of the lesion, suggesting a papillomatous dermal nevus. **B,** Confluent intraepidermal proliferation of melanoma cells is a striking feature of verrucous melanoma.

making up NM, at least in the superficial part of the lesion and perhaps throughout, are generally polygonal or epithelioid cells (mimicking the so-called type-A or epithelioid nevus cells) and sufficiently small to suggest nevus cells (Fig. 10-22C). They nonetheless demonstrate definite but sometimes subtle nuclear enlargement, pleomorphism, and often hyperchromatism; rather prominent nucleoli may be present (Figs. 10-22C and 10-23D). As mentioned, many NM may suggest maturation—that is, diminished cytoplasmic and nuclear diameters with depth and a transition to smaller type-B, or lymphocyte-like cells, and perhaps type-C, or Schwann-like cells. At

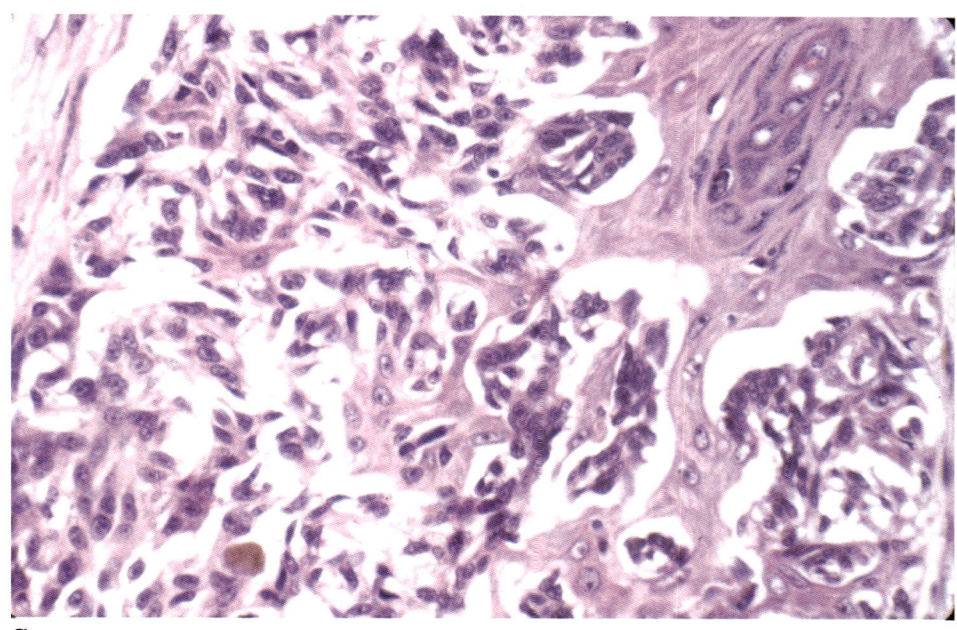

FIGURE 10-24 *Continued.* **C,** Higher magnification of panel B showing irregular confluent intraepidermal nesting of pleomorphic melanoma cells. (Courtesy of Dr. K. Blessing, University of Aberdeen, UK.)

the same time, the latter transition may be accompanied by diminished cellularity with deph and loss of pigment synthesis. Nonetheless, major clues to diagnosis of NM are the presence of definite nuclear pleomorphism and, in particular, irregular nuclear contours, hyperchromatism, and nucleoli as well as continued pigment synthesis in the deepest parts of the dermal component (Figs. 10-22C and 10-23D). Commonly, one observes well-defined nests of relatively small cuboidal cells in the deepest portions of NM with the latter characteristics.

One of the most important and sometimes the single most important criterion for diagnosis is the presence of mitoses in the dermal component (222,231,233,234). The latter finding is often the first clue to considering melanoma in the differential diagnosis. The presence of one or a small number of dermal mitoses does not constitute sufficient evidence for diagnosis of melanoma, but it should prompt the histopathologist to search for additional criteria for melanoma and to either confirm or exclude the diagnosis (if possible). Mitoses are present in virtually all cases, and their absence should provoke skepticism about melanoma. The mitotic rate in commonly relatively low, often < 6/mm². Increasing mitotic rate, deeply situated mitoses, and atypical forms also provide progressively more support for NM. We have found that the presence or absence of mitotic figures in the deepest portion of a lesion can be a decisive factor in confirming or ruling out NM (93) (Fig. 10-22C).

Ancillary Techniques

Because of the profound difficulty of these lesions, one must marshal all resources available in the assessment of such tumors. Unfortunately, methodologies such as analysis of DNA-ploidy and nucleolar organizer regions or use of various immunomarkers usually provide no better answers than conventional microscopy at present (229,236). Some authors thus have studied the gradient of immunostaining with HMB-45 and proliferative activity with Ki-67 of the dermal component of lesions suspicious for NM. In a small number of NM, some but not all have showed comparable degrees of expression of the latter markers in both the upper- and lower-most portions of the lesions. Perhaps in the near future, cDNA microarray analysis may disclose more objective information in resolving this problem.

Differential Diagnosis The principal lesions to be distinguished are compound or dermal nevi, possibly with papillomatous or verrucous surface morphology, that often demonstrate one or more of the following: high cellular density of nevus cells in the dermis, confluence of nevus cells in dermis, lack of complete maturation, nuclear pleomorphism, mitotic figures, and inflammation and partial regression (Table 10-21). Because of the profound heterogeneity of nevi and melanomas (as with any tissue and organ system), there are variations on this theme too numerous to expound on. Thus a number of

TABLE 10-21 Comparison of nevoid melanoma and melanocytic nevus.

Nevoid melanoma	Melanocytic nevus
Clinical features	
Older age	Younger age
Larger size, 1–2 cm	Smaller size, < 6 mm
Some variation in color	More homogenous color
Greater asymmetry	Less asymmetry
Histopathological features	
Greater asymmetry	Symmetry
Less well circumscribed	Well circumscribed
Greater likelihood of pagetoid spread	Little or no pagetoid spread
Intraepidermal basilar melanocytic proliferation common	Basilar proliferation, less common
Infiltration of adnexae	Usually no infiltration of adnexae
Little or no maturation	Maturation
Mitoses in dermis	Usually no dermal mitoses
Atypical mitoses, variable	No atypical mitoses
Deep infiltration of dermis	No deep infiltration

other features—including lesional diameter, presence of asymmetry or not, lesional heterogeneity, presence of pagetoid spread or not, characteristics of the epidermis such as effacement and thinning, age of the patient, location of the lesion, clinical history of a changing lesion, and gross morphologic features—usually figure into this complex deliberation as to whether a lesion can be categorized as a benign nevus, a biologically indeterminate lesion, or as melanoma. Features often shared by nevi and NM, which usually provide no discriminatory value include relative small diameter (e.g., 3–6 mm), symmetry, well-circumscribed appearance, some apparent maturation, and a limited intraepidermal component with little or no pagetoid spread. One's confidence in rendering a diagnosis of nevoid melanoma directly correlates with the number of abnormal features present.

In our experience, the following attributes are of critical importance for distinguishing NM from a nevus. (a) Dermal mitoses, usually muliple and scattered throughout the lesion, are probably mandatory for the diagnosis. The higher the absolute mitotic rate and the more deeply located the mitoses, the more certain is the diagnosis. However, the presence of rare mitoses particularly in nevi in young or pregnant individuals and in nevi without atypia must be interpreted with caution and are not proof of NM. (b) Dermal aggregates or fascicles of melanocytes showing high density and confluence, having a sheetlike appearance throughout, or showing both features are suggestive. The dermal population often demonstrates a monotonous appearance. (c) Cytologic atypia of the melanocytes is mandatory for the diagnosis. By definition, there are lesser degress of atypia than in conventional melanomas. Careful scrutiny at higher magnifications is necessary to establish the presence of cytologic atypia. In general, the melanocytes may be relatively small compared to the usual enlarged epithelioid melanoma cells and thus the resemblance to a nevus.

Atypical Halo or Halo-Like Nevi

In our experience, a major problem is the differentiation of atypical halo or halo-like nevi from NM. The former group of lesions commonly demonstrates asymmetry, thinning and effacement of the epidermis, confluent nests and fascicles of atypical melanocytes along the dermoepidermal junction, dermoepidermal separation, and cytologic atypia of melanocytes. Some component of large Spitz-like melanocytes may be present in some lesions, partial regression in some, and occasional mitoses may be seen in the dermal component. Features favoring a halo or halo-like nevus include the overall nested organizational pattern of a nevus, maturation of the dermal component, and a well-defined horizontal lower-most margin; a large majority of melanocytes with uniformly dispersed chromatin patterns and without thickening of nuclear membranes; and, generally, the development of the lesions on the backs of children, adolescents, and young adults. A subset of such lesions can be categorized only as biologically indeterminate because of the degree of atypia present and managed accordingly.

Metastatic Melanoma

Metastatic melanoma, particularly the epidermotropic forms, may in fact be nevoid or closely resemble a nevus (117). The distinction of a primary from a metastatic lesion may be impossible in a proportion of cases without clinical information. Such metastases often appear as multiple small pink papules in the region of an antecedent primary melanoma. Histologically, they are often small (e.g. 2–4 mm in diameter), have a predominately dermal localization, and consist of monomorphous spheroid aggregates of melanocytes.

Verrucous Melanoma

Although verrucous melanoma was initially described in his classification of melanoma in 1967, Clark (9) subsequently discarded the term since he believed that its features could be present in any of the major subtypes of melanoma (10). In his depiction of verrucous melanoma, Clark (9) called attention to its striking keratotic surface and prominent epidermal hyperplasia on histologic examination. Since the 1990s or so, additional cases of verrucous melanoma have been reported (223,232), some under a number of closely related terms such as verrucous and pseudonaevoid melanoma (223,224), verrucous-keratotic melanoma (225), and verrucous naevoid and keratotic melanoma (226). All of the latter reports have emphasized the prominent clinical and histologic verrucous features of such melanomas and the difficulty in classifying many of these lesions. Some authors have also called attention to the striking resemblance to papillomatous dermal nevi. The latter features thus suggest that some or many of these melanomas might also be classified as nevoid melanoma.

According to Kuehl-Petzoldt et al. (225), verrucous melanomas have the same biologic behavior and prognosis as conventional melanomas when matched pairs are analyzed. It should be noted, however, that tumor depth may be inappropriately thick in many cases because of epidermal hyperplasia or papillomatous configuration. Anatomic level thus may provide a more accurate assessment of the biologic potential of the tumor.

Clinical Features Some studies have reported a greater frequency of these lesions on the lower extremities of women (225,232) (Table 10-22). However, this has not been corroborated in all studies, since the backs of men may also be commonly affected (226). The majority of patients have been in their 6th decade at the time of diagnosis (225,226,232). Most lesions are described as well circumscribed; 1–2 cm in diameter; and characterized by a dark brown, black, or grayish appearance and hyper-keratotic verrucous surface. Whitish or bluish color suggesting regression is distinctly uncommon (225,232). Many such lesions are diagnosed clinically as seborrheic keratosis or papillomatous nevi (226,232).

Histopathologic Features The most striking feature at scanning magnification is the prominent papillomatous or verrucoid epidermal hyperplasia suggesting a seborrheic keratosis, epidermal nevus, verruca, or papillomatous melanocytic nevus (223–226,228,232–234) (Figs. 10-17 and 10-24; Table 10-22). Many such lesions also exhibit some degree of symmetry, although this feature should not be as common as in a benign process. Hyperkeratosis and parakeratosis may also be prominent (232). The degree of epidermal hyperplasia may be marked and have a pseudoepitheliomatous pattern in some instances (226). The intraepidermal melanocytic component may vary from minimal or none to pagetoid spread (Fig. 10-20B,C). Also in common with pagetoid melanoma is the frequent presence of a laterally extending intraepidermal component (226). As noted by Levene, some of these tumors may show a contiguous basilar and suprabasilar proliferation of atypical melanocytes, often involving adnexal epithelium (223) (Fig. 10-24). In common with nevoid melanoma, the dermal component in some melanomas may show a startling resemblance to a dermal nevus. The cell type in the latter tumors resembles a small nevus cell, but careful inspection should disclose prominent cellular pleomorphism, little or no maturation, and cells dispersed in confluent nests and sheets without orderly infiltration of stroma. The presence of mitotic figures (e.g., more than two or three per section)

TABLE 10-22 Verrucous melanoma.

Clinical features
  50–60 years
  Women > men
  Location anywhere but lower extremities favored
  Well circumscribed
  1–2 cm
  Dark brown, black, grayish
  Verrucous hyperkeratotic surface
  Ulceration uncommon
Histopathologic features
  Hyperkeratosis
  Papillomatous epidermal hyperplasia
  Pseudoepitheliomatous hyperplasia, occasionally
  Symmetry, occasionally
  Epidermal involvement
    None
    Pagetoid spread
    Contiguous basilar melanocytic proliferation
    Involvement of adnexal structures
  Dermal component
    Striking nevus-like appearance, occasionally
    Little or no maturation
    Confluent sheets or nests of cells
  Mitoses in dermis
  Necrotic cells
  Little or no inflammation common
  May resemble any other histogenetic type of melanoma
Differential diagnosis
  Papillomatous dermal nevus
Prognosis
  Same as other types of melanoma

and necrotic cells in the dermal component also argues against a benign process.

Differential Diagnosis On cursory examination, verrucous melanoma may suggest nonmelanocytic tumors, such as seborrheic keratosis, verruca, and epidermal nevus. However, the melanocytic nature of the lesion should become clear with careful inspection. Of particular concern is the potential misdiagnosis of verrucous melanoma as a benign nevus, especially a papillomatous dermal nevus (96). Many of the same characteristics as outlined in Table 10-22 must be weighed in assessing problematic lesions. A host of factors are potentially relevant (see discussion for nevoid melanoma): age of the patient (older age more common in melanoma), size of the lesion (size > 6 mm and especially > 10 mm), clinical asymmetry, variegation of color, histologic asymmetry, pagetoid or contiguous basilar melanocytic proliferation, confluent sheets of cells in dermis, lack of maturation, and dermal mitoses.

Small Cell Melanoma

The term *small cell melanoma* has been introduced into the literature to describe a heterogenous assortment of melanomas from several settings perhaps linked only by the common thread of a population of *small* melanoma cells. This term has been used to refer to rare melanomas developing in children and adolescents on the scalp; melanomas developing in congenital melanocytic nevi of children and adolescents (223,234); melanomas developing in any setting, but particularly adults, that resemble small round cell malignancies, such as Merkel cell carcinoma (238,239); melanomas developing in sun-damaged skin of older individuals in a setting of solar melanocytic neoplasia or atypical lentiginous nevi (236,237); and melanomas in adults that have the characteristics of nevoid melanoma, as described above. Small cell melanomas occurring in children and adolescents are discussed in Chapter 9. Since the there is considerable overlap of small cell melanomas and nevoid melanomas in adults (see above), this section deals only with two entities (Table 10-23): exceptionally rare melanomas that mimic high-grade small round cell malignancies and small cell melanomas arising predominately in sun damaged skin of elderly individuals.

Small Cell Melanoma Mimicking Merkel Cell Carcinoma (Neuroendocrine Carcinoma)
Variants of small cell melanoma that mimic Merkel cell carcinoma are so rare that one can make only anecdotal remarks about them (238,239). Perhaps they have been most commonly recognized as metastases presumably indicating progression or dedifferentiation to high-grade blastlike tumors.

Nonetheless, primary tumors occur in adults. The lesions are primarily defined by a small round cell population arranged in nests, cords, and sheets (Fig. 10-25). Melanin and intrepidermal involvement may or may not be pres-

TABLE 10-23 Small cell melanoma

Clinical features
  Small cell melanoma mimicking Merkel cell carcinoma
    Extremely rare
    Adults (any age)
    Any site
    0.4–2 cm, often
    Amelanotic papule or nodule, often
  Small cell melanoma arising in predominately sun-damaged skin
    > 50 years of age, often (range 18–91)
    Men > women (2:1)
    Backs of men, legs of women
    > 1 cm, usually
    Variegated color
    Tan, brown, black, gray, often

Histopathologic features
  Small cell melanoma mimicking Merkel cell carcinoma
    Melanin and intraepidermal involvement may or may not be present
    Cohesive nests, cords, sheets of small round cells, often
    Cells with scant cytoplasm
    Round to oval nuclei
    Prominent mitotic rate and necrosis
  Small cell melanoma arising in predominately sun-damaged skin
    Intraepidermal component often extensive, lentiginous and nested
    Some pagetoid spread, usually
    Elongated epidermal rete ridges, common
    Effacement and thinning of epidermis, common
    Small cuboidal melanocytes with scant cytoplasm
    Melanocytes larger that those in nevi
    Nuclear pleomorphism
    Irregular nuclear contours
    Dense chromatin
    Prominent nucleoli
    Dermal nests often large, nodular, cohesive, anatomosing
    Absence of maturation, often
    Continued pigment synthesis with depth
    Mitotic figures, rare
    Solar elastosis
    Host response with fibroplasia, partial regression, common

Differential diagnosis
  Small cell melanoma mimicking Merkel cell carcinoma
    Metastatic melanoma
    Primary and metastatic neuroendocrine carcinoma
    Metastatic small cell carcinoma
    Lymphoma
    Other small round cell malignancies
  Small cell melanoma arising in predominately sun-damaged skin
    Atypical lentiginous nevi of sun-exposed skin

ent. These tumors feature cells with scant cytoplasm, round to oval nuclei, high mitotic rates, and scattered necrotic cells. Amelanotic tumors resemble neuroendocrine carcinoma, primary or metastatic; lymphoma; other small cell carcinomas; and metastatic small cell carcinoma of the lung. Immunohistochemisty is of fundamental importance for confirming a melanocytic origin versus the other entities mentioned above. In particular, neuroendocrine carcinoma, metastatic small cell carcinoma of the lung, and other small cell carcinomas may show intraepidermal involvement including nesting and pagetoid spread.

Small Cell Melanomas Arising Predominately in Sun-Damaged Skin of Elderly Individuals Another variant of small cell melanoma, that also might be subsumed under the general category of nevoid melanoma, occurring in sun-damaged skin of individuals generally over the age of 50 years has been proposed by Kossard and Wilkinson (236,237). A series of 131 such cases constituting 7% of all melanomas from the Skin and Cancer Foundation in Sydney, Australia, was the subject of their reports. While undoubtedly some proportion of or many these lesions may in fact be melanoma, the banal appearance of and resemblance of such lesions to lentiginous nevi, a negligible mitotic rate, and the lack of follow-up call into question the diagnosis of melanoma. Thus the group of 131 cases may possibly include an admixtue of atypical nevi, biologically indeterminate lesions, and melanomas. Although we are confident that this entity exists, it is certain that these lesions as a group require further study.

Clinical Features In our experience and that of Kossard and Wilkinson such lesions generally develop in sun-exposed skin of older individuals, with about 80% being 50 years or older (range, 18–91 years) (236,237) (Table 10-23). Men outnumber women by a ratio of about 2:1. These tumors are most common on the backs of men and the lower extremities of women. The lesions are often more than 1 cm in diameter and clinical diagnoses include melanoma, nevus, and basal cell carcinoma.

Histopathological Features The essential histopathological criteria include the following (236,237) (Figs. 10-26 and 10-27; Table 10-23):

- A predominance of small melanoma cells that are generally cuboidal with scant cytoplasm and hyperchromatic nuclei.
- An intraepidemal component that is often extensive, is predominantly lentiginous and nested, usually exhibits limited pagetoid spread, and is composed of small hyperchromatic melanocytes.
- Dermal nests that are often large, nodular, and confluent; show tubular anastomosing features; have an absence of typical maturation; often display continued pigment synthesis with depth; and are composed of small cuboidal melanocytes with hyperchromatic nuclei.
- Frequent solar elastosis and host response changes, including fibrosis, lymphocytic infiltrates, and pigment incontinence consistent with partial regression in the superficial dermis.
- Melanocytic nuclei that are generally larger than those present in nevi, exhibit pleomorphism, have dense nuclear chromatin, and have irregular nuclear contours; some may contain prominent nucleoli.

The intraepidermal component is often 1 cm or more in diameter and demonstrates thinning and effacement of the epidermis, but at the same time the epidermal rete may be elongated in other portions of the lesion. It shows varying features of both solar melanocytic neoplasia (lentigo maligna) and atypical lentiginous junctional or compound nevi, referred to above (Fig. 10-26). In the latter circumstance one may observe well-defined nests of small cuboical melanocytes that vary considerably in size and shape. These features are often subtle and important attribute, suggesting melanoma is the cause of some pagetoid spread; however, pronounced pagetoid spread is noted in only a minority of cases. Aggregates of melanocytes are often dispersed throughout a zone of fibrosis in the dermis with little or no maturation.

Differential Diagnosis Distinguishing such lesions from atypical lentiginous compound nevi is the major challenge; some lesions prove so difficult that they can be categorized only as biologically indeterminate. Unfortunately, since dermal mitoses are generally rare or absent, a major aid to diagnosis is lacking. Of particular use is the recognition of melanoma in situ and contiguity of the latter with the dermal component. Effacement and thinning of the epidermis, confluent nesting of melanocytes along the dermoepidermal junction, some pagetoid spread, and sufficient atypia of the melanocytes allow for a diagnosis of intraepidermal melanoma.

Spitzoid Melanoma

Although it can justifiably be argued that some proportion of melanomas (perhaps large) resemble Spitz tumors and the converse, the term *Spitzoid melanoma*, if used at all, should be reserved for melanomas that truly have a striking morphologic resemblance to Spitz tumors (240–242). The term probably best describes a rare group of tumors often developing in young individuals that are diagnosed as melanoma only in retrospect—that is, after

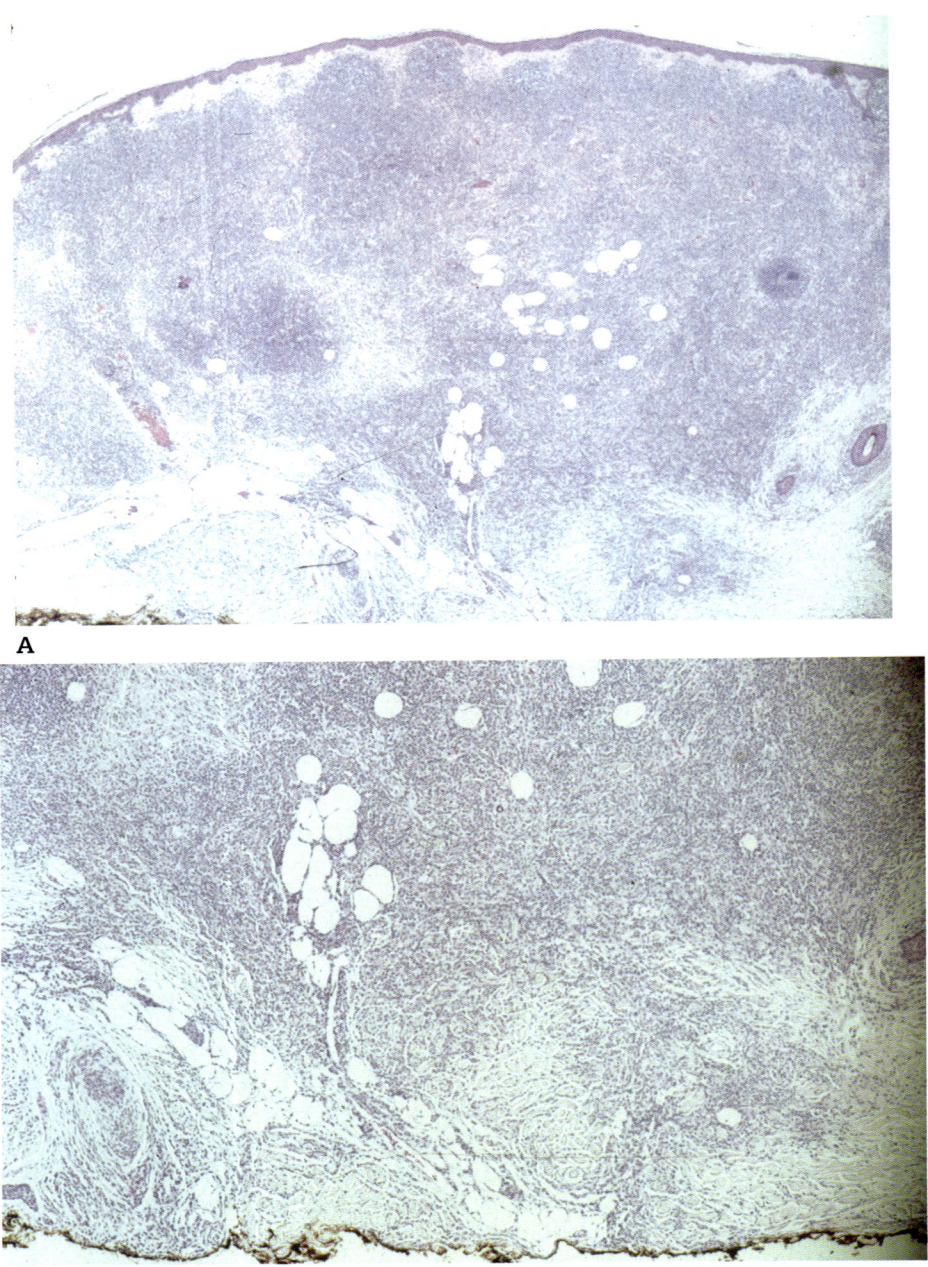

FIGURE 10-25 Small cell melanoma arising de novo on the back of an elderly female. **A,** At scanning magnification, the lesion suggests a dermal nevus, lymphoid infiltrate, or possibly another type of small round-cell malignancy. There is virtually no melanin present; however, the lesion expressed S-100 protein, Mart-1, and HMB-45. **B,** The base of the lesion shows some diminished cellular density with depth suggesting a nevus.

the development of metastases and an aggressive course. Given the profound difficulty of distinguishing some Spitz and Spitz-like tumors from melanoma, we discourage the use of the term *Spitzoid melanoma*, since it may result in the indiscriminate labeling of a heterogeneous group of lesions, including benign Spitz tumors, lesions that are biologically indeterminant, conventional melanomas, and a rare controversial group of tumors previously termed metastasizing Spitz nevus/tumor. The latter group of lesions includes some that have given rise to sin-

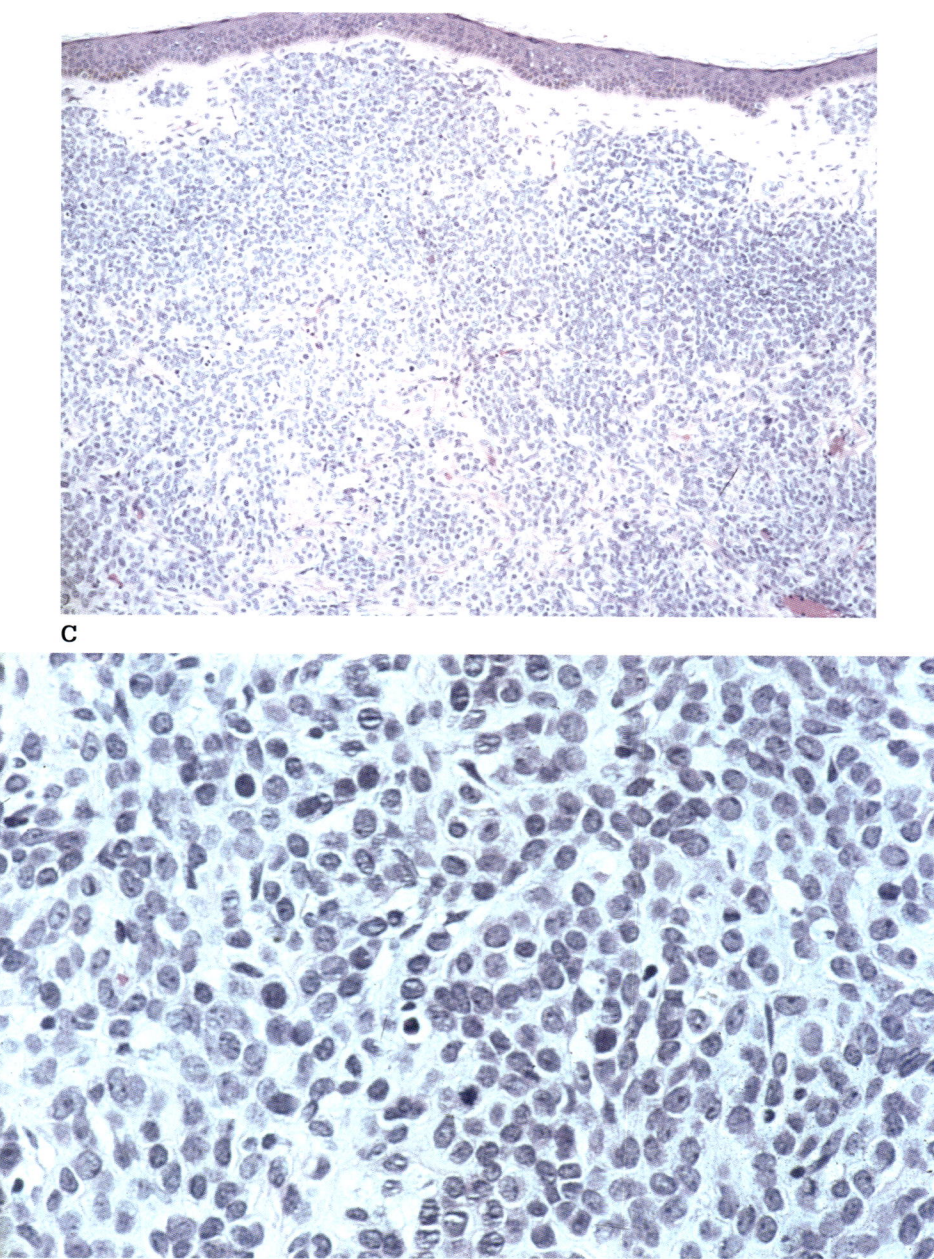

FIGURE 10-25 *Continued.* **C,** In this field there is no epidermal involvement. A monomorphous population of small round cells fills the dermis in a confluent pattern without maturation. **D,** High magnification reveals high cellular density of tumor cells. The small cuboidal cells contain scant cytoplasm and exhibit nuclear pleomorphism and hyperchromatism. The mitotic rate is high.

gle lymph node metastases without subsequent recurrence of melanoma on long-term follow-up.

It cannot be overemphasized that, as a group, all of these unusual Spitz-like tumors require more detailed study as to their biologic nature. We recommend such melanocytic proliferations be categorized, if at all possible, into one of the following groups: (a) Spitz tumor, (b) Spitz-like melanocytic tumor with atypical features (atypical Spitz tumor) and indeterminate biologic potential (describing the abnormal features present such as large size, deep involvement, ulceration, lack of maturation, mitotic rate, presence of deep mitoses), or (c) melanoma.

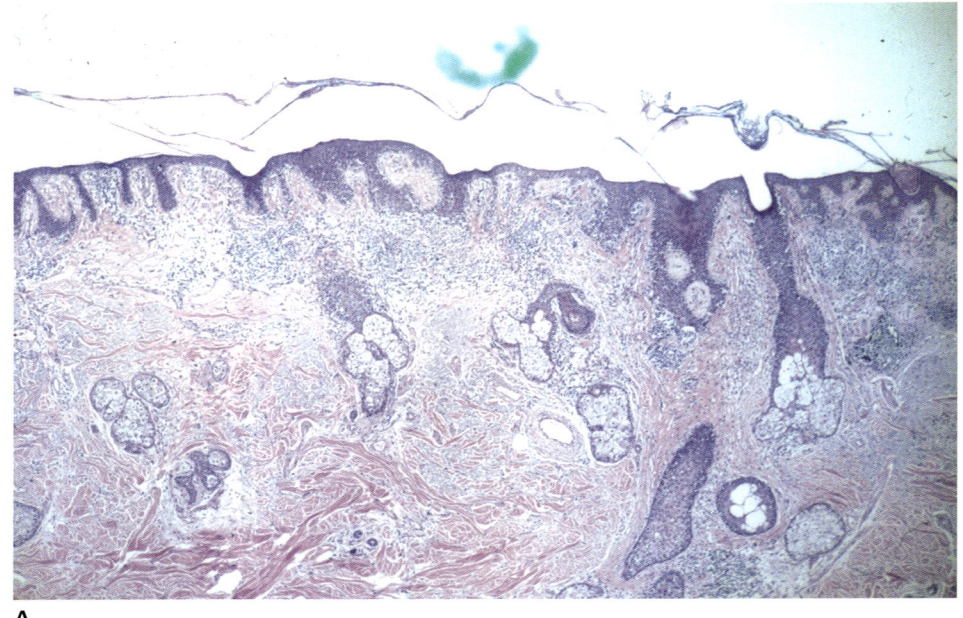

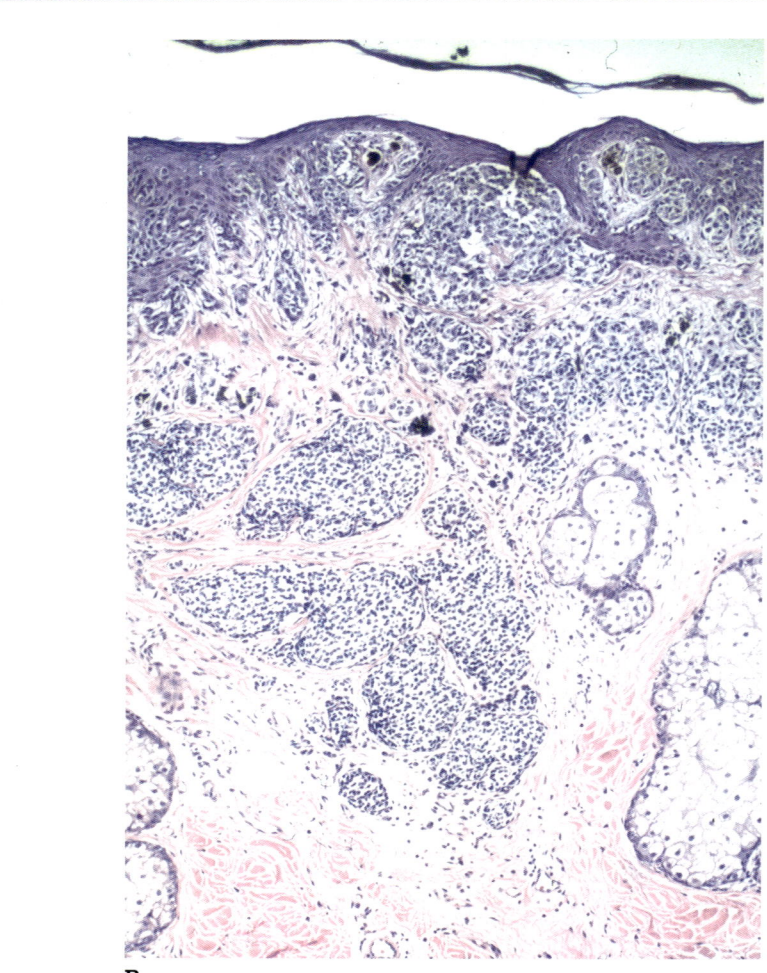

FIGURE 10-26 Small cell melanoma variant arising in sun-exposed skin of older individuals. **A,** Note the asymmetry and large size of the lesion and diffuse intraepidermal proliferation of the melanocytes in lentiginous and nested arrangements. **B,** Note the disordered intraepidermal nesting of atypical melanocytes with some resemblance to a melanocytic nevus. Small cuboidal cells extend into dermis.

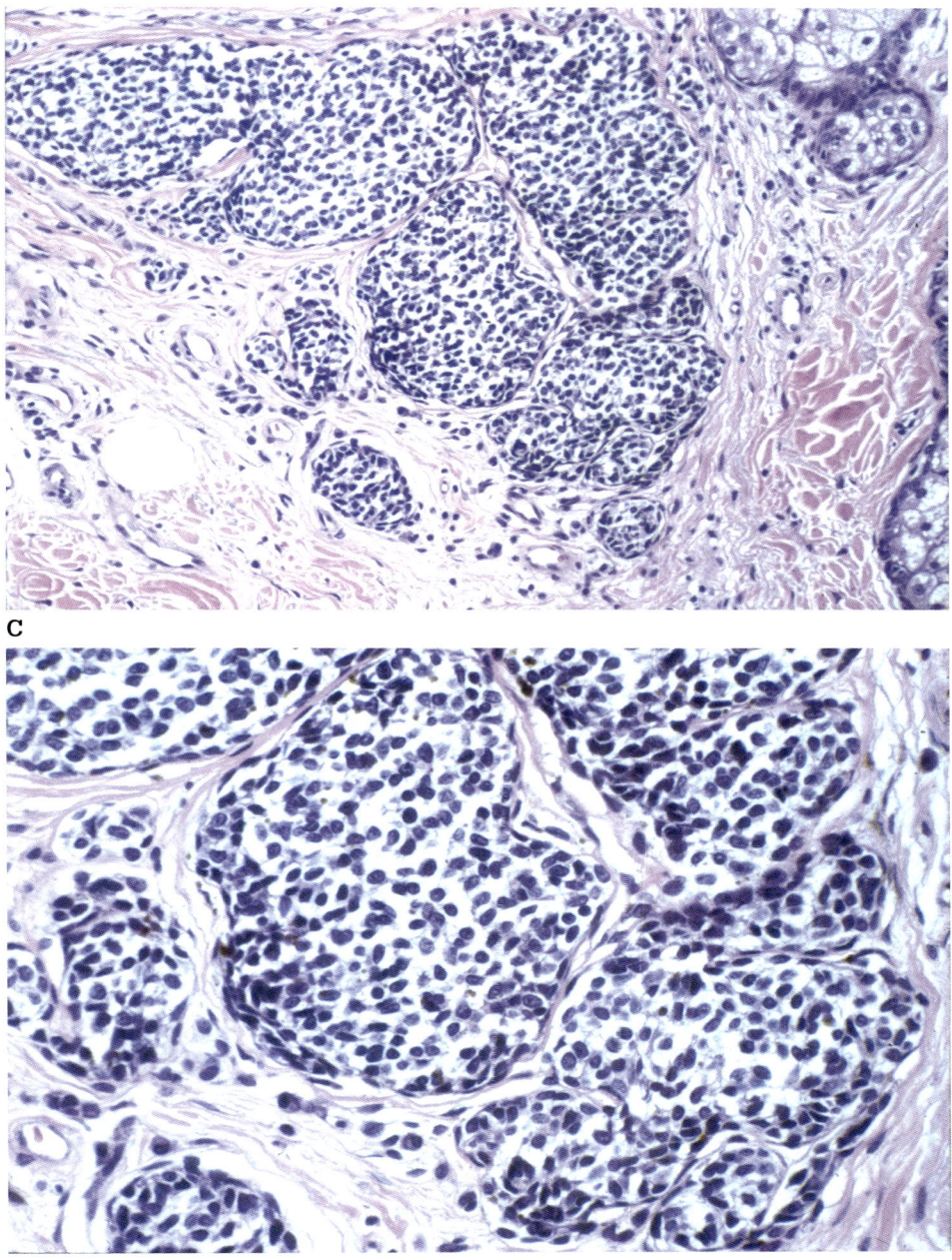

FIGURE 10-26 *Continued.* **C,** Large confluent rests of small cuboidal melanocytes in dermis are seen. Although the nests suggest a nevus, there is no maturation and the melanocytes demonstrate nuclear pleomorphism and hyperchromatism. **D,** High magnification shows monomorphous nature of small melanoma cells with nuclear atypia. A rare mitotic figure is present.

Clinical Features In general, there are no distinctive clinical features; in our experience, such Spitzoid melanomas often have abnormal clinical attributes such as size > 5 mm, asymmetry, and irregular coloration, suggesting an atypical nevus or melanoma. Some such lesions may suggest a Spitz tumor clinically but it must be recalled that the clinical diagnosis of a Spitz tumor is rather imprecise (Chapter 7).

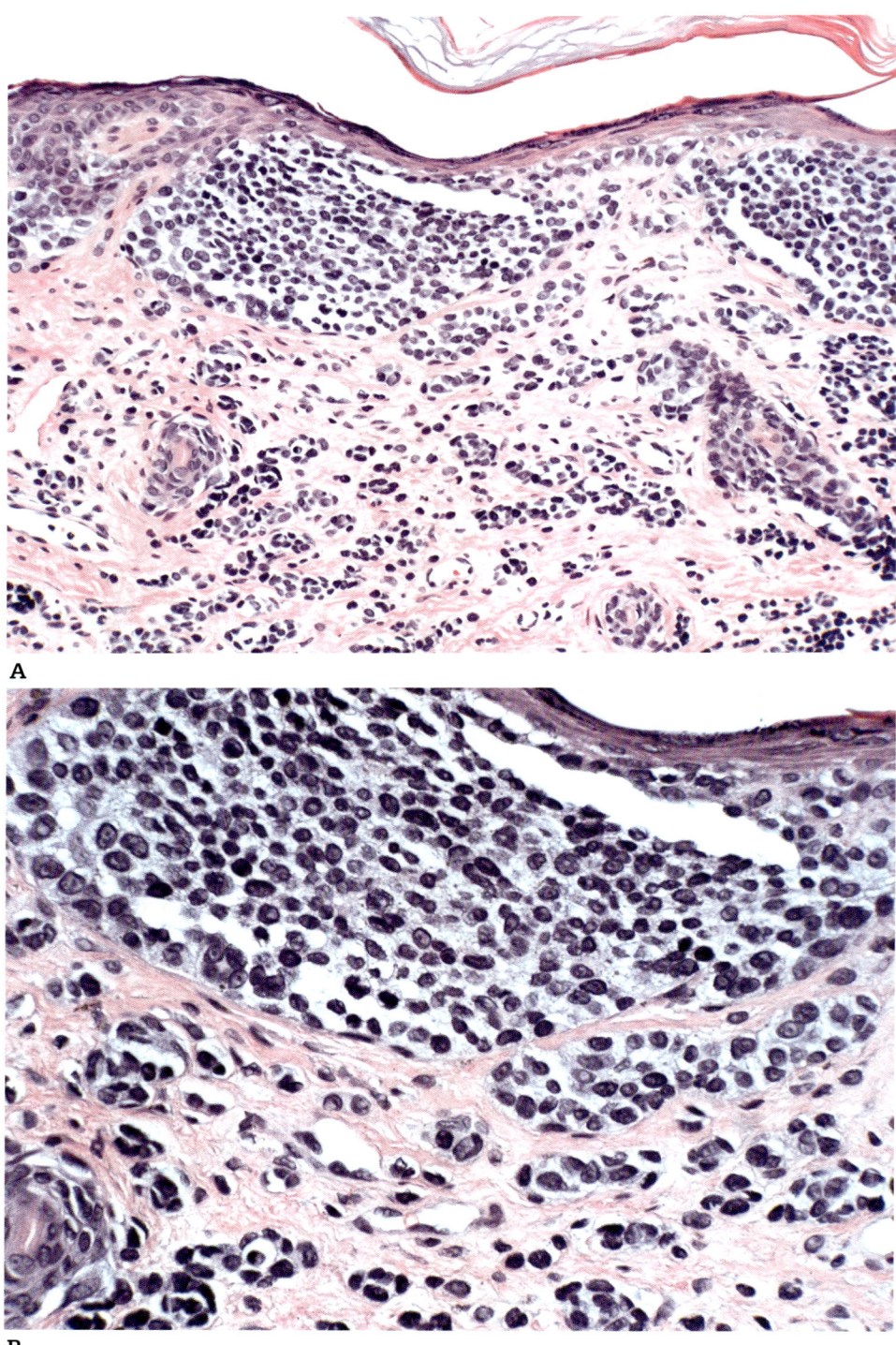

FIGURE 10-27 Small cell melanoma variant arising in sun-exposed skin of older individuals. **A,** Large confluent nests of small melanocytes within epidermis. There is some effacement and thinning of epidermis. **B,** The melanocytes display high nuclear to cytoplasmic ratios, significant nuclear pleomorphism, and hyperchromatism. The tumor extends into the dermis as confluent aggregates.

Histopathologic Features The diagnosis of a melanoma as Spitzoid, as mentioned above, is based on the striking architectural and cytologic resemblance to a Spitz tumor (Fig. 10-28). Thus such features potentially include any of the following: dome-shaped, plaque-like, or wedge-shaped morphololgy; little or no asymmetry; epidermal hyperplasia; clefting about intrapidermal nests of melanocytes; presence of dull pink or Kamino bodies; some evidence of zonation or maturation; and especially a population of enlarged epithelioid and/or fusiform melanocytes with abundant opaque or ground glass cytoplasm.

As discussed extensively in Chapter 7 and in Table 10.7, the pathologist is generally able distinguish the two entities with careful attention to all histopathologic and clinical criteria. Such Spitzoid melanomas are thus often larger (> 5–6 mm, often > 10 mm) and may have significant depth. They may demonstrate asymmetry (or greater asymmetry), poor circumcription, heterogeneity of cellular populations, more disordered intraepidermal proliferative patterns of melancytes without clefting, extensive pagetoid spread, irregular epidermal alterations including thinning and effacement, significant melanocytic density and confluence, and the lack of zonation or diminished cellular density with depth (maturation) (Fig. 10-28B,C). The lack of uniformity or homogeneity of cell type along comparable strata (from side to side) of the tumor cannot be overemphasised as a major criterion favoring melanoma. Similarly, the failure of a tumor to show progressive dispersion of melanocytes to smaller aggregates and particularly to single melanocytes (among apparently unaffected collagen bundles) in the deepest part of the lesion also suggests melanoma (Fig. 10-28D). Usually, a concomitant alteration with depth is the uniform diminution of cellular and nuclear sizes and regular spacing of melanocytes in a Spitz tumor; the failure to observe the latter feature should prompt consideration of melanoma. Cytologic features favoring (but not necessarily diagnostic of) melanoma include heterogeneity of cell type throughout the lesion, particularly in an asymmetrical or haphazard pattern; high nuclear/cytoplasmic ratios; granular or dusty cytoplasm versus the ground glass cytoplasm of Spitz melanocytes; absence of delicate or dispersed chromatin patterns with thickening of nuclear membranes; a large proportion of melanocytes with hyperchromatic nuclei; and the presence of large eosinophilic nucleoli.

Much has been written about assessing mitotic rate in Spitz tumors versus melanoma. As discussed in Chapter 7, the greater the absolute rate (per square millimeter) and number of deeply located (dermal) mitoses, the more evidence one has favoring melanoma; atypical mitoses and necrotic cells favor melanoma but there are exceptions. Although many lesions can be categorized as melanoma or Spitz tumor after careful application of criteria, there remains a subset of lesions that presently cannot be confidently classified as benign or malignant, as discussed above, and should be designated as biologically indeterminate. As noted throughout this book, appropriate management should include adequate excision, follow-up, and potential consideration of sentinel lymph node biopsy.

Differential Diagnosis Acknowledging that this differential diagnosis is one of the most difficult in melanoma pathology, there are circumstances that make it even more exasperating if not impossible. In particular, trauma and significant host response often introduce abnormal features such as asymmetry, heterogeneity, and cytologic abnormality, suggesting the greater likelihood of melanoma. It must be kept in mind that the nuclei in Spitz tumors are delicate and that any artifact, such as tissue compression or overstaining or significant host response may introduce alterations, suggesting greater cytologic atypicality. In the latter circumstances, the pathologist must carefully consider all of the available criteria before rendering an interpretation. When entertaining the possibility of a Spitzoid melanoma, one must always consider a Spitz nevus with overlapping features of pigmented spindle cell nevus and one with phenotypic heterogeneity (combined nevus). Pigmented spindle cell nevi show considerable overlap with Spitz tumors and may introduce features suggesting melanoma, such as greater pagetoid spread, expansile papillary dermal nests, and the absence ground glass cytoplasm (see Chaper 7). Spitz tumors with phenotypic heterogeneity (combined nevus) may exhibit asymmetry and heterogeneity, two attributes suggesting melanoma. One must assess each component of such a lesion individually with the criteria already mentioned (Table 10.7).

Melanoma Arising in Association with Dermal Nevi

The development of melanoma in the dermal component of an acquired nevus is a rare event judging from the number of cases reported to date (243–245) (Table 10-24). This phenomenon may overlap to some degree with nevoid melanoma and verrucous melanoma. It is also possible that some of these melanomas may originate from adnexal-associated nevus elements.

Clinical Features Most patients reported thus far have been 40–60 years of age and the most common site of involvement has been the head and neck area (243–245) (Table 10-24). The general clinical appearance is usually rather innocuous and in fact rather similar to that of a

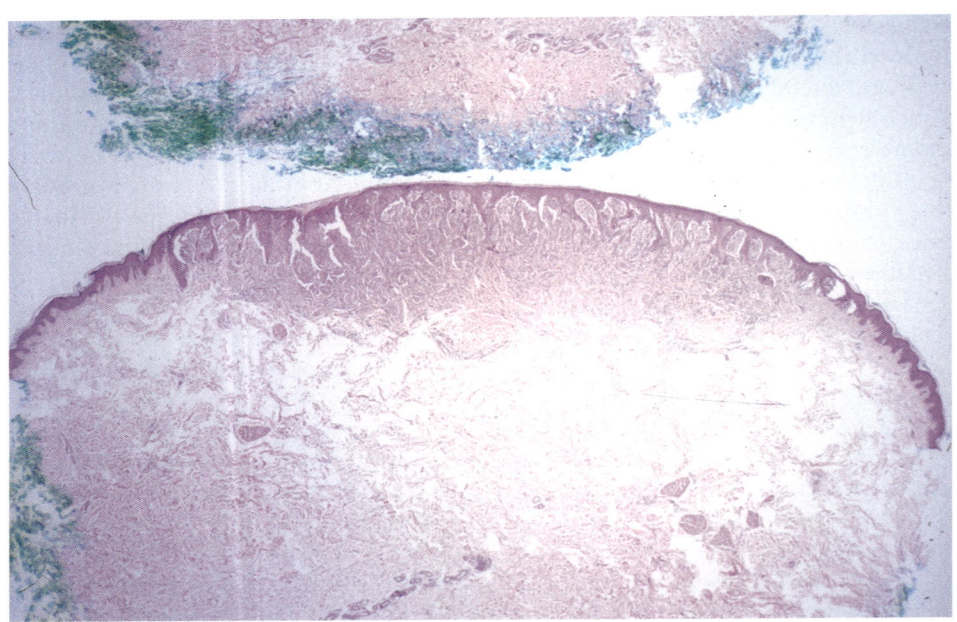

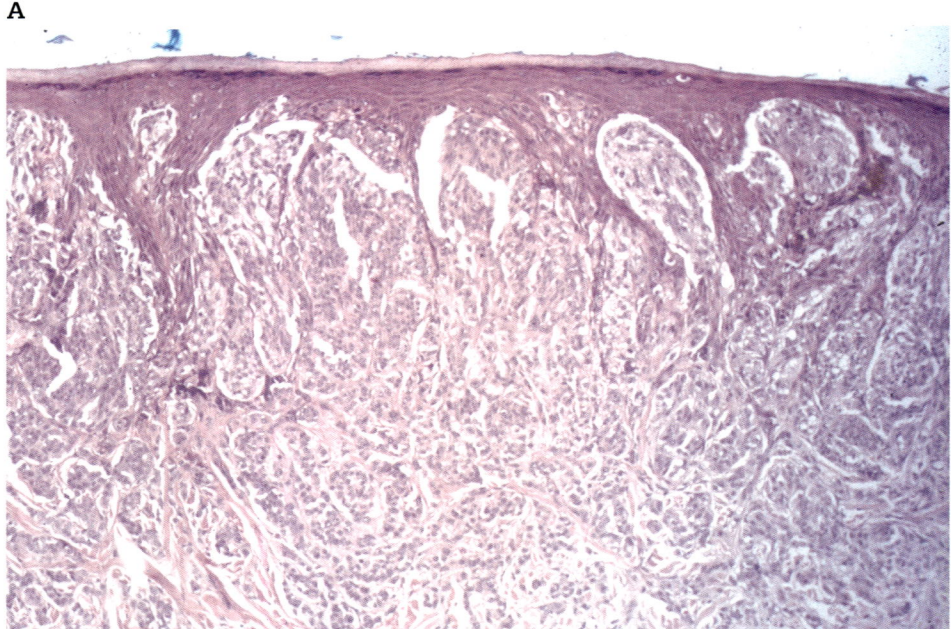

FIGURE 10-28 Spitzoid melanoma on the thigh of a young woman; a diagnosis of Spitz nevus was rendered. The lesion subsequently resulted in lymph node metastases about 1 year later. **A,** The profile of the tumor at scanning magnification suggests a Spitz nevus based on the relative small diameter of the lesion, the general symmetry, and the rather sharp circumscription present. **B,** Epidermal hyperplasia and clefting about nests of spindled melanocytes suggest a Spitz nevus; however, note the high cellular density and confluence of melanocytes.

dermal nevus (e.g., uniform pink or tan color). However, the lesions are often larger than ordinary dermal nevi (e.g., 1–2 cm), and there is usually a history of recent change or enlargement.

Histopathologic Features Usually within an otherwise ordinary dermal nevus, one encounters a distinct nodule of cytologically atypical melanocytes (243–245) (Fig. 10-29; Table 10-24). The latter nodule is characterized by

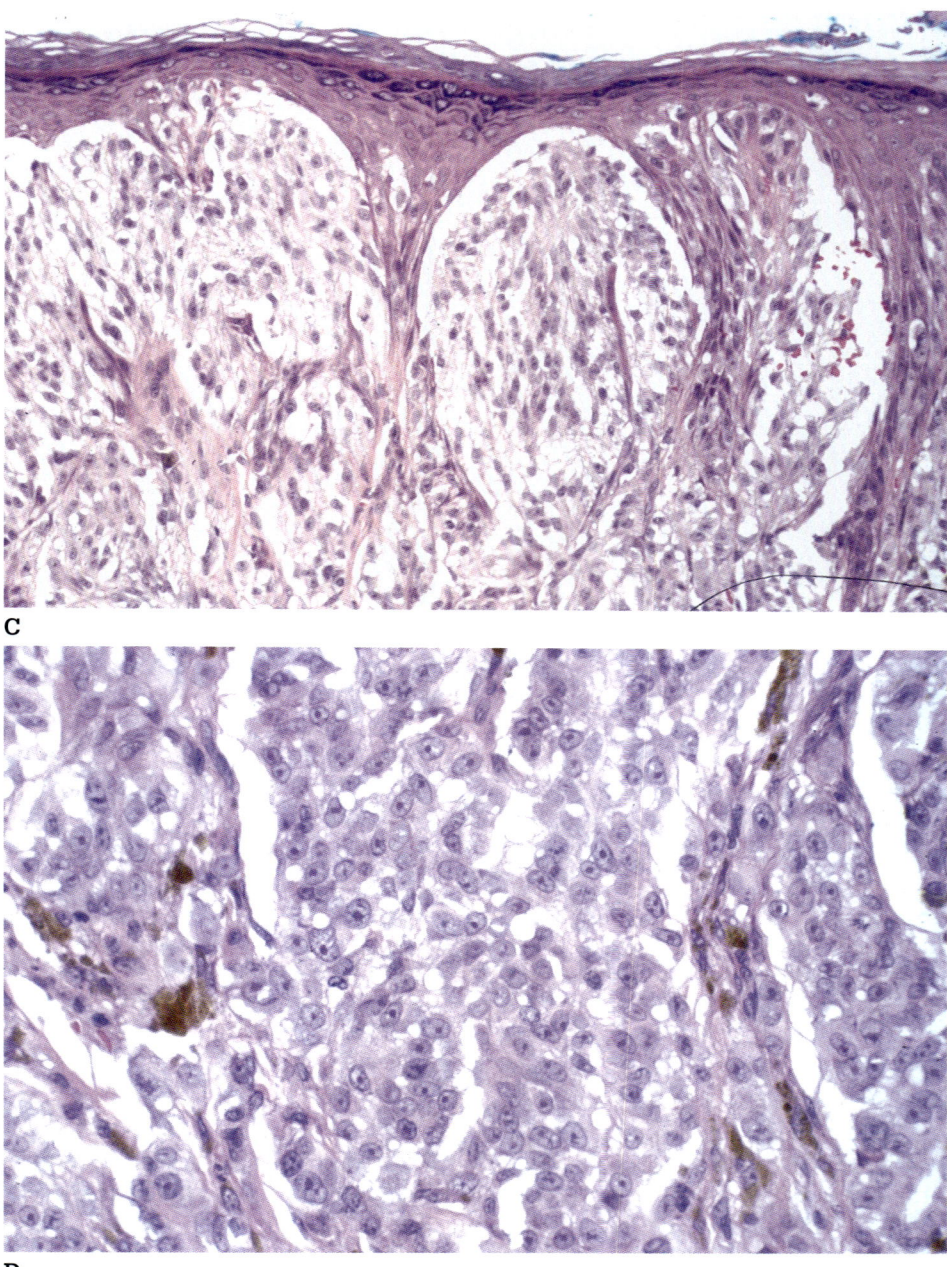

FIGURE 10-28 *Continued.* **C,** Large, somewhat discohesive nests of spindle cells efface and replace the epidermis, which are abnormal characteristics. **D,** Large epithelioid polyhedral cells in the dermis show striking confluence and high density. The melanocytes demonstrate nuclear pleomorphism and contain large nucleoli, providing strong support for melanoma.

a monomorphous and crowded appearance with high cellular density of melanocytes and absence of maturation. There is usually a fairly abrupt transition from the ordinary dermal nevus component to the nodular aggregate of atypical cells (Fig. 10-29A) but there are exceptions. The latter cells are most commonly enlarged with abundant cytoplasm and some may have some resemblance to spitzoid melanocytes. The cells generally demonstrate a high nuclear/cytoplasmic ratio and pleomorphic nuclei. The nuclear membranes are usually thickened, and prominent nucleoli may be evident. Mitotic figures are critical to the diagnosis and are usually easily found within

TABLE 10-24 Melanoma arising in association with dermal nevus.

Clinical features
   40–60 years
   Head and neck, most common sites
   0.5–2 cm, often
   Resembles dermal nevus
   Uniform pink, tan, or brown, often
   History of recent enlargement, often
Histopathologic features
   Focal cohesive nodules of atypical melanocytes
   Background of ordinary dermal nevus
   Monomorphous cells in nodules
   Cellular and nuclear enlargement
   Nuclear pleomorphism
   Melanin content variable
   Mitotic figures, usually present
Differential diagnosis
   Dermal nevus
   Nevus with phenotypic heterogeneity (combined, inverted type A, clonal nevus)

the nodule. Inflammatory cell infiltrates are often present, and there may be partial regression.

Differential Diagnosis The most obvious dilemma is the differentiation of a focus of melanoma from dermal nevus (especially a nevus with cytologically bizarre nevus cells, as in ancient schwannoma), a distinct focus of epithelioid or fusiform cells (as in a nevus with phenotypic heterogeneity, or a so-called combined nevus, inverted type-A nevus, or clonal nevus), or an inflamed nevus with reactive yet atypical features (211,246,247). First, the nodular area in question should demonstrate a cohesive or expansile aggregate of cells with unequivocal cytologic atypia. Although these melanocytic cells will usually have a monomorphous or clonal appearance, inspection of individual cells should disclose substantial nuclear pleomorphism and often prominent nucleoli and hyperchromatism. Mitotic figures should also be present in this focus. A dermal nevus with bizarre or ancient cytologic features will usually show only rare or no mitoses. One should also consider clinical factors, such as age of the patient (melanoma usually in persons > 40 years of age), size (such lesions are often > 1 cm in diameter), and history of recent change or enlargement. On the other hand, so-called nevi with phenotypic heterogeneity or combined nevi are often present in younger individuals, are characterized by a small dark nodule or papule in a relatively small symmetric nevus, and usually show low-grade or no cytologic atypia of the epithelioid/fusiform cells. Often, the latter cells display prominent melaninization of melanocytes and are accompanied by melanophages.

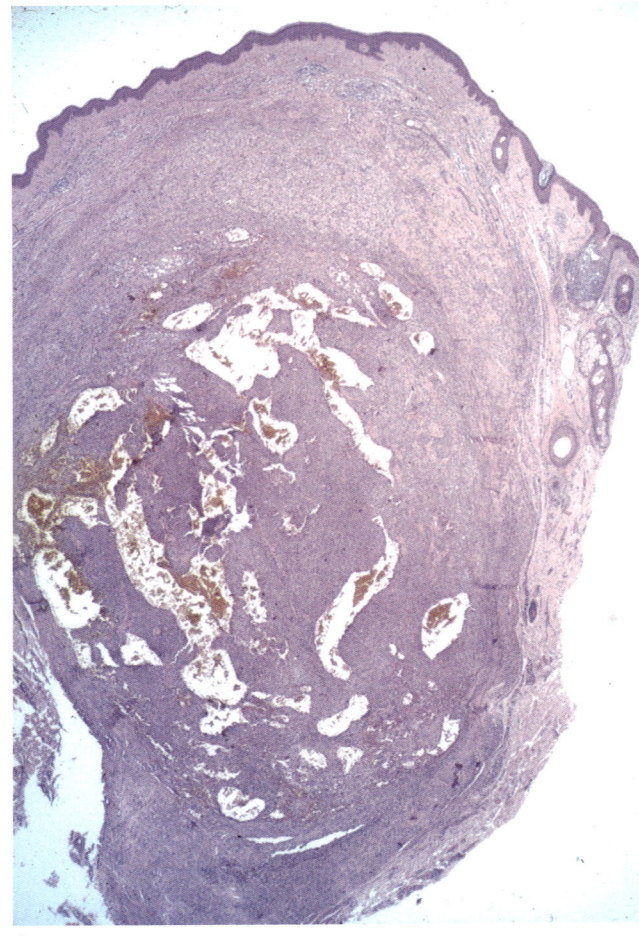

A
FIGURE 10-29 Melanoma arising in the dermal component of a nevus. **A,** A dome-shaped cohesive nodule in the dermis with surrounding dermal nevus. The blood-filled spaces and lack of pigment suggest a vascular tumor, such as a glomus tumor.

Melanoma Arising in or Resembling a Blue Nevus: Malignant Blue Nevus

The biologic characteristics and natural history of atypical and malignant melanocytic lesions originating from or resembling blue nevi remain poorly understood at present and are still being defined (248–280). This conclusion is based on the extreme rarity of such malignancies and the lack of longitudinal studies of cellular blue nevi (CBN), particularly those with atypical features (281–284). In the ensuing discussion, we consider all such malignancies that have been termed malignant blue nevus to be a variant of malignant melanoma.

Allen and Spitz (249) first proposed the term *malignant blue nevus* (MBN) in their description of six patients with melanomas associated with a CBN remnant. Since that report, the term MBN has been applied to melanomas

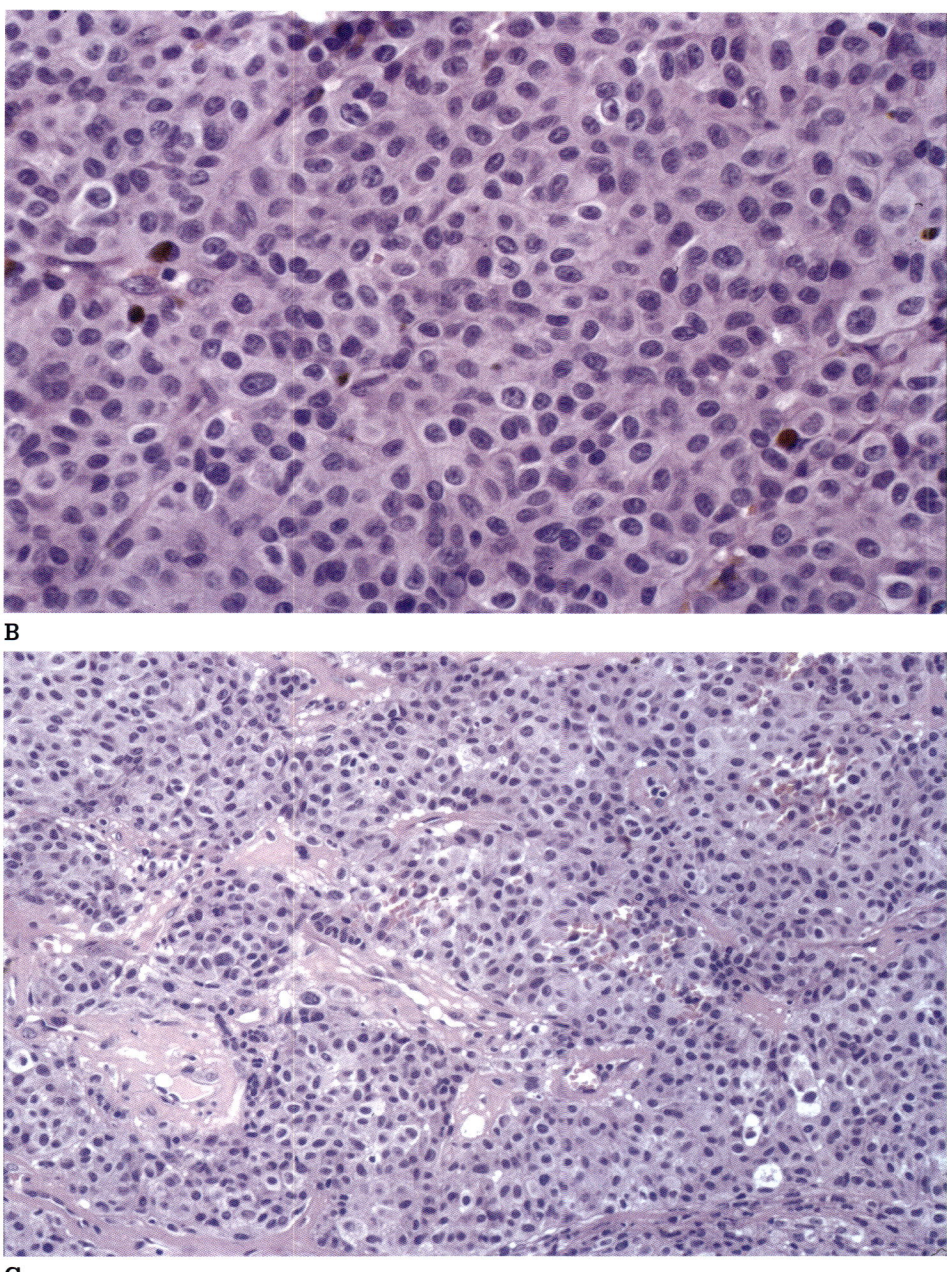

FIGURE 10-29 *Continued.* **B,** The nodule contains confluent cords of cuboidal cells demonstrating high cellularity, nuclear pleomorphism, and mitotic activity. **C,** There is strikingly high cellular density of melanoma cells. Note the marked nuclear pleomorphism.

without an intraepidermal component arising in (a) congenital or acquired CBN; (b) congenital or acquired ordinary blue nevi; (c) nevus of Ota, Ito, and related lesions; (d) the site of a previously biopsied or excised blue nevus; and (e) de novo melanomas resembling CBN but lacking an obvious blue nevus component. It is not difficult to recognize overtly malignant tumors with a clearcut benign blue nevus remnant, especially those that have metastasized. However, it may be impossible to distinguish a so-called de novo MBN (melanoma resembling a CBN) from metastatic melanoma without specific clinical information, if at all. Thus the latter diagnosis should be made with caution. Some proportion of MBN seem to lack overt criteria for malignancy and thus suggest CBN with atypia. The latter lesions are often recognized as melanoma only in retrospect—after recurrences and/or metastases have ensued. The latter dilemma is further exacerbated by the fact that rare MBN may develop metastases after intervals as long as 20 years (277,280).

Another particular problem is the entity referred to in the literature as CBN with "benign" lymph node metastases (249,285–288). Allen and Spitz (249) first reported four young individuals with CBN located on the extremites that were associated with small discrete metastases involving the marginal sinuses of inguinal or axillary lymph nodes. These and other similar patients have been reported to have had no subsequent disease progression (287,288); however, the the lack of sufficient follow-up in many instances may preclude making any authoritative statements about the nature of all such lymph node deposits until more definitive studies are available.

Approximately 80 cases of MBN have thus far been reported in the literature, and the largest series has included only 12 patients (270). The average age at diagnosis is 46.1 years (range, 5–69 years), two thirds of the patients are men, and the commonest site of origin is the scalp. The overwhelming majority of MBN originate from CBN, and a significant percentage of the nevi are congenital. These melanomas are unique since they develop in the dermis or subcutis rather than along the dermoepidermal junction. A high proportion of cases are associated with satellite metastases, and the most common sites of metastasis are the regional lymph nodes.

Malignant blue nevus are regarded as highly aggressive based on the large proportion of cases reported that result in metastasis and death. It must be pointed out that such lesions are usually advanced at the time of diagnosis—that is, they have significant thickness. Furthermore, many originate from the scalp, a site generally associated with a worse prognosis. In addition, the published cases have been highly selected; it is possible that there is a cohort of lesions perhaps categorized under terms such as *CBN with atypia* or *atypical CBN* (which may be indistinguishable from some MBN) that have a more indolent course.

Clinical Features Malignant blue nevi most frequently present as blue or blue-black plaques or nodules, ranging from 0.3 to 24 cm (mean, 2.9 cm) (270) that are often multinodular (265) (Table 10-25). There is usually a history of recent growth, enlargement, or change, such as bleeding or ulceration in a previously stable blue nevus. Satellite lesions or metastases are distinct clinical findings in a proportion of cases.

Histopathologic Features The essential criteria for diagnosis include sparing of the epidermis; demonstration

TABLE 10-25 Malignant blue nevus (melanoma arising in or resembling a blue nevus).

Clinical features
  Mean age 46.1 years
  Men > women
  Scalp most common site
  1–24 cm (mean 2.9 cm; usually > 3 cm)
  Blue or blue-black plaque or nodules
  Multinodular
  Recent change in stable blue nevus, often
  Satellite lesions may be present

Histopathologic features
  Sparing of epidermis
  Nodular or multinodular aggregates of spindle cells
  Polygonal cells, occasionally
  Highly variable cytologic atypia
  Two variants
    Distinctly malignant component of severely atypical epithelioid and/or spindle cells with prominent nucleoli
    Sheetlike arrangements of atypical spindle cells, not obviously malignant
  Pigmentation in one third of cases
  Necrosis in one third of cases
  Mitotic figures infrequent (often $\sim$ 2/mm^2)
  Component of cellular blue nevus and less often ordinary blue nevus or dermal melanocytosis

Differential diagnosis
  Cellular blue nevus and atypical variants
  Nodular melanoma
  Clear cell sarcoma
  Metastatic melanoma

of a benign component of blue nevus or a similar lesion, a history of a stable blue nevus at the site of melanoma, or a melanoma resembling a blue nevus; and exclusion of metastatic melanoma (Fig. 10-30). (Table 10-25) MBN usually presents in one of three patterns (249–280):

- A lesion with an overtly malignant component juxtaposed to a benign blue nevus component, usually a CBN.
- A more subtle sarcoma-like presentation (without florid benign and malignant components), initially suggesting CBN but exhibiting large densely cellular fascicles or nodules of spindle cells that, on closer inspection, have sufficient atypicality for malignancy and are distinctly more abnormal that the usual small fascicular or alveolar patterns in CBN.
- A lesion suggesting a benign CBN with additional atypical features—such as large diameter, asymmetry, prominent cellular density, nuclear pleomorphism, and some mitotic activity at least focally—but not obviously malignant that subsequently results in malignant behavior (we term such lesions biologically indeterminate).

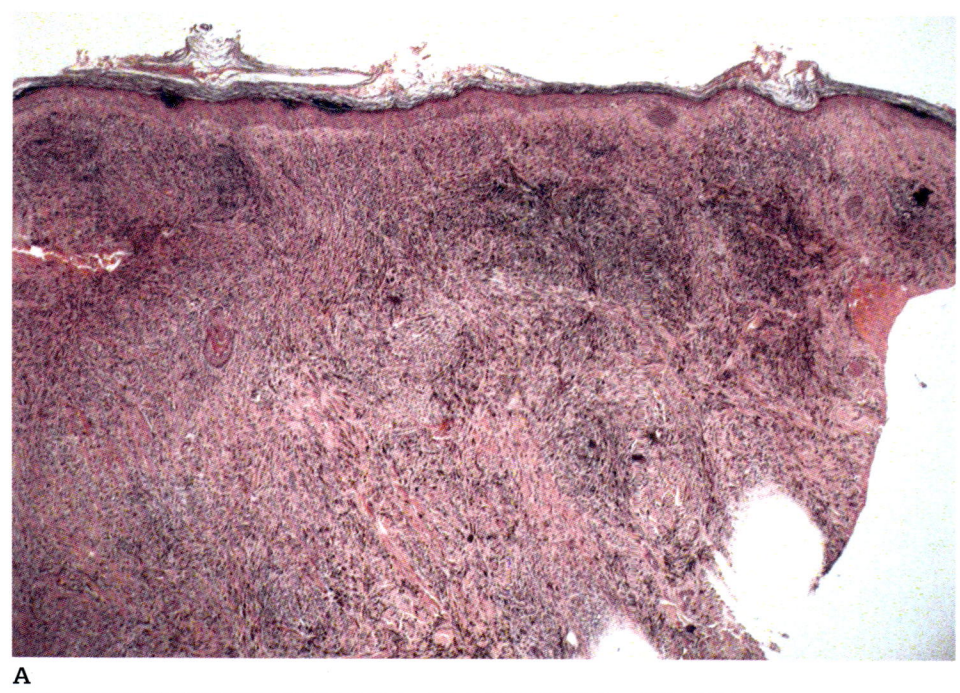

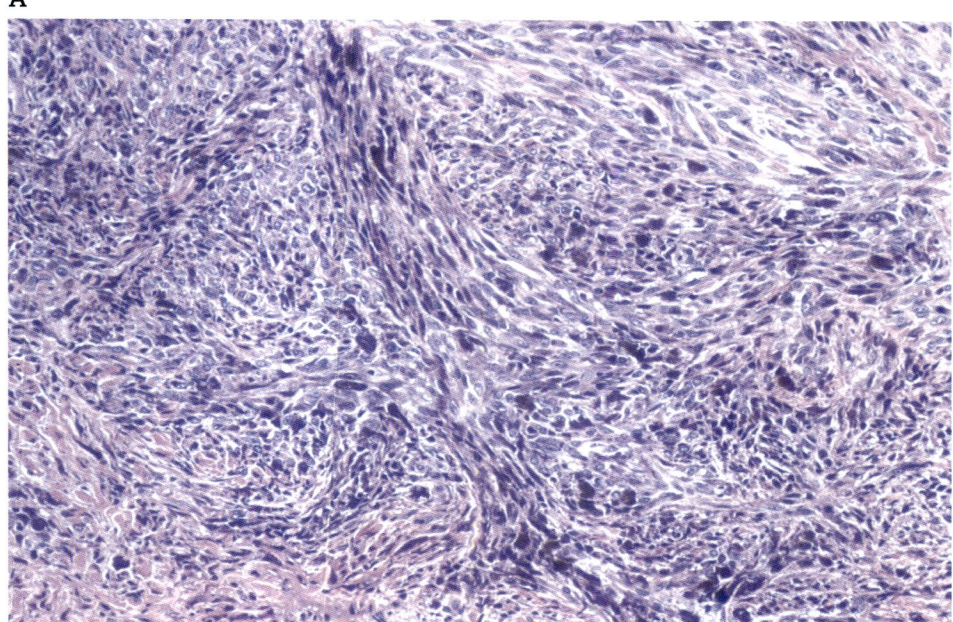

FIGURE 10-30 Malignant blue nevus (malignant melanoma arising in association with blue nevus). **A,** Malignant melanoma occupies the dermis without connection to the overlying epidermis. This melanoma can be distinguished from conventional melanoma only by the association with or history of a previous blue nevus at this site. **B,** Note the fascicular arrangements of spindle cells, many of which contain melanin.

In the most common presentation MBN are characterized by generally large and asymmetrical nodular or multinodular aggregates or fascicles of spindle cells in the dermis and often the subcutis with rounded contours at the base reminescent of a CBN (Fig. 10-30B). Distinctly malignant components may occupy any proportion of the tumor and may be made up of pleomorphic spindle cells with hyperchromatic nuclei and/or ep-

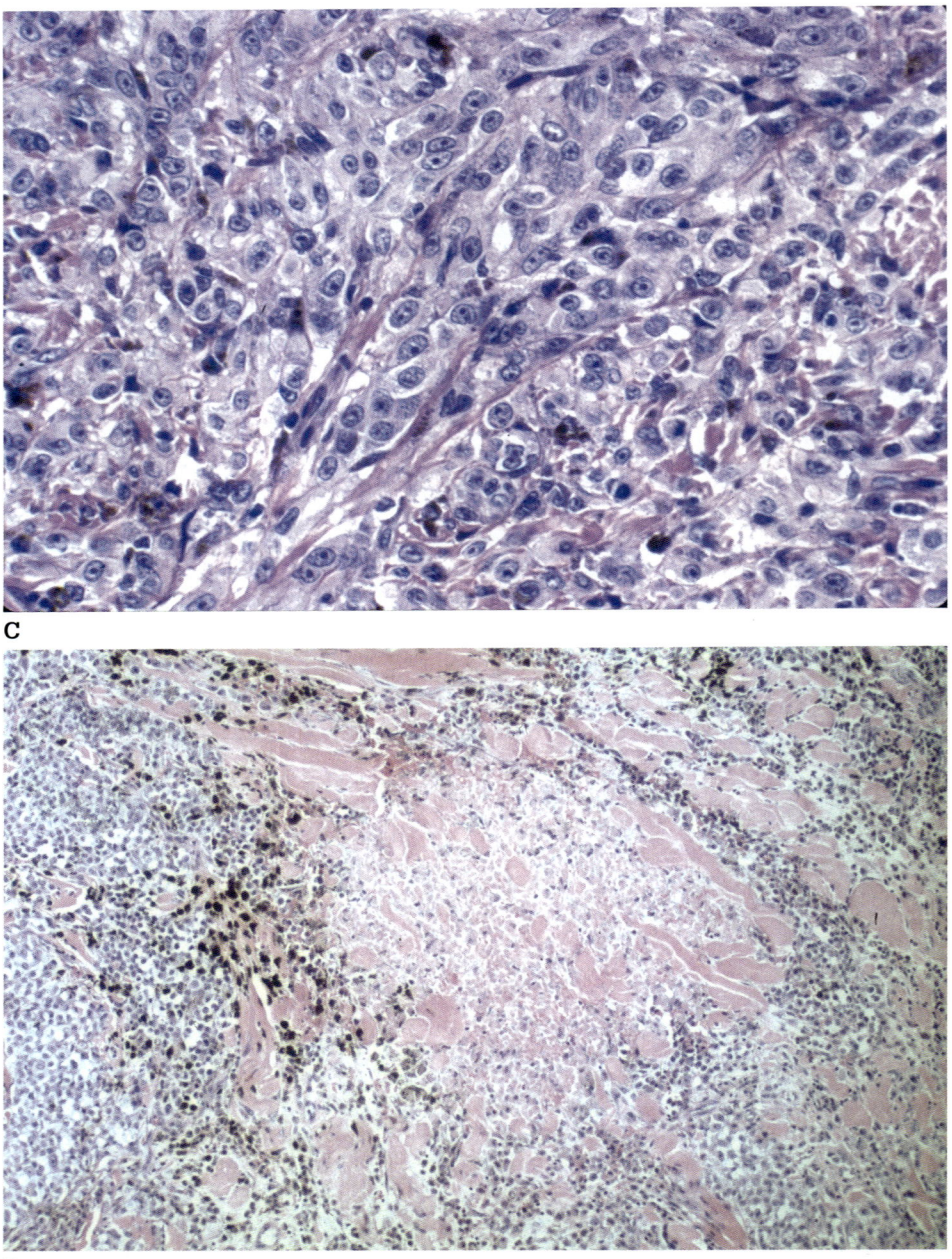

FIGURE 10-30 *Continued.* **C,** High magnification showing compact aggregates of plump fusiform cells and epithelioid melanoma cells. Marked cytologic atypia is present. **D,** Note the highly atypical epithelioid cells with confluent zones of necrosis.

ithelioid cells with prominent nucleoli (Fig. 10-30C–E). There also may be striking vacuolization of cytoplasm. Multinucleate giant cells are encountered on occasion. Necrosis may be prominent but is present in only about a third of cases (Fig. 10-30D,E). The mitotic rate is commonly low (e.g., in the order of 1–2/mm^2) in the majority of cases (270,280). Atypical mitotic figures have been proposed as one of the most sensitive features for MBN; however, they do not occur in all instances and are a rather subjective finding. Significant melanin pigment is noted in up to 67% of cases (270). Most MBN have a component of CBN, often at the peripheries, but elements of ordinary blue nevus (pigmented dendritic melanocytes, fibrosis, and melanophages) and, rarely, other dermal melanocytoses such as nevus of Ota may be observed (251,270).

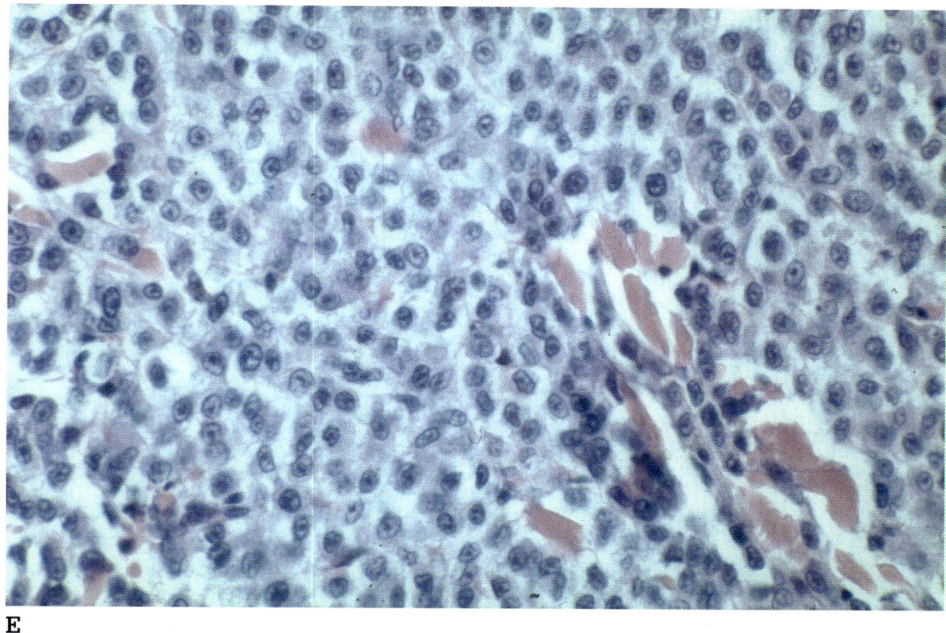

E
FIGURE 10-30 *Continued.* **E,** Higher magnification showing epithelioid melanoma cells with prominent nucleoli.

Differential Diagnosis Malignant blue nevus must be distinguished from CBN with or without atypical features (so-called atypical variants of CBN) (281–283), a primary or metastatic melanoma, and clear-cell sarcoma. The discrimination of MBN from CBN is based on clinical and histologic characteristics. MBN are usually > 3 cm in longest diameter, whereas CBN are usually < 2 cm (254). MBN are often typified by a markedly irregular, asymmetric, and frequently multinodular appearance in contrast to the more symmetric and regular CBN. Histologically, MBN usually display greater asymmetry, hypercellularity, frankly malignant cytologic characteristics, and more mitoses and necrosis than found in CBN. Atypical mitoses are characteristic of MBN but not present in all. Less commonly, MBN may demonstrate rather banal cytologic features, and occasional CBN with atypical features show necrosis. Distinction of MBN from CBN with atypical features may be exceedingly difficult or impossible (in a minority of cases). Lesions designated as CBN with atypical features should, therefore, have adequate surgical margins and long-term follow-up (110).

Because there are no histologic features specific for MBN, a contiguous remnant of blue nevus should be identified or a history of an antecedent blue nevus documented to distinguish MBN from either NM or metastatic melanoma (270,280–283). MBN are considered by many to be highly aggressive with metastasis to lymph nodes and a variety of visceral sites in 82% of the 33 cases mentioned above (270).

Clear-Cell Sarcoma (Malignant Melanoma of Soft Parts)

Clear-cell sarcoma (CCS) of tendons and aponeuroses is a rare tumor of soft tissue first decribed in 1965 by Enzinger (289–290). These tumors are closely related to conventional malignant melanoma because of shared histomorphologic attributes; melanin synthesis; ex-pression of markers such as S-100 protein, HMB-45, Mart-1, MITF, and tyrosinase; and the ultrastructural demonstration of external lamina and cytoplasmic premelanosomes (291–299). On occasion, CCS is confused with metastatic melanoma with unknown primary. As a result, CCS has also been termed malignant melanoma of soft parts. Nonetheless CCS is now recognized as a distinct clinicopathologic entity, particularly because of an apparently tumor-specific translocation involving chromosomes 12 and 22 in 60–75% of cases. The latter translocation is characterized by the fusion of a portion of the activating transcription factor 1 (ATF-1) gene on the long arm of chromosome 12 (12q13.1-13.2) and the Ewing sarcoma oncogene (EWS) on chromosome 22 (22q13). This translocation has not been identified in conventional melanoma when studied by reverse transcriptase polymerase chain reaction (RT-PCR) and FISH (293–295)

Clear-cell sarcoma are recognized as aggressive tumors of soft tissue; the 5-year survival rates are about 50%. Nevertheless patients with tumors measuring < 2 cm in diameter may be associated with a more favorable course; in contrast, those with tumors > 5 cm may have mortality rates of 80% (294). Local recurrences and regional lymph node metastases are frequent: 70% of patients in one series experienced at least one recurrence during a mean period of 4.2 years (290), whereas among 29 patients reported from the Netherlands, 45% developed regional lymph node metastases. The recurrences are often multiple. Distant metastases almost inevitably follow local recurrences and regional lymph node metastases. The preferred sites are the lungs, followed by the bones, distant lymph nodes, the brain, etc. All forms of the disease may relapse after intervals as long as 10–20 years.

Clinical Features Clear-cell sarcoma develops in young adults between the ages of 20 and 40 (range, 2–95 years; median, 30 years) with a predilection for the distal extremities (the foot and ankle being the most common region followed by the hand) but may also involve the knee, thigh, forearm, and elbow (289–299) (Table 10-26). Men and women are equally affected. The tumor typically presents as a slowly enlarging deep-seated mass because of its association with tendons, aponeuroses, and fascia, and there may be occasional tenderness or pain. The tumors are 2–5 cm in diameter at the time of diagnosis. The overlying skin is generally unaffected, although there may be upward extension of the tumor into the subcutaneous fat and dermis.

TABLE 10-26 Clear-cell sarcoma.

Clinical features
  20–40 years
  Women ≥ men
  Distal extremities, the foot most commonly involved
  Deep location, tendons and aponeuroses
  Slowly enlarging mass
  Tenderness, pain
Histopathologic features
  Multilobulated tumor
  Oval or fusiform cells in nests and fascicles
  Fibrous trabeculae separate cellular aggregates
  Clear or eosinophilic cytoplasm
  Multinucleate giant cells
  Melanin in over half of cases
Immunohistochemistry
  S-100 protein+
  HMB-45+
Electron microscopy
  Premelanosomes
  Melanosomes
Differential diagnosis
  Metastatic melanoma
  Cellular blue nevus and atypical variants
  Malignant blue nevus
  Malignant peripheral nerve sheath tumor
  Epithelioid sarcoma
  Synovial sarcoma
  Fibrosarcoma

Histopathologic Features The tumor is characterized by a well-circumscribed, multilobulated appearance (289–299) (Table 10-26). Oval or fusiform cells with clear or eosinophilic granular cytoplasm are arranged in well-defined nests and fascicles (Figs 10-31). Tumor aggregates are generally compartmentalized by fibrous tissue of variable thickness that merges with aponeurotic or tendinous structures (Fig. 10-31). There is variation in nuclear size and shape, and the nuclei are notable for vesicular qualities and prominent nucleoli. Distinctive multinucleate giant cells occur in about two thirds of cases (113,114). The mitotic rate is generally low (often < 3 mitoses/10 hpf). Melanin may be detected in approximately half of these tumors. Special stains will yield more tumors containing melanin. As mentioned above, most tumors react with antibodies to vimentin, S-100 protein, HMB-45, Mart-1, tyrosinase, and neuron-specific enolase (291, 295). There may be some expression of cytokeratins of low molecular weight. There is no staining with antibodies against epithelial membrane antigen or leukocyte common antigen (291). Melanosomes and premelanosomes are noted on electron microscopy (291).

Differential Diagnosis Clear-cell sarcoma may be confused with CBN with or without atypia, MBN, metastatic melanoma, a malignant peripheral nerve sheath tumor, epithelioid sarcoma, synovial sarcoma, and fibrosarcoma (289–299). The tumor probably most closely resembles CBN with atypia and MBN, but the latter do not usually occur in soft tissue. CCS is distinguished by the typical clinical presentation in young adults, involvement of distal extremities, deep soft tissue involvement, typical histology, and immunohistochemistry. If necessary the EWS-ATF1 fusion gene in CCS can be identified through the use of RT-PCR or FISH. Epithelioid sarcoma, and synovial sarcoma immunostain with cytokeratin and epithelial membrane antigen but not with S-100 protein, with some exceptions for synovial sarcoma, and HMB-45.

UNUSUAL OR RARE VARIATIONS OF MELANOMA AND PARTICULAR HISTOMORPHOLOGIC ALTERATIONS

The capacity of melanoma for the expression of highly diverse histomorphologic patterns is simply without parallel in pathology. Thus melanoma can mimic a wide range of carcinomas, sarcomas, and even lymphomas. This is especially true for advanced, recurrent, and metastatic melanoma. Some of these unusual and rare manifestations of melanoma not previously mentioned are discussed in this section and Chapter 11 (Table 10-27).

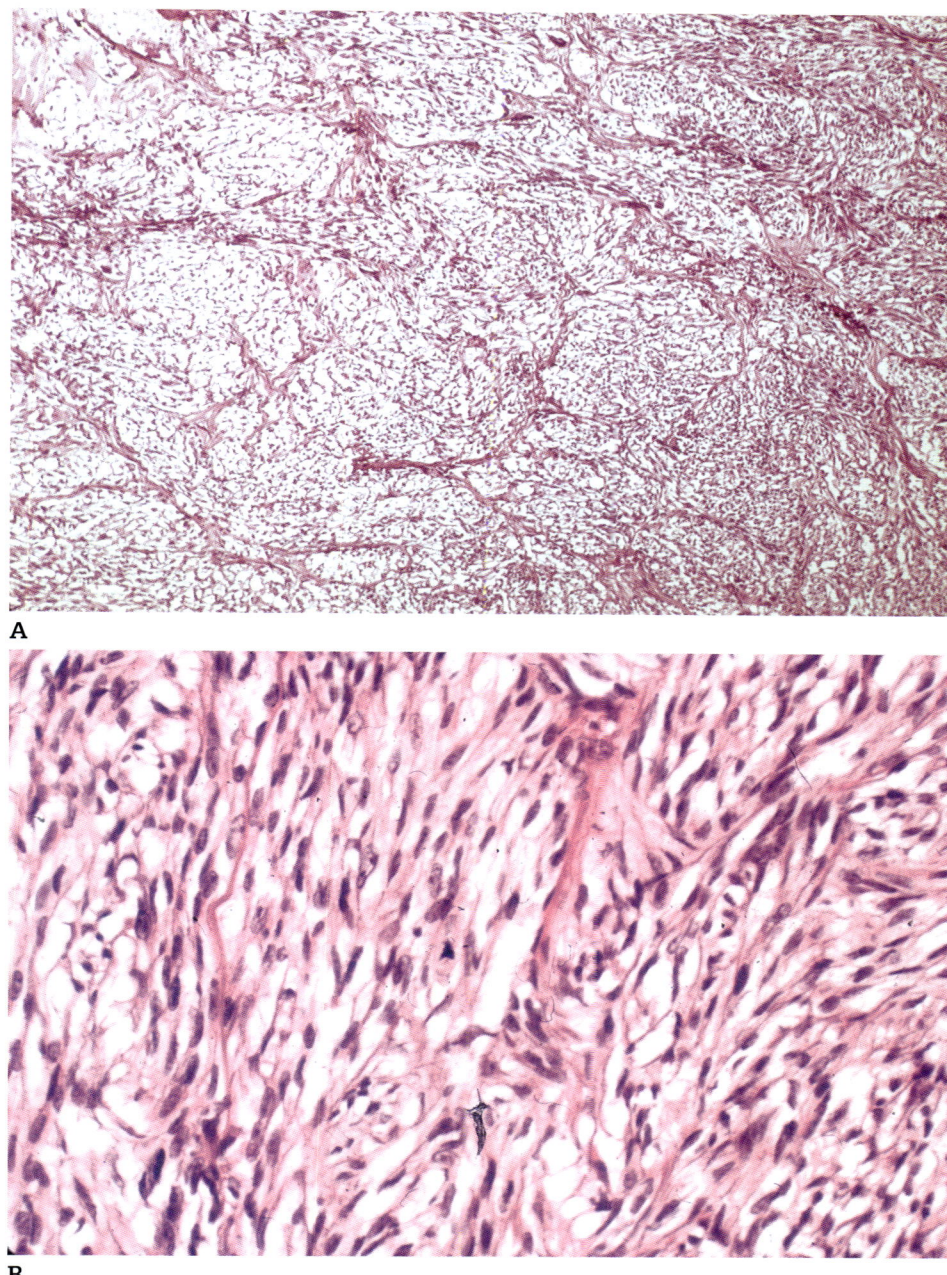

FIGURE 10-31 Clear-cell sarcoma. **A,** The tumor is remarkable for intersecting fascicles of spindle cells, compartmentalized by fibrous tissue focally. **B,** The spindle cells are characterized by clear cytoplasm. The nuclei are pleomorphic with hyperchromatism.

Polypoid Configuration of Melanoma

Melanomas occasionally are polypoid (Figs. 10-11 and 10-14). In a large series from Australia, 21.5% were polypoid (302), either pedunculated or sessile. Virtually all of the tumor is located above the epidermal surface in pedunculated melanomas, whereas sessile tumors have more than half the tumor above the epidermal surface (Fig. 10-6). Polypoid tumors usually have an ulcerated, friable surface and epidermal collarettes at the tumor base. Approximately two thirds are of nodular type (302). Originally, an adverse prognosis was assigned to polypoidal melanoma, but subsequent studies have failed to confirm this.

TABLE 10-27 Unusual or rare variants of melanoma.	
Feature	Reference(s)
Variation in cytoplasmic features	
Balloon cells	304–306
Clear cells	306,312
Pseudolipoblastic cells	301
Rhabdoid cells	316
Signet-ring cells	313–315
Variation in nuclear features	
Binucleation and multinucleation	301
Intranuclear inclusions	301
Lobation	301
Plasmacytoid appearance	300,301
Variation in architectural arrangements	
Pseudoglandular pattern	300,301
Pseudopapillary pattern	300,301
Pseudofollicular pattern	301
Pseudorosette pattern	300,301
Hemangiopericytoma pattern	300
Angiomatoid/pseudoangiosarcomatous pattern	317
Glomeruloid vascular pattern	301
Metaplastic variations	
Schwannian	301
Fibroblastic	301
Myofibroblastic	301
Smooth muscle	301
Rhabdomyoblastic	301
Osteocartilaginous	318,319
Ganglionic	301
Gangioneuroblastic	301

Amelanotic Melanoma

Uncommonly, primary melanomas develop without associated pigmentation: 1.8% in a series of 2881 melanoma (303). Most such tumors are invasive bulky "nodular" melanomas and in particular subungual and desmoplastic–neurotropic melanomas are often amelanotic (Fig. 10-25). However, an amelanotic invasive component may supervene with any type of on a pigmented intraepidermal component. Very rarely in situ or microinvasive melanoma may also be devoid of pigment. Such tumors are difficult to diagnose clinically because they lack important clues, such as variegated pigmentation.

In fact, melanin pigment is almost always present in some portion of a primary melanoma and careful scrutiny of tumors apparently lacking pigment, will often demonstrate finely granular melanin in some tumor cells. Special silver stains such as the Fontana-Masson stain, will frequently yield a positive result with even small amounts of melanin. Finally, immunohistochemistry will verify the melanocytic nature of a tumor (see Chapter 2). Metastatic melanoma is amelanotic much more frequently than primary melanoma and thus often enters into the differential diagnosis of metastatic cancer.

Balloon Cell Melanoma

Analagous to balloon cell nevus (see Chapter 5), balloon cell melanoma (BCM) is defined by a distinctive cellular alteration—that is, ballooning in at least 50% of the melanoma cells (304–306). The individual "balloon cells" have abundant vacuolated cytoplasms that impart a clear-cell appearance. Although BCM is extremely rare, knowledge of BCM is important for its distinction from the much more common balloon cell nevus and from other clear-cell tumors of the skin. The prognosis in BCM appears to be directly related to tumor thickness and to be no different from conventional melanoma. In a series of 34 cases of BCM, the 5-year survival was 37.5% (close to half of the tumors were > 2.0 mm in thickness) (305). BCM is reported to have a particular propensity for multiple skin and subcutaneous metastases (304).

Clinical Features In a series of 34 cases of BCM, the median age of patients was 54 years (range 19–91) (305) (Table 10-28). BCM is most commonly located on the head, neck, and upper trunk. Compared to conventional melanoma, there are no distinctive clinical features of BCM. These lesions have ranged in size from 3 to 35 mm.

Histopathologic Features The characteristic balloon cells are large, round, or polygonal cells with clear or eosinophilic, slightly granular cytoplasm (304,305) (Table 10-28). The nuclei are irregularly placed and exhibit only slight to moderate atypia. Mitotic activity is also generally low. The balloon cells occasionally are associated with pagetoid spread in the epidermis (Fig. 10-32A,B) and often form large nodular aggregates and nests in the dermis. Melanin has been noted in about a quarter of cases (305). Metastases from BCM often show balloon cell change but maybe difficult to diagnose because they are amelanotic and fail to exhibit nesting. Virtually all BCM studied thus far show positive immunostaining with S-100 protein and HMB-45 (305). A small number may be positive for carcinoembryonic antigen.

Causes The balloon cell change has been attributed to (a) degeneration and coalescence of melanosomes, (b) defective melanosome formation and subsequent generation of large membrane-bound vesicles, (c) blocked melanin synthesis and subsequent accumulation of protyrosinase vesicles, (d) lipoidal degeneration of melanocytes, and (e) glycogen (305,306). Ultrastructural studies have provided evidence supporting the first three and the fifth explanation. In addition, the presence of abundant RNA in the balloon cells and immunostaining with HMB-45 suggest that the cells are metabolically active rather than degenerative (305). A recent study has suggested that melanomas comprised of 30% or more of balloon cells

TABLE 10-28 Balloon cell melanoma.
Clinical features
Exceedingly rare
Median age, 54 years
Head, neck, and upper trunk most common sites
No distinctive clinical features
0.3–5 cm
Histopathologic features
Enlarged polygonal cells containing vacuolated (clear) cytoplasms in ≥ 50% of melanoma
Pagetoid spread of balloon cells, occasionally
Large nodular aggregates of balloon cells in dermis
Irregular placement of nuclei
Slight to moderate variation in nuclear characteristics and mitotic activity, generally
Multinucleate balloon giant cells occur
Immunohistochemistry
S-100 protein+
HMB-45+
Neuron-specific enolase+ (weak)
Carcinoembryonic antigen+ (2/7 tumors)
Differential diagnosis
Balloon cell nevus
Clear-cell sarcoma (malignant melanoma of soft parts)
Xanthoma
Hibernoma
Metastatic clear cell carcinomas
Renal cell carcinoma
Clear-cell carcinoma of lung, ovary, and endometrium
Granular cell tumor
Malignant eccrine acrospiroma
Clear-cell syringoma
Sebaceous carcinoma
Clear-cell squamous cell carcinoma
Atypical fibroxanthoma
Lepromatous leprosy
Prognosis
No different from conventional melanomas, directly related to tumor thickness
Degree of balloon cell change does not alter prognosis
5-year survival, 37.5% (melanomas of all thicknesses)

contain significant deposits of glycogen in the latter cells based on diastase-sensitive PAS staining (306).

Differential Diagnosis Because of the striking clear-cell appearance and low-grade cellular atypia, BCM may be confused with balloon cell nevus, xanthoma, hibernoma, granular cell tumor, metastatic clear-cell carcinomas (such as renal cell or adenocarcinoma), liposarcoma, and clear-cell appendage tumors (304,305) (Table 10-27). Clinical correlation is critical since most balloon cell melanomas have the gross morphology of melanoma. Perhaps, the greatest problem is distinction of BCM from balloon cell nevus. Careful attention to the overall characteristics of the tumor should allow distinction of BCM from a balloon cell nevus. In general, balloon cell nevi occur in young individuals (< 30 years), show "maturation" of nevus cells (decreased size of cells and nuclei with depth), the presence of multinucleate giant cells (see Chapter 5), in contrast to BCM, which tends to develop in older patients, to lack maturation of melanoma cells, and to have cellular atypia and mitotic activity (305).

Myxoid Melanoma

In rare instances, both primary and metastatic melanoma may demonstrate prominent myxoid alteration of the tumor stroma (307–309) (Fig. 10-33). Such mucin deposition may be focal or diffuse and be associated with any type of melanoma. The association with desmoplastic–neurotropic melanoma has already been discussed. Since the lesions are so rare, no distinctive clinical features have thus far been reported with the exception that most are amelanotic. Primary tumors may demonstrate a lobular configuration with pushing borders. Poorly defined septa composed of delicate fibrovascular tissue may separate the tumor lobules. The melanoma cells are often arranged in cords, may form pseudoglandular structures, or occur as single cells; there may be a perivascular or paraseptal localization of tumor cells. The tumor cells are commonly spindled or stellate but also may be large epithelioid cells. Vacuolated cells resembling lipoblasts may be present. As already mentioned, melanin may be minimal or absent. The tumor stroma may contain pools of mucin and are relatively vascular. The mucin usually stains with Alcian blue at pH 2.5.

Differential Diagnosis Myxoid melanoma must be distinguished from other myxoid tumors, including a melanocytic nevus; myxoid appendageal tumors, such as cutaneous mixed tumor, mucinous or colloid carcinoma; metastatic adenocarcinoma; squamous cell carcinoma; basal cell carcinoma; focal dermal mucinosis; myxoma; angiomyxoma; neurofibroma; schwannoma; nerve sheath myxoma (neurothekeoma); myxoid atypical fibroxanthoma (malignant fibrous histiocytoma); myxoid malignant peripheral nerve sheath tumors; myxoid liposarcoma; myxoid extraskeletal chondrosarcoma; and other myxoid sarcomas. The demonstration of an atypical intraepidermal melanocytic component or melanoma in situ; melanin pigment (by Fontana-Masson stain if necessary); and immunoreactivity with melanocytic markers such as S-100 protein, HMB-45, Mart-1, MITF, and tyrosinase favors melanoma over the latter entities. Metastatic melanoma should be excluded if an intraepidermal component is absent.

Atypical Dermal Melanocytic Tumor Similar to Spontaneous and Induced Melanoma in Animals (Animal-Type Melanoma)

Clark et al. (310) drew attention to an unusual and controversial heavily pigmented melanocytic tumor rarely

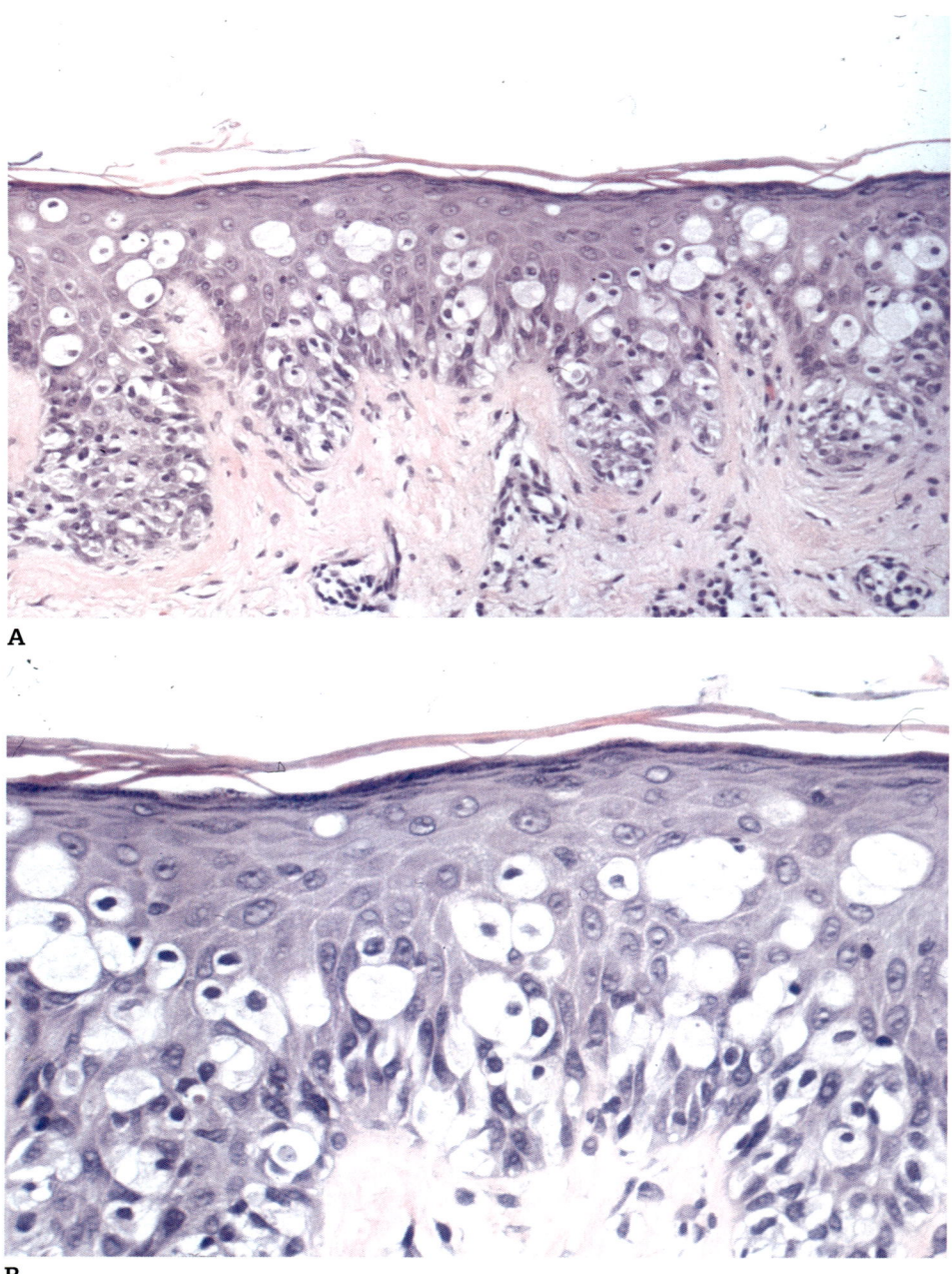

FIGURE 10-32 Balloon cell melanoma. **A,** Note the pagetoid spread of balloon cells in this melanoma in situ. **B,** Balloon melanoma cells are enlarged with abundant clear cytoplasm and pleomorphic nuclei. (Courtesy of Dr. T.-Y. Wong.)

occurring in humans that closely mimics melanomas developing spontaneously or induced in animals. To describe such tumors Clark coined the rather colorful term *animal-type melanoma;* however, at the same time, he emphasized that the biologic potential of such tumors remained largely unknown, and that they should not be categorized as frank melanoma. Among 20 cases accrued by Clark, only 2 developed regional lymph node metastases, and both patients were disease-free with follow-up of about 5 and 15 years. Heavily pigmented nodular neoplasms had long been recognized in horses and described under the term *equine melanotic disease* (311). In general, the latter tumors are associated with a rather nonaggressive course, but they nonetheless may result in metastases.

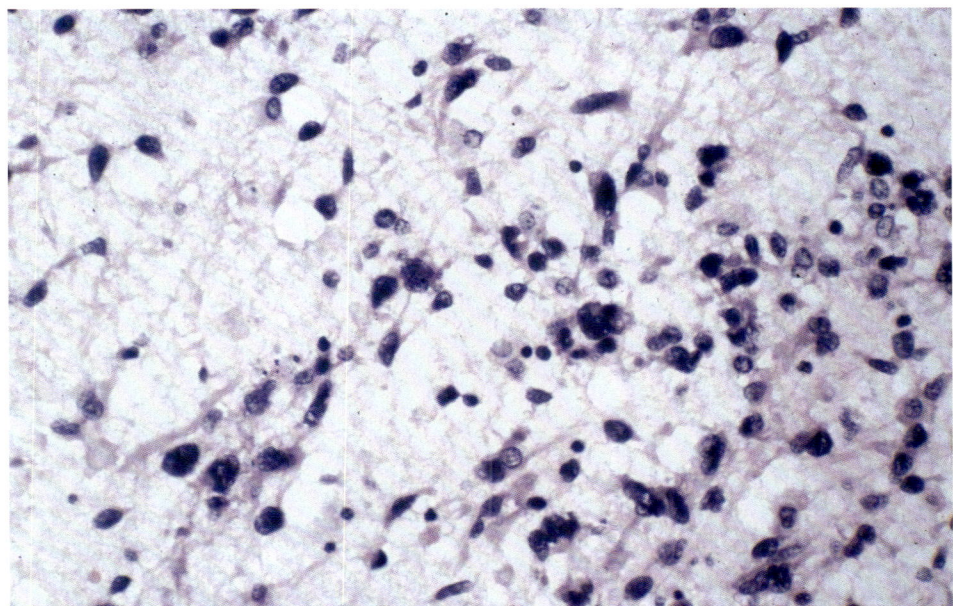
FIGURE 10-33 In myxoid melanoma, the melanoma cells are dispersed in an abundant mucinous stroma. (Courtesy of Dr. M. Wick,)

With his introduction of the term *melanosarcoma* to depict dermal pigmented spindle cell melanocytic tumors in humans (in fact a description of CBN), Darier (311) perhaps first recognized the similarities among these peculiar animal lesions and comparable human tumors.

Because of the extreme rarity of such tumors and their potential relationship to or confusion with CBN and CBN with atypical features, malignant blue nevus (melanoma arising in or closely mimicking blue nevus), so-called deep penetrating nevus, and possibly partially or largely regressed melanoma (tumoral melanosis), one may call into question the existence of this entity (Fig. 10-34). We advise the adoption of strict criteria for diagnosis and the study of additional cases with long-term follow-up to better define the entity and its biologic potential. We recommend that, unless overt malignant features are present in the context of the criteria outlined below, such tumors should be categorized as biologically indeterminate. Patients should undergo appropriate excision and should be closely monitored for disease recrudescence.

Clinical and Histopathologic Features According to Clark, such lesions develop slowly as black nodules with a rough surface and circular but irregular borders (Table 10-29). Applying strict histopathologic criteria, such tumors are defined as follows: (a) They lack an intraepidermal component. (b) They are composed of confluent dermal nodular collections of predominately heavily melaninized polygonal melanocytes that, on initial inspection, suggest melanophages. (c) They exhibit nuclei that are generally obscured by melanin, but the nuclei that can be observed generally have condensed chromatin peripherally, clear nucleoplasm, and prominent nucleoli. (d) Mitoses are generally uncommon. (e) There is an absence of blue nevus remnants. (f) Metastatic melanoma is ruled out (Fig. 10-34). Bleaching tissue sections with potassium permanganate may be useful to study cytologic detail. Immunohistochemistry with melanocytic and histiocytic markers is essential to verify that the overwhelming majority of cells are melanocytes.

Differential Diagnosis The principal entity entering into the differential diagnosis and potentially having some relationship to animal-type melanoma is tumoral melanosis—that is, completely or largely regressed melanoma (see below). (Table 10-29) In some instances, epithelioid cell variants of blue nevus and malignant blue nevus must be considered and may share some features in common. The identification of a typical blue nevus component with organoid configuration, dendritic melanocytes, and non-scarring fibrosis distinguishes the latter two conditions from animal-type melanoma.

Clear-Cell Melanoma

Clear-cell melanomas, in addition to typical balloon cell melanomas as discussed above, must be distinguished from various clear-cell carcinomas, including those from the breast, kidney, large bowel, lung, salivary gland, and thyroid and from adnexal tumors (particularly syringoma),

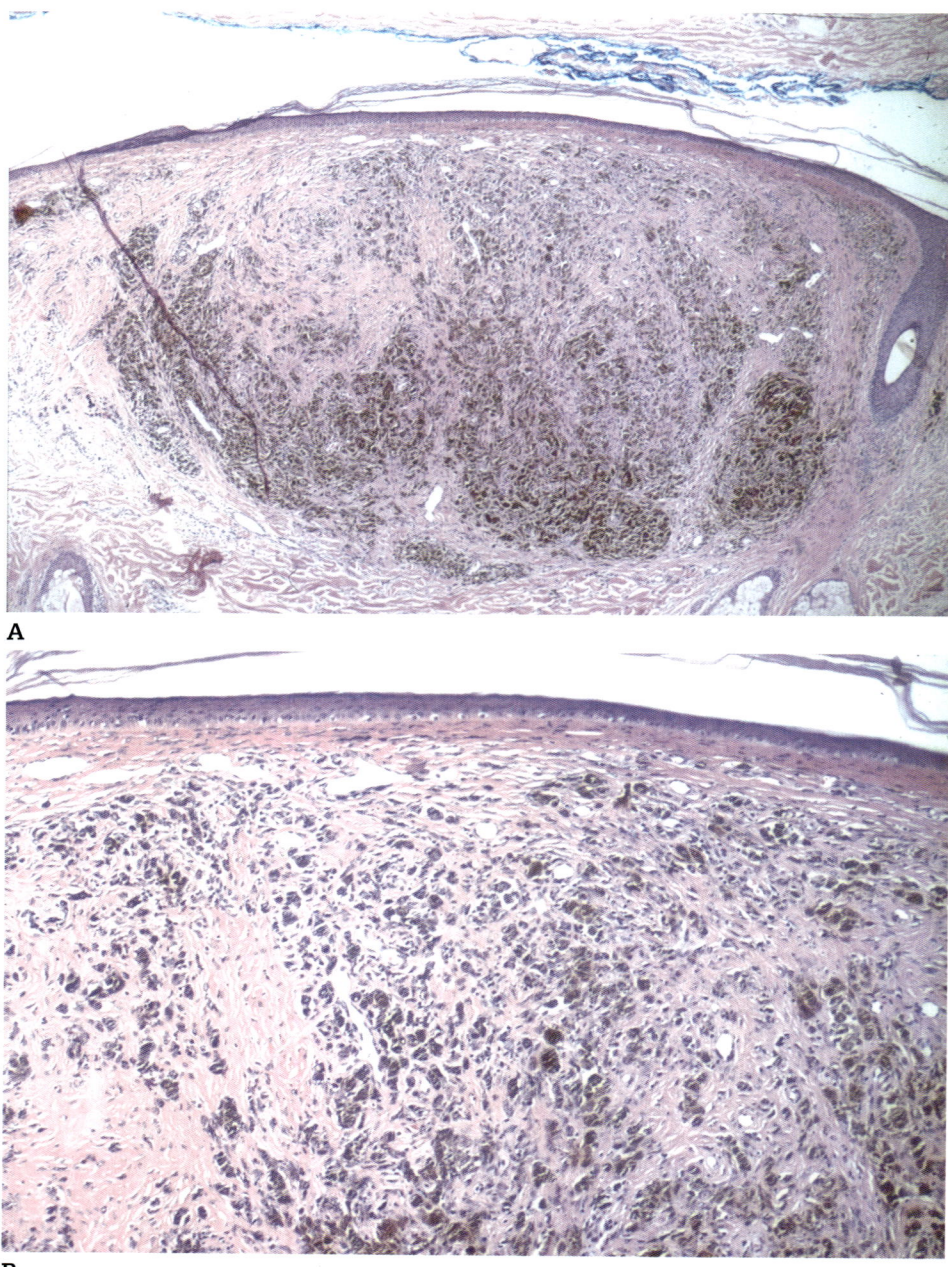

FIGURE 10-34 Tumoral melanosis. **A,** Note the asymmetrical nodular aggregates of heavily pigmented polygonal cells in the dermis accompanied by fibrosis. **B–D,** Many of the cells are melanophages, whereas a small number of melanoma cells are scattered throughout the pigmented nodule, as verified by expression of melanoma markers.

basal cell carcinoma, various clear-cell eccrine carcinomas, sebaceous carcinoma, and seminoma (301,312).

Signet-Ring Cell Melanoma

Primary and metastatic melanomas composed of signet cells evoke a wide differential diagnosis, including signet-ring cell nevi, mucin-producing adenocarcinoma, liposarcoma, lymphoma, squamous cell carcinoma, vascular tumors, and epithelioid cell smooth muscle tumors. The cytoplasmic vacuoles in such signet-ring cell melanomas do not contain mucin, lipid, or glycogen and ultrastructurally seem to contain intermediate filaments that are most likely vimentin; they nonetheless appear as empty spaces (301,313–316) (Figs. 10-24 and 10-25).

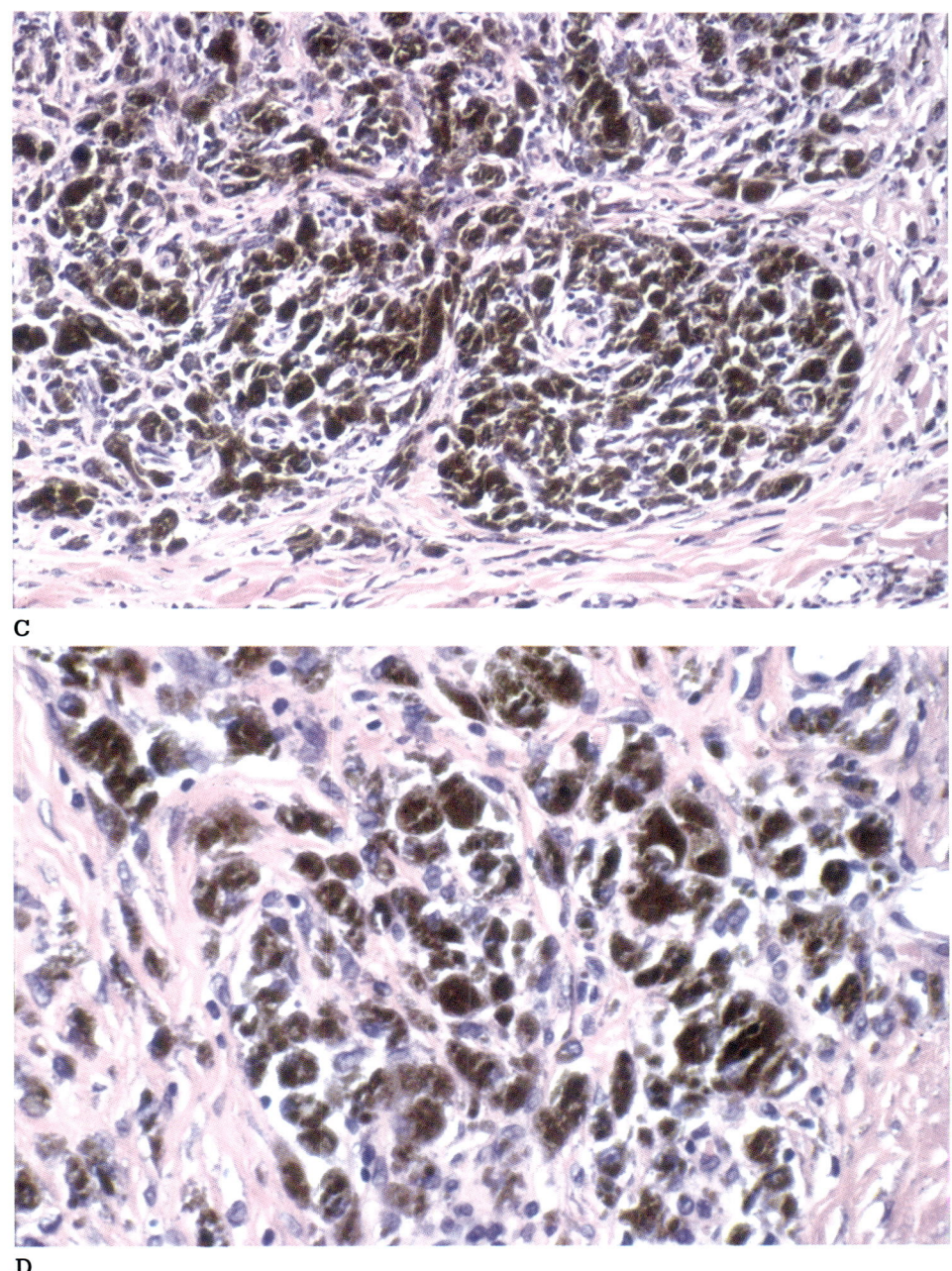

FIGURE 10-34 *Continued.* Tumoral melanosis.

Mucosal Melanoma

Primary melanomas of mucosal sites, such as the oral cavity, nasal cavity, esophagus, vulva, vagina, urethra, and anorectum, are relatively rare and account for 3–4% of all melanomas, with an annual incidence of 0.15/100,000 (320–331). They often share clinical and histopathologic features in common with acral melanoma (Fig. 10-35) (see above). In general, many of these mucosal melanomas appear to develop from atypical lentiginous melanocytic proliferations of mucosal epithelium and often subsequently exhibit lentiginous intraepithelial growth phases (Fig. 10-35B). The most common cell type making up these lesions is a pleomorphic spindled or dendritic melanocyte; however, epithelioid and small cells are observed often (Fig. 10-35C). Some mucosal melanomas also show intraepithelial pagetoid spread. "Nodular" melanomas—that is, melanomas without any apparent adjacent intraepithelial component—may involve mucosal surfaces and, as with all such nodular melanomas, must be distinguished from metastatic melanoma. The

TABLE 10-29 Animal-type melanoma.
Clinical features
Extremely rare
Any age
Any site
1–2 cm or more, often
Black nodule with rough surface
Circular but irregular borders
Histopathologic features
Intraepidermal component, usually absent
Confluent dermal nodular aggregates of heavily melaninized polygonal melanocytes, suggesting melanophages
Nuclei obscured by melanin
Condensed chromatin peripherally
Prominent nucleoli
Mitotic figures uncommon
Differential diagnosis
Metastatic melanoma
Cellular blue nevus and atypical variants
Malignant blue nevus
Tumoral melanosis

invasive component of mucosal melanoma is often composed of pleomorphic or small round cells, but spindle cells and epithelioid cells are also observed. As with other lentiginous melanomas, the invasive component is not uncommonly desmoplastic–neurotropic (see above). In general, mucosal melanomas are diagnosed at an advanced stage but are nonetheless considered aggressive tumors and are associated with a dismal prognosis. For example, patients with vulvar melanoma from Sweden have a 47% 5-year survival versus 80% on average for patients with cutaneous melanoma. As with cutaneous melanoma, prognosis is generally directly related to tumor thickness.

REGRESSION

Melanoma is notable for its frequency of spontaneous regression (45,103,104,332–340). The prevalence of histologic regression varies according to the definition of regression used and the thickness range of the melanomas reported (45,104,334). In a study of 563 cases of primary melanoma, histologic regression was noted in 46% of thin (< 1.5 mm), 32% of intermediate (1.5–3.0 mm), and 9% of thick (> 3.0 mm) melanomas (334). McGovern et al. (335) recorded regression in 58% of melanomas < 0.70 mm in thickness. Complete regression of melanoma is uncommon and has been reported to occur with a frequency of 2.4–8.7% (335,336). Many cases of metastatic melanoma with unknown primary are thought to be explained by spontaneous regression of the primary melanoma (332,341).

Regression is thought to be immunologically mediated because of mononuclear cell infiltrates containing T lymphocytes, plasma cells, and monocyte/macrophages at the site of regression (337). Regression is seen most often in microinvasive melanoma and is present as focal, partial, and rarely complete regression of the tumor

FIGURE 10-35 Vulvar melanoma. **A,** Ulcerated advanced vulvar melanoma demonstrating highly cellular nodule of amelanotic melanocytes.

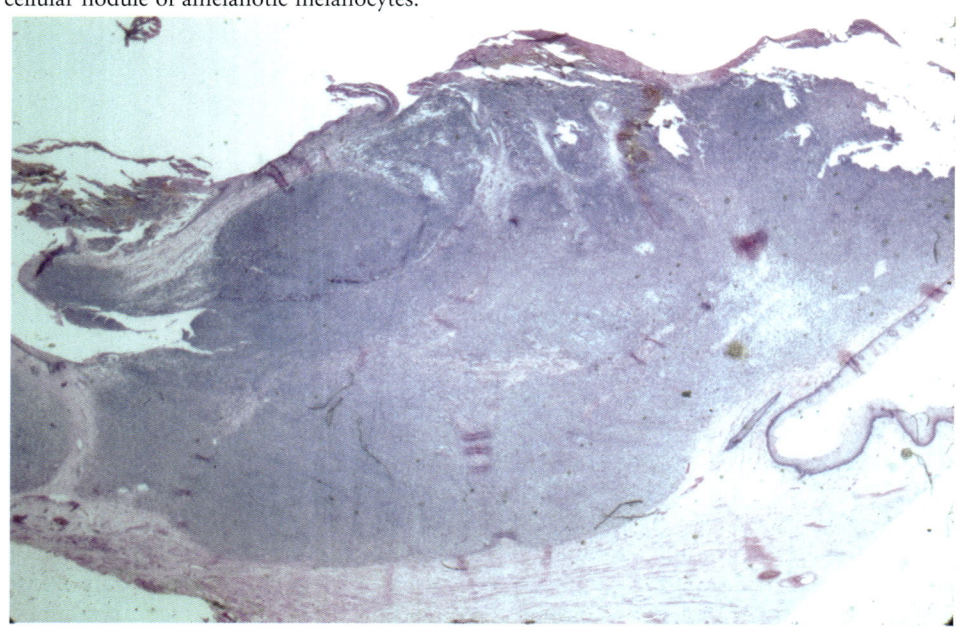

A

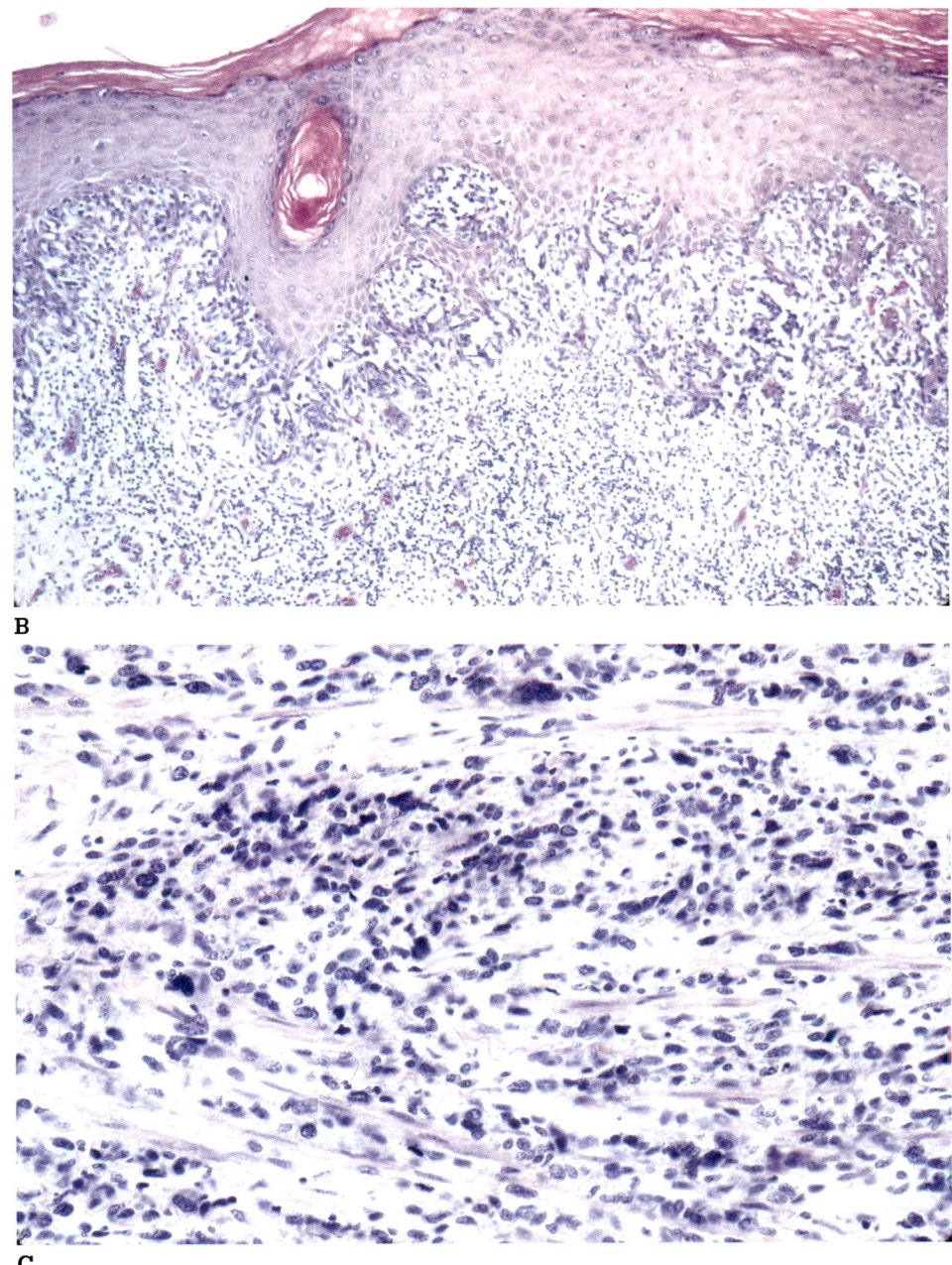

FIGURE 10-35 *Continued*. **B,** Note the lentiginous pattern of this vulvar melanoma. The melanoma cells show striking confluence along the basal layer without significant pagetoid spread. **C,** The invasive component of a vulvar melanoma. The tumor cells are small, round to elongate amelanotic cells with striking nuclear variation and hyperchromatism.

(45,103,104). The changes of regression form a continuum and may be arbitrarily categorized into three stages (104) (Table 10-30). Early regression shows a rich mononuclear infiltrate closely associated with the invasive dermal melanoma (Fig. 10-36). It is necessary that actual tumor cell destruction is demonstrated, and careful inspection will usually disclose lymphoid cells closely opposed to tumor cells (satellitosis) in a pattern reminiscent of graft versus host disease. There may also be epidermal infiltration by the mononuclear cells.

Intermediate regression is characterized by loss or dropout of tumor, in the papillary dermis, epidermis,

TABLE 10-30 Stages of histological regression of malignant melanoma.

Stage	Comments
Early (or active)	Zone of papillary dermis and epidermis within a recognizable melanoma characterized by dense infiltrates of lymphocytes disrupting or replacing nests of melanoma cells within the papillary dermis and possibly the epidermis, compared to adjoining zones of tumor. Degenerating melanoma cells should be recognizable. There is no obvious fibrosis.
Intermediate	Zone of papillary dermis and epidermis within a recognizable melanoma characterized by reduction (loss) in the amount of tumor (a disruption in the continuity of the tumor) or absence of tumor in papillary dermis and possibly within the epidermis, compared to adjacent zones of tumor. Replacement by varying admixtures of lymphoid cells and increased fibrous tissue (compared to normal papillary dermis) in this zone. Variable telangiectasia (and new blood vessel formation) and melanophages may also be present.
Late	Zone of papillary dermis and epidermis within a recognizable melanoma characterized by marked reduction in the amount of tumor compared to adjacent areas of tumor or absence of tumor in this zone. Replacement and expansion of the papillary dermis in this zone by extensive fibrosis (usually dense fibrous tissue, horizontally disposed). Also seen are variable telangiectasia (and new blood vessel formation), melanophages, sparse or no lymphoid infiltrates, and effacement of the epidermis (other than fibrosis, the latter features are frequently present but not essential for recognizing regression).

or both, and continued host response (104) (Fig. 10-36B,C; Table 10-30). The loss of tumor is associated with variable thickening and fibroplasia (scarring) of the papillary dermis, mononuclear cell (lymphocytes and plasma cells) infiltrates, prominent vascularity, and melanin-containing macrophages. In general, there is some diminution in the intensity of the infiltrate at this stage, and there may be effacement of the epidermal rete pattern.

Late-stage regression shows prominence of papillary dermal fibrosis or scarring (104) (Fig. 10-36D,E; Table 10-30), characterized by dense layering of coarse fibrous tissue similar to scarring. There is absence of tumor in both epidermis and dermis and often complete effacement of the epidermal rete pattern. Residual single melanoma cells or small nests of cells may remain at the dermoepidermal junction or entrapped in the fibrosis. Mononuclear cell infiltrates are minimal or absent at this

FIGURE 10-36 Three stages of regression in melanoma. **A,** Early regression demonstrating dense mononuclear cell infiltrates in the papillary dermis and apoptotic cells near the dermoepidermal junction.

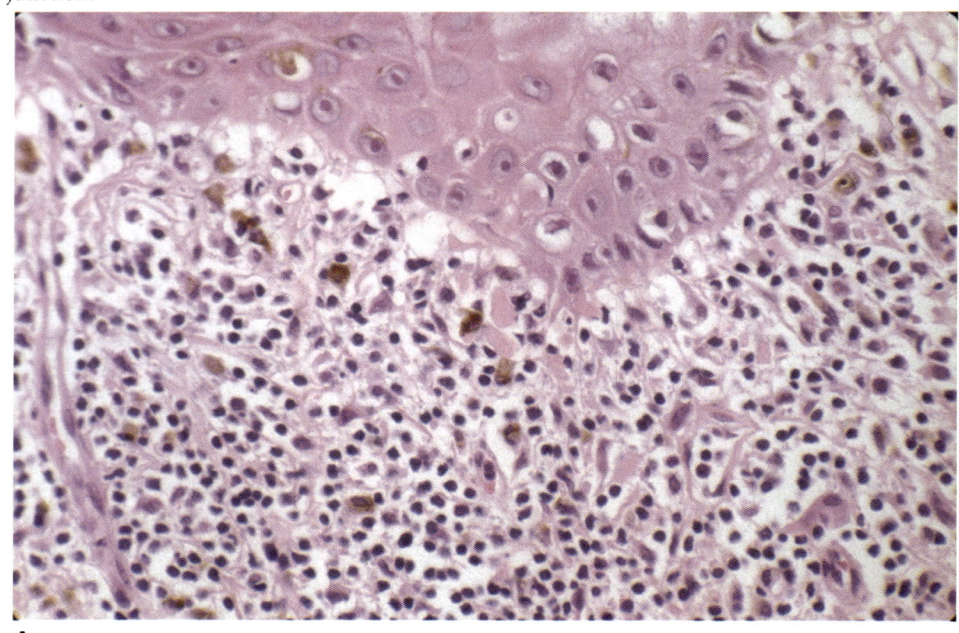

A

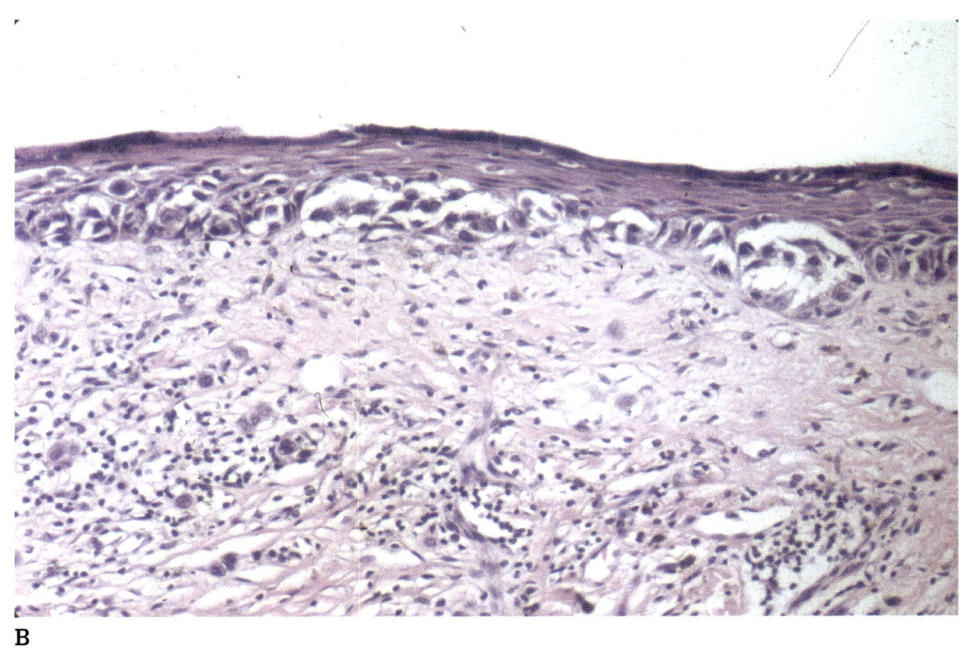

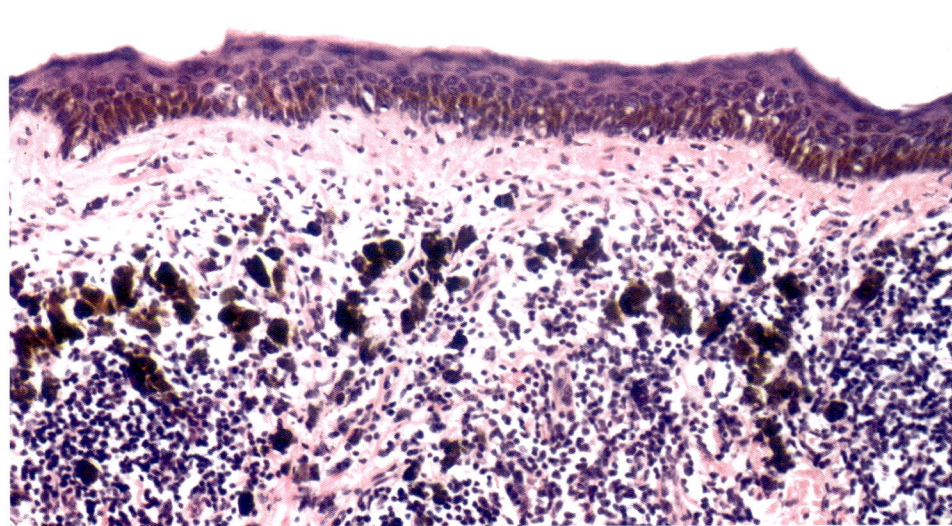

FIGURE 10-36 *Continued.* **B,** In intermediate regression there is effacement of epidermis, but residual melanoma is present within both epidermis and dermis. Fibrosis of the papillary dermis and patchy mononuclear infiltrates can also be observed. **C,** In intermediate to late regression, the papillary dermis contains relatively dense lymphoid infiltrates and aggregates of melanophages. There is virtually complete absence of melanoma.

stage. There may be remarkable angiogenesis and ectasia of vessels in these zones of regression (338) and melanophages may be present to a variable extent.

The changes of regression vary considerably from tumor to tumor and within a single tumor (104). The proportion of the melanoma involved may range from a small focus (most common) to complete regression. All phases of regression may be found within the same tumor, resulting in several distinctive presentations of melanoma that are important to recognize (45). Melanoma

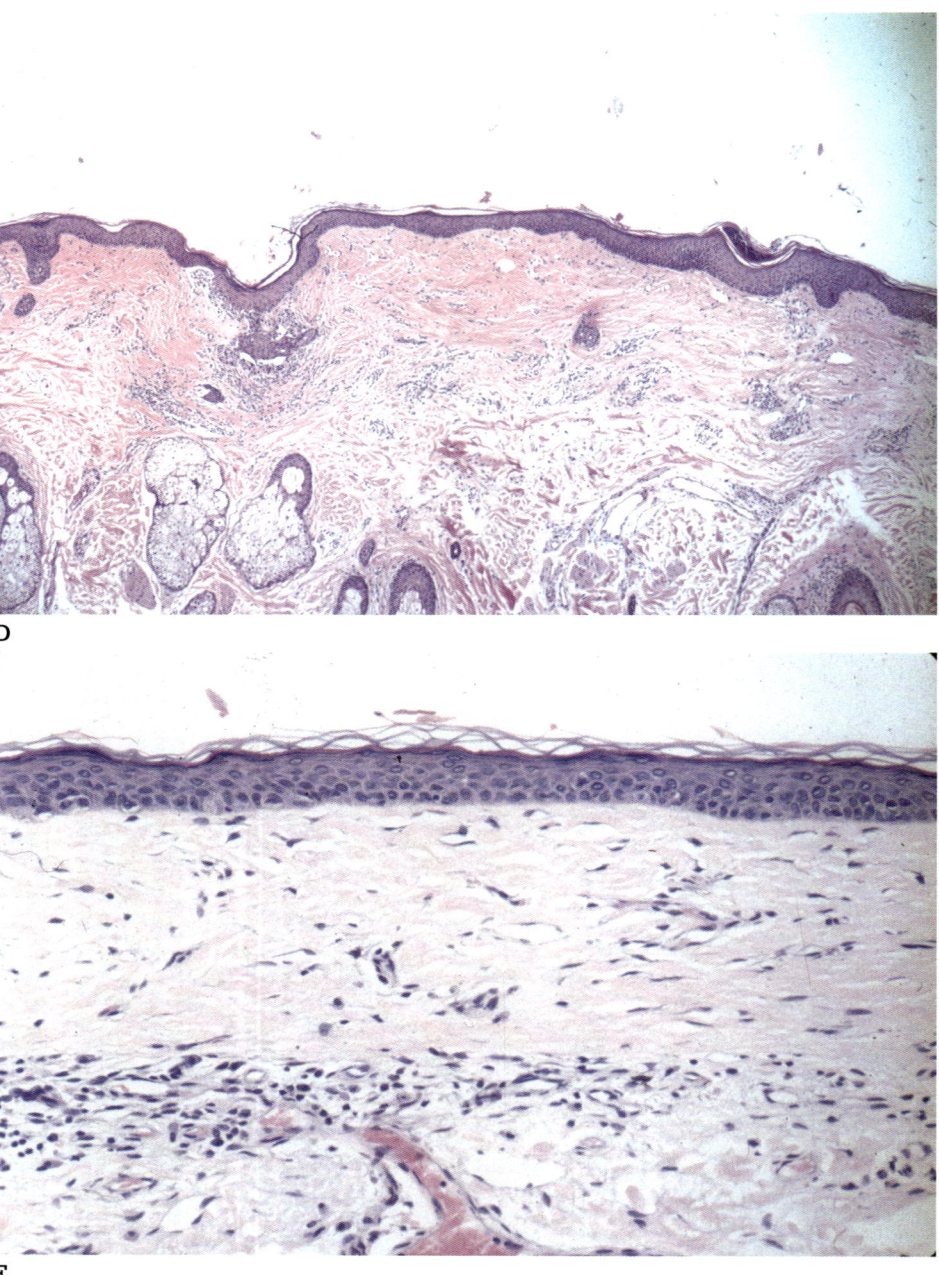

FIGURE 10-36 *Continued.* **D,** In late-stage regression there is almost complete absence of melanoma, effacement of the epidermal rete ridges, and thickening and fibrosis of the papillary dermis. **E,** Note the fibrosis of dermis and complete absence of melanoma in late-stage regression.

with prominent mononuclear cell infiltrates (early regression) may simulate a halo nevus clinically and histologically (see below).

Regression of the intraepidermal component of melanoma leaving residual melanoma in the dermis, may strongly suggest metastatic melanoma or local satellites, solitary or multifocal (45). Complete obliteration of the dermal component of melanoma occasionally leaves persistent junctional nests and dermal fibrosis, simulating in situ or microinvasive melanoma and falsely suggesting an excellent prognosis, when in reality the patient has a greater risk for metastasis.

Complete Regression of Primary Melanoma

Uncommonly, primary melanoma may undergo complete regression, and its recognition usually follows the development of metastases and a search for primary melanoma. Metastatic melanoma with an unknown primary accounts for about 2.5% of all melanomas (341). Completely regressed melanoma may present in the following scenarios (45,339,340).

Hypopigmented or Vitiligo-Like Lesion Hypopigmented or vitiligo-like lesion is probably the most common manifestation of completely regressed melanoma (340). The patient presents clinically with a solitary circumscribed usually asymmetrical hypopigmented or depigmented patch. Histologically, there is little if any melanin pigment present either in the basal layer of the epidermis (usually a complete loss of melanin) or near the dermoepidermal junction, owing to the destruction of melanoma cells and some normal basilar melanocytes. The epidermis is usually effaced and atrophic. The papillay dermis is thickened by a variable combination of dermal fibroplasia, bandlike yet often sparse lymphoplasmacellular infiltrates, melanophage accumulation, and increased vascularity without any residual melanoma. The fibroplasia may be loose and edematous or scar-like.

Differential Diagnosis Hypopigmented regressed melanoma must be distinguished from vitiligo, postinflammatory hypopigmentation or hyperpigmentation, resulting from an antecdent inflammatory process (such as fixed drug eruption) and a completely regressed halo nevus (340). In general, the approach to the problem of regression requires the following measures: (a) obtaining detailed clinical information about the patient, the nature of the clinical lesion, its duration and evolution, any evidence of metastatic or systemic disease, and history of drug ingestion or exposure to other external or environmental agents and (b) step sectioning of the tissue block in an effort to identify residual melanoma or another process. The presence of plasma cells and scarring in regressed melanoma usually allows for a distinction from vitiligo and other primary inflammatory dermatitides. A completely regressed halo nevus may prove to be more challenging. However, in many instances the clinical findings alone provide sufficient evidence for the distinction from melanoma. Halo nevi usually exhibit a well-defined and symmetrical, round or oval annulus of hypopigmentation or depigmentation about a small central nevus; the borders of both the halo and the nevus are almost always regular. Moreover, almost all halo nevi develop on the trunk (commonly the upper back) of young individuals (children and adolescents) and are much more prevalent than halo-like melanomas. On the other hand, hypopigmented regressed melanomas virtually always demonstrate asymmetrical macular hypopigmentation or depigmentation. In the case of a halo-like melanoma, there is clinically residual obvious melanoma present. Microscopically, the regression in melanoma is usually distinct from inflammatory regression of melanocytic nevi. Halo nevi are characterized by delicate fibroplasia and stromal mucinous alterations that differ from the dense, coarse fibrosis and linear scarring and by the presence of plasma cells in melanoma (340). Moreover, completely regressed halo nevi generally display depigmentation at the peripheries of the lesion, compared to a more diffuse depigmentation in melanoma.

Lichenoid Pattern As mentioned above, regressing/regressed melanoma may present with a dense bandlike lymphoid infiltrate occupying the papillary dermis (early to intermediate stage regression), which may be confused with a lichenoid dermatitis (340). The histologic findings often shared in common among these entities include infiltrates containing predominately lymphocytes but also histiocytes and plasma cells; considerable melanin pigment (both free and in melanophages), in many instances; and the frequent presence of apoptotic keratinocytes (colloid or Civatte bodies) (Fig. 10-36A,C).

Differential Diagnosis The primary considerations for differential diagnosis include lichen planus, lichenoid drug eruption, contact dermatitis, connective tissue disease with lichenoid pattern, lichenoid keratosis, and rarely other regressing neoplasms such as pigmented basal cell carcinoma and mycosis fungoides (340). The clinical presentation will usually allow the immediate distinction of a lichenoid dermatitis from regression of melanoma. However, solitary lesions, such as a lichenoid keratosis, cutaneous lupus erythematosus, lichen planus, and a lichenoid drug eruption or contact dermatitis may prove exceedingly difficult to discriminate from regressed melanoma. The lichenoid (lichen planus-like) keratosis may pose the greatest challenge, since a priori it is almost always solitary, occurs in older individuals, and is often localized to sun-exposed skin. This keratosis often demonstrates a residual portion of solar lentigo or seborrheic keratosis at the peripheries, some melanin in the basal layer, and usually an absence of scarring, allowing discrimination from melanoma. However, the same approach as outlined above for possible regression of melanoma should be pursued. In some percentage of cases, regression of melanoma cannot be ruled out and thus complete excision of the lesion and close monitoring of the patient are necessary.

Cutaneous lupus erythematosus is usually distinguished from regressed melanoma by basement membrane thickening, the presence of basal layer melanin, dermal mucin deposition, perivascular and periadnexal lymphoid infiltrates that involve the deep reticular dermis, and absence of scarring. Lichenoid drug eruptions and contact dermatitis contain eosinophils within the infiltrates and display basal layer melanin, dermal perivascular lymphoid infiltrates, and an absence of scarring. Clinical information and step sections are necessary to confirm the regression of other neoplastic processes such as pigmented basal cell carcinoma or mycosis fungoides. We have observed complete regression of melanoma at the site of a compound nevus.

Tumoral Melanosis (Tumoral Melanophagocytosis, Nodular Melanosis, Melanophagic Dermatitis and Panniculitis) Tumor melanosis is a rare but distinctive process characterized by cohesive aggregates of heavily melaninized large polyhedral cells in the superficial dermis, forming a nodule or plaque that suggests a primary "nodular" melanoma (339,340) (Figs. 10-34 and 10-37; Table 10-31). These tumors often show epidermal hyperplasia and the papillary dermis is expanded by masses of large cells packed with melanin. There may be focal epidermal involvement by the latter component of cells. Fibrosis, lymphoplasma cellular infiltrates, and zones of prototypic regression may be present. Cytologic and nuclear details are obscured by melanin pigment. The latter findings and immunohistochemisty confirming the presence of melanophages are consonant with a regressing/regressed melanoma. Often such lesions are associated with metastases (Fig. 10-37). Such a tumor also may occur in the deep dermis or subcutaneous fat, suggesting the regression of a metastasis. There may or may not be residual intraepidermal or dermal melanoma present.

Differential Diagnosis Other entities to be considered include heavily pigmented melanocytic tumors, such as atypical dermal melanocytic tumor similar to spontaneous and induced melanomas in animals, epithelioid cell blue nevus and related lesions, cellular blue nevus and atypical variants, malignant blue nevus (melanoma arising in or resembling blue nevus), and finally regressed nonmelanocytic tumors (e.g., basal cell carcinoma) that may rarely result in tumoral melanosis (Table 10-31) (342). The heavily pigmented tumor resembling animal melanomas may have considerable overlap with tumoral melanosis and thus may constitute a regressing form of melanoma in some cases (310,311). A critical finding providing evidence for tumoral melanosis is the presence of conventional regression with scarring. All such tumors should be assessed carefully for residual melanoma and the changes of regression by step sections, bleaching, and immunohistochemistry with melanocytic and histiocytic markers.

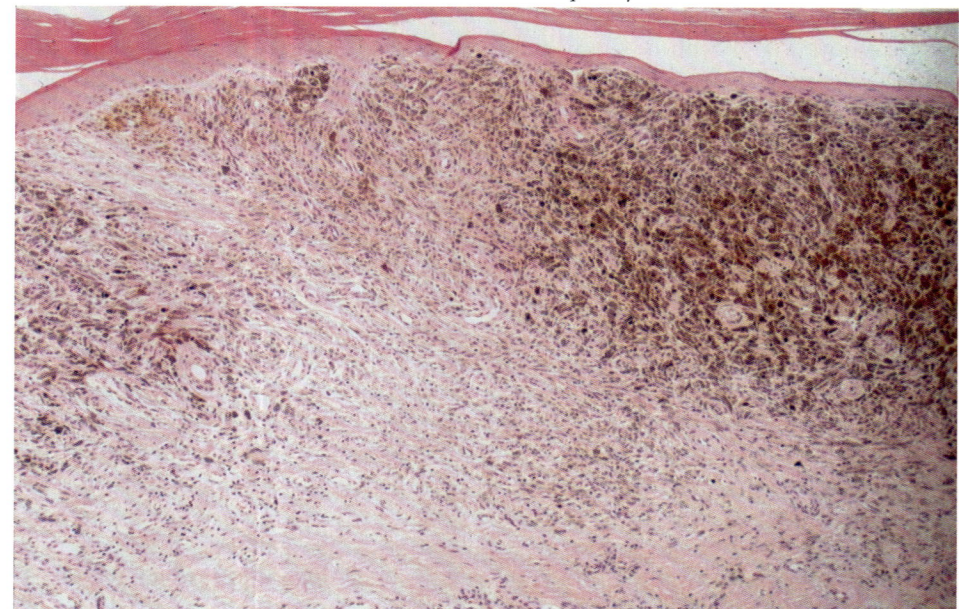

FIGURE 10-37 Tumoral melanosis. A raised asymmetrical tumoral lesion demonstrating dense aggregates of melanophages and variable degrees of dermal fibrosis. There was no evidence of residual melanoma upon evaluation with immunohistochemistry. This patient presented initially with metastatic melanoma, and this cutaneous lesion was subsequently found on examination of the skin.

TABLE 10-31 Tumoral melanosis.

Clinical features
- Extremely rare
- Any age
- Any site
- 1–5 cm, often
- Black, blue-black nodule

Histopathologic features
- Epidermal hyperplasia, often
- Intraepidermal component may be focally present
- Confluent dermal nodular aggregates of heavily melaninized polygonal cells, suggesting melanophages
- Nuclei obscured by melanin
- Fibroplasia, focally present
- Lymphoplasma cellular infiltrates, often
- Focal conventional regression may be present
- Focal residual melanoma may or may not be present
- Mitotic figures, uncommon

Differential diagnosis
- Metastatic melanoma
- Cellular blue nevus and atypical variants
- Epithelioid blue nevus
- Melanocytic nevi with phenotypic heterogeneity (combined nevi) and heavily pigmented component
- Malignant blue nevus
- Atypical melanocytic tumor (animal-type)

Completely Regressed Melanoma with Residual Benign Nevus Remnant

Completely regressed melanoma with residual benign nevus remnant is an extremely rare phenomenon in which melanoma in continuity with a nevus regresses completely, leaving behind the hallmarks of regression and an unscathed nevus (340). The diagnosis can be made confidently only in retrospect, after the development of metastases.

Differential Diagnosis Host response changes commonly occurring in melanocytic nevi must be distinguished from regressed melanoma. The composite findings of depigmentation, scarring, and plasma cells consonant with regression of melanoma are usually not observed in nevi.

DIAGNOSIS AND MANAGEMENT OF THE BORDERLINE OR CONTROVERSIAL LESIONS SUGGESTING MELANOMA

In this and other chapters we discuss at length particular lesions or histopathologic findings that suggest or mimic primary melanoma on a regular basis. Accordingly, a major goal of this book is to provide clinical, histopathologic, and other criteria that are as precise as possible to aid the physician in resolving or at least managing these problems.

The aims of this section are to list in one place the most common borderline lesions one is likely to encounter and to offer advice about their management. Because each borderline lesion is to some degree unique, it is simply not possible to exhaustively recount all of the potential scenarios or variations, since they are myriad (if one has seen one borderline melanocytic lesion, one has seen one).

As has been emphasized throughout this chapter and book, the histopathologist must recognize his or her limitations; not all melanocytic lesions at present can be classified as benign or malignant. Thus the histopathologist should marshall all resources available to interpret as precisely as possible a difficult melanocytic lesion and to place it into one of three categories: (a) benign, (b) biologically indeterminate, or (c) malignant, for the optimal communication to and management of the patient. A biologically indeterminate lesion is defined as one that has some potential (uncertain) risk for local recurrence and metastasis but cannot be interpreted as malignant using all criteria currently available. The diagnostic exercise should be comprehensive and include collecting information such as age, gender, site, clinical characteristics, presence or absence of ulceration, diameter, thickness, mitotic rate per square millimeter, and possibly immunostaining for proliferative rate (e.g., with Ki-67) and other markers to quantify as much as possible the abnormalities present that favor or argue against melanoma. The diagnostic evaluation of such a difficult lesion should probably include obtaining the opinion of a recognized authority in the field.

Nomenclature

The nomenclature of borderline lesions should be kept as simple as possible to facilitate lucid communication and management (Table 10-32). The four broad scenarios are discussed.

Atypical Intraepidermal Melanocytic Proliferation with Indeterminate Biological Potential

Lesions with Upward Migration or Pagetoid Spread of Melanocytes

Atypical intraepidermal lesions with upward migration probably cause considerable difficulty when distinguishing between benign simulants and melanoma (Figs. 10-27A,B). One must rely on other histologic criteria, such as the presence or absence of asymmetry, large size, poor circumscription, maturation, age of the patient, clinical appearance, and anatomic site (Table 10-32). The principal melanocytic lesions entering into the differential diagnosis include melanocytic nevi in children, congenital nevi (particularly in the 1st year of life), spindle and epithelioid cell (Spitz) nevi, pigmented spindle cell nevi (Fig. 10-28A), nevi from acral surfaces, recurrent melanocytic nevi, and nevi with reactive changes from solar irradiation and other external agents.

TABLE 10-32 Management of biologically indeterminate melanocytic lesions.

Lesion	Management[a]
Atypical intraepidermal melanocytic proliferations with indeterminate biologic potential	
Atypical (dysplastic) nevus with pagetoid spread	Surgical margins: ~5 mm
Intraepidermal epithelioid cell pagetoid melanocytic proliferation	Follow-up: every 6 months
Pagetoid Spitz tumor	
Pigmented spindle cell nevus with pagetoid spread	
Pigmented spindle cell nevus with prominent nested pattern	
Acral nevus with pagetoid spread	
Recurrent melanocytic nevus with pagetoid spread and atypia	
Melanocytic nevus with pagetoid spread and atypia, not otherwise specified	
Solar lentiginous melanocytic proliferation with atypia	
Acral lentiginous melanocytic proliferation with atypia	
Atypical intraepidermal and dermal melanocytic proliferations with indeterminate biologic potential (< 1 mm thickness)	
Atypical (dysplastic) compound nevus vs. melanoma, invasive	Surgical margins: 5–10 mm
Compound Spitz tumor with atypical features	Follow-up: every 6 months
Compound pigmented spindle cell nevus with atypical features	
Halo-like nevus with atypical features	
Compound nevus with small cells and atypical features vs. nevoid melanoma	
Acral compound nevus with atypical features	
Genital nevus with atypical features	
Atypical intraepidermal and dermal melanocytic proliferations with indeterminate biologic potential (> 1 mm thickness)	
Atypical (dysplastic) compound nevus vs. melanoma, invasive	Surgical margins: 5–10 mm
Compound Spitz tumor with atypical features	Follow-up: every 3–6 months
Compound pigmented spindle cell nevus with atypical features	Consider sentinal lymph node biopsy
Halo-like nevus with atypical features	
Compound nevus with small cells and atypical features vs. nevoid melanoma	
Acral compound nevus with atypical features	
Genital compound nevus with atypical features	
Atypical dermal melanocytic proliferations with indeterminate biologic potential (> 1 mm thickness)	
Spitz-like tumor with prominent dermal nodular proliferation	Surgical margins: 5–10 mm or more
Dermal nodular melanocytic proliferation arising in conventional compound or dermal nevus, acquired	Follow-up: every 3–6 months
Dermal nodular melanocytic proliferation arising in conventional compound or dermal nevus, congenital	Consider sentinal lymph node biopsy
Dermal epithelioid cell nodular melanocytic proliferation arising in halo-like compound or dermal nevus, acquired	
Plexiform pigmented and/or epithelioid cell spindle cell melanocytic proliferation with atypical features	
Cellular blue nevus with atypical features	

[a]Management individualized for each patient; there is currently no consensus about such management. Sentinel lymph node biopsy is considered by many an experimental procedure reserved for patients with melanomas generally > 1 mm in thickness in the context of a clinical trial. Recently sentinel lymph node (SLN) biopsy has been carried out for such biologically indeterminate melanocytic tumors. However, the use of the latter technique remains controversial for such lesions. Although the finding of large deposits meeting established criteria for malignancy in lymph nodes provides confirmatory evidence for true metastatic disease, the biological significance of small, often bland cellular aggregates in SLNs from such lesions has not been established and requires further study. Thus we urge caution in the recommendation of SLN biopsy for patients with such tumors and also in its interpretation, if performed.

Melanocytic nevi in children and adolescents may have prominent pagetoid spread of cells (48,49). The upward migration of melanocytes is independent of age, sex, or type of nevus. The pagetoid spread in such nevi is notable for limitation usually to the lower-most epidermis; aggregates of cells predominate over single cells, and cytologic atypia is low grade or absent. Other architectural characteristics will generally be present and include overall symmetry, small size, well-circumscribed margins, and maturation. A particular problem is the evaluation of small or partial biopsies in which other architectural parameters cannot be adequately assessed. In this circumstance, the histologic diagnosis should be deferred until the entire lesion can be fully evaluated. The clinical setting is also of paramount importance since melanoma in childhood is rare.

The same comments are generally applicable to presence of pagetoid spread in congenital nevi, spindle and epithelioid cell nevi, pigmented spindle cell nevi, and acral nevi. Congenital nevi will usually show an overall symmetry and orderly transmigration of cells. There is also maturation of nevus cells in the dermal component, if present. Spitz nevi/tumors and pigmented spindle cell nevi are also characterized by a usually orderly upward migration of cells, the predominance of nests over cells, an overall orderly and symmetric pattern within the epidermis, and the lack of marked cytologic atypia (Fig. 10-31).

Recurrent melanocytic nevi on occasion have a disorderly pattern of junctional nesting with some upward migration of cells. However, these nevi are distinguished from melanoma because of the confinement to the intraepidermal proliferative elements to the epidermis above the scar, and the presence of little or no cytologic atypia. The typical arrangement of intraepidermal nests above a fibrotic dermis and the original dermal nevus remnant provides the characteristic features of recurrent nevus.

Nonmelanocytic tumors that enter into the differential diagnosis of this pattern include squamous cell carcinoma in situ, mammary or extramammary Paget disease, sebaceous carcinoma, epidermotropic eccrine carcinoma, neuroendocrine carcinoma, and cutaneous T cell lymphoma.

Nested Pattern of Melanocytic Proliferation
Melanocytic nevi including pigmented spindle cell nevus may exhibit prominent nesting of atypical melanocytes that strongly suggests melanoma (see earlier discussion in this chapter).

Lentiginous Pattern of Melanocytic Proliferation
The lentiginous pattern, describing single-cell proliferation along the dermoepidermal junction, is the predominant type of proliferation observed in SIMP (lentigo maligna), acral, and mucusal melanomas (Figs. 10-9 and 10-11). Occasional lentigines and AMN may present this change and suggest melanoma. The criteria favoring melanoma include the various architectural features described in Table 10-32. The patterns noted in melanoma include contiguous proliferation of melanocytes along the dermoepidermal junction reaching confluence and a uniformity of marked cytologic atypia. This frequency of melanocytic proliferation is not present in lentigines and usually not in AMN. SIMP furthermore is notable for nesting of atypical cells with diminished cohesion and the basilar proliferation of melanocytes in appendageal epithelium. Acral melanoma has epidermal hyperplasia and presence of strikingly enlarged melanoma cells possessing prominent dendrites.

Atypical Intraepidermal and Dermal Melanocytic Proliferation with Indeterminate Biologic Potential (< 1 mm)

Large Confluent Nests of Atypical Melanocytic Cells Disposed along the Dermoepidermal Junction
Atypical (dysplastic) nevus and other related nevi, superficial (plaque-like) Spitz nevus/tumor, and pigmented spindle cell nevus are most likely to be confused with melanoma because of large confluent nests of atypical melanocytic cells of the dermoepidermal junction. Melanoma is characterized by effacement of the epidermal rete pattern, whereas the typical configuration of the epidermis is maintained in the other three entities. AMN generally has elongated rete, an organized nesting pattern, and discontinuous cytologic atypia (Fig. 10-29). Compound Spitz nevus/tumor and pigmented spindle cell nevus may on occasion have prominent horizontally disposed fascicles of cells. However, there is an overall orderly and regular placement of nesting within the epidermis consistent with a benign process. The majority of cells in the latter lesions are fairly uniform with delicate chromatin patterns.

Distinction of Melanoma in the Dermis from Dermal Nevus Cells
One of the most perplexing diagnostic problems encountered by the histopathologist is the discrimination of melanoma from nests of dermal nevus cells. Specific situations in which this dilemma is encountered are nests of nevus-appearing cells either in continuity or discontiguous with invasive melanoma, entrapped in a fibrotic dermis of markedly atypical (dysplastic) nevus, halo nevi with atypia (Fig. 10-30A,B), and in areas of regression.

Probably the easiest of these three problems posed above is the discrimination of dermal melanoma cells from a discontiguous nevus-appearing focus. The presence of two distinct, spatially separate components, one clearly melanoma and the other suggesting nevus, is probably the best evidence favoring a remnant of dermal nevus. However, other characteristics of dermal nevus cells include envelopment of individual nevus cells and cellular aggregates by collagenous fibers (as well as other basement membrane elements), lack of expansile qualities of the nests, lack of striking nuclear hyperchromasia, relatively low nuclear to cytoplasmic ratios of nevus cells, fairly uniform nuclei with inconspicuous or absence of nucleoli, and the usual absence of mitoses and necrotic cells. Melanoma cells may on occasion display such pronounced nevus differentiation that careful consideration of all the above criteria is needed for separation of nevus from melanoma.

Certain (nevoid) melanomas demonstrate "maturation" or a gradient of increasing nevus differentiation of melanoma cells with depth in the dermis. The latter phenomenon refers to contiguous cells that appear most nevus-like in the lower-most portions of the dermal component (Fig. 10-31C). Because the entire cellular mass is continuous, it is assumed (and seems logical to conclude) that all elements are melanoma (Fig. 10-31C). This gradient in differentiation may in fact represent stages of tumor progression or possibly the inductive effects of stroma on the tumor cells. However, if the deepest portion of the nevomelanocytic proliferation qualifies as fully benign, then the atypical cells above this area should not necessarily be considered malignant.

Nests of atypical melanocytic cells entrapped in a fibrotic matrix must be assessed in the overall context of the lesion. In the case of an atypical (dysplastic) nevus, the intraepidermal findings will usually support a benign diagnosis: maintenance of rete patterns, cohesive junctional nesting of variably atypical melanocytic cells, and overall orderly pattern with usually little or no pagetoid spread (Fig. 10-31A,B). The presence of residual nests of cells in the setting of regression may prove to be exceedingly difficult if the cells are not obvious melanoma or nevus cells. One must weigh all of the characteristics referred to above for discrimination of melanoma from nevus cells in the dermis.

Atypical Intraepidermal and Dermal Melanocytic Proliferation with Indeterminate Biologic Potential (> 1 mm)
See discussions in the sections above and below.

Atypical Dermal or Subcutaneous Melanocytic Proliferation with Indeterminate Biologic Potential (> 1 mm)

Lesions with Dermal Cohesive Cellular Nodules Cohesive cellular aggregates are occasionally noted in Spitz tumors/nevi, pigmented spindle cell nevi, the dermal component of both acquired and congenital nevi, halo nevi, and cellular blue nevi and are considered architecturally atypical (Fig. 10-30). Although the overall histologic picture may suggest a benign process, a focal nodular proliferation may indicate focal transformation to melanoma. Features strongly suggesting melanoma include hypercellularity and crowding of nuclei within the nodule, abrupt transition from the nodule to the surrounding cellular elements rather than a gradual transition, an expanding or pushing quality with disregard of surrounding stroma, a uniformity of cytologic atypia, marked cytologic atypia, high nuclear to cytoplasmic ratios, easily found mitotic figures including atypical mitoses, and necrotic cells.

Management
There is currently no consensus about the management of such proliferations with the exception that one should do no harm to the patient and a conservative approach should be taken. Guidelines for the management of borderline lesions are outlined in Table 10-32. It must be emphasized that the management should be individualized for each patient. Lesions confused with in situ and mi-

TABLE 10-33 Histopathological reporting of malignant melanoma.

Essential features	
Site:	Skin: back or right thigh, etc.
Specimen type:	Biopsy or excision
Diagnosis:	Malignant melanoma in situ or invasive
Breslow thickness:	Measured in mm, e.g.: 1.0 mm
Clark level*:	II, III, IV, or V
Ulceration*:	Absent or present (may be measured in mm)
Microscopic satellitosis*:	Absent or present
Margins:	Peripheral and/or deep margins involved or not involved (distance to closest margin in mm)
*Other prognostic factors***	
Mitotic rate:	Number/mm^2
Lymphocytic response:	Absent, present (corresponding to "non-brisk"), marked ("brisk")
(Tumor infiltrating lymphocytes, response at base of tumor, or both)	
Regression:	Absent or present (<50%, or >50% of melanoma)
Angiotropism:	Absent or present
Vascular/lymphatic invasion:	Absent or present
Desmoplasia:	Absent or present
Neurotropism:	Absent or present

*Features influencing new AJCC staging.

**Factors influencing prognosis in some publications and potentially important in future prognostic assessment of melanoma. Other prognostic factors have been reported but all are not included here.

croinvasive melanoma situ probably pose little threat to the patient except for possible recurrence and evolution to melanoma. We advise complete excision with margins of about 5 mm for the first group and between 5 and 10 mm for the second group, with follow-up about every 6 months. For dermal proliferative lesions > 1 mm in thickness there is potentially greater risk to the patient for metastatic disease. We recommend margins between 5 and 10 mm and often up to 1 cm, with possible consideration of sentinel lymph node biopsy. Follow-up should be individualized, but it is usually every 3–6 months for at least 5 years.

HISTOPATHOLOGIC REPORTING OF MELANOMA

The pathology report (see Table 10-33) should include the following minimum information: diagnosis (i.e., malignant melanoma, in situ or invasive), depth of tumor invasion (in millimeters) measured vertically from the

TABLE 10-34 Histopathological reporting of melanoma.

Essential information
  Diagnosis: malignant melanoma, in situ or invasive
  Measured depth (in millimeters)
  Adequacy of surgical margins
Other prognostic information
  Histologic ulceration
  Mitotic rate (per square millimeter)
  Angiotropism
  Desmoplasia, neurotropism, or both
  Marked or virtually complete regression
  Vascular/lymphatic invasion
  Anatomic level (I, II, III, IV, V)
  Tumor-infiltrating lymphocytes
  Microscopic satellites

granular layer of the epidermis or from the surface of an ulcer with an ocular micrometer), and the adequacy of and proximity of surgical margins (Table 10-34). The following histologic features should also be reported or mentioned if present: mitotic rate per square millimeter, ulceration, angiotropism, desmoplasia or neurotropism, marked or virtually complete regression, microscopic satellites, and true vascular/lymphatic invasion. Other prognostic factors, such as anatomic level, host response, and tumor-infiltrating lymphocytes might be reported as well (see Chapter 12 for additional discussion).

REFERENCES

1. Berwick M. Epidemiology: current trends, risk factors, and environmental concerns In: Balch CM, Houghton AN, Sober AJ, Soong S-J, eds. Cutaneous Melanoma. 3rd ed. St. Louis: Quality Medical, 1998:551–1.
2. Berwick M. Why are people still dying of from melanoma? Arch Dermatol 1999;135:1534–6.
3. Lipsker DM, Hedelin G, Held E, et al. Striking increase of thin melanomas contrasts with stable incidence of thick melanomas. Arch Dermatol 1999;135:1451–6.
4. Roush GC, Schymura MJ, Holford TR. Risk for cutaneous melanoma in recent Connecticut birth cohorts. Am J Public Health 1985;75:679–82.
5. Roush GC, Holford TR, Schymura MJ, et al. Cancer risk and incidence trends: Connecticut Perspective. Washington DC: Hemisphere 1987.
6. Sondik EJ, Kessler LG, Ries LAG. Cancer statistics review, 1973–1987 [Publ. No. NIH 90-2789]. Washington, DC: U.S. Government Printing Office, 1990.
7. Miller RW, Young JL Jr, Novakovic B. Childhood cancer. Cancer 1995;75(Suppl 1):395-405.
8. Goldstein AM, Tucker MA. Genetic epidemiology of cutaneous melanoma. A global perspective. Arch Dermatol 1999;137:1493–6.
9. Clark WH Jr. A classification of malignant melanoma in man correlated with histogenesis and biologic behavior. In: Montagna W, Hu F, eds. Advances in the Biology of the Skin. New York: Pergamon, 1967;8:621–47.
10. Clark WH Jr, From L, Bernardino EA, Mihm MC. The histogenesis and biologic behavior of primary human malignant melanomas of the skin. Cancer Res 1969;29:705–27.
11. McGovern V, Mihm MC Jr, Bailly C, et al. The classification of malignant melanoma and its histologic reporting. Cancer 1973;32:1446–57.
12. Mishima Y. Melanocytic and nevocytic malignant melanoma. Cellular and subcellular differentiation. Cancer 1967;20:632–49.
13. Ten Seldam R, Helwig E, Sobin L, et al. Histological typing of skin tumours. In: Histological Typing of Skin Tumours. International Histological Classification of Tumors [No. 12]. Geneva: World Health Organization, 1974.
14. Mishima Y, Matsunaka J. Pagetoid premalignant melanosis and melanoma: differentiation from Hutchinson's freckle. J Invest Derm 1975;65:434–40.
15. Price NM, Rywlin AM, Ackerman AB. Histologic criteria for the diagnosis of superficial spreading malignant melanoma: Formulated on the basis of proven metastatic lesions. Cancer 1976;38:2434–41.
16. Ackerman AB. Malignant melanoma: a unifying concept. Hum Pathol 1980;11:591–5.
17. Elder DE, Jucovy PM, Tuthill RJ, Clark WH Jr. The classification of malignant melanoma. Am J Dermatopathol 1980;2:315–20.
18. Heenan PJ, Holman CDJ. Nodular malignant melanoma: a distinct entity or a common end stage? Am J Dermatopathol 1982;4:477–8.
19. Vollmer R. Pathology of melanoma. In: Seigler H, ed. Clinical Management of Melanoma. The Hague: Nijhoff, 1982: 9–40.
20. Holman CDJ, Armstrong B, Heenan P. A theory of the etiology and pathogenesis of human cutaneous malignant melanoma. J Natl Cancer Inst 1983;71:651–6.
21. Reed RJ. The pathology of human cutaneous melanoma. In: Costanzi JJ, ed. Malignant Melanoma I. The Hague: Nijhoff, 1983;85–116.
22. Clark WH Jr, Elder DE, Van Horn M. The biologic forms of malignant melanoma. Human Pathol 1984;17:443–50.
23. Clark WH Jr, Elder DE, Guerry D IV, et al. A study of tumor progression: the precursor lesions of superficial spreading and nodular melanoma. Hum Pathol 1984;15:1147–65.
24. Heenan PJ, Matz LR, Blackwell JB, et al. Inter-observer variation between pathologists in the classification of cutaneous malignant melanoma in western Australia. Histopathology 1984;8:717–29.
25. Holman CDJ, Armstrong BK. Cutaneous malignant melanoma and indicators of total accumulated exposure to the sun: An analysis separating histogenetic types. J Natl Cancer Inst 1984;73:75–82.

26. English DR, Heenan PJ, Holman CD, et al. Melanoma in Western Australia in 1980–81: incidence and characteristics of histological types. Pathology 1987;19:383–92.
27. Heenan PJ, Armstrong BK, Engligh DE, et al. Pathological and epidemiological variants of cytaneous malignant melanoma. In: Elder DE, ed. Pathobiology of Malignant Melanoma. Basel: Karger, 1987:107–46.
28. Herlyn M, Clark WH, Rodeck U, et al. Biology of tumor progression in human melanocytes. Lab Invest 1987; 56:461–74.
29. Clark WH Jr, Elder DE, Guerry D IV, et al. Model predicting survival in stage I melanoma based on tumor progression. J Natl Cancer Inst 1989;81:1893–904.
30. Clark WH. Tumor progression and the nature of cancer. Br J Cancer 1991;64:631–644.
31. Clark WH Jr, Evans HL, Everett MA, et al. Early melanoma: histologic terms. Am J Dermatopathol 1991; 13:579–82.
32. Barnhill RL, Mihm MC, Jr. The histopathology of cutaneous malignant melanoma. Semin Diag Pathol 1993;10: 47–75.
33. Barnhill RL. Pathology of Melanocytic Nevi and Malignant Melanoma. Boston: Butterworth-Heinemann, 1995.
34. Barnhill RL, Mihm MC Jr. Histopathology of malignant melanoma and its precursor lesions. In: Balch CM, Houghton AN, Sober AJ, Soong S-J, eds. Cutaneous Melanoma. 3rd ed. St. Louis: Quality Medical, 1998:103–133.
35. Walter SD, King WD, Marrett LD. Association of cutaneous malignant melanoma with intermittent exposure to ultraviolet radiation: results of a case-control study in Ontario, Canada. Int J Epidemiol 1999;28:418–427.
36. Barnhill RL. Malignant melanoma, dysplastic melanocytic nevi, and Spitz tumors: histologic classification and characteristics. Clin Plast Surg 2000;27:331–60.
37. Barnhill RL. The histological diagnosis of melanoma. Clin Lab Med Pathol2001;20:645–65.
38. Gruber SB, Barnhill RL, Stenn KS, Roush GC. Nevomelanocytic proliferations in association with cutaneous malignant melanoma: a multivariate analysis. J Am Acad Dermatol 1989;21:773–80.
39. Barnhill RL, Roush GC, Duray PH. Correlation of histologic architectural and cytoplastic features with nuclear atypia in atypical (dysplastic) nevomelanocytic nevi. Hum Pathol 1990;21:51–58.
40. Barnhill RL. Current status of the dysplastic melanocytic nevus. J Cutan Pathol 1991;18:147–59.
41. Dubow BE, Ackerman AB. Malignant melanoma in situ: the evolution of a concept. Mod Pathol 1990;3:734–44.
42. Cox NH, Aitchison TC, Sirel JM, Mackie RM. Comparison between lentigo maligna melanoma and other types of malignant melanoma of the head and neck. Brit J Cancer 1996;73:940–44.
43. Mihm MC Jr, Fitzpatrick TB, Brown MM, et al. Early detection of primary cutaneous malignant melanoma. A color atlas. N Engl J Med 1973;289:989–96.
44. Barnhill RL, Fitzpatrick TB, Fandrey K, et al. The Pigmented Lesion Clinic: A Color Atlas and Synopsis of Benign and Pigmented Lesions. New York: McGraw-Hill, 1995.
45. McGovern VJ. Spontaneous regression of melanoma. Pathology 1975;7:91–9.
46. Fallowfield ME, Cook MG. Pagetoid infiltration in primary cutaneous melanoma. Histopathology 1992;20: 417–20.
47. Cotton DWK. Pagetoid infiltration in primary cutaneous melanoma. Histopathology 1993;94.
48. Haupt HM, Stern JB. Pagetoid melanocytosis: histologic features in benign and malignant lesions. Am J Surg Pathol 1995;19:792–7.
49. Stern JB, Haupt HM. Pagetoid melanocytosis: tease or tocsin? Semin Diagn Pathol 1998;15:225–9.
50. Megahed M, Schon M, Selimovic D, Schon MP. Reliability of diagnosis of melanoma in situ. Lancet 2002;359: 1921–2.
51. Kamino H, Kiryu H, Ratech H. Small malignant melanomas: clinicopathologic correlation and DNA ploidy analysis. J Am Acad Dermatol 1990;22:1032–8.
52. Gonzalez A, West A, Pitha J, Taira J. Small-diameter invasive melanomas: clinical and pathologic characteristics. J Cutan Path 1996;23:126–32.
53. Barnhill RL, Barnhill MA, Berwick M, Mihm MC Jr. The histologic spectrum of pigmented spindle cell nevus: a review of 120 cases with emphasis on atypical variants. Hum Pathol 1991;22:52–8.
54. Busam KJ, Barnhill RL. Pagetoid Spitz nevus: intraepidermal Spitz tumor with prominent pagetoid spread. Am J Surg Pathol 1995;19(9):1061–7.
55. Hutchinson, J. Notes on the cancerous process and on new growth in general. Arch Surg (London) 1892;3:315–22.
56. Hutchinson J. On tissue dotage. Arch Surg (London) 1892;3:315–22.
57. Hutchinson J. On cancer. Arch Surg (London) 1893;4: 61–3.
58. Hutchinson J. Lentigo-melanosis: a further report. Arch Surg (London) 1894;5:253–6.
59. Hutchinson J. President's address at the Third International Congress of Dermatology. Arch Surg (London) 1896;7:297–317.
60. Dubreuilh MW. Lentigo malin des vieillards. Ann Dermatol Syphil (Paris) 1894;5:1092–9.
61. Dubreuilh MW. De la melanose circonscrite precancereuse. Ann Dermatol Syphil 1912;3:129–51, 205–30.
62. Sachs W, MacKee GM, Schwartz OD, et al. Junction nevus: nevocarcinoma. J Am Med Assoc 1947;135:216–8.
63. Becker SW. Critical evaluation of the so-called "junctional nevus." J Invest Dermatol 1954;22:217–23.

64. Mishima Y. Melanosis circumscripta praecancerosea (Dubreuilh): a non-nevoid premelanoma distinct from junction nevus. J Invest Dermatol 1960;34:361–75.
65. Trapl J, Palecek L. Ebel J, et al. Origin and development of skin melanoblastoma on the basis of 300 cases. Acta Derm Venereol (Stockh) 1964;44:377–80.
66. Clark WH Jr. Mihm MC Jr. Lentigo maligna and lentigo maligna melanoma. Am J Pathol 1969;55:39–67.
67. Silvers DN. Focus on melanoma: the therapeutic dilemma of lentigo maligna (Hutchinson's freckle). J Dermatol Surg Oncol 1976;2:301–3.
68. Finan MC, Perry HO. Lentigo maligna: a form of melanoma in situ. Geriatrics 1982;37(12):113–5.
69. Greene A, Little JH, Weedon D. The diagnosis of Hutchinson's melanotic freckle (lentigo Maligna) in Queensland. Pathology 1983;15:33–5.
70. Cramer SF, Kiehn CL. Sequential histology study of evolving lentigo maligna melanoma. Arch Pathol Lab Med 1982;106:121–125.
71. Cohen LM. Lentigo maligna and lentigo maligna melanoma. J Am Acad Dermatol 1995;33:923–36.
72. Cohen LM. The starburst giant cell is useful for distinguishing lentigo maligna from photo damaged skin. J Am Acad Dermatol 1996;35:962–67.
73. Somach SC, Taira FW, Pitha FV, Everett MA. Pigmented lesions in actinically damaged skin. Histopathologic comparison of biopsy and excisional specimens. Arch Dermatol 1996;132:1297–302.
74. Weyers W, Bonczkowitz M, Weyers I, et al. Melanoma in situ versus melanocytic hyperplasia in sun-damaged skin. Assessment of the significance of histopathologic criteria for differential diagnosis. J Am Acad Dermatol 1996;18:560–66.
75. Cox NH, Aitchison TC, Mackie RM. Extrafacial lentigo maligna: analysis of 71 cases and comparison with lentigo maligna melanoma of the head and neck. Br J Dermatol 1998;139:439–43.
76. Acker S, Nicholson JH, Rust PF, Maize JC. Morphometric discrimination of melanoma in situ of sun-damaged skin from chronically sun-damaged skin. J Am Acad Dermatol 1998;39:239–45.
77. Allan SJ, Dicker AJ, Tidman MJ, et al. Amelanotic lentigo maligna and amelanotic lentigo maligna melanoma: a report of three cases mimicking intraepidermal squamous carcinoma. J Eur Acad Dermatol Venereol 1998;11:78–81.
78. Flotte TJ, Mihm MC. Lentigo maligna and malignant melanoma in situ, lentigo maligna type. Hum Pathol 1999; 30:533–36.
79. Tannous ZS, Lerner LH, Duncan LM, et al. Progression to invasive melanoma from malignant melanoma, lentigo maligna type. Hum Pathol 2000;31:705–8.
80. Lewis MG. Malignant melanoma in Uganda (the relationship between pigmentation and malignant melanoma on the soles of the feet). Br J Cancer 1967;21:483–96.
81. Lewis MG, Kiryabwire JWN. Aspects of behavior and natural history of malignant melanoma in Uganda. Cancer 1968;21:876–87.
82. Reed RJ. Acral lentiginous melanoma. In: Reed RJ, ed. New Concepts in Surgical Pathology of Skin. New York: Wiley, 1976:89–90.
83. Arrington JH III, Reed RJ, Ichinose H, Krementz ET. Plantar lentiginous melanoma: a distinctive variant of human cutaneous malignant melanoma. Am J Surg Pathol 1977;1: 131–43.
84. Clark WH Jr, Bernardino EA, Reed RJ, Kopf AW. Acral lentiginous melanomas including melanomas of mucous membranes. In: Clark WH Jr, Goldman LI, Mastrangelo MJ, eds. Human Malignant Melanoma. New York: Grune & Stratton, 1979:109–24.
85. Coleman WP III, Loria PR, Reed RJ, Krementz ET. Acral lentiginous melanoma. Arch Dermatol 1980;116:773–6.
86. Krementz ET, Reed RJ, Coleman WP III, et al. Acral lentiginous melanoma. A clinicopathologic entity. Ann Surg 1982;195:632–45.
87. Feibleman CE, Stoll H, Maize JC. Melanomas of the palm, sole, and nailbed. Cancer 1980;46:2492–504.
88. Collins FJ. Melanoma in the Chinese of Hong Kong. Cancer 1984;54:1482–8.
89. Mishima Y, Nakanishi T. Acral lentiginous melanoma and its precursor–heterogeneity of palmo-plantar melanomas. Pathology 1985;17:258–65.
90. Scrivner D, Oxenhandler RW, Lopez M, Perez-Mesa C. Planter lentiginous melanoma. A clinicopathologic study. Cancer 1987;60:2502–9.
91. Saida T, Yoshida N, Ikegawa S, et al. Clinical guidelines for the early detection of plantar malignant melanoma. J Am Acad Dermatol 1990;23:37–40.
92. Stevens NG, Liff JM, Weiss NS. Plantar melanoma: is the incidence of melanoma of the sole of the foot really higher in blacks than whites? Int J Cancer 1990;45:691–93.
93. Tuominer L, Strengell L. Melanoma of palms, soles, and nail-beds. Scand J Plast Reconstr Hand Surg 1992;26:287–92.
94. Dwyer PK, Mackie RM, Watt DC, Aitchison TC. Plantar malignant melanoma in a white population. Br J Dermatol 1993;128:115–20.
95. Kato T, Seutake T, Sugiyama Y, et al. Improvement in the survival rates of patients with acral melanoma observed in the past 22 years in Sendai, Japan. Clin Exp Dermatol 1993;18:107–10.
96. Ridgeway CA, Hieken TJ, Ronan SG, et al. Acral lentiginous melanoma. Arch Surg 1995;130:88–92.
97. Kato T, Seutake T, Sugiyama Y, et al. Clinicopathology study of acral melanoma in situ in 44 Japanese patients. Dermatology 1996;193:192–7.
98. Harmelin ES, Holcombe RN, Goggin JP, et al. Acral lentiginous melanoma. J Foot Ankle Surg 1998;37:540–45.
99. Kato T, Seutake T, Sugiyama Y, et al. Epidemiology and

prognosis of plantar melanoma in 62 Japanese patients over a 28-year period. Int J Dermatol 1999;38:515–9.
100. Kuchelmeister C, Schaumburg-Lever G. Garbe C. Acral cutaneous melanoma in caucasians: clinical features, histopathology and prognosis in 112 patients. Br J Dermatol 2000;143:275–80.
101. Cho KH, Han KH, Minn KW. Superficial spreading melanoma arising in a longstanding melanocytic nevus on the sole. J Dermatol 1998;25:337–40.
102. Saida T. Malignant melanoma on the sole: how to detect the early lesions. Pigment Cell Res 2000;13(Suppl 8):135–9.
103. Guitart J, Lowe L, Piepkorn M, et al. Histologic characteristics of thin metastasizing melanomas: a case-control study of 43 cases. Arch Dermatol 2002;138:603–8.
104. Kang S, Barnhill RL, Mihm MC, Sober AJ. Regression in malignant melanoma: an interobserver concordance study. J Cutan Pathol 1993;20:126–9.
105. Day CL Jr, Harrist TJ, Gorstein F, et al. Malignant melanoma. Prognostic significance of "microscopic satellites" in the reticular dermis and subcutaneous fat. Ann Surg 1981;194:108–12.
106. Barnhill R, Dy K, Lugassy C. Angiotropism in cutaneous melanoma: a prognostic factor strongly predicting risk for metastasis. J Invest Dermatol. 2002;119:705–6.
107. Fitzpatrick JE. The histologic diagnosis of intraepithelial pagetoid neoplasms. Clin Dermatol 1991;9:255–9.
108. Gillman SL, Morrison RG, Hurt MA. Epidermotropic neuroendocrine carcinoma. J Cutan Pathol 1991;18:120–7.
109. Cochran AJ, Wen D-R. S-100 protein as a marker for melanocytic and other tumors. Pathology 1985;17:340–5.
110. Schmitt FC, Bacchi CE. S-100 protein: Is it useful as a marker in diagnostic immunocytochemistry? Histopathology 1989;15:281–8.
111. Gown AM, Vogel AM, Hoak D, et al. Monoclonal antibodies specific for melanocytic tumors distinguish subpopulations of melanocytes. Am J Pathol 1986;123:195–203.
112. Busam KJ, Chen YT, Old LJ, et al. Expression of melan-A (Mart-1) in benign melanocytic nevi and primary cutaneous malignant melanoma. Am J Surg Pathol 1998;22:976–92.
113. Busam KJ, Iversen K, Coplan KC, Jungbluth AA. Analysis of microphthalmia transcription factor expression in normal tissues and tumors, and comparison of its expression with S-100 protein, gp100, and tyrosinase in desmoplastic malignant melanoma. Am J Surg Pathol 2001;25:197–204.
114. Boyle JL, Haupt HM, Stern JB, Multhaupt HAB. Tyrosinase expression in malignant melanoma, desmoplastic melanoma, and peripheral nerve tumors: an immunohistochemical study. Arch Pathol Lab Med 2002;126:816–822.
115. Makin CA, Bobrow LG, Bodmer WF. Monoclonal antibody to cytokeratin for use in routine histopathology. J Clin Pathol 1984;37:975–83.
116. Gullick WJ, Berger MS, Bennett PL, et al. Expression of the C-erb B_2 protein in normal and transformed cells. Int J Cancer 1987;40:246–54.
117. Elder DE. Metastatic melanoma. In: Elder DE, ed. Pigment Cell. Basel: Karger, 1987;8:182–204.
118. Stern JB, Peck GL, Haupt HL, et al. Malignant melanoma in xeroderma pigmentosum: search for a precursor lesion. J Am Acad Dermatol 1993;28:591–94.
119. Barnhill RL, Flotte T, Fleischli M, Perez-Atayde AR. Childhood melanoma and atypical Spitz-tumors Cancer 1995;76:1833–45.
120. Weinstock MA, Sober AJ. The risk of progression of lentigo maligna to lentigo maligna melanoma. Br J Dermatol 1987;116:303–10.
121. Michalik EE, Fitzpatrick TB, Sober AJ. Rapid progression of lentigo maligna to lentigo maligna melanoma. Report of two cases. Arch Dermatol 1983;119:831–5.
122. Kelly JW. Following lentigo maligna may not prevent the development of life-threatening melanoma. Arch Dermatol 1992;128:657–60.
123. Gilchrest BA, Blog FB, Szabo G. Effects of aging and chronic sun exposure on melanocytes in human skin. J Invest Dermatol 1979;73:141–3.
124. Montagna W, Kirchner S, Carlisle K. Histology of sun-damaged human skin. J Am Acad Dermatol 1989;21:907–18.
125. Zimarowski MJ, Harrist TJ, Crowson AN, et al. Atypical melanocytic hyperplasia in fibrous papules mimicking lentigo maligna. Lab Invest 1994;70:51A.
126. Bastian BC, Kashani-Sabet M, Hamm H, et al. Gene amplifications characterize acral melanoma and permit the detection of occult tumor cells in the surrounding skin. Cancer Res 2000;60:1968–73.
127. Lewis MG, Johnson K. The incidence and distribution of pigmented nevi in Ugandan Africans. Br J Dermatol 1968;82:362–6.
128. Nogita T, Wong TY, Ohhara K, et al. Atypical melanosis of the foot: a report of three cases in Japanese population. Arch Dermatol 1994;130:1042–5.
129. Saida T. Heterogeneity of the site of origin of malignant melanoma in ungula areas: "subungual" malignant melanoma may be a misnomer. Br J Dermatol 1992;126:529.
130. Hutchinson J. Melanosis often not black: melanotic whitlow. Br Med J 1886;1:491.
131. Patterson RH, Helwig EB. Subungual malignant melanoma: a clinical-pathologic study. Cancer 1980;46:2074–87.
132. Daly JM, Berlin R, Urmacher C. Subungual melanoma: a 25-year review of cases. J Surg Oncol 1987;35:107–112.
133. Saida T, Ohshima Y. Clinical and histopathologic characteristics of early lesions of subungual malignant melanoma. Cancer 1989;63:556–60.

134. Blessing K, Kernohan NM, Park KGM. Subungual malignant melanoma: clinicopathological features of 100 cases. Histopathology 1992;19:425–9.
135. Rigby HS, Briggs JC. Subungual melanoma: A clinicopathological study of 24 cases. Br J Plast Surg 1992;45:275–8.
136. Krige JEJ, Hudson DA, Johnson CA, et al. Subungual melanoma. S Afr J Surg 1995;33:10–14.
137. Kato T, Seutake T, Sugiyama Y, et al. Epidemiology and prognosis of subungual melanoma in 34 Japanese patients. Br J Dermatol 1996;134:383–7.
138. Quinn MJ, Thompson JE, Crotty K, et al. Subungual melanoma of the hand. J Hand Surg 1996;21:506–11.
139. Glat PM, Spector JA, Roses DF, et al. The management of pigmented lesions of the nail bed. Ann Plast Surg 1996;37:125–34.
140. Levit EK, Kagen MH, Scher RK, et al. The ABC rule for clinical detection of subungual melanoma. J Am Acad Dermatol 2000;42:269–74.
141. Baran R, Kechijian P. Longitudinal melanonychia (melanonychia striata): diagnosis and management. J Am Acad Dermatol 1989;21:1165–75.
142. Baran R, Kechijian P. Hutchinson's sign: a reappraisal. J Am Acad Dermatol 1996;34:87–90.
143. Caron GA. Familial congenital pigmented nevi of nails. Lancet 1982;1:508–9.
144. Kato T, Usuba Y, Takematso H, et al. Rapidly growing nail streak resulting in diffuse melanosis of the nail: a possible sign of subungual melanoma in situ. Cancer 1989;64:2191–7.
145. Kichuki, I, Inoue S, Sakaguchi E, One R. Regressing nail melanosis in childhood. Dermatology 1993;186:88–93.
146. Pomerance J, Kopf AW, Ramos L, et al. A large pigmented nail bed lesion in a child. Ann Plast Surg 1994;33:80–2.
147. Conley J, Lattes R, Orr W. Desmoplastic malignant melanoma (a rare variant of spindle cell melanoma). Cancer 1971;28:914–36.
148. Labrecque PG, Hu C, Winkelmann RK. On the nature of desmoplastic melanoma. Cancer 1976;38:1205–13.
149. Valensi QJ. Desmoplastic malignant melanoma. A report of two additional cases. Cancer 1977;39:286–92.
150. Valensi QJ. Desmoplastic malignant melanoma. A light and electron microscopic study of two cases. Cancer 1979;43:1148–55.
151. Valensi QJ. Desmoplastic malignant melanoma: study of a case by light and electronmicroscopy. J Dermatol Surg Oncol 1979;5:31–5.
152. Bryant E, Ronan SG, Felix EL, Manaligod JR. Desmoplastic malignant melanoma. A study by conventional and electron microscopy. Am J Dermatopathol 1982;4:467–74.
153. From L, Hanna W, Kahn HJ, et al. Origin of the desmoplasia in desmoplastic malignant melanoma. Hum Pathol 1983;14:1072–80.
154. Reiman HM, Goellner JR, Woods JE, Mixter RC. Desmoplastic melanoma of the head and neck. Cancer 1987;60:2269–74.
155. Egbert B, Kempson R, Sagebiel R. Desmoplastic malignant melanoma. A clinico-histopathologic study of 25 cases. Cancer 1988;52:2033–41.
156. Walsh NM, Roberts JT, Orr W, Simon GT. Desmoplastic malignant melanoma. A clinico-pathologic study of 14 cases. Arch Pathol Lab Med 1988;112:922–7.
157. Beenken S, Byers R, Smith JL, et al. Desmoplastic melanoma. Histologic correlation with behavior and treatment. Arch Otolaryngol Head Neck Surg 1989;115:374–9.
158. Jain S, Allen PW. Desmoplastic malignant melanoma and its variants. A study of 45 cases. Am J Surg Pathol 1989;13:358–73.
159. Smithers BM, McLeod GR, Little JH. Desmoplastic, neural transforming and neurotropic melanoma: A review of 45 cases. Aust N Z J Surg 1990;60:967–72.
160. Bruijn JA, Mihm MC Jr, Barnhill RL. Desmoplastic melanoma. Histopathology 1992;20:197–205.
161. Bruijn JA, Salasche SJ, Sober AJ, et al. Desmoplastic melanoma: clinicopathologic aspects of six cases. Dermatology 1992;185:3–8.
162. Anstey A, McKee P, Wilson Jones E. Desmoplastic malignant melanoma: a clinicopathologic study of 25 cases. Br J Dermatol 1993;129:359–71.
163. Carlson JA, Dickerson GR, Sober AJ, Barnhill RL. Desmoplastic neurotropic malignant melanoma: A clinicopathologic analysis of 28 cases. Cancer 1995;75:478–94.
164. Baer SC, Schultz D, Synnestvedt M, Elder DE. Desmoplasia and neurotopism: prognostic variables in patients with stage I melanoma. Cancer 1995;76:2242–7.
165. Skelton HG, Smith KJ, Laskin WB, et al. Desmoplastic malignant melanoma. J Acad Dermatol 1995;32:717–25.
166. Longacre TA, Egbert BM, Rouse RV. Desmoplastic and spindle cell malignant melanoma. An immunohistochemical study. Am J Surg Pathol 1996;20:1489–500.
167. Kilpatrick SC, White WL, Browne JD. Desmoplastic malignant melanoma of the oral mucosal: an underrecognized diagnostic pitfall. Cancer 1996;78:383–9.
168. Tsao H, Sober AJ, Barnhill RL. Desmoplastic neurotropic melanoma. Semin Cutan Med Surg 1997;16:131–6.
169. Quinn MJ, Crotty KA, Thompson JF, et al. Desmoplastic and desmoplastic neurotropic melanoma: experience with 280 patients. Cancer 1999;83:1128–35.
170. Reed RJ, Leonard DD. Neurotropic melanoma: a variant of desmoplastic melanoma. Am J Surg Pathol 1979;3:301–11.
171. Kossard S, Doherty E, Murray E. Neurotropic melanoma. A variant of desmoplastic melanoma. Arch Dermatol 1987;123:907–12.
172. Barnhill RL, Fine J, Roush GC, Berwick M. Predicting five-year outcome from cutaneous melanoma in a population-based study. Cancer 1996;78:427–32.

173. Kanik AB, Yaar M, Bhawan J. p75 nerve growth factor receptor staining helps identifiy desmoplastic and neurotropic melanoma. J Cutan Pathol 1996;23:205–10.
174. Iwamoto S, Burrows RC, Agoff SN, et al. The p75 neurotrophin receptor, relative to other Schwann cell and melanoma markers, is abundantly expressed in spindled melanomas. Am J Dermatopathol 2001;23:288–94.
175. Warner TCS, Hafez GR, Finch RE, Schwann cell features in neurotropic melanoma. J Cutan Pathol 1981;8:177–87.
176. DiMaio SM, Mackay BM, Smith JL, Dickerson GR. Neurosarcomatous transformation in malignant melanoma. Cancer 1982; 50:2345–54.
177. Gentile RD, Donovan DT. Neurotropic melanoma of the head and neck. Laryngoscope 1985;85:1161–6.
178. Mack EE, Gomez EC. Neurotropic melanoma. J Neuro-Oncol 1992;13:165–71.
179. Barnhill RL, Sagebiel RW, Lugassy C. Angiotropic melanoma: report of seven additional cases J Cutan Pathol. 2000;27:548.12
180. Barnhill RL, Bolognia JL. Neurotropic melanoma with prominent melanization. J Cutan Pathol 1995;22:450–9.
181. Warner TF, Lloyd RV, Hafez GR, Angevine JM. Immunocytochemistry of neurotropic melanoma. Cancer 1984;53:254–57.
182. Anstey A, Cerio R, Rammarain N, et al. Desmoplastic malignant melanoma, an immunocytochemical study of 23 cases. Am J Dermatopathol 1994;16:14–22.
183. Eng W, Tschen JA. Comparison of S-100 versus hematoxylin and eosin staining for evaluating dermal invasion and peripheral margins by desmoplastic malignant melanoma. Am J Dermatopathol 2000;22:26–9.
184. Wick MR, Swanson PE, Rocamora A. Recognition of malignant melanoma by monoclonal antibody HMB-45. An immunohistochemical study of 200 paraffin-embedded cutaneous tumors. J Cutan Pathol 1988;15:201–7.
185. AL-Alousi S, Carlson JA, Blessing K, et al. Expression of basic fibroblast growth factor in desmoplastic neurotropic malignant melanoma. J Cutan Pathol 1996;23:118–25.
186. Xu X, Chu AY, Pasha TL, et al. Immunoprofile of MITF, tyrosinase, Melan-a, and MAGE-1 in HMB45-negative melanomas. Am J Surg Pathol 2002;26(1):82–7.
187. Gartner MFRM, Fearns C, Wilson EL, et al. Unusual growth characteristics of human melanoma xenografts in the nude mouse: a model for desmoplasia, dormancy and progression. Br J Cancer 1992;64:487–90.
188. Fearns C, Dowdle EB. The desmoplastic response: induction of collagen synthesis by melanoma cells in vitro. Int J Cancer 1992;50:621–7.
189. Gutzmer R, Herbst RA, Mommert S, et al. Allelic loss at the neurofibromatosis type 1 (NF1) gene locus is frequent in desmoplastic neurotropic melanoma. Hum Genet 2000;107:357–61.
190. Smithers BM, McLeod GR, Little JH. Desmoplastic melanoma: patterns of recurrence. World J Surg 1992;16:186–90.
191. Jaroszewski DE, Pockaj BA, DiCaudo DJ, Bite U. The clinical behavior of desmoplastic melanoma. Am J Surg 2001; 186(6):590–5.
192. Payne WG, Kearney R, Wells K, et al. Desmoplastic melanoma. Am Surg 2001;67:1004–6.
193. Mihm MC, Googe PB. Problems in various subtypes of malignant melanoma. In: Mihm MC, Googe PB, eds. Problematic Pigmented Lesions—A Case Method Approach. Philadelphia: Lea & Febiger, 1990:279–370.
194. Barr RJ, Morales RV, Graham JH. Desmoplastic nevus. A distinct histologic variant of mixed spindle cell and epithelioid cell nevus. Cancer 1980;46:557–64.
195. Barnhill RL, Mihm MC. Cellular neurothekeoma: a distinctive variant of neurothekeoma mimicking nevomelanocytic tumors. Am J Surg Pathol 1990;14:113–20.
196. Kaneishi ND, Cockerell CJ. Histologic differentiation of desmoplastic melanoma from cicatrices. Am J Dermatopathol 1998;20:128–34.
197. Robson A, Allen P, Hollowood K. S 100 expression in cutaneous scars: a potential diagnostic pitfall in the diagnosis of desmoplastic melanoma. Histopathology 2002;38:135–40.
198. Recamier JCA. Recherches sur le Traitement du Cancer. Paris: Gabon, 1829.
199. Lugassy C, Escande JP. The hematogenous theory of metastasis: Recamier did not propose it. Virchows Arch 1997;431:371.
200. Handley WS. The pathology of melanotic growths in relation to their operative treatment. Lancet 1907;927: 996–8.
201. Lugassy C, BP Eyden, L Christensen, JP Escande. Angiotumoral complex in human malignant melanoma characterised by free laminin: ultrastructural and immuno-histochemical observations. J Submicrosc Cytol Pathol 1997;29:19–28.
202. Lugassy C, Christensen L, Le Charpentier M, et al. Ultrastructural and immunohistological observations concerning laminin in B16 melanoma: is an amorphous form of laminin promoting a non hematogenous migraton of tumor cells? J Submicrosc Cytol Pathol 1998;30:137–44.
203. Lugassy C, Christensen L, Le Charpentier M, et al. Angiotumoral laminin in murine tumors derived from human melanoma cell lines. Immunohistochemical and ultrastructural observations. J Submicrosc Cytol Pathol 1998; 30(2):231–7.
204. Lugassy C, Dickersin GR, Christensen L, et al. Ultrastructural and immunohistochemical studies of the periendothelial matrix in malignant melanoma: evidence for an amorphous matrix containing laminin. J Cutan Pathol 1999;26:78–83.
205. Lugassy C, Shahsafaei A, Bonitz P, et al. Tumor microvessels in melanoma express the beta-2 chain of

laminin. Implications for melanoma metastasis. J Cutan Pathol 1999;26:222–6.
206. Moreno A, Espanol I, Romagosa V. Angiotropic malignant melanoma. Report of two cases. J Cutan Pathol 1992;19:325–9.
207. Shea CR, Kline MA, Lugo J, McNutt NS. Angiotropic metastatic malignant melanoma. Am J Dermatopathol 1995;17:58–62.
208. Saluja A. Moncy N, Zivony DI, Solomon AR. Angiotropic malignant melanoma: a rare pattern of local metastases. J Am Acad Dermatol 2001;44:829–32.
209. Lugassy C, Kleinman HK, Fernandez PM, et al. Human melanoma cell migration along capillary-like structures in vitro: a new dynamic model for studying extravascular migratory metastasis. J Invest Dermatol 2002;119:703–4.
210. Lugassy C, Haroun RI, Brem H, et al. Pericytic-like angiotropism of glioma and melanoma cells. Am J Dermatopathol 2002;24:473–8.
211. Reed RJ, Ichinose H, Clark WH Jr, Mihm MC Jr. Common and uncommon melanocytic nevi and borderline melanomas. Semin Oncol 1975;2:119–47.
212. Reed RJ. Consultation case. Am J Surg Pathol 1978;2:215–20.
213. Hendrickson MR, Ross JC. Neoplasms arising in congenital giant nevi: morphologic study of seven cases and a review of the literature. Am J Surg Pathol 1981;5:109–35.
214. Muhlbauer JE, Margolis RJ, Mihm MC Jr, Reed RJ. Minimal deviation melanoma: a histologic variant of cutaneous malignant melanoma in its vertical growth phase. J Invest Dermatol 1983;80(Suppl):63S–5S.
215. Phillips ME, Margolis RJ, Merot Y, et al. The spectrum of minimal deviation melanoma: a clinicopathologic study of 21 cases. Hum Pathol 1986;17:796–806.
216. Reed RJ. Minimal deviation melanoma. In: Mihm MC Jr, Murphy GF, Kaufman N, eds. Pathobiology and Recognition of Malignant Melanoma. Baltimore: Williams & Wilkins, 1988:110–52.
217. Reed RJ, Webb S, Clark WH Jr. Minimal deviation melanoma (halo nevus variant). Am J Surg Pathol 1990;14:53–68.
218. Larsen TE, Grude TH. A retrospective histologic study of 669 cases of primary cutaneous malignant melanoma in clinical stage I: II. The relation of cell type, pigmentation, atypia, and mitotic count to histologic type and prognosis. Acta Pathol Microbiol Scand A 1978;86:513–22.
219. Day CL, Harrist TJ, Lew RA, Mihm MC Jr. Classification of malignant melanoma according to the histologic morphology of melanoma nodules. J Dermatol Surg Oncol 1982;8:874–5, 900.
220. Baak JP, Tan G. The adjuvant prognostic value of nuclear morphometry in stage I malignant melanoma of the skin: a multivariate analysis. Anal Quant Cytol Histol 1986;68:241–4.
221. Sorensen FB. Objective histopathologic grading of cutaneous malignant melanomas by stereologic estimation of nuclear volume. Cancer 1989;63:1784–98.
222. Schmoeckel C, Castro CE, Braun-Falco O. Nevoid malignant melanoma. Arch Dermatol Res 1985;277:362–9.
223. Levene A. On the histological diagnosis and prognosis of malignant melanoma. J Clin Pathol 1980;33:101–24.
224. Suster S, Ronnen M, Bubis JJ. Verrucous pseudonevoid melanoma. J Surg Oncol 1987;36:134–7.
225. Kuehnl-Petzoldt C, Berger H, Wiebelt H. Verrucous-keratotic variations of malignant melanoma. A clinicopathological study. Am J Dermatopathol 1982;4:403–10.
226. Blessing K, Evans AT, Al-Nafussi A. Verrucous nevoid and keratotic malignant melanoma: a clinico-pathological study of 20 cases. Histopathology 1993;23:453–8.
227. Wong TY, Duncan LM, Mihm MCJ. Melanoma mimicking dermal and Spitz's nevus ("nevoid" melanoma). Semin Surg Oncol 1993;9:188–93.
228. Wong TY, Suster S, Duncan LM, et al. Nevoid melanoma: a clinicopathological study of seven cases of malignant melanoma mimicking spindle and epithelioid cell nevus and verrucous dermal nevus. Hum Pathol 1995;26:171–9.
229. McNutt NS, Urmacher C, Hakimian J, et al. Nevoid malignant melanoma: morphologic patterns and immunohistochemical reactivity. J Cutan Pathol 1995;22:502–17.
230. McNutt NS. "Triggered trap": nevoid malignant melanoma. Semin Diagn Pathol 1998;15:203–9.
231. Zembowicz A, McCusker M, Chiarelli C, et al. Morphological analysis of nevoid melanoma: a study of 20 cases with a review of the literature. Am J Dermatopathol 2001;23:167–75.
232. Steiner A, Konrad K, Pehamberger H, Wolff K. Verrucous malignant melanoma. Arch Dermatol 1988;124:1534–7.
233. Barnhill RL. Childhood melanoma. Semin Diagn Pathol 1998;15:189–94.
234. Spatz A, Barnhill RL. Small cell melanoma in childhood. Pathol Case Rev 1999;4:102–6.
235. Blessing K, Grant JJH, Sanders SDA, et al. Small cell malignant melanoma: a variant of naevoid melanoma. Clinicopathological features and histological differential diagnosis. J Clin Pathol 2000;53:591–5.
236. Kossard S, Wilkinson B. Nucleolar organizer regions and image analyis nuclear morphometry of small cell (nevoid) melanoma. J Cutan Pathol 1995;22:132–6.
237. Kossard S, Wilkinson B. Small cell (naevoid) melanoma: a clinicopathologic study of 131 cases. Austral J Dermatol 1997;38(Suppl):S54–8.
238. Siegelman-Danieli N, Cohen HI, Ben-Izhack O. Malignant skin lesions. Case 1: nevoid malignant melanoma of the breast presenting as a contralateral breast metastasis. J Clin Oncol 1999;17:3850–2.
239. House N, Fedok F, Maloney ME, Helm KF. Malignant

239. melanoma with clinical and histologic features of Merkel cell carcinoma. J Am Acad Dermatol 1994;31:839–42.
240. Okun MR. Melanoma resembling spindle and epithelioid cell nevus. Arch Dermatol 1979;115:1416–20.
241. Busam KJ, Barnhill RL. Spitz nevus and spitzoid melanoma. In: Kirkham N, Lemoine N. Progress in Pathology. Churchill Livingstone, 1995;2:31–46.
242. Barnhill RL, Argenyi ZB, From L et al. Atypical Spitz nevi/tumors: lack of consensus for diagnosis, discrimination from melanoma, and prediction of outcome. Hum Pathol 1999;30:513–20.
243. Okun M, Bauman L. Malignant melanoma arising from an intradermal nevus. Arch Dermatol 1965;92:69–72.
244. Okun MR, Di Mattia A, Thompson J, Pearson SH. Malignant melanoma developing from intradermal nevi. Arch Dermatol 1974;110:599–601.
245. Benisch B, Peison B, Kannerstein M, Spivack J. Malignant melanoma originating from intradermal nevi. A clinicopathologic entity. Arch Dermatol 1980;116:696–8.
246. Ball NJ, Golitz LE. Melanocytic nevi with focal atypical epithelioid cell components: a review of seventy-three cases. J Am Acad Dermatol. 1994;30:724-9.
247. Collina G, Deen S, Cliff S, et al. Atypical dermal nodules in benign melanocytic naevi. Histopathology 1997;31: 77–101.
248. Coffey RJ, Berkeley WT. Prepubertal malignant melanoma. J Am Med Assoc 1951;147:846–9.
249. Allen A, Spitz S. Malignant melanoma. A clinicopathological analysis of the criteria for diagnosis and prognosis. Cancer 1953;6:1–45.
250. Fisher ER. Malignant blue naevus. Arch Dermatol 1956; 74:227–31.
251. Kerstin DW, Caro MR. Cellular blue nevus of Ota followed for 22 years. AMA Arch Derm 1956;74:539–47.
252. Kwittken J, Negri L. Malignant blue nevus: case report of a Negro woman. Arch Dermatol 1966;94:64–9.
253. Leopold JG, Richards DB. Cellular blue naevi. J Pathol Bacteriol 1967;94:247–55.
254. Rodriguez HA, Ackerman LV. Cellular blue nevus. Cancer 1968;21:393–405.
255. Merkow LP, Burt RC, Hayeslip DW, et al. A cellular and malignant blue nevus. A light and electron microscopic study. Cancer 1969;24:888–96.
256. Mishima Y. Cellular blue nevus: melanogenic activity and malignant transformation. Arch Derm 1970;101:104–10.
257. Hourihane DO'B. Malignant blue nevus with metastasis to regional lymph node. Ir J Med Sci 1971;140:169–75.
258. Silverberg G, Kadin MF, Dorfman RF, et al. Invasion of the brain by a cellular blue nevus of the scalp: a case report with light and electron microscopic studies. Cancer 1971;27:349–55.
259. Hernandez JF. Malignant blue nevus: a light and electron microscopic study. Arch Dermatol 1973;107:741–4.
260. Speakman JS, Phillips MJ. Cellular and malignant blue nevus complicating oculodermal melanosis (nevus of Ota syndrome). Can J Ophtalmol 1973;8:539–47.
261. Levene A. On the natural history and comparative pathology of the blue naevus. Ann R Coll Surg 1980;62:327–34.
262. Rubinstein N, Kopolovic J, Wexler MR, Peled IJ. Malignant blue nevus. J Dermatol Surg Oncol 1985;11:921–3.
263. Wetherington GM, Norin AL, Sadove AM. Locally invasive cellular blue nevus of the scalp. Plast Reconstr Surg 1987;79:114–7.
264. Temple-Camp CRE, Saxe N, King H. Benign and malignant cellular blue nevus: a clinicopathologic study of 30 cases. Am J Dermatopathol 1988;10:289–96.
265. Goldenhersh MA, Savin RC, Barnhill RL, Stenn KS. Malignant blue nevus. Case report and literature review. J Am Acad Dermatol 1988;19:712–22.
266. Kuhn, A, Groth W. Garmann H, Steigleder GK. Malignant blue nevus with metastases to the lung. Am J Dermatopathol 1988;10(5):436–41.
267. Shallman RW, Hoehn JL, Lawton BR, Dickson KB. Malignant cellular blue nevus: unusual case of a rare tumor. Wisc Med J 1988; 87:16–8.
268. Modly C, Wood C, Horn T. Metastatic malignant melanoma arising from a common blue nevus in a patient with subacute cutaneous lupus erythematosus. Dermatological 1989;178:171–5.
269. Boi S, Barbareschi M, Vigl E, Cristofolini M. Malignant blue nevus: report of four new cases and review of the literature. Histol Histopathology 1991;6:427–34.
270. Connelly J, Smith JL Jr. Malignant blue nevus. Cancer 1991;67:2653–7.
271. Mehregan DA, Gibson LE, Mehregan AH. Malignant blue nevus: a report of eight cases. J Dermatol Sci 1992;4: 185–92.
272. Pich A, Chiusa L, Margaria E, Aloi F. Proliferative activity in the malignant cellular blue nevus. Hum Pathol 1993; 24:1323–9.
273. Pathy AL, Helm TN, Elston D, et al. Malignant melanoma arising in a blue nevus with features of pilar neurocristic hamartoma. J Cutan Pathol 1993;20:459–64.
274. Scott GA, Trepeta R. Clear cell sarcoma of tendons and aponeuroses and malignant blue nevus arising in prepubescent children: report of two cases and review of the literature. Am J Dermatopathol 1993;15:139–45.
275. Aloi E, Pich A, Pippione M. Malignant cellular blue nevus: a clinicopathological study of 6 cases. Dermatology 1996;192:36–40.
276. Koch H, Cerroni L, Soyer HP, Kera H. Zelger B. Malignant blue nevus: malignant melanoma in association with blue nevus. Eur J Dermatol 1996; 6:335–8.
277. Spatz A, Zimmermann U, Bachollet B, et al. Malignant blue nevus of the vulva with late ovarian metastatis. Am J Dermatopathol 1998;20:408–12.

278. Calista D, Schianchi S, Landi C. Malignant blue nevus of the scalp. Int J Dermatol 1998;37:126–7.
279. Duteille F, Duport G, Larregue M, et al. Malignant blue nevus: three new cases and a review of the literature. Ann Plast Surg 1998;41:674–8.
280. Granter SR, McKee PH, Calonje E, et al. Melanoma associated with blue nevus and melanoma mimicking cellular blue nevus: a clinicopathologic study of 10 cases on the spectrum of so-called 'malignant blue nevus'. Am J Surg Pathol 2001;25:316–23.
281. Avidor I, Kessler E. "Atypical" blue nevus—a benign variant of cellular blue nevus. Dermatologica 1977;154:39–44.
282. Goette DK, Robinson JW. Atypical cellular blue nevus. J Assoc Militar Dermatol 1980;4(1):6–8.
283. Tran TA, Carlson JA, Basaca B, Mihm MC Jr. Cellular blue nevus with atypia (atypical cellular blue nevus): a clinicopathologic study of nine cases. J Cutan Pathol 1998;25:252–8.
284. Busam KJ, Woodruff JM, Erlandson RA, Brady MS. Large plaque-type blue nevus with subcutaneous cellular nodules. Am J Surg Pathol 2000;24(1):92–9.
285. Lamovec J. Blue nevus of the lymph node capsule: report of a new case with review of the literature. Am J Clin Pathol 1984;81:367–72.
286. Epstein JI, Erlandson RA, Rosen PP. Nodal blue nevi: a study of three cases. Am J Surg Pathol 1984;8:907–15.
287. Lambert WC, Brodkin RH. Nodal and subcutaneous cellular blue nevi: A pseudometastasizing pseudomelanoma. Arch Dermatol 1984;120:367–70.
288. Sterchi JM, Muss HB, Weidner N. Cellular blue nevus simulating metastatic melanoma: report of an unusually large lesion associated with nevus-cell aggregates in regional lymph nodes. J Surg Oncol 1987;36:71–5.
289. Enzinger FM. Clear-cell sarcoma of tendons and aponeuroses: an analysis of 21 cases. Cancer 1965;18:1163–74.
290. Chung EB, Enzinger FM. Malignant melanoma of soft parts: a reassepagetoid melanomaent of clear-cell sarcoma. Am J Surg Pathol 1983;7:405–13.
291. Swanson PE, Wick MR. Clear cell sarcoma. An immunohistochemical analysis of six cases and comparison with other epithelioid neoplasms of soft tissue. Arch Pathol Lab Med 1989;113:55–60.
292. Sara AS, Evans HL, Benjamin RS. Malignant melanoma of soft parts (clear cell sarcoma): a study of 17 cases, with emphasis on prognostic factors. Cancer 1990;65:367–74.
293. Zucman J, Delattre O, Cesmaze C, et al. EWS and ATF-1 gene fusion induced by t(12;22) translocatio in malignant melanoma of soft parts. Nat Genet 1993;4:341–5.
294. Van Roggen JFG, Mooi WJ, Hogendoorn PCS. Clear cell sarcoma of tendons and aponeurosis (malignant melanoma of soft parts) and cutaneous melanoma: exploring the histogenetic relationship between these two clinicopatholgical entities. J Pathol 1998;186:3–7.
295. Deenik W, Mooi WJ, Rutgers EJ, et al. Clear cell sarcoma (malignant melanoma) of soft parts: a clinicopathologic study of 30 cases. Cancer 1999;86:969–75.
296. Finley JW, Hanypsiak B, McGrath B, et al. Clear cell sarcoma: the Roswell Park experience. J Surg Oncol 2001;77:16–20.
297. Langezaal SM, van Roggen JFG, Cleton-Jansen AM, et al. Malignant melanoma in genetically distinct from clear cell sarcoma of tendons and aponeurosis (malignant melanoma of soft parts). Br J Cancer 2001;84:535–538.
298. Panagopoulos I, Mertens F, Debiec-Rychter M, et al. Molecular genetic characterization of the EWS/AFT1 fusion gene in clear cell sarcoma of tendons and aponeuroses. Int J Cancer. 2002;99:560–7.
299. Ferrari A, Casanova M, Bisogno G, et al. Clear cell carcinoma of tendons and aponeurosis in pediatric patients: a report from the Italian and German soft tissue sarcoma cooperative group. Cancer 2002;94:3269–76.
300. Nakhleh RE, Wick MR, Rocamora A, et al. Morphologic diversity in malignant melanomas. Am J Clin Pathol 1990;93:731–40.
301. Banerjee SS, Harris M. Morphological and immunphenotypic variations in malignant melanoma. Histopathology 2000;36:387–402.
302. McGovern VJ, Shaw HM, Milton GW. Prognostic significance of a polypoid configuration in malignant melanoma. Histopathology 1983;7:663–72.
303. Giuliano AE, Cochran AJ, Morton DL. Melanoma from unknown primary site and amelanotic melanoma. Semin Oncol 1982 9:442–447.
304. Peters MS, Su WPD. Balloon cell malignant melanoma. J Am Acad Dermatol 1985;13:351–4.
305. Kao GF, Helwig EB, Graham JH. Balloon cell malignant melanoma of the skin: a clinicopathologic study of 34 cases with histochemical, immunohistochemical, and ultrastructural observations. Cancer 1992;69:2942–52.
306. Novak MA, Fatteh SM, Campbell TE. Glycogen-rich malignant melanoma and glycogen-rich balloon cell melanoma. Arch Pathol Lab Med 1998:122:353–60.
307. Bhutta S, Mirra JM, Cocharan AJ. Myxoid malignant melanoma: a previously undescribed histologic pattern noted in metastatic lesions and a report of four cases. Am J Surg Pathol 1986;10:203–11.
308. Sarode VR, Joshi K, Ravichandran P, Das R. Myxoid variant of primary cutaneous malignant melanoma. Histopathology 1992;20:186–7.
309. Prieto VG, Kanik A, Salob S, McNutt NS. Primary cutaneous myxoid melanoma: Immunohistologic clues to a difficult diagnosis. J Am Acad Dermatol 1994;30:335–9.
310. Clark WH Jr, Elder DE, Guerry D IV. Dysplastic nevi and malignant melanoma. In: Farmer ER, Hood AF, eds. Pathology of the Skin. Norwalk, Appleton & Lange, 1990:684–756.
311. Crowson AN, Magro CM, Mihm MC Jr. Malignant mel-

311. anoma with prominent pigment synthesis: "animal type" melanoma—a clinical and histological study of six cases with a consideration of other melanocytic neoplasms with prominent pigment synthesis. Hum Pathol 1999;30:543–50.
312. Macak J, Krc I, Elleder M, Lukas Z. Clear cell melanoma of the skin with regressive changes. Histopathology 1991;18:276–7.
313. Sheibani K, Battifora H. Signet-ring cell melanoma. Am J Surg Pathol 1988;12:28–34.
314. Al-Talib RK, Theaker JM. Signet-ring cell melanoma: light microscopic, immunohistochemical and ultrastructural features. Histopathology 1991;18:572–5.
315. LiVolsi VA, Brooks, JJ, Soslow R, et al. Signet cell melanocytic lesions. Mod Pathol 1992;4:515–20.
316. Borek BT, CmKee PH, Freeeman FA, et al. Primary malignant melanoma with rhaboid features: a histologic and immunocytochemical study of three cases. Am J Dermatopathol 1998;20:123–7.
317. Baron JA, Monzon F, Galaria N, Murphy GF. Angiomatoid melanoma: a novel pattern of differentiation in invasive periocular desmoplastic malignant melanoma. Hum Pathol 2000;31:1520–2.
318. Toda S, Heasley DD, Mihm MC. Osteogenic melanoma: stromal metaplasia in association with subungual melanoma. Histopathology 1997;31:293–5.
319. Hoorweg JJ, Loftus BN, Hilgers FJM. Osteoid and bone formation in a nasal mucosal melanoma and its metastasis. Histopathology 1997;31:465–8.
320. Ross MI, Stern SJ. Mucosal melanoma. In: Balch CM, Houghton AN, Sober AJ, Soong S-J, eds. Cutaneous Melanoma. 3rd ed. St. Louis: Quality Medical, 1998; 195–206.
321. Piura B, Egan M, Lopes A, Monaghan JM. Malignant melanoma of the vulva: a clinicopathologic study of 18 cases. J Surg Oncol 1992;50:234–40.
322. Ragnarsson-Olding B, Johansson H, Rutquist L-E, Ringborg U. Malignat melanoma of the vulva and vagina. Trends in incidence, age distribution, and long-term survival among 245 consecutive cases in Sweden 1960–1984. Cancer 1993;71:1893–7.
323. Weinstock MA. Gynecology: malignant melanoma of the vulva and vagina in the United States: patterns of incidence and population-based estimates of survival. Am J Obstet Gynecol 1994;171:1225–30.
324. Raeber G, Mempel V, Jackish C, et al. Malignant melanoma of the vulva: report of 89 patients. Cancer 1996;78:2353–8.
325. Egan CA, Bradley RR, Logsdon VK, et al. Vulvar melanoma in childhood. Arch Dermatol 1997;133:345–8.
326. DeMatos P, Tyler D, Seigler H. Mucosal melanoma of the female genitalia: a clinicopathologic study of 43 cases at Duke University Medical Center. Surgery 1998;124:38–48.
327. Gorsky M, Epstein JB. Melanoma arising from the mucosal surfaces of the head and neck. Oral Surg Oral Med Oral Pathol 1998:715–9.
328. Prasad ML, Patel S, Hoshaw-Woodard S, et al. Prognostic factors for malignant melanoma of the squamous mucosa of the head and neck. Am J Surg Pathol 2002;26:883–92.
329. Pandey M, Mathew A, Abraham EK, et al. Primary malignant melanoma of the mucous membranes. Eur J Surg Oncol 1998;24:303–7.
330. Larsson KBM, Shaw HM, Thompson JF, et al. Primary mucosal and glans penis melanomas: the Sydney melanoma unit experience. Aust NZ J Surg 1999;69:121–6.
331. Oliva E, Quinn TR, Amin MB, et al. Primary malignant melanoma of the urethra. A clinicopathological analysis of 15 cases. Am J Sur Pathol 2000;24(6):785–96.
332. Pack GT, Miller TR. Metastatic melanomas with indeterminate primary site. J Am Med Assoc 1961;176:55–6.
333. Smith JL Jr, Stehlin JS Jr. Spontaneous regression of primary malignant melanomas with regional metastases. Cancer 1965;18:1399–415.
334. McGovern VJ. Melanoma—growth patterns, multiplicity and regression. Paper presented at the International Cancer Conference, Sydney, 1972.
335. McGovern VJ, Shaw HM, Milton GW. Prognosis in patients with thin malignant melanoma: influence of regression. Histopathology 1983;7:673–80.
336. Blessing K, McLaren KM. Histological regression in primary cutaneous melanoma: Recognition, prevalence and significance. Histopathology 1992;20:315–22.
337. Tefany FJ, Barnetson RS, Halliday GM, et al. Immunocytochemical analysis of the cellular infiltrate in primary regressing and non-regressing malignant melanoma. J Invest Dermatol 1991;97:197–202.
338. Barnhill RL, Levy MA. Regressing thin cutaneous malignant melanomas (≤ 1.0 mm) are associated with angiogenesis. Am J Pathol 1993;143:99–104.
339. Barr RJ, White GM, Kiao SY. Tumoral melanophagocytosis: a rare and confusing pattern of regressed melanoma. J Cutan Pathol 1990;17:287.
340. Barr RJ. The many faces of completely regressed malignant melanoma. Pathology 1994;2:359–70.
341. Sagebiel R. Pigmented lesion pathology: the specimen and its report. A personal and probably biased approach. Pathology 1994;2:281–98.
342. Flax SH, Skelton HG, Smith KJ, Lupton GP. Nodular melanosis due to epithelial neoplasms. A finding not restricted to regressed melanomas. Am J Dermatopathol 1998;20:118–22.

CHAPTER 11

Metastatic Malignant Melanoma

Klaus J. Busam and Raymond L. Barnhill

After treatment of the primary tumor, melanoma will recur in approximately one third of patients (1,2). The pattern of recurrence is unpredictable, and any site of the body may be involved. Melanoma can spread hematogenously, through an intralymphatic or perilymphatic route, extension along anatomic structures such as vascular channels or nerves, or by direct local invasion. Metastases are more frequent to skin, subcutaneous tissue, and lymph nodes (nonvisceral sites) than to visceral organs (2). The site of initial recurrence is an important predictor of survival (2–10). Patients who recur with regional lymph node metastasis and undergo lymphadenectomy have reported 5-year survival rates ranging from 20 to 50%. If the recurrence is at a distant site, 5-year survival is only 5%.

Accurate diagnosis of metastatic disease is important for staging. Pathologic parameters are key determinants of clinical outcome (9,10). From a clinical staging point of view, metastases are divided into locoregional and distant metastases.

LOCOREGIONAL METASTASES (AMERICAN JOINT COMMITTEE ON CANCER STAGE III DISEASE)

Locoregional metastases include tumor deposits in regional lymph nodes and regional cutaneous or soft tissue deposits between the primary tumor and the regional nodes (10). The latter have historically been divided into satellite and in-transit metastases. Satellite metastases represent tumor aggregates that are separated from the invasive tumor component by normal tissue but confined to a radius of ≤ 2 cm from the primary tumor (11). In-transit metastases are located outside the radius of 2 cm (11). The cutoff value separating satellite and in-transit metastases is arbitrary and has been changed over the past decades. Both imply increased risk for further recurrences (12–16). Although pathophysiologically and prognostically satellite and in-transit metastases represent a similar process, they had been separated in past American Joint Committee on Cancer (AJCC) staging systems (satellite metastasis implied T4b, whereas in-transit represented N2b disease) (11). Available data show no substantial difference in survival outcome between satellite and in-transit metastases (9,12,15), which is why both have been assigned the same prognostic value in the newly proposed AJCC staging system (10). They are classified as N2c in the absence of synchronous nodal metastases because both imply a prognosis similar to multiple nodal metastases. Patients with nodal and regional cutaneous or soft tissue metastases have a worse prognosis than with either event alone. They have been assigned as having N3 disease (10). The reported incidences of satellite and in-transit metastases vary. For example, Elder et al. (16) reported in a study on re-excisions of melanomas that satellites were found in 22% of tumors thicker than 2 mm. At Memorial Sloan-Kettering Cancer Center, we have found that the incidence of satellite metastases in re-excisions for melanomas thicker than 2 mm is only 3.6%.

The status of the regional lymph nodes has been established as an important prognostic parameter (17–19). Sentinel lymph node biopsy (SLNB) and mapping have been highly accurate in staging nodal basins at risk for regional melanoma metastases. This surgical procedure has become standard at cancer centers in the United States for staging patients with primary cutaneous melanomas with a Breslow thickness of ≥ 1 mm or extension into the reticular dermis (Clark level IV). Metastases are detected in 15–20% of these patients (17–19). The status of the SLN has become established as the most powerful predictor of outcome in patients with cutaneous melanoma

(17–19). Accordingly, pathologic examination of the SLN is important.

For best results, the SLN is to be split in half along the longitudinal axis in the plane of the hilum. Most pathology laboratories examine more than one level of hematoxylin and eosin-stained sections of the lymph nodes and also use immunohistochemistry for at least S-100 protein; at some institutions two or three melanocyte differentiation markers are used to facilitate recognition of small metastatic tumor deposits (20). Antibodies to gp100, Mart-1, Melan-A, or tyrosinase are superior to anti-S-100 protein in detecting solitary metastatic tumor cells in the lymph node. In contrast to anti-S-100 protein, they do not stain nonmelanocytic cells like follicular dendritic cells, which allows a more straightforward interpretation of staining results.

Immunohistochemical studies likely increase the yield of detection of micrometastatic disease, although it is unclear how much of the increased sensitivity is due to immunohistochemistry and how much due to the fact that overall more tissue sections were examined. In the vast majority of metastases, tumor cells can be detected by careful analysis of hematoxylin and eosin (H&E) stained sections. However, there are cases, in which rare tumor cells become apparent only on immunostains. It is unknown at the current time whether there is a prognostic difference between a tumor volume that is readily detected by routine H&E sections and a minimal volume that requires immunohistochemistry.

It is clear, however, that the sensitivity of detecting melanocytes in the lymph node can be increased by molecular studies (21). Reverse transcriptase polymerase chain reaction (RT-PCR) studies for tyrosinase mRNA expression have documented that this gene can be detected in up to two thirds of patients undergoing SLNB. Studies have shown that the lack of detectable tyrosinase mRNA implies a favorable outcome, which has led to proposals for molecular staging of patients with cutaneous melanoma (21). However, the prognostic value of molecular data is still subject to further investigation, and they do not yet play a part in the AJCC staging system.

DISTANT METASTASES (AMERICAN JOINT COMMITTEE ON CANCER STAGE IV DISEASE)

Distant metastases may occur at any site. Because of the prognostic significance of the site of initial recurrence, the AJCC has proposed changes in the classification of metastatic disease (M classification). Patients with nonvisceral metastases (soft tissue, distant nodal) have been reported to have longer survival rates than patients with visceral metastases. They are classified as having M1 disease (10). Since some series have suggested better survival with pulmonary metastases than with visceral metastases at other sites, these patients are being classified as having M2 disease. Patients with nonpulmonary visceral metastases are classified as having M3 disease (10). Irrespective of the site of distant recurrence, elevated serum levels of lactate dehydrogenase (LDH) have been found to imply a poor prognosis. According to the AJCC guidelines, patients with elevated LDH are also classified as having M3 disease (10).

Much of what has been written in the literature about the distribution of visceral metastases is based on autopsy series (22, 23). While virtually any organ can be involved, certain sites are preferred for metastatic spread. As reviewed by Lee (23), involvement of the lungs is most commonly seen. It has been documented to occur in 70–87% of postmortem examinations of individuals with metastatic melanoma. Next in frequency are liver (54–77%), brain (39–54%), bone (23–49%), intestine (26–58%), heart (40–45%), pancreas (38–53%), adrenals (36–54%), kidney (35–48%), and thyroid (25–39%) (22–24).

To the clinician, the information as to which organ site the first metastases can be expected may be more relevant than the clinical end stage or postmortem anatomic distribution of metastases. The most common first sites of visceral metastases reported in clinical studies are lung (14–20%), liver (14–20%), brain (12–20%), bone (11–17%), and intestine (1–7%), whereas first metastases at other sites are very rare (< 1%) (23).

PITFALLS IN THE DIAGNOSIS OF METASTATIC MELANOMA

The pathologic diagnosis of metastatic melanoma poses a number of pitfalls and challenges. The diagnostic problems depend on the anatomic site of involvement. At any

TABLE 11-1 Histologic features of metastatic melanoma.

Location
   Melanocytic growth in unexpected sites (e.g., subcutis, lymph nodes, viscera)
Growth pattern
   Nodular, circumscribed, or infiltrative
Cellular arrangements
   Nests, sheets, fascicles or dispersed single cells
Cytology
   Melanin pigment
   Epithelioid and/or spindle cells
     Nuclear pseudoinclusions
     Large eosinophilic or amphophilic nucleoli
Host response
   Sparse lymphocytic infiltrate
   Mild fibrosis

site, metastatic melanoma needs to be distinguished from other primary or metastatic tumor types. Additional problems arise in the skin, mucosal sites, and lymph nodes. In lymph nodes, metastatic melanoma needs to be distinguished from nodal nevi. At mucosal and cutaneous sites, epitheliotropic metastatic melanoma may be confused with a new primary melanoma. On rare occasions, a deceptively bland metastatic melanoma to the skin may mimic a nevus (nevoid metastasis). Rendering the correct diagnosis in these instances is critical because of the serious implications for treatment and prognosis.

Typical Morphology of Metastatic Melanoma

Features commonly seen in metastatic malignant melanoma are listed in Table 11-1. Like primary invasive melanoma, metastatic melanoma has a tendency to grow in nests, sheets, or fascicles (Figs. 11-1 and 11-2). Cytologically, epithelioid and/or spindle cells are commonly found in metastatic melanoma. In particular, a combination of both cell types (Fig. 11-2) is typical of melanoma but can also be seen in other tumors, such as meningiomas, sarcomatoid carcinomas, and sarcomas. Large epithelioid cells with abundant cytoplasm (Fig. 11-1B) and nuclear atypia (Fig. 11-3), characterized, for example, by prominent eosinophilic or amphophilic nucleoli and nuclear cytoplasmic pseudoinclusions are not uncommon. Such cytologic features suggest melanoma but are not specific.

Melanin pigment may be apparent (Fig. 11-2), subtle, or absent on H&E-stained sections (amelanotic melanoma). The presence of melanin greatly facilitates the recognition of a metastatic melanoma.

Metastatic Melanoma Versus Nonmelanocytic Tumor

Metastatic melanoma may assume a great variety of morphologic appearances and may mimic a number of primary

FIGURE 11-1 Malignant melanoma metastatic to lung. **A,** Nests of metastatic epithelioid cells are seen in lung parenchyma. **B,** Many of their nuclei show prominent nucleoli.

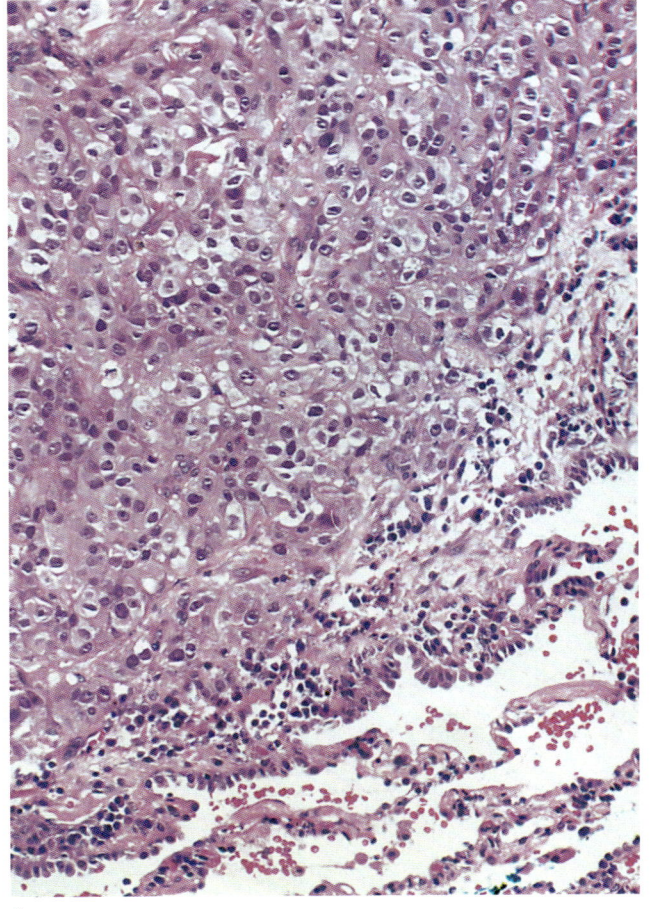
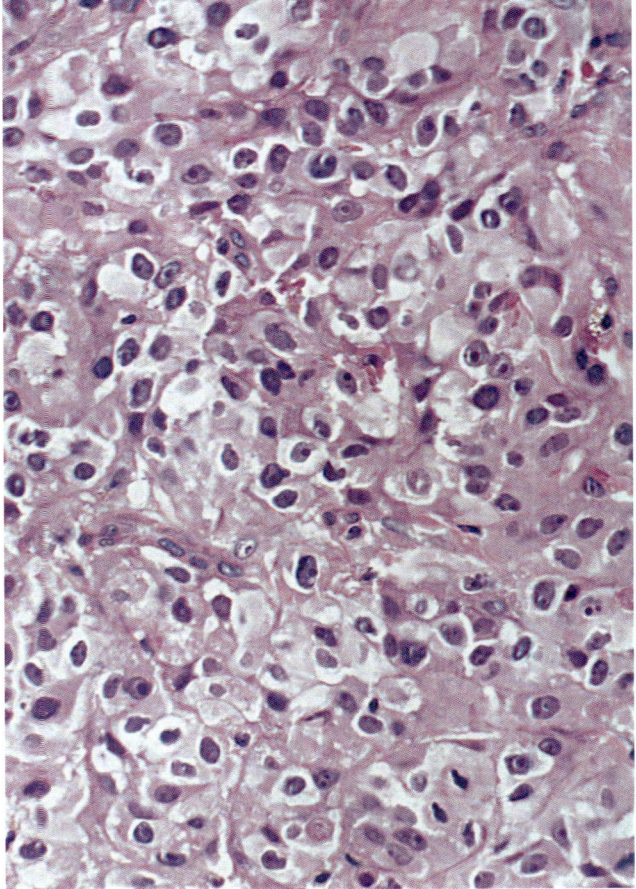

A

B

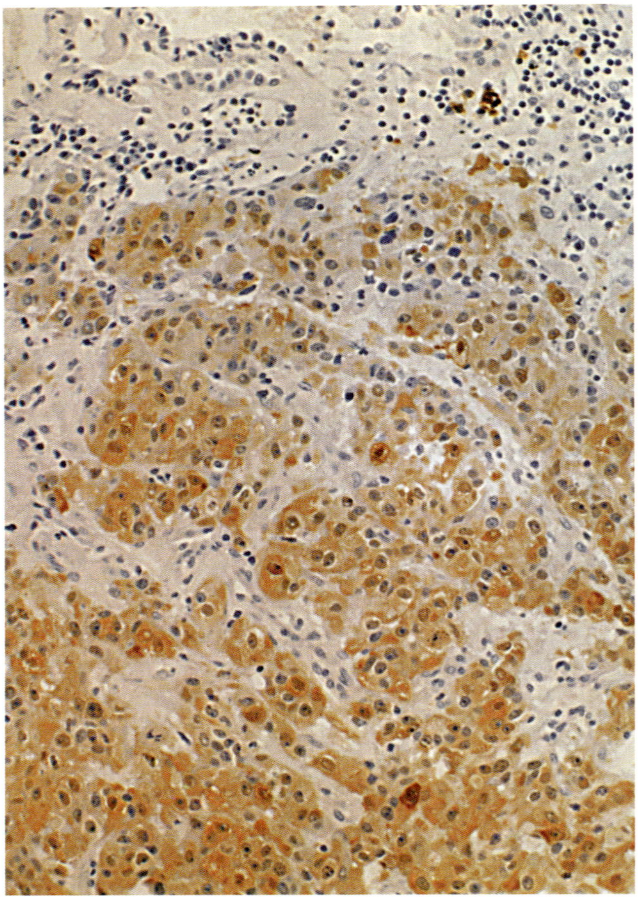

C

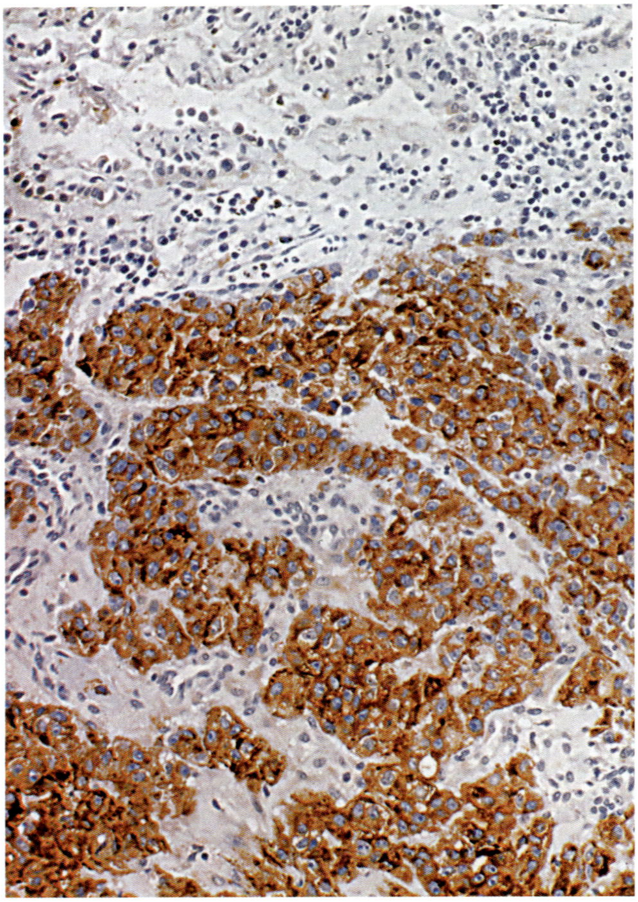

D

FIGURE 11-1 *Continued.* Immunoreactivity for S-100 protein (**C**) and HMB-45 (**D**) are also shown.

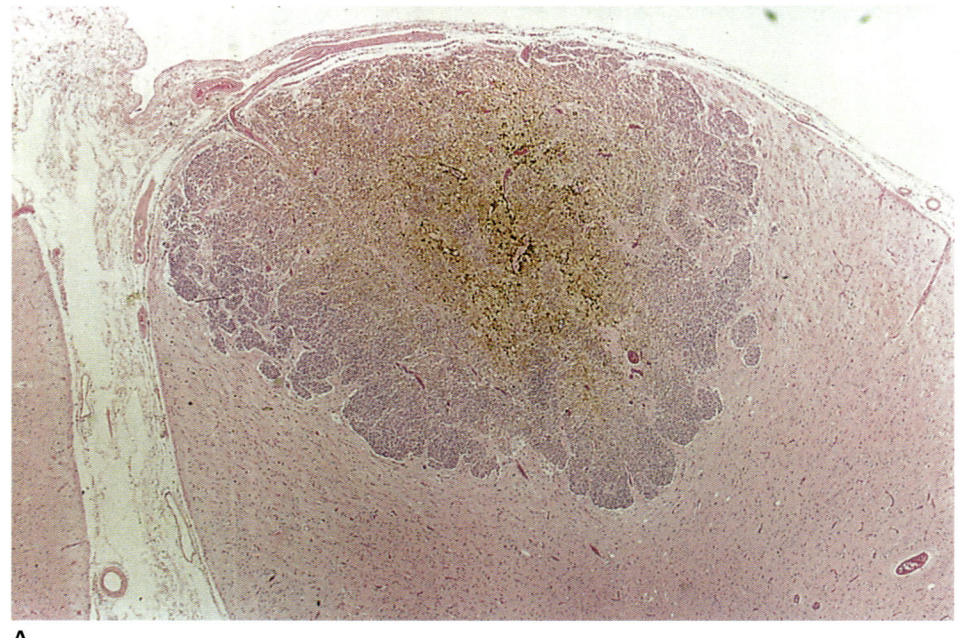

A

FIGURE 11-2 Metastatic melanoma. **A,** Malignant melanoma metastatic to brain.

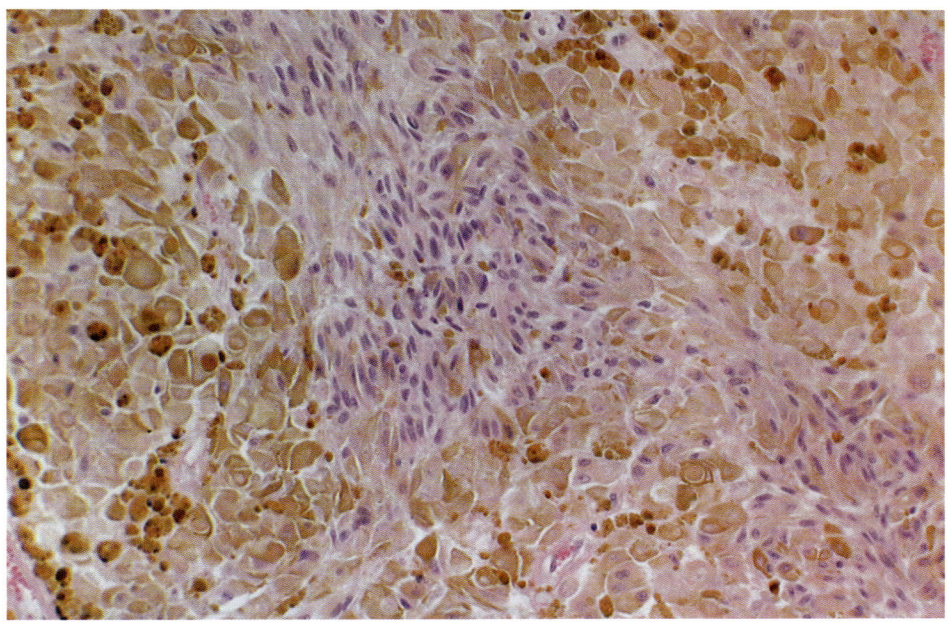

FIGURE 11-2 *Continued.* **B,** The metastati lesions is composed of both spindle and epithelioid cells. Abundant melanin is present.

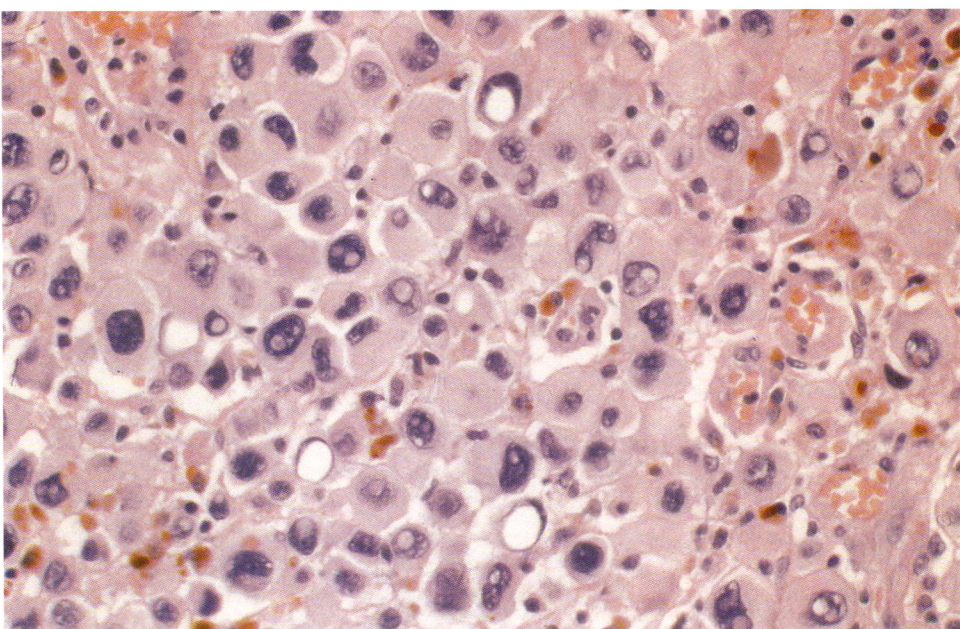

FIGURE 11-3 Malignant melanoma metastatic to brain. Pleomorphic epithelioid cells are present, exhibiting marked irregularity in nuclear shape, size, and chromaticity. Many cells have nuclear pseudoinclusions; some show signet-ring morphology.

or metastatic nonmelanocytic tumors, such as lymphoma, carcinoma, and sarcoma (25). If melanin pigment is absent, immunohistochemical studies using antibodies against melanocytic differentiation antigens are invaluable.

When melanoma assumes an undifferentiated or unusual morphology, a major danger lies in the fact that the possibility of a melanoma may not be considered at all in the differential diagnosis. A variety of morphologic features that have been reported to occur in metastatic melanoma are listed in Table 11-2 (25,26).

Epithelioid cell morphology is the most common appearance of melanomas in metastases (Figs. 11-1 to 11-4). This type of melanoma needs primarily to be distinguished from poorly differentiated carcinomas of various primary sites or large-cell anaplastic lymphoma. If melanoma has prominent or exclusive *spindle cell morphology* (Fig. 11-6) it needs to be distinguished from sarcomas or sarcomatoid carcinomas (25–27). Immunohistochemical studies usually allow a clear diagnosis, with rare exceptions. They are of little or no help in the distinction of melanoma from a primary or metastatic pigmented peripheral nerve sheath tumor. Both types of tumors may show similar morphologic and immunohistochemical features. Ultrastructural studies may be helpful. If prominent basal lamina is present, a nerve sheath tumor is favored (28). Likewise, the gross appearance of the tumor may provide important clues. A tight association of the tumor with a nerve trunk and a firm appearance of the tumor's cut surface favor a nerve sheath origin. Immunohistochemical studies are also of little help in distinguishing a nodule derived from a cutaneous melanoma from melanoma of soft parts (clear cell sarcoma) (Fig. 11-7). Cytogenetics for the t(11,22) translocation or molecular studies for the EWS-ATF1 fusion gene are invaluable for this distinction (29,30).

Signet-ring cell morphology is seen in some primary or metastatic melanomas (Fig. 11-3), sometimes even with diastase-resistant periodic acid-Schiff (PAS) positive material (31). Mucicarmine stains are typically negative in such cases. The differential diagnostic work-up needs primarily to rule out adenocarcinoma and signet-ring cell lymphoma, which can easily be accomplished by immunohistochemistry.

Balloon cell morphology has been reported to occur in metastatic melanoma (31–33). If macrovacuolar cytoplasmic changes are well developed, the presence of a liposarcoma may be suggested. Prominent cytoplasmic clear-cell appearance may resemble a metastatic renal cell carcinoma (31).

Disassociation of tumor cells with adherence of tumor cells to the surrounding fibrovascular stroma may architecturally mimic alveolar rhabdomyosarcoma (24,25,34). Large sheets or lobules of discohesive tumor cells may mimic malignant lymphoma (24,25). Dissociation of tumor cells may also lead to irregular empty spaces and sometimes an adenoid/pseudopapillary pattern (24,25,34) or a pattern mimicking angiosarcoma.

Some metastatic melanomas may develop a promi-

TABLE 11-2 Metastatic melanoma simulating other neoplasms.

Morphologic feature of tumor cells	Differential diagnosis
Epithelioid cell	Carcinoma
	Anaplastic large cell lymphoma
	Angiosarcoma
	Epithelioid sarcoma
Spindle cell	Sarcoma (fibrous, myofibroblastic, smooth muscle, peripheral nerve sheath, vascular, undifferentiated)
	Meningiomas
Signet-ring cell	Adenocarcinoma
	Lymphoma
Balloon cell	Clear-cell carcinoma (sebaceous, renal cortical)
Macrovacuolization	
Clear-cell changes	
Disassociation of tumor cells	
Sheet-like/lobular	Lymphoma
Pseudoalveolar	Alveolar rhabdomyosarcoma
Adenoid/pseudopapillary	Adenocarcinoma, mesothelioma
Myxoid stromal changes	Myxoid variants of sarcomas
	Pleomorphic adenoma
	Malignant sweat gland tumor
Staghorn vascular pattern	Hemangiopericytoma, synovial sarcoma
Multinucleated giant cells	Giant cell–rich sarcoma, giant cell–rich carcinoma

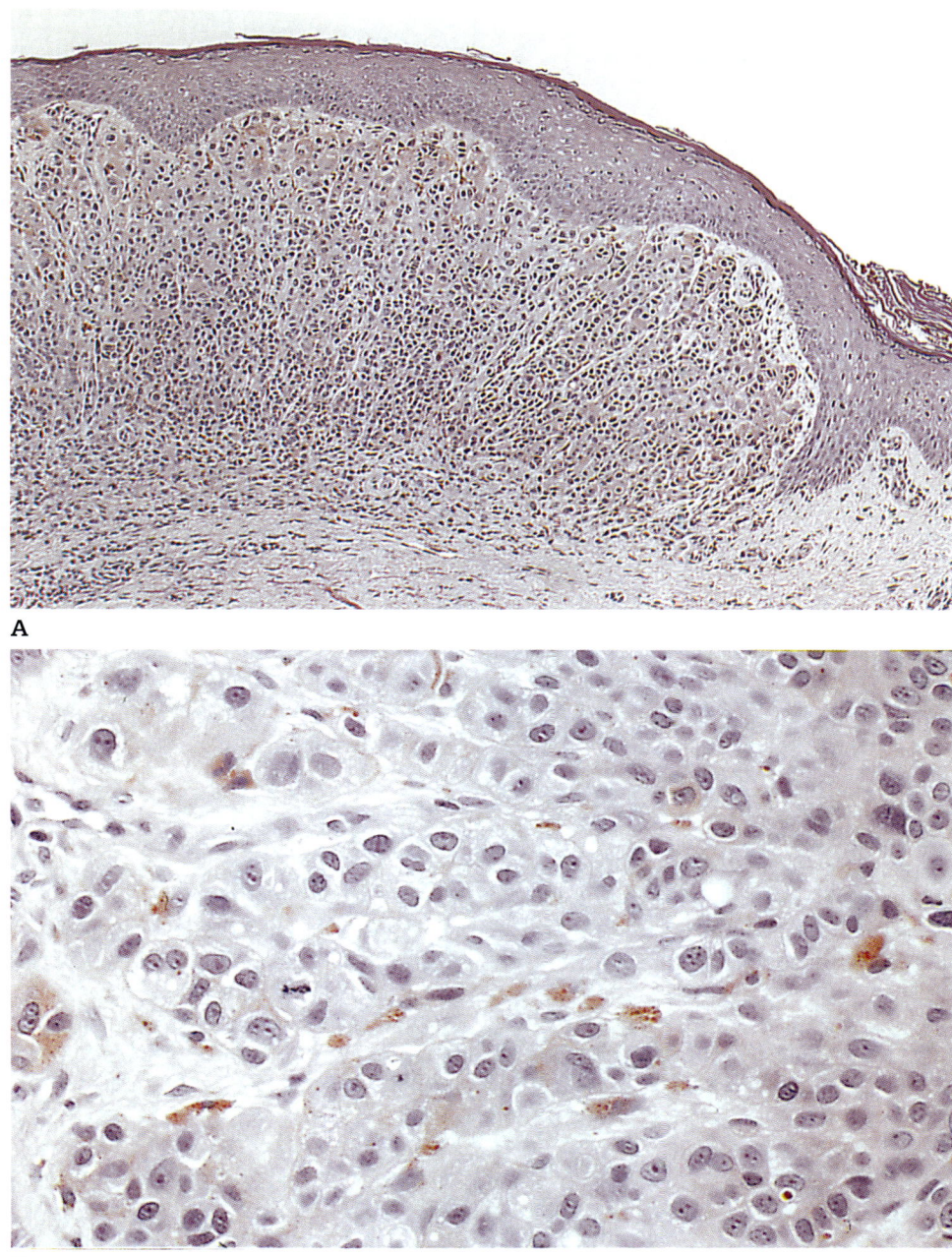

FIGURE 11-4 A, Malignant melanoma metastatic to skin. **B,** Higher magnification. Epithelioid cells are present in the dermis and arranged in a pattern similar to a dermal nevus. They are lined laterally by an epidermal collarette. No epidermal involvement is seen.

nent *myxoid stromal reaction,* as seen in various myxoid tumors (myxofibrosarcoma, liposarcoma, chondrosarcoma, rhabdomyosarcoma, malignant sweat gland tumors, pleomorphic adenoma, or others) (35–37). A *"staghorn"-like vascular pattern* of prominent branching thin-walled blood vessels, mimicking the vascular pattern of a hemangiopericytoma, may occur in some metastatic melanomas (25). A number of other unusual patterns have been described in melanomas, such as a small-cell variant of melanoma (25), melanoma resembling a neuroendocrine neoplasm, and melanoma with numerous giant cells mimicking a giant cell malignant fibrous histiocytoma.

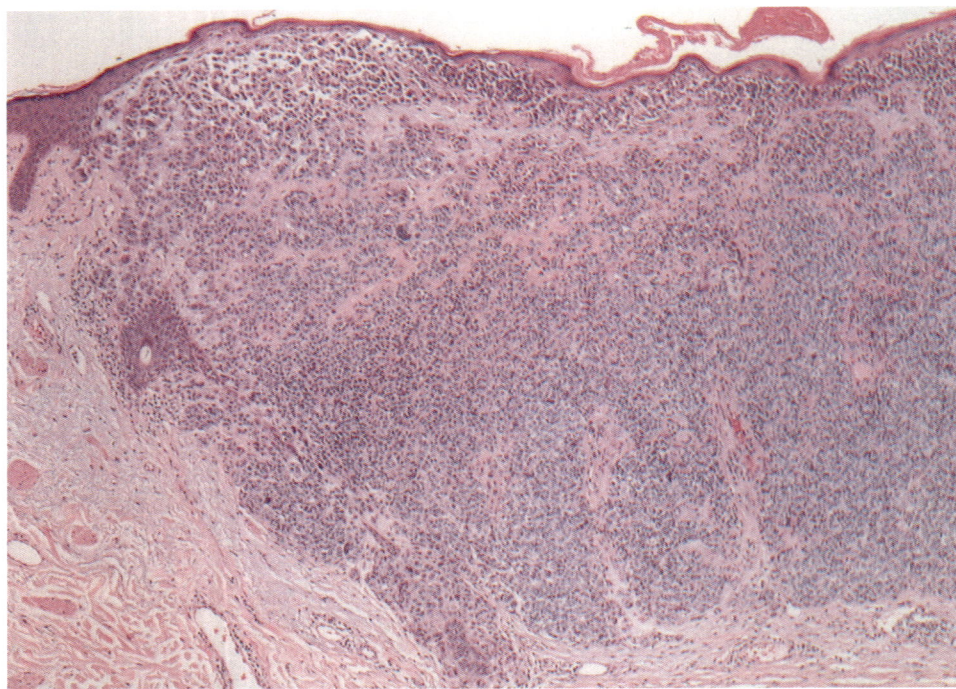

FIGURE 11-5 Epidermotropic cutaneous melanoma metastasis. Uniformly atypical epithelioid cells are seen in the dermis and at the dermoepidermal junction.

Primary Cutaneous Melanoma Versus Metastatic Melanoma to the Skin

The distinction between a primary cutaneous melanoma and a skin metastasis has obvious prognostic significance. A number of features have been suggested to differentiate histologically a cutaneous metastasis from a primary tumor (Table 11-3).

Solid histologic evidence for a primary tumor is the presence of a broad in situ component or the presence of an associated nevus component. In the absence of a noninvasive precursor lesion, other parameters provide some guidance. Cutaneous metastases usually present as nodules within the reticular dermis or subcutis and only rarely involve the overlying epidermis (4,15) (Fig. 11-4). In cases of metastatic melanoma that do show epidermotropism (38,39), the volume of the epidermal component is usually relatively small compared to the dermal mass (Fig. 11-5). If the dermal metastasis is very superficially located, the overlying epidermis may be thinned and the lateral borders may show hyperplastic elongated rete ridges turned inward forming a *collarette*. Tumor cells within vascular lumina are more likely to be found in and around a metastatic lesion than near a primary tumor (38,39).

After evaluating the location and architecture of the lesion, the cytologic features of the tumor cells may provide additional clues, in making a distinction between a primary and secondary tumor (38). Mitotic figures tend to be more frequent in metastatic than in primary tumors.

Primary tumors generally display more pleomorphism than metastatic lesions, which often appear as an atypical, but rather monomorphous population of cells. Primary tumors tend to show more variation in the overall composition of the lesion. There is often more fibrosis and more of an inflammatory host response. The reliability of the guidelines listed in Table 11-3 has been questioned for a number of cases in which the histologic features of a presumed primary lesion did not fit the patient's clinical history (39). When deciding whether a melanocytic tumor is a metastasis or a primary lesion, it is always important to weigh the histologic appearance against a careful and detailed clinical history to arrive at the correct diagnosis.

Primary Mucosal Melanoma Versus Metastatic Melanoma

Primary mucosal melanomas are rare tumors and they may be confused with a metastasis to a mucosal site derived from a primary extramucosal (usually cutaneous) melanoma. In the absence of a prior history of melanoma at another site, the presence of a dominant mass at a mucosal site favors a primary mucosal tumor. The primary nature of the melanoma is supported histologically by the presence of a broad in situ component. A histologically detectable in situ component, however, may be absent, for example, due to ulceration. In contrast, metastases to mucosal sites usually occur in the setting of known clin-

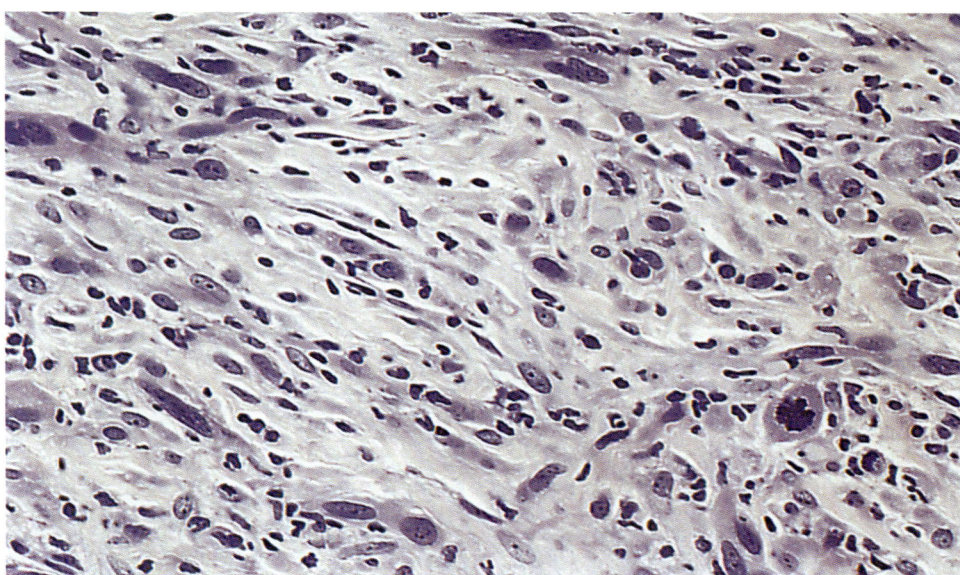

FIGURE 11-6 Metastatic melanoma with spindle cell morphology. Amelanotic malignant spindle cells and few epithelioid cells with mitoses are present.

ically advanced melanoma. The probability of a mucosal site being the first site of metastatic disease is extremely low. When metastases occur to mucosal sites, they usually present as multiple nodules associated with lymphatic tumor emboli. Metastatic nodules are typically located in the deep tissue of a mucosal wall, but they may extend to the surface. Primary mucosal tumors are usually large and show phenotypic heterogeneity of the tumor cells, whereas metastatic tumors tend to be more homogenous in their cytologic appearance. Rarely, epitheliotropic mucosal metastases can occur. In those instances, especially, if one deals only with a small biopsy samples, knowledge of the clinical findings and patterns of lymphatic spread, if present, are important to avoid a diagnostic pitfall.

Cutaneous Nevus Versus Metastasis

Sometimes a small cutaneous metastasis has a nevic silhouette and must be distinguished from a dermal or

FIGURE 11-7 Malignant melanoma of soft parts (clear-cell sarcoma) metastatic to bone. Epithelioid cells, some of which have clear cytoplasm, are arranged in nests. Their nuclei show prominent nucleoli.

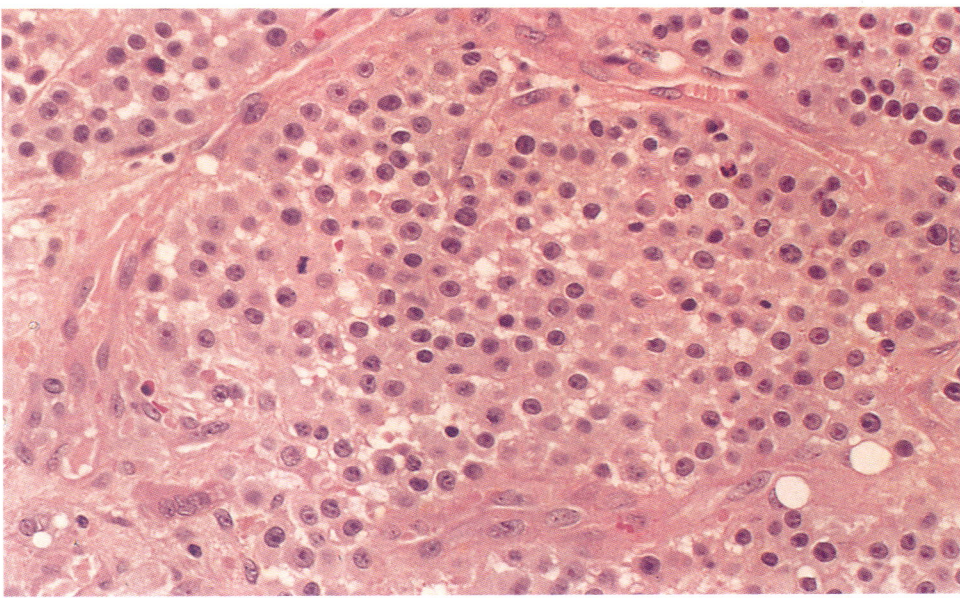

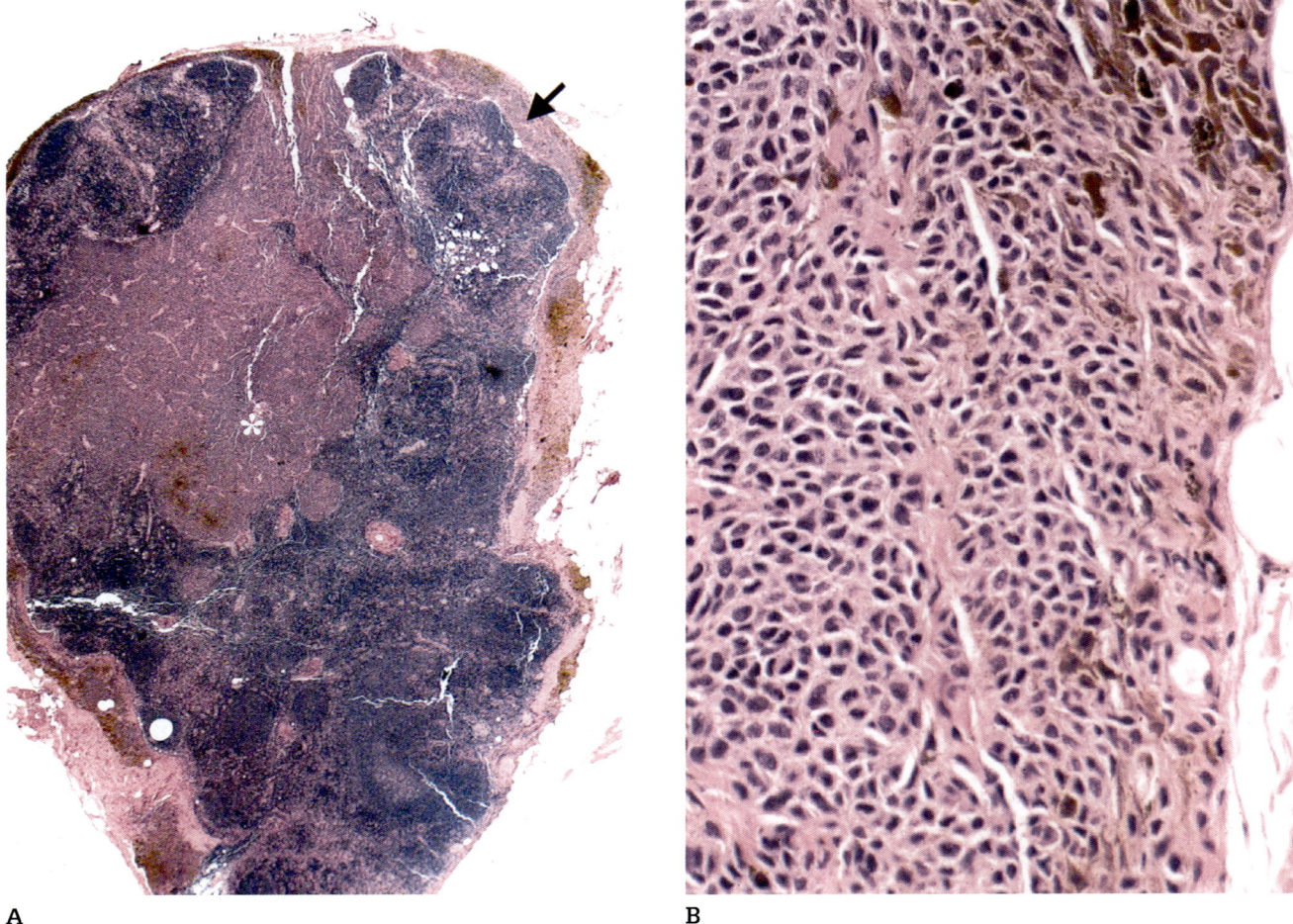

FIGURE 11-8 Large nodal nevus. **A,** Aggregates of nevomelanocytes are present in the fibrous capsule (*arrow*) and in the lymph node (star). This lymph node was obtained during a radical mastectomy procedure with axillary lymph node dissection for invasive mammary duct carcinoma. **B,** Higher magnification shows cytologically bland melanocytes.

compound nevus. For the latter discrimination, the pathologist must carefully assess the lesion for cytologic atypia, presence or absence of maturation, and mitotic figures, particularly atypical ones. Cutaneous melanoma metastases can mimic a variety of nevi (nevoid metastases), usually epithelioid cell nevi but also blue nevi (Fig. 11-9). Metastatic melanoma simulating blue nevus has been reported for both cutaneous and ocular melanoma (40,41).

Nodal Nevus Versus Metastasis

The distinction of nevi from metastases not only applies to the skin but is also relevant for the examination of lymph nodes. Collections of small melanocytes are occa-

TABLE 11-3 Primary cutaneous melanoma versus cutaneous metastasis.

Feature	Primary melanoma	Cutaneous metastasis
Location of tumor	Both dermis and epidermis, usually	Dermis and/or subcutis
If epidermal involvement	Prominent, usually; pagetoid horizontal and vertical spread, commonly present	Usually < dermal involvement; pagetoid spread less common
Epidermal collarette	Less likely present	More likely present
Cytology	Polymorphous, usually	Monomorphous, usually
Reactive fibrosis	May be marked	Mild, usually
Vascular invasion	Rarely seen	More likely present

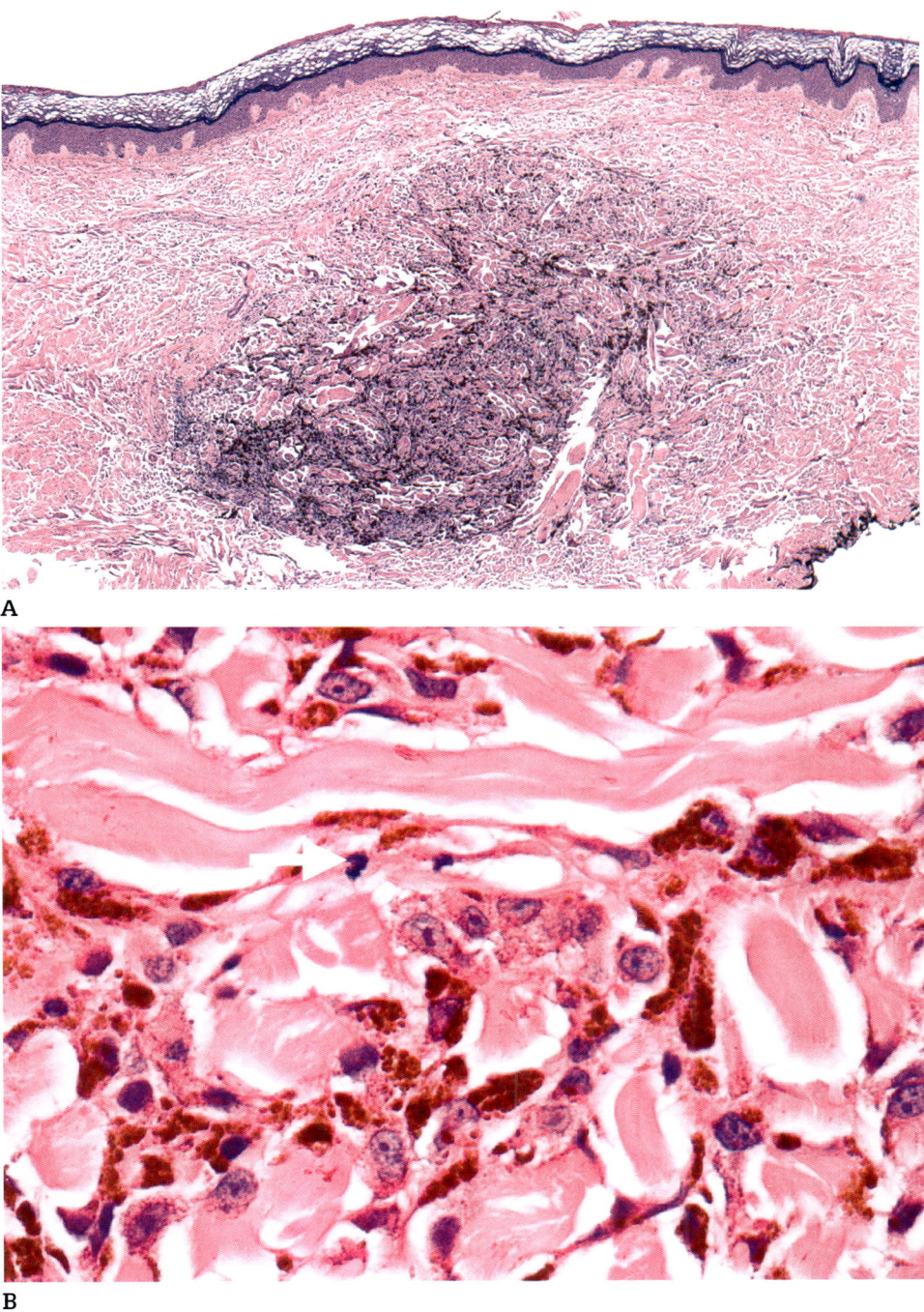

FIGURE 11-9 Metastatic melanoma simulating blue nevus. **A,** An in-transit metastasis from a patient with primary acral melanoma. The growth pattern resembles a blue nevus. **B,** Higher magnification reveals epithelioid atypia and a mitotic figure (*arrow*).

sionally seen within lymph nodes draining the skin (Fig. 11-8). They were first described by Stewart and Copeland (42) in 1931. These melanocytic or nevus cell aggregates are usually small and inconspicuous (43–50). However, they may rarely occupy most of the lymph node (49,50) (Fig. 11-8). They are usually located in the fibrous capsule of the node rather than the marginal sinus (47), but rarely can be found in the lymphatic tissue proper (47,50). They usually resemble architecturally and cytologically melanocytes of dermal nevi composed of small spindle and/or epithelioid cells. Nodal blue nevi have also been described (48), including cellular variants (49). Their bland appearance and their predominent location in the fibrous capsule of the lymph node help distinguish them from micrometastases. However, especially in frozen sections or in the rare situation of intranodal location, the presence of melanocytic aggregates in lymph nodes may lead to diagnostic confusion. Distinction of nodal nevi from melanoma can be facilitated by comparing the cytology of the nodal melanocytes with the cells of the invasive component of the primary tumor. On occasion, immunohistochemical studies may be helpful (50). Nodal melanocytes are usually strongly and homogenously positive for S-100 protein, Mart-1/Melan-A, or tyrosinase. Although they may be focally immunopositive with HMB-45, they usually lack strong and diffuse staining with this antibody (50). The use of MIB-1 has also been suggested for the distinction of nodal nevi from metastatic melanoma. Nodal nevi usually do not stain for MIB-1 (0 or < 1% of cells may be positive), but positive MIB-1 labeling is usually readily detected in metastatic melanoma, although the range of positive staining may vary from < 5% to > 70% of tumor cells (50).

The prevalence of melanocytic aggregates lymph nodes varies, ranging from ≤ 1% in axillary lymph nodes of patients undergoing surgery for breast carcinoma (45,46), to 3.9% in patients with primary cutaneous melanoma undergoing sentinel lymph node biopsy (47). Whether these nodal melanocytic lesions derive from aberrant migration of melanoblasts from the neural crest during embryogenesis or represent lymphatic spread from a benign cutaneous nevus has been the subject of much debate. The proponents of the theory of aberrant migration point out that the melanocytic aggregates are usually located in the fibrous capsule rather than intranodal (44). The view that lymphatic spread may account for the phenomenon of melanocytic nodal aggregates is usually defined by the argument that intranodal deposition of a variety of extranodal tissue, such as endometrium or endosalpinx, has been reported. Moreover, lymphatic invasion by melanocytes have been documented to occur in the setting of melanocytic aggregates in lymph nodes draining the area of a dermal nevus (43).

Primary Melanoma of Soft Parts Versus Metastatic Melanoma to Soft Tissue

Melanoma of soft parts is a distinct variant of melanoma that does not arise at the dermoepidermal junction or in association with a nevus. It has historically been termed clear-cell sarcoma, but it has become apparent that its differentiating features—such as the presence of melanin pigment and melanocytes differentiation antigens—place this tumor in close relationship with melanoma. In contrast, however, to cutaneous melanomas, this tumor has a balanced translocation t(11,22) (29,30). This is of diagnostic help. If the question arises whether a melanoma nodule in the deep soft tissue in the absence of a known primary melanoma represents a metastasis or primary melanoma of soft parts, RT-PCR studies may be helpful. The demonstration of the presence of the fusion gene EWS-ATF1 provides an unequivocal diagnosis of melanoma of soft parts.

Multiple Melanomas

The incidence of multiple primary melanomas has been reported to be between 1 and 4% of all patients with malignant melanoma (51). At large referral centers, the incidence of patients with multiple melanomas may be as high as 14%. A strong correlation between multiple primary tumors and familial melanoma has been suggested. Before a diagnosis of multiple primary melanomas is made, the possibility of metastatic lesions needs to be excluded. Histologic guidelines (Tables 11-1 and 11-3) assist in the diagnostic decision. However, they are not absolute. The final diagnosis depends on a good clinicopathologic correlation, taking into account not only the morphologic features of the tumors but also the time course of their development and their anatomic distribution.

Metastatic Melanoma with Unknown Primary Site

In as many as 4–12% of melanoma cases, a metastatic lesion is found without a clinically apparent primary tumor (52–55). While it is possible that some melanomas may arise de novo within a lymph node or visceral site, it is generally believed that the phenomenon of an unidentified primary site is related to complete regression of a cutaneous melanoma that becomes clinically undetectable (54). Metastatic melanomas with unknown primary site are twice as common in men as in women, which is in agreement with the observation that tumor regression is more commonly observed in men than in women.

The most common site of presentation is in lymph nodes (64%) (Fig. 11.6), in particular in the axillary, inguinal and neck region. Another site is the subcutis (15%), most often on the trunk. About 21% of the cases presented with visceral metastases, most often to the lung and brain (52–55).

A diagnosis of metastatic melanoma with unknown primary site obviously should be rendered only after careful diagnostic evaluation has failed to disclose a primary cutaneous, mucosal, or ocular melanoma or melanomas of other sites (Fig. 11-10). The search for potential cutaneous primary sites can be facilitated with a Wood's UV lamp to detect areas of depigmentation. Ophthalmoscopic and radiographic studies may be indicated, if the clinical situation suggests a potential extracutaneous primary melanoma. The relative frequencies of sites of pri-

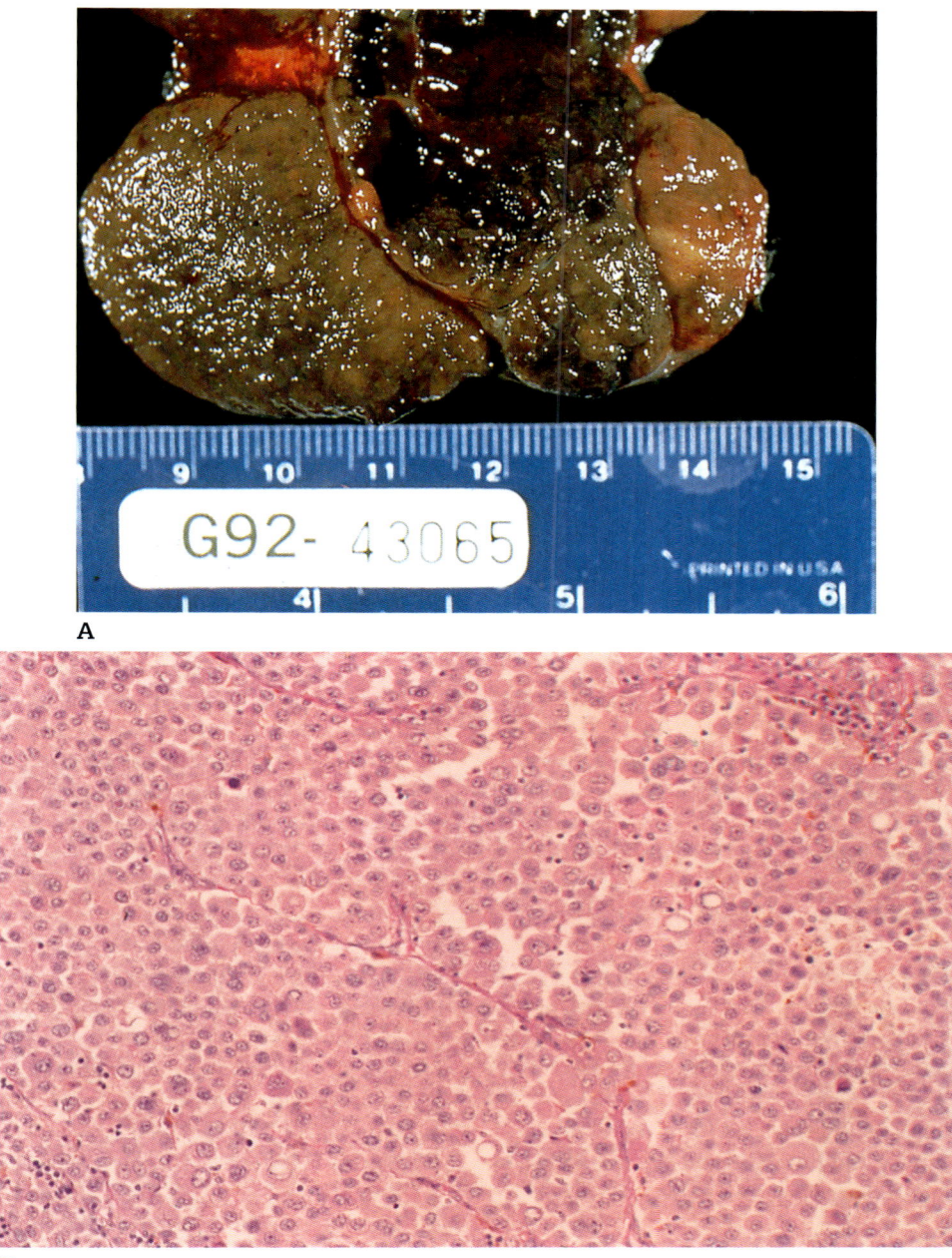

FIGURE 11-10 Metastatic malignant melanoma of unknown primary site. **A,** The brown and enlarged pelvic lymph node. **B,** The lymph node contained pleomorphic epithelioid melanoma cells. No primary site was identified in this patient. The only pigmented lesion that was clinically detected and biopsied was a vulvar lentigo.

mary extracutaneous melanoma according to the Third National Cancer Survey of the United States (56) were: eye (78.9%), vulva (7.2%), soft tissues (2.5%), anorectum (2.3%), vagina (2.1%), upper respiratory tract (1.6%), gums and mouth (1.2%), and gastrointestinal tract (0.7%). Other visceral sites accounted for < 0.5% each.

Melanosis in Metastatic Melanoma

Diffuse cutaneous or generalized melanosis is a rare complication of metastatic melanoma characterized by slate blue to gray or brown discoloration of the skin. The German pathologist E. Wagner and co-workers (57) were the first to report the occurrence of this phenomenon in 1864.

Diffuse melanosis may be limited to the skin or generalized, involving the internal organs. It may be associated with melanuria, melanoptysis, and dark brown discoloration of the serum. Histologically, the skin involved by diffuse melanosis usually shows increased pigment deposition in the dermis and subcutis, predominantly within macrophages. The epidermis may or may not show hyperpigmentation. Various hypotheses have been proposed to explain melanosis (58–63). It is thought that the dermal melanin pigment results from lysis of heavily pigmented tumor cells. Tumor-derived pigment is presumably carried and deposited via the circulation. In some cases, there may also be increased melanin pigment production by epidermal melanocytes in response to circulating melanin-synthesis-stimulating factors (63).

REFERENCES

1. Reintgen DS, Vollmer R, Tso CY, Seigler HF. Prognosis for recurrent stage I malignant melanoma. Arch Surg 1987;122:1338–42.
2. Allen PJ, Coit DJ. The role of surgery for patients with metastatic melanoma. Curr Opin Oncol 2002;14:221–6.
3. Markowitiz JS, Cosimi LA, Carey RW, et al. Prognosis after initial recurrence of cutaneous melanoma. Arch Surg 1991;126:703–7.
4. Coit DG, Rogatko A, Brennan MF. Prognostic factors in patients with melanoma metastatic to axillary or inguinal lymph nodes: a multivariant analysis. Ann Surg 1991;214:627–36.
5. Morton DL, Wanek L, Nizze JA, et al. Improved long-term survival after lymphadenectomy of melanoma metastatic to regional lymph nodes: analysis of prognostic factors in 1134 patients from John Wayne Cancer Clinic. Ann Surg 1991;214:491–9.
6. Amer MH, Al Sarraf M, Vaitkevicius VK. Clinical presentation, natural history and prognostic factors in advanced malignant melanoma. Surg Gynecol Obstet 1979;149:687–92.
7. Roses DF, Karp NS, Oratz R, et al. Survival with regional and distant metastasis from cutaneous malignant melanoma. Surg Gynecol Obstet 1992;172:262–8.
8. Barth A, Wanek LA, Morton DL. Prognostic factors in 1,521 melanoma patients with distant metastases. J Am Coll Surg 1995;181:193–201.
9. Balch CM, Soong SJ, Gershenwald JE, et al. Prognostic factors analysis of 17,600 melanoma patients: validation of the American Joint Committee on Cancer melanoma staging system. J Clin Oncol 2001;19:3622–34.
10. Balch CM, Buzaid AC, Soon SJ, et al. Final version of the American Joint Committee of Cancer staging system for cutaneous melanoma. J Clin Oncol 2001;19:3635–48.
11. American Joint Committee on Cancer. Manual for Staging of Cancer. Philadelphia: Lippincott, 1992.
12. Buzaid AC, Ross MI, Balch CM, et al. Critical analysis of the current AJCC staging system for cutaneous melanoma and proposal to a new staging system. J Clin Oncol 1997;15:1039–51.
13. Day CJ, Harrist T, Gorstein F, et al. Malignant melanoma: prognostic significance of microscopic satellites in reticular dermis and subcutaneous fat. Am Surg 1981;194:108–12.
14. Leon P, Daly JM, Synnestadt M, et al. The prognostic implications of microscopic satellites in patients with clinical stage I melanoma. Arch Surg 1991;126:1461–68.
15. Coit DG. Recurrent regional metastases and their management. In: Balch CM, Houghton AN, Sober AJ, Soong S-J, eds. Cutaneous Melanoma. St. Louis: Quality Medical, 1998:301–9.
16. Elder DE, Guerry DI, Heiberger R, et al. Optimal resection margins for cutaneous malignant melanoma. Plast Reconstr Surg 1983;71:66–72.
17. Gershenwald J, Thompson W, Mansfield P, et al. Multi-institutional melanoma lymphatic mapping experience: the prognostic value of sentinel lymph node status in 612 stage I or II melanoma patients. J Clin Oncol 1999;17:976–83.
18. Clary BM, Brady MS, Lewis JJ, Coit DG. Sentinel lymph node biopsy in the management of patients with primary cutaneous melanoma: review of a large single-institutional experience with an emphasis on recurrence. Ann Surg 2001;233:250–8.
19. McMasters KM, Reintgen DS, Ross MI, et al. Sentinel lymph node biopsy for melanoma: controversy despite widespread agreement. J Clin Oncol 2001;19:2851–5.
20. Yu LL, Flotte TJ, Tanabe KK, et al. Detection of microscopic melanoma metastases in sentinel lymph nodes. Cancer 2999;86:677–87.
21. Sung J, Li W, Shivers S, Reintgen D. Molecular analysis in evaluating the sentinel node in malignant melanoma. Ann Surg Oncol 2001;8:29S–30S.
22. Balch C, Milton G. Diagnosis of metastatic melanoma at distant sites. In: Balch CM, Milton GW, eds. Cutaneous Melanoma. Clinical Management and Treatment Results Worldwide. Philadelphia: Lippincott, 1985:221–50.
23. Lee Y. Malignant melanoma. Patterns of metastasis. Can J Physicians 1980;30:69–75.
24. Nakhleh R, Wick M, Rocamora A, et al. Morphologic diversity in malignant melanoma. Am J Clin Pathol 1990;93:731–40.
25. Mooi W, Krausz T. Cutaneous melanoma. In: Mooi W, Krausz T, eds. Biopsy Pathology of Melanocytic Disorders. London: Chapman & Hall, 1992:215–303.
26. Wick M, Fitzgibbon J, Swanson P. Cutaneous sarcomas and sarcomatoid neoplasms of the skin. Semin Diagn Pathol 1993;10:148–58.
27. Silvis N, Swanson P, Manviel J, et al. Spindle-cell and pleo-

morphic neoplasms of the skin. Am J Dermatopathol 1988; 10:9–19.
28. Dickersin GR. Schwannoma and other nerve sheath neoplasms. In: Dickersin GR, ed. Diagnostic Electron Microscopy. New York: Igaku-Shoin, 1991:238.
29. Fletcher J, Kozakewich H, Hoffer F, et al. Diagnostic relevance of clonal cytogenetic aberrations in malignant soft tissue tumors. N Engl J Med 1991;324:436–43.
30. Peulve P, Michot C, Vannier J-P, et al. Clear cell sarcoma with t(11;22) (q13-14;q12). Genes Chrom Cancer 1991;3:400–2.
31. Akslen L, Myking A. Balloon cell melanoma mimicking clear cell carcinoma. Pathol Res Pract 1989;184:548–50.
32. Sheibani K, Battifora H. Signet-ring cell melanoma. Am J Surg Pathol 1988;12:28–34.
33. Gardner W, Vazquez M. Balloon cell melanoma. Arch Pathol 1970;89:470–2.
34. Lodding P, Kindblom L, Angervall L. Metastases of malignant melanoma simulating soft tissue sarcoma. A clinicopathological, light ane electron microsocpic and immunohistochemical study of 21 cases. Virchow Arch A Pathol Anat 1990;417:377–88.
35. Urso C, Gianotti B, Bondi R. Myxoid melanoma of the skin. Arch Pathol Lab Med 1990;114:527–8.
36. Nottingham J, Slatter D. Malignant melanoma: a new mimic of colloid adenocarcinoma. Histopathology 1988;13:576–8.
37. Bhuta S, Mirra J, Cochran A. Myxoid malignant melanoma. Am J Surg Pathol 1986;10:203–211.
38. Kornberg R, Harris M, Ackerman A. Epidermotropically metastatic malignant melanoma. Arch Dermatol 1978;114:67–9.
39. Bengoechea-Beeby M, Velasco-Oses A, Fernandez F, et al. Epidermotropic metastatic melanoma. Cancer 1993;72:1909–13.
40. Busam KJ. Metastatic melanoma to the skin simulating blue nevus. Am J Surg Pathol 1999;23:276–82.
41. Wieselthier JS, White WL. Cutaneous metastasis of ocular malignant melanoma. An unusual presentation simulating blue nevi. Am J Dermatopathol 1996;18:298–95.
42. Stewart F, Copeland M. Neurogenic sarcoma. Am J Cancer 1931;15:1235–320.
43. Von Alberti M. Sur un cas de neuro-naevus avec metastase ganglionaiere de meme caractere. Bull Soc Fr Dermatol Syphil 1935;42:1273–8.
44. Ioannides G. Lymph nodes with aggregates of nevus cells: a thesis. In: Ackerman AB, ed. Pathology of Malignant Melanoma. New York: Masson, 1981:297–300.
45. Ridolfi R, Rosen P, Thaler H. Nevus cell aggregates associated with lymph nodes: estimated frequency and clinical significance. Cancer 1977;39:164–71.
46. Andreola S, Clemente C. Nevus cells in axillary lymph nodes from radical mastectomy specimens. Pathol Res Pract 1985;179:616–8.
47. Carson KF, Wen DR, Li PX, et al. Nodal nevi and cutaneous melanomas. Am J Surg Pathol 1996;20:834–40.
48. Epstein J, Erlandson R, Rosen P. Nodal blue nevi: a study of three cases. Am J Surg Pathol 1984;8:907–15.
49. Sterchi JM, Muss HB, Weidner N. Cellular blue nevus simulating metastatic melanoma: report of an unusually large lesion associated with nevus-cell aggregates in regional lymph nodes. J Surg Oncol 1987;36:71–5.
50. Lohmann CM, Iversen K, Jungbluth AA, et al. Expression of melanocytic differentiation markers and Ki-67 in nodal nevi, and comparison of Ki-67 expression in nodal nevi with metastatic melanoma. Am J Surg Pathol 2002;26:1351–7.
51. Moseley H, Guiliano A, Storm F, et al. Multiple primary melanoma. Cancer 1979;43:939–44.
52. Das Gupta T, Bowden L, Berg J. Malignant melanoma of unknown primary origin. Surg Gynecol Obstetr 1963;117:341–5.
53. Giuliano A, Cochran AJ, Morton D. Melanoma from unknown primary site and amelanotic melanoma. Semin Oncol 1982;9:442–7.
54. Smith J, Stehlin J. Spontaneous regression of primary melanomas with regional metastases. Cancer 1965;18:1399–415.
55. Reintgen D, McCarty K, Woodard B, et al. Metastatic malignant melanoma with an unknown primary. Surg Gynecol Obstet 1983;156:335–40.
56. Scotto J, Graumen J, Lee J. Melanomas of the eye and other noncutaneous sites: epidemiologic aspects. J Natl Cancer Inst 1976;56:489–91.
57. Wagner E. Ein Fall von Kombination eines Pigmentkrebses mit einer reinen Pigmentgeschwulst. Arch Heilkunde 1864;5:280–4.
58. Fitzpatrick TB, Montgomery H, Lerner AB. Pathogenesis of generalized dermal pigmentation secondary to malignant melanoma and melanuria. J Invest Dermatol 1954;22:163–72.
59. Silberberg I, Kopf A, Gumport S. Diffuse melanosis in malignant melanoma. Arch Dermatol 1968;97:671–7.
60. Pierard G. Melanophageic dermatitis and panniculitis. A condition revealing an occult metastatic malignant melanoma. Am J Dermatopathol 1988;10:133–6.
61. Eide J. Pathogenesis of generalized melanosis with melanuria and melanoptysis secondary to malignant melanoma. Histopathology 1981;5:285–94.
62. Rowden G, Sulicca V, Butler T, Manz H. Malignant melanoma with melanosis. Ultrastructural and histological studies. J Cutan Pathol 1980;7:125–39.
63. Boehm M, Schiller M, Nashan D, et al. Diffuse melanosis arising from metastatic melanoma: pathogentic function of elevated melanocyte peptide growth factors. J Am Acad Dermatol 2001;44:747–54.

CHAPTER 12

Prognostic Factors in Cutaneous Malignant Melanoma

Michael Piepkorn and Raymond L. Barnhill

As with all malignant tumors, the biological potential of any given primary melanoma is encrypted in the genome of the clone of malignant cells giving rise to that tumor. At present, the code is indecipherable at the systems biology level that coordinately executes the tumor's behavior within the host. Thus one must resort to surrogate phenotypic prognostic markers, which, it is hoped, may accurately reflect the status of the neoplastic genotype. Interest in prognostic factors as determined by the phenotypic characteristics of melanomas relates to critical aspects of diagnosis and management. Foremost among these is the obvious need for reliable information with which to counsel patients regarding the likelihood of disease progression. Prognostic factors constitute the essential basis of clinicopathologic staging of disease in patients, from which clinical prognostications are made and are used as the principal guide for definitive surgical management following initial diagnosis. As interest has increased in the application and testing of adjuvant therapies for melanoma, accurate staging based on dependable prognostic indicators has become an essential component in the identification of individuals likely to benefit from adjuvant treatments, such as interferon and melanoma vaccines. Moreover, cohorts of melanoma patients are staged from multiple prognostic factors in ongoing clinical trials so that the potential efficacy of newer therapies can be more reliably ascertained.

Recent times have experienced a surge in interest in the identification and testing of newer and putative phenotypic indicators of prognosis, as well as in the further testing and refinement of older criteria. Advances in newer clinical technologies, such as sentinel lymphatic mapping, has led in similar directions, and indeed that technique has given rise to novel strategies in the design and implementation of prognostic criteria. As discussed in detail in this chapter and elsewhere in this text, the impetus provided by lymphatic mapping has yielded important new information on the prognostic power of molecular markers in melanoma assayed by techniques ranging from immunohistochemistry to reverse transcriptase polymerase chain reaction (RT-PCR). These new diagnostic strategies have been applied to characterizing phenotypic aspects of primary tumors and to detecting and evaluation markers of melanoma cells in the systemic circulation. The availability of larger and well-characterized databases with long-term follow-up of patients at many institutions has facilitated the rigorous evaluation of new technologies, which now demands the use of multivariate analysis according to the Cox proportional hazard regression model for validation (1–3). Collectively, the widespread efforts of many groups of investigators have in recent years considerably refined our ability to more precisely stage patients with melanoma and thus to predict survival from the disease.

Regardless of the appeal of newer technologies for evaluating prognosis, one must interpret the emerging literature with caution. In any given report, extrapolation of the data may be constrained by a limiting number of patients or by insufficient follow up (3). The well-known tendency of melanoma for late recurrences, even after 10 years from original diagnosis, may further confound attempts to extrapolate from existing datasets.

Emphasis is placed in this chapter on existing and emerging prognostic factors in localized (American Joint Committee on Cancer stage I and II) melanoma; however, factors relevant to regional (stage III) and distant (stage IV) disease will also be addressed (Tables 12-1 and 12-2).

TABLE 12-1 Staging system for melanoma (American Joint Committee on Cancer) pathologic staging[a]

Stage grouping	T	N	M
0	Tis	N0	M0
IA	T1a	N0	M0
IB	T1b/T2a	N0	M0
IIA	T2b/T3a	N0	M0
IIB	T3b/T4a	N0	M0
IIC	T4b	N0	M0
III A-C	Any T	N1a-N3	M0
IV	Any T	Any N	Any M1

Source: Adapted and condensed from Balch et al. (2001) (4).

[a]Tumor (microstaging of primary tumor): Tis, in situ; T1, ≤ 1.0 mm (a = without ulceration; b = with ulceration or level IV/V); T2, 1.01–2.0 mm (a = without ulceration; b = with ulceration); T3, 2.01–4.0 mm (a = without ulceration; b = with ulceration); T4, > 4.0 mm (a = without ulceration; b = with ulceration). Nodes (pathologic staging of regional lymph node basin): N1, 1 node involved (a = micrometastasis; b = macrometastasis); N2, 2–3 nodes (a = micrometastasis; b = macrometastasis; c = in transit or satellite metastases); N3, 4 or more nodes. Metastases: M1a–M1c, distant skin, lung, or other visceral/distant metastasis, respectively.

PROGNOSTIC FACTORS FOR STAGE I AND II MELANOMA

New phenotypic variables continue to be introduced and analyzed in efforts to better refine staging and prognosis in the management of melanoma patients. Across most databases, however, the thickness of the primary tumor remains the single most important prognostic criterion in clinically localized disease to which many, if not most, other phenotypic criteria are linked (1–3,5). Indeed, other factors, such as Clark level and often ulceration, may be confounded by their correlation with tumor thickness (5).

Irrespective of the overriding prognostic effect of primary tumor thickness, combinations of prognostic factors can provide more precise estimates of the hazard of tumor progression (2). Thus in some large databases, gender, site of the primary tumor, level of invasion, and thickness are all highly significant as independent prognostic factors in multivariate analysis (6). These inde-

TABLE 12-2 Prognostic factors in stage I and II malignant melanoma.

Factors	Effect on prognosis
Pathologic	
Thickness	Worse prognosis with increasing thickness
Clark level	Worse prognosis with deeper levels
Ulceration	Worse prognosis with presence of ulceration (but may be secondary to mitotic rate)
Mitotic rate	Worse prognosis with increasing mitotic rate
Growth phase	Greater likelihood of metastasis with vertical growth phase
Regression	Increased risk for metastasis in tumors < 1.0 mm with marked regression
Vascular invasion	Worse prognosis with vascular invasion
Angiotropism	Worse prognosis
Microscopic satellites	Worse prognosis and increased risk for local, regional, and distant recurrences when present
Host lymphoid response	Worse prognosis with diminished lymphoid infiltrates
Histogenetic type	Contested better prognosis for lentigo maligna, worse prognosis for acral lentiginous melanoma
Cell type	Better prognosis for tumors composed of spindle cells versus other cell types
Tumor vascularity	Not consistently confirmed at this time
Tumor volume	Worse prognosis with increasing volume
Cross-sectional profile	Worse prognosis with polypoid or verrucous configuration
Neurotropism and desmoplasia	Worse prognosis with neurotropism
Clinical factors	
Age	Worse prognosis with increasing age
Anatomic site	Extremity lesions have more favorable prognosis versus head and neck areas, palms, and soles
Gender	Women have better prognosis than men
Stage	Worse prognosis with more advanced stage
Pregnancy	No clear effect
Local recurrence	Worse prognosis with local recurrence
Other	
Volume-weighted mean nuclear volume	Worse prognosis with increasing nuclear volume
DNA content	Worse prognosis with increasing DNA aneuploidy
Nucleolar organizer regions	Worse prognosis with increasing AgNOR[a] counts
Proliferation and tumor cell motility indices	Worse prognosis with increased values of these indices
Circulating melanoma cells	Worse prognosis with RT-PCR or immunochemical evidence of circulating melanoma cells

[a]AgNOR, silver-staining nucleolar organizer region.

pendent effects have fostered efforts toward developing multifactorial prognostic models (7) that have emerged as potentially useful in the stratification of disease risk.

New and established phenotypic variables are evaluated in datasets stratified according to staging schema that have incorporated the major prognostic factors. In a revision of the traditional staging schema, efforts under the auspices of the American Joint Committee on Cancer (AJCC) resulted in a new staging paradigm that places major emphasis on thickness and ulceration in the T category as the pre-eminent prognostic factors in clinicopathologically localized melanoma. In the new scheme, localized disease historically assigned to clinical stage I is now stratified into stages I and II, with stratification based on thicknesses of ≤ 1.0 or ≥ 1.01 mm, respectively, and modified by the presence or absence of ulceration (4) (Table 12-1). In the following sections, the prognostic factors are described in the context of the current AJCC staging system, which has been validated in independent databases (8,9).

Pathologic Factors

Tumor Thickness The collective experiences of melanoma investigators over many years have firmly established the pre-eminence of tumor thickness as the principal prognostic indicator in melanoma (1–3,5,8,10–13). This central tenet has been reinforced in population-based studies (14,15) and in very large databases, such as the recent multivariate analysis of 17,600 patients from 13 cancer centers with complete follow up information, wherein thickness and ulceration constituted the most powerful predictors of disease progression (16). For patients without evidence of nodal or distant metastasis at the time of prospective enrollment into that collated database, the risk ratio for disease progression attributable to Breslow thickness was 1.558 (95% CI 1.473–1.647, $p < .00001$) and that attributable to ulceration was 1.901 (95% CI 1.735–2.083, $p < .00001$) (16). The status of these two factors as the most significant predictors of outcome was consistent across the individual cancer centers contributing to the database.

Allen and Spitz (17) originally observed that superficial melanomas had a better prognosis than more deeply invasive tumors. Subsequently, other investigators established the inverse correlation between depth of invasion and likelihood of survival from melanoma (18–21) (Table 12-3). To improve both the reproducibility and accuracy of assessing the extent of tumor invasion, Breslow (10) introduced a quantitative method of directly measuring tumor thickness with an ocular micrometer (Fig. 12-1). According to his recommendations, tumors are measured in the vertical dimension from the epidermal granular cell layer to the deepest observed penetration of neoplastic cells into the dermis or subcutaneous fat.

Although it may seem surprising, for many years it was believed that the relationship between melanoma thickness and clinical outcome was not a linear function but rather was a stepwise phenomenon with several "natural" breakpoints at reliable tumor thickness intervals (22). Breslow (10), for example, reported a 100% rate of 5-year survival for people with tumors < 0.76 mm in thickness, compared to a poor prognosis for those with tumors > 3 mm in thickness. Other investigators reported different breakpoint intervals (23,24). More recent studies, however, call the existence of natural breakpoints into question (24). Breakpoints may depend on statistical factors unique to each dataset. For example, Buttner et al. (25) characterized a dataset of > 5000 melanoma patients and found an almost linear relationship to 6 mm. These results taken in conjunction with other large databases (26) now make it reasonably clear that the biologic relationship between tumor thickness and disease outcome is almost certainly a continuous function, as originally suggested by Breslow, rather than interrupted or stepwise as postulated by others.

It is evident that in some situations tumor thickness does not always accurately predict biologic behavior of

TABLE 12-3 Early studies concerning depth of tumor invasion and prognosis.

Depth of invasion	5-year survival	Reference
Superficial	74.1% (5–12 years)	17
Superficial	75%	18
Invasion of reticular dermis	28%	19
Superficial		20
Stage 1 (in situ)	100%	
Stage 2 (invasive without "tumor" formation)	82.3%	
Stage 3 (invasion of reticular dermis)	50.7%	
Stage 1 (superficial invasion)	77.6%	21
Stage 2 (invasion of reticular dermis)	38.6%	
Stage 3 (invasion of subcutaneous fat)	8.0%	

FIGURE 12-1 Breslow thickness and anatomic levels of invasion. As described by Breslow (10), the greatest depth of melanoma invasion is measured in the vertical dimension from the granular layer (or top of an ulcerated surface) to the point of deepest tumor invasion. The anatomic level of invasion (Clark) refers to the extent of melanoma incursion into the papillary dermis, reticular dermis, and subcutaneous tissue.

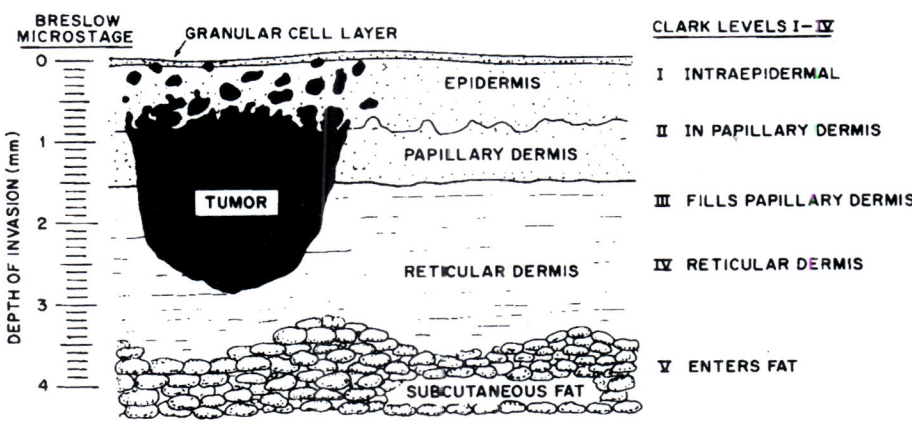

melanoma (2). On one hand, ~5% of patients with melanomas < 1 mm thick develop metastases (2), and on the other, thick melanomas with Breslow value > 4 mm can be survivable. Thus there has been a continued search for other factors of combinations thereof that may better predict outcome. The major independent prognostic factor for thick melanomas emerging from multivariate analyses is the presence or absence of micrometastatic disease by SLN (27,28). SLN status and ulceration of the primary tumor independently predicted 5-year survival status for melanomas > 3 mm in thickness in one analysis, but no other characteristics of the primary tumor were predictive (29), whereas thickness, ulceration and mitotic rate were all independently predictive in one database (30). For melanomas > 4 mm in thickness, vascular involvement, Breslow depth, and ulceration have proved to be independent predictors of survival by multivariate analysis (28,31).

Regardless of newer technologies and special situations, such as discussed above, more recent multivariate analyses of large databases confirm tumor thickness as the major independent prognostic factor in melanoma (6,16,32,33). These analyses also underscore the emerging importance of tumor ulcerations as a principal prognostic factor meriting incorporation into newer staging schema (discussed later in this chapter) (16,33).

Anatomic Level Clark et al. (34) extended the work of their predecessors (21) and defined five levels of tumor invasion in the dermis and subcutis (Fig. 12-1), presenting evidence that increasing level of invasion correlated inversely with the rate of survival. Univariate analysis has assigned prognostic power to level of invasion, and while levels retain some power on multivariate analysis (1–3,5), thickness according to Breslow predominates substantially over level in most multivariate analyses). In some reports, Clark levels have no independent prognostic effects after adjustment for thickness (14,25), although in other reports tumors < 1 mm in thickness could be significantly stratified for metastatic hazard by levels. In one of these analyses, which involved a large database compiled from four German medical centers, Clark level III as compared to level II imparted a relative risk of 3.5 for disease progression in melanomas ≤ 1.0 mm (25). The very large database of 17,600 patients collated from 13 cancer centers also found that Clark levels were predictive in thin melanomas (≤ 1.0 mm), such that the risk ratio associated with levels by multivariate regression analysis was 1.451 (95% CI 1.253–1.680, $p < .00001$); this hazard was second only to ulceration in predictive value in the thin melanoma group (16). In a case series of 9 patients with thin (< 0.76 mm in thickness) melanomas with aggressive clinical behavior, there was a greater than expected rate of Clark level III or IV in the primary tumor (35). Similar data were reported in a Scandinavian population-based dataset (36). In some situations, therefore, anatomic level may more accurately predict stage of tumor progression (2) or may add important prognostic information to the Breslow thickness (37).

As a prognostic indicator, anatomic levels are confounded by several limitations. For one, heterogeneity exists within given Clark levels (11). For example, thick polypoid level III tumors have an overall worse prognosis than thin level III lesions. This can be explained by the greater mass of tumor in polypoid tumors. A more practical limitation is that the assessment of levels can be quite subjective (38), especially in the distinctions among levels II and III and between III and early level IV. One factor bearing on the subjectivity is that the papillary-reticular dermal interface is often indistinct histologically; this is especially true for acral skin, and assessment of levels is not possible for mucosal surfaces (38). Consequently, there are limitations in the interobserver reproducibility in the assignment of Clark's levels. In one study, the overall rate of agreement was 71.6% for level I, 66.7% for level II, 67.3% for level III, 69.1% for level IV, and 80% for level V (39).

Ulceration As an independent prognostic factor in some, but not all, multivariate analyses, ulceration is a histologic criterion that is generally reproducible among observers, as reflected in a κ value of 0.65 (40). It is strongly linked with tumor thickness (3,16,41) and in some studies weakly correlated with both anatomic site and gender (42). It was found not to be an independent risk factor in a population-based dataset (15). Nonetheless, it is independently associated with the hazard of disease progression in many reports (8,33,39), including a very large database (17,600 patients) wherein it was shown to be one of two major prognostic factors, the other being tumor thickness (16). Ulceration has consequently been incorporated as a major criterion into a newly revised staging scheme for melanoma (4). The prognostic significance of the criterion may be abrogated, however, in the subset of patients with lymph node metastasis (8).

Mitotic Rate Reflecting the proliferative capacity of tumors, the mitotic rate correlates inversely with survival (3,43). There has been, however, no standardization or consensus in the manner by which the criterion is reported in much of the older literature. The recent trend has been to report the density of mitotic figures per square millimeter in histologic section. This practice is limited by sampling error in conjunction with regional variation in the frequency of mitotic activity within tumors. Thus mitotic "hot spots" are generally quantified.

The mitotic rate is linked to tumor thickness by multivariate analysis (3), but remains an independent factor in some reports (2). If mitotic rate is excluded from analysis, ulceration becomes an independent prognostic factor in some datasets (15). A refinement has been suggested by incorporating thickness along with mitotic rate in a "prognostic index," defined as the product of mitotic rate times thickness (44,45). A marker of proliferation, Ki-67, has been assessed in immunohistochemical studies using monoclonal antibody markers such as MIB-1 directed against that cell cycle–related molecule. Melanomas > 1.5 mm in Breslow thickness that had metastasized were more strongly immunolabeled with MIB-1 compared to those tumors that had not metastasized (46). Another report evaluating the marker failed to confirm either labeling intensity with Ki-67 or mitotic rate as having significant independent prognostic value above that provided by thickness alone (47). Consequently, the prognostic value of mitotic rate remains uncertain, at least insofar as it is assessed by current methods.

Phase of Tumor Progression Radial and vertical growth phases are central components of a tumor progression model that dichotomizes the natural history of melanoma into discrete risk categories assigned by histologically assessed patterns of growth, in which it is hypothesized that tumors in the radial phase have no potential for metastasis, whereas vertical growth phase tumors do possess that potential (2,48). The proponents of the concept have observed that the survival rate is 100% at 8 years for patients with tumors < 1 mm in thickness and restricted to the radial growth phase (2,48). Because only 30% of melanomas exhibiting vertical phase growth in the database of Clark et al. have metastasized (2,22), the general utility of the concept may be limited. Correlation of growth phase of tumor progression with tumor thickness has similar implications. Moreover, interobserver concordance in assigning growth phase has not yet been accurately quantified. A case-control study of 43 metastasizing thin (< 1 mm) melanomas reported 10 "nontumorigenic" radial growth phase melanomas, including two in situ lesions, that metastasized (49). Similar results in another large case-control study of thin (< 1 mm) metastasizing melanomas have been reported, in which 41% of metastasizing lesions were in the radial growth phase at the time of original diagnosis (50). Two additional instances of metastasizing radial growth phase melanomas were independently described (51). Thus the clinical reliability and predictive value of the criterion of growth phase, or its definition, should be viewed with caution.

Regression Controversy has long existed regarding the effects of regression on prognosis in melanoma (52–66). The original observations of several independent groups suggested that thin melanomas (< 0.76 mm) with regression have greater than expected risk for metastasis (2,54,61–63,65,66). Other analyses failed to confirm the association on long term follow up (35,59,64,67).

Definitive conclusions as to the role of regression in assignment of prognosis are limited by lack of standardization of criteria for its diagnosis, by extrapolation from small datasets, and by limited follow up observation. One particular difficulty is the distinction of regression from tumor stromal reactions (58). According to studies that quantified the interobserver κ value for regression to be 0.32, the histologic diagnosis of regression is poorly reproducible among observers (40).

Table 12-4 summarizes the studies correlating the frequency of regression in thin melanomas with prognosis. According to a more recent study of melanomas < 1.5 mm in thickness, regression, in conjunction with thickness, and the absence of tumor infiltration were predictors of disease progression (68). In a case-control analy-

TABLE 12-4 Frequency of histologic regression in thin melanomas and its effect on prognosis.

Number of patients	Number with regression	Number without regression	Metastasis Number with regression	Metastasis Number without regression	Effects of regression on prognosis	Reference
121	23 (19%)	98	5 (21.7%)	2 (2%)	Adverse	53
36	11 (30%)	25	5 (45.5%)	3 (12%)	Adverse	54
116	41 (36.3%)	75	1 (1.3%)	0	None	55
353	205 (58%)	148	17 (8%)	3 (5%)	None	56
90	NA[a]	NA	3/8	5/8	None	57
48 (extremities)	11 (23%)	37	0	0	None	58
251	69 (27%)	185	5 (7.2%)	7 (3.8%)	None	59
486	85 (17%) slight active 66 (14%) marked active 122 (25%) past	213	NA	NA	Adverse[b]	61
649	NA	NA	17/20	3	Adverse	62
103	30 (29%)	73	6 (>77% regression)	0	Adverse	63
846	518 (61%)	328	41 (7.9%)	20 (6.1%)	None	64
681	Mild 14.65% Moderate 18.2% Severe 19.8%		40%	17%	Adverse for severe regression	65
555	13/26 metastasis 1/40 no recurrence		NA	NA	Adverse	66
287	249 (86.8%)	38	NA	NA	None	68
85	20 (23.5%)	65	18 (42%)	25	Adverse	49
110	44 (40%)	66	27 (50%)	27	N/A	50

[a]Not available.
[b]There was 79% 10-year survival for past regression versus 95% for no regression.

sis of metastasizing thin (< 1mm in Breslow thickness) melanomas, extensive regression was present in 42% of the cases, compared to 5% of cases of thin melanoma without metastasis (p = .001) (49). Another case-control study of thin melanomas found regression in 50% of metastasizing lesions and 30.4% of nonmetastasizing controls (p = .036) (50). Evaluating the literature collectively, therefore, it is likely that extensive regression with involution of virtually the entire primary tumor has an adverse prognostic effect.

Vascular Invasion The presence of melanoma cells within vascular or lymphatic channels correlates with reduced survival. One analysis showed a 35.3% survival at 8 years versus 73.9% for comparable vertical growth phase (VGP) tumors without vascular invasion (2). In another dataset, relapse-free survival was 26.1 months without vascular invasion and 10.2 months with invasion (p < .001), and overall survival was 54.2 months versus 32.6 months, respectively (p = .001); the adverse effect of the phenomenon persisted under multivariate analysis, being equivalent to the effect of ulceration and second only to tumor thickness in prognostic power (69). Vascular invasion correlated as an independent factor predicting reduced survival in other multivariate analyses, but it was linked to tumor thickness, diameter, and ulceration (70,71). The utility of the criterion, however, is limited by its infrequent occurrence and by false-positive mimicry due to the artifact of tissue shrinkage (38).

Microscopic Satellites As a criterion, the histologic assessment of microscopic satellites is constrained by both arbitrary definition and by mimicry from direct extension of the primary tumor in histologic sections—that is, pseudopod-like extensions of the melanoma mass in which the connecting cells happen not to be displayed in the planes of section. In regard to the former constraint, how large must a tumor cell mass be for diagnosis and how far from the primary tumor must it be to qualify as a satellite? Without supportive empirical data, any attempt at an objective definition would be arbitrary. Nevertheless, conventional definition requires an aggregate of at least 0.05 mm in diameter that is localized to the der-

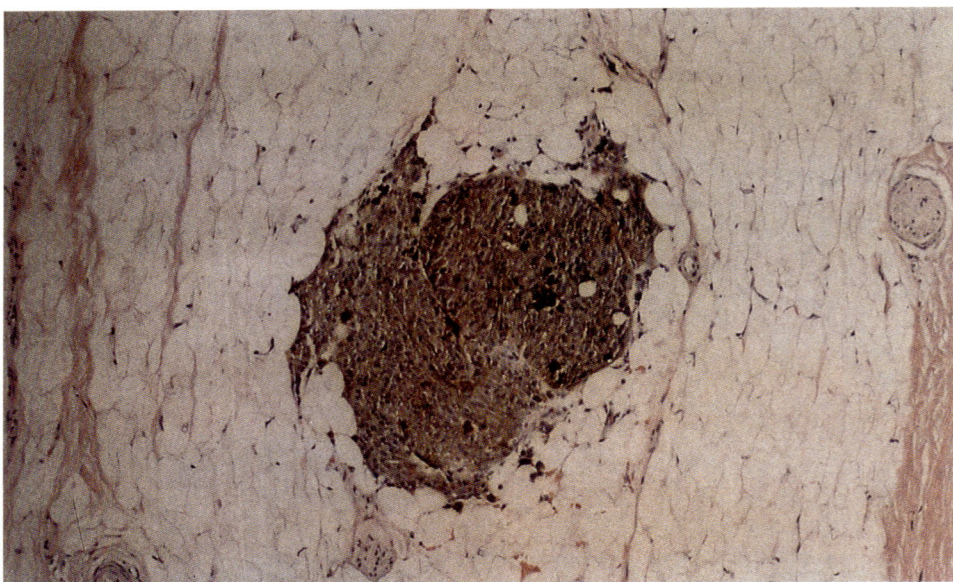

FIGURE 12-2 Microscopic satellite in subcutaneous fat. The primary melanoma measured 8.19 mm in thickness.

mis, subcutis, or intravascular sites and separated in two-dimensional histologic section from the primary tumor by normal tissue (72,73) (Fig. 12-2). Conceptually, the development of satellites may be related to vascular invasion, which would account for the correlation with lymph node and visceral metastasis (73). Thus on univariate analysis they are associated with decreased survival—40% at 8 years compared to 75.2% without satellites (2)—but the effect generally disappears with adjustment for the major prognostic factors on multivariate analyses, with the exception of some studies (74,75).

Host Response and Lymphocytic Infiltration The notion that host cell–mediated immunity exerts an appreciable effect in preventing or constraining the development of malignancy has long held conceptual appeal. As with the criterion of regression, however, there has been no objective consensus definition for the grading and reporting of host response (76). Investigators variously base their assessments on lymphocytic infiltrates at the base of the tumor, at the lateral perimeter, and within the tumor mass itself. The reproducibility of the criterion is thus in question and the results not surprisingly contradictory (38,73,77–81). There is, nonetheless, some evidence that a lymphocytic response at the base of a melanoma tumor exerts a favorable effect on prognosis (2,82). The association is limited by the well-recognized inverse correlation of lymphocytic response with tumor depth (82), which raises questions as to its independent prognostic value.

After adjustment for other parameters, such as thickness, the presence of tumor-infiltrating lymphocytes (TILs) has been reported to be a significant factor (2). In that study, TILs were defined as "brisk" if lymphocytes permeated the melanoma tumor and the entire base of the lesion. Brisk TILs proved to be one of the most significant criteria in a multifactorial model of prognosis. Subsequent support for the prognostic power of the lymphocytic response emerged from a multivariate analysis that employed "strict" standards for definition of the criterion (67). *Brisk* TILs required lymphocytes to be present throughout the substance of the VGP or across its entire base, *nonbrisk* required lymphocyte aggregates at one or more foci within or at the periphery of the tumor, and *absent* denoted no lymphocytic infiltration of the tumor (67). In that analysis, only thickness and TILs were independent factors by multivariate analysis among the histologic criteria. The 5-year overall survival rates were, respectively, 55%, 45%, and 27% for brisk, nonbrisk, and absent TILs (67). Quantification of the lymphocytic infiltration in histologic section has refined the use of this criterion in one detailed analysis (83). The independent prognostic effect of TILs was lost on multivariate analysis in another database (15). The presence of plasma cells and macrophages within the infiltrate has been suggested to have adverse prognostic effects (84,85).

Histogenetic Type The concept that melanomas develop as distinctive histogenetic types led to attempts to classify melanomas into qualitatively discrete categories based on recognition of differences in the cytologic and histologic phenotype of tumors. As a result of these attempts, it was considered for some time that melanomas of lentigo maligna type portend a better prognosis than is associated with superficial spreading and nodular melanomas (12,34). Subsequent studies suggested that any differences in overall prognosis were simply explained by differences in average tumor thicknesses (2,3,86), as reflected in declining average thicknesses of tumor types in the following order: nodular melanoma > superficial spreading melanoma > lentigo maligna melanoma (82).

This theme has been repeated in later reports, which have found no association of prognosis with type of melanoma (14) and particularly no difference associated with diagnosis of the lentigo maligna subtype as compared with superficial spreading and nodular melanomas by multivariate analysis (87). The poor prognosis of acral lentiginous melanomas has been explained by the adverse effect of location at acral, glabrous (non-hair-bearing) sites (88). Moreover, imprecise interobserver concordance has been observed in the classification of melanoma type, with a κ value reported to be 0.52 (40).

Tumor Cell Type Various investigators have evaluated the prognostic significance of the predominant cell population making up the invasive component of melanoma, whether of spindle, epithelioid, nevoid, or small cell type (80,89–92). It has been held that melanomas composed of a spindle cell population have a better than expected prognosis compared to epithelioid or other types (1,93,94), and although the spindled phenotype has had a favorable prognostic influence on univariate analysis, the effect has not persisted in multivariate analyses (2,30,38). The concept of the *minimal deviation melanoma* has been invoked to reflect the less-aggressive course associated with a well-differentiated, or nevoid, cell type; but the concept has not gained general acceptance. Morphometry and related techniques of image analyses have been introduced to quantify cell type more precisely (95). A general limitation to the use of melanoma cell type as a prognostic indicator is that heterogeneity of cell populations is rather common within melanoma tumors, particularly with respect to a combination of spindled and epithelioid cell types. The problem is further confounded by the lack of reproducible definitions of the different cell types. Thus stratification of risk on the basis of tumor cell type has not at present gained general acceptance.

Tumor Vascularity Angiogenesis is considered necessary for growth of tumors beyond a diameter of 1–2 mm (96). Recent times have experienced increased interest in the application of vascular parameters as predictors of outcome. Preliminary evidence was presented that tumor vascularity (expressed as percent vascular area) may be a significant prognostic factor, with greater vascularity correlating with higher risk of metastasis (97), and in another study increased vascular area was significantly higher in metastasizing melanomas of intermediate thickness (98), but other results have not been confirmatory (99). More recent investigations have employed immunostaining of tissue sections with endothelial markers as a means to enhance precision in evaluating the density of tumor vascularity. In one such study, high vascular density assessed by CD31 staining correlated with improved survival in univariate analysis, but it was not an independent prognostic factor by multivariate analysis (100). Combined vessel immunolabeling with CD105, vascular endothelial growth factor (VEGF) receptor, and factor VIII as measures of microvessel density in primary tumors and in metastases indicated that labeling with CD105 and factor VIII, but not with VEGF receptor, correlated with disease progression (101).

Tumor Volume The original objective of Breslow was to measure the volume of the primary tumor as a prognostic factor for melanoma. Because of the practical limitations associated with conventional, two-dimensional histologic analysis, he simply resorted to thickness as a surrogate measure of tumor volume (10). Because it remains likely that tumor volume confers more prognostic information than unidimensional thickness alone, efforts have periodically been made to implement computerized methods to approximate tumor volume. In one small study ($n = 25$), volume indeed proved to be more discriminatory of outcome than was thickness: the survival rate was 91.4% for tumor volume < 200 mm^3 versus 16.7% for volume > 200 mm^3 (102).

Cross-Sectional Profile Cross-sectional profile refers to the topologic growth pattern of a tumor as reflected in its two-dimensional silhouette in vertical section. The silhouette may be plaque-like or dome shaped, or it may present a polypoid or verrucous profile, as two of the more common patterns among the melanoma variants that have been linked to reduced survival by multivariate analysis (94). It is not clear, however, that prognostic information related to the cross-sectional profile is entirely independent of the effects of tumor thickness (103).

Neurotropism and Desmoplasia The propensity of certain types of melanoma to percolate along the tissue planes of the perineurium is referred to as neurotropism. Desmoplasia is defined as an exaggeration of the usual fibrosis associated with the host stromal response to melanoma. Both features have been incriminated as factors responsible for a greater risk of local recurrence, in part due to difficulties at the clinical and histologic levels with adequately defining the peripheral extension of the primary tumor. Moreover, neurotropism, but not desmoplasia, has been associated as an independent risk factor with reduced survival in one large database (104).

Clinical Factors

Age Both the incidence and the thickness of melanoma increase directly with age (105). Some investigators have posited an independent, adverse effect of increasing age on prognosis after adjustment for the major risk factors (106). Other hazard models have not confirmed this association (2). Age did remain a significant factor in the multivariate analysis of Austin et al. (107), wherein age > 65 years and thickness were the only independent predictors of adverse outcome.

Anatomic Site The location of the primary melanoma may have an independent effect on prognosis (2,3), but location is clearly a covariate with gender (i.e., legs in women and trunk in men are the principal gender-dependent sites of predisposition) and to a lesser degree thickness and ulceration (3,42). Large multivariate analyses have, nonetheless, confirmed the independent effect of site on survival (2). Extremity melanomas have a better than expected prognosis compared to other sites (2), whereas scalp and the glabrous skin of the acra are considered prognostically adverse sites (88). Additional multivariate analyses have shown an unfavorable prognosis associated with location on the scalp, neck, and trunk (14) and with sites on the thorax, upper arm, neck, and scalp (TANS) (108). A potential explanation for these empirical observations is that extremity melanomas upon relapse are more prone to local recurrence or regional nodal metastasis, whereas axial melanomas have a greater propensity for visceral metastasis with its higher attendant risk of mortality (109).

Gender In some multivariate analyses, female gender imparts an independent and favorable prognostic outlook (2). The effect of gender, however, has not been robust in other datasets and analyses, in part because gender is confounded by an association with thickness, ulceration, and, most important, predilection for anatomic sites on the extremities (42). Nevertheless, a study from Duke University determined that female gender accounted for a ∼22% survival advantage after adjustment for thickness and other covariates (32). Similarly robust results for a favorable prognostic effect of female gender emerged from analysis of a Swedish database, wherein women had a 33% lower relative hazard than men (14), and from the studies of Karakousis and Driscoll (110), who determined by multivariate analysis that gender was more predictive of outcome than was site.

Pathologic Stage Clinically occult, microscopic metastasis to lymph nodes (AJCC stage III) markedly reduces survival probability from melanoma. Survival at 5 years is 42% with microscopic metastasis (5,111,112), versus > 80% for all stage I–II patients (5). Risk is further stratified on the basis of extent of nodal involvement, so that clinically overt and clinically occult (i.e., microscopic) metastasis is associated with 21% versus 44% 5-year survival, respectively (113). Within the group of patients with macroscopic nodal involvement, the prognosis is related to size of the metastatic deposit(s) and numbers of nodes involved, as well as by characteristics of the primary tumor, particularly the Breslow thickness (111). The prognostic effects of Breslow thickness in microscopic stage III disease vary inversely with the extent of nodal involvement (111).

Pregnancy Status The influence of pregnancy and hormonal status on survival from melanoma has been a controversial subject, with studies showing favorable effects, adverse effects, or no effects at all (114–125) (Table 12-5). There is no consistent association between risk of melanoma and history of oral contraceptive use (117). Definitive conclusions as to the prognostic effects of pregnancy, if any, have been hampered by the small size of the datasets available for analysis and insufficient control for the effects of the major prognostic factors, especially Breslow thickness. The preponderance of the larger study populations has failed to conclusively establish an adverse effect of pregnancy (120–122,125). In a large case-control study, early childbearing and multiparity were associated

TABLE 12-5 Prognostic effect of pregnancy on outcome of stage I melanoma.

Number of patients	5-year survival	Effect of pregnancy on survival	Effect of pregnancy on disease-free interval	Effect of pregnancy on interval to nodal metastasis	Reference
20	80%	None	None	NA[b]	120
58	∼90%[a]	None	Significantly shortened	NA	118
66	86%	None	None	NA	121
23	∼85%[a]	None	None	NA	122
100	∼82%[a]	None	Significantly shortened	Significantly shortened	123, 124
92	∼80%[a]	None	None	None	125

[a]Estimate of 5-year survival rates from actuarial survival curves.
[b]Not available.

with a 5-year, ~8–16% reduced risk of melanoma (127). A retrospective, controlled study determined that the mean thickness of pregnancy-associated melanomas was significantly greater than that of non–pregnancy-associated tumors (2.28 versus 1.22 mm, respectively, $p < .007$) (128), suggesting that any apparent effects of pregnancy on outcome may be explained by differences in thickness of the primary tumor at time of diagnosis. The case-control study of Slingluff et al. (123,124), nonetheless, determined that median disease-free intervals and time to development of lymph node metastases were shorter in pregnant patients and that pregnancy was significantly associated with the development of metastatic disease by multivariate analysis, but that pregnancy by itself was not a risk factor for overall patient mortality.

Local Recurrence The development of local recurrence from a melanoma at the site of original treatment is an uncommon event, occurring in only 1.3% of patients in one large population-based dataset and in from 1 to < 10% of patients in a review of the literature (129). It has long been taken as a grave prognostic indicator. Analyses of the prognostic effects of local recurrence, however, have not been consistent across multiple independent datasets. Local recurrence had no overriding, detrimental effect on survival in one study, being associated with a 28% fatality rate at a median follow up of 8 years (129). In contrast, investigators from Duke University determined that local recurrence had grave implications, with a 48.5% mortality rate at 5 years (130). More ominous were observations from long-term follow-up of the Intergroup study sponsored by the National Cancer Institute. In that database, local recurrence was a strong independent factor on multivariate analysis, being associated with a 9% 5-year and a 5% 10-year survival rate, compared to an 86% rate of survival in the absence of local recurrence (131). Confirmatory results by multivariate analysis of the adverse prognostic effects of local recurrence, independent of the effects of ulceration and tumor thickness, emerged from an Australian study, wherein local recurrence signified progressive disease and was associated with a 41% mortality rate at 5 years (132).

One explanation for the apparent discrepancies with respect to the adverse effects of local recurrence derives from differences in operational definition. Depending on how the phenomenon is defined, local recurrence could represent persistence of the primary tumor due to inadequate margin control at the time of original diagnosis and treatment, or it could represent the development of local satellitosis in the immediate environment of the primary site. Because satellitosis is considered to signify the pending systematization of melanoma, the two processes should have vastly different prognostic implications.

Other Factors

Melanocytic Nuclear Volume Stereologic techniques have been used to calculate volume-weighted mean nuclear volume in 71 stage I–II melanoma patients, leading to the observation that the calculated values had greater prognostic significance than either nuclear DNA content or tumor thickness (133). An independent study of 32 thin melanomas (< 0.76 mm) confirmed the association of nuclear volume with metastatic probability (134). In a study of thick melanomas, morphometric analysis of nuclear area and shape factors correlated with prognosis (135).

DNA-Ploidy As a prognostic factor, the significance of DNA content within melanoma cells is unsettled because of conflicting data (136–138). Interpretation of results has been constrained by the confounding effects of tumor thickness and by methodologic variations, such as use of flow versus image cytometry, fresh versus formalin-fixed tissue, nonstandardized instrumentation, and methodologic differences in data analysis and interpretation (137,138). DNA aneuploidy was found to be a significant, independent prognostic factor in an analysis of 177 stage I–II patients (136), but the association was not as robust in a separate analysis (137) and was not substantiated by critical review of the literature (138). The applicability of DNA-ploidy analysis is further limited by observations suggesting that up to two thirds of melanomas lack aneuploidy and that aneuploidy when present is a covariate of Breslow thickness.

Since the first edition of this textbook, interest has substantially increased in the evaluation of DNA-ploidy and S-phase analysis as clinically useful prognostic indicators. A multivariate analysis of melanoma patients with metastatic disease found that ploidy and S-phase DNA fraction were independently related to survival, such that median survival times were 45 months for diploid melanomas, 18 months for aneuploid tumors, 45 months for S-phase fraction > 5%, and 19 months for fraction > 10% (139). Aneuploidy also correlated with worse overall survival in a population with regional lymph node metastasis in another analysis (140). The S-phase fraction, as well as the mitotic index, independently correlated with poor overall survival in a multivariate analysis of a Finnish dataset of stage I–II patients followed up for a mean of 6.4 years (141). Contrarily, although correlations existed between aneuploidy and advanced stage, ploidy studies were suggested to be not useful for predicting the metastatic potential of primary melanoma in a separate study comparing DNA content by flow and image cytometry between melanoma tumors of different clinical stage (142).

Nucleolar Organizer Regions Nucleolar organizer regions (NORs) are circular arrangements of chromosomal DNA within nucleoli that encode for ribosomal RNA and that when visualized as black dots by silver stains are designated AgNORs (143). Among 98 melanoma patients with disease clinically restricted to the primary site, the mean number of AgNORS (2.792 ± 0.901) was significantly less in patients without metastasis than the mean number (4.889 ± 1.403) in patients with metastasis (144). AgNOR counts > 3.62 were associated with an 82% probability of developing metastasis in that dataset (144). The reliability of this method of prognostication requires validation by other studies, but unfortunately interest in AgNOR counts has diminished in more recent times.

Proliferation and Motility Digital image analysis has been employed as a means of quantifying the contributions of proliferation and motility to outcome in melanoma (145,146). Proliferation rate is currently often assessed by immunolabeling of Ki-67, which is a nuclear molecule expressed in cells actively transiting the cell division cycle. In one study, quantification of the mitotic rate and immunolabeling of Ki-67, taken in conjunction with a morphologic measure of tumor invasiveness, correlated significantly with overall and disease-free survival (146). Labeling for either Ki-67 or proliferating cell nuclear antigen (PCNA; another marker for proliferation) has also correlated significantly with disease-free and overall survival by univariate analysis (147). Another confirmatory study found that Ki-67 labeling of primary melanoma tumors retained prognostic significance by multivariate analysis (148).

Circulating Melanoma Cells In recent years, interest has increased in developing methods by which to detect evidence of melanoma cells in the systemic circulation, the objective being the implementation of more reliable, prospective indicators of clinical relapse. Much of the effort has focused on the amplification by RT-PCR of mRNA sequences that are unique to cells of melanocytic lineage within the general vascular circulation (149–160). Tyrosinase mRNA, which has been the principle focus of these effects, was first reported to be a sensitive method to detect circulating melanoma cells in blood samples by Smith et al. (149). A later case-control study that examined RT-PCR signals for tyrosinase in the blood of melanoma cases and matched controls found a 3.8-fold increased risk of disease relapse associated with the presence of a positive signal (150). In later analyses, odds ratios for disease progression and/or an overall decrease in survival ranged from 2.4 to 4.33 (151–156). Illustrative studies that have correlated the percentages of cases positive for tyrosinase RT-PCR signals with stage of disease are listed in Table 12-6. Not all results, however, have been entirely consistent across independent analyses (159). In one dataset, RT-PCR of blood tyrosinase failed to detect the likelihood of clinical relapse, prompting the investigators to conclude that the technique is presently not adequate for monitoring melanoma progression (160). In a study that screened for multiple circulating melanoma antigen markers, p97, MUC18, and Melan-A, but not tyrosinase, were found to be independently associated with prognosis (151). Demonstrating the variability in the literature, other investigators have found in their databases that tyrosinase RT-PCR (153) or multimarker RT-PCR (tyrosinase, MAGE-3, MUC-18, p97) (152) constituted a significant, independent prognostic marker signifying increased risk of relapse. Nonetheless, detection of tyrosinase transcripts by RT-PCR cannot be considered at present a reliable marker for melanoma progression.

Other strategies have included assay for serum levels of S-100 protein by immunochemical methods. S-100 protein is not normally found in significant levels within the blood, and increased levels can be taken as a presumptive indicator of circulating melanocytic cells. Indeed, the detection of serum S-100 protein has correlated with reduced survival from melanoma (161). In a later study of patients with metastatic melanoma, elevated S-100 protein levels correlated with reduced survival on univariate but not multivariate analysis (162). Levels did

TABLE 12-6 Correlation of rate of blood tyrosinase RT-PCR positivity with stage of disease.

	Percent of patients tyrosinase RT-PCR positive			
Stage I	Stage II	Stage III	Stage IV	Reference
			50%	150
	2.3%[a]	0%	27.3%	157
	0%[a]	0%	38%	158
	13%[a]	17%	44%	159
31%	39%	49%	75%	151
19%	31%	29%	52%	154
11%	18%	31%	67%	153
34%	51%	50%	65%	206

[a]Combined stages I and II.

correlate with metastatic events in another database, yielding a specificity for detection of metastasis of 0.96 but a low sensitivity of 0.32; the impact of serum S-100 protein assay on survival time was thus considered to require further study (163).

S-100B protein, a putatively more specific serum marker for circulating melanoma cells, was tested by Hauschild et al. (164), who found that S-100B protein levels ≥ 0.2 μg/L in patients with stage IV melanoma significantly predicted reduced survival. The adverse prognostic effect persisted on multivariate analysis (165). In a large group of melanoma patients ($n = 1007$), serum S-100B protein levels by luminescence immunoassay proved to be the strongest independent prognostic marker by multivariate analysis in patients with regional or distant metastatic disease, but the levels were not significant predictors in melanoma clinically localized to the primary site, wherein tumor thickness remained the strongest prognostic factor (166).

Miscellany By cytogenic criteria, the number of chromosome 9p markers that were deleted correlated directly with adverse outcome, but multivariate analysis was not employed in the study design (167). The significance of this observation rests with the assignment of the major melanoma tumor suppressor gene, CDKN2A/p16, to chromosome 9p (168). Cyclin A, which acts in the cell-division cycle as a regulatory subunit in molecular complexes with CDK4 (168), is a candidate protooncogene. By immunohistochemical labeling, the protein levels of cyclin A and the proliferation marker Ki-67 increased with increasing stage of melanoma, such that the levels of expression significantly correlated as independent predictors of adverse outcome (169). Micropthalmia transcription factor (MITF) is a factor that is embryologically required for melanocytic development and differentiation. By immunolabeling, increased expression of MITF was associated by multivariate analysis with improved overall and disease-free survival in intermediate (1–4 mm) thickness melanomas (170). Similarly, high levels of expression of the melanocytic marker Melan A (Mart-1) correlated with favorable survival by Kaplan-Meier analysis (171).

The major pathologic and clinical prognostic factors that have been evaluated in multivariate analyses that included > 450 cases and > 5 years mean follow-up are summarized in Table 12-7.

PROGNOSTIC FACTORS FOR STAGE III MELANOMA

The revised AJCC staging system for cutaneous melanoma assigns cases with metastasis to regional lymphatic basins to revised clinical stage III, which is further subclassified based on numbers of involved nodes and whether the metastatic deposits are clinically occult or overt (4,172) (Table 12-1). The importance of regional lymph node metastasis is reflected in the statistic that lymph nodes constitute the first site of relapse in > 50% of all patients who develop recurrent disease (173). More significantly, however, overall survival from melanoma decreases to 30–50% at 5 years once nodal relapse has occurred, but there is considerable heterogeneity with respect to outcome, depending on the extent of nodal involvement (2,12,111,174–176). In general, survival following nodal relapse becomes largely independent of the primary tumor characteristics (8,173), however, outcome in patients with nodal relapse can be influenced by histologic characteristics of the primary tumor, especially thickness and to a lesser degree ulceration (16) and anatomic site (Table 12-8). Prognosis is particularly influenced by tumor thickness in cases with limited node involvement, for example in the situation of occult (i.e., microscopic) metastasis (111), but nodal factors dominate the prognostic models with clinically manifest node involvement.

The most important nodal prognostic factors relate to the degree of lymph node involvement and whether metastatic disease is clinically manifest (16). The number of positive nodes is the single most important variable across most databases at this stage of disease (8,112). The large database described by Balch et al. (16) reported number of nodal metastases to be the most significant predictor of outcome in stage III patients, with a χ^2 value of > 57 and a risk ratio of 1.257 ($p < .0001$). The 5-year survival rate was 61% for one microscopically involved node (46% for one macroscopically involved node) and 35% for more than four microscopically involved nodes (24% for more than four macroscopically involved nodes). In other studies, patients with three or fewer involved nodes had a 45% 5-year survival versus 21% survival for patients with four or more positive nodes (112), and the 5-year overall survival rates corresponding to one, two to four, and more than 4 involved nodes were 58%, 25%, and 11%, respectively (177). Involvement of three or more nodes, or the presence of palpable nodes, conferred significantly adverse prognosis in yet another study by multivariate analysis (178). In addition to the preeminent effect of number of positive nodes, other measures of tumor burden, including size of metastatic deposits relative to total nodal mass, have prognostic value in certain situations (179). Some analyses have shown that the thickness of the primary tumor, along with the number of nodes involved, constitutes the major, statistically significant prognostic factor on multivariate analysis, irrespective of size of the nodal deposits (180,181). In the collated database of Balch et al. (16) including patients followed for > 5 years, the three major independent prognostic factors once nodal metastasis had occurred

TABLE 12-7 Multivariate studies of prognostic factors in stage I–II melanoma, including > 450 cases and ≥ 5 years mean or median follow-up[a]

n	Accrual period	Breslow thickness	Ulceration	Site of primary	Gender	Age at diagnosis	Mitosis	Clark level	Regression	Histogenic type	Source
747	1967–75	+	—	NS	+	NS	—	NS	—	NS	Cascinelli (1980)
1931	1949–78	+	+	+	NS	NS	+	+	+	NS	Söndergaard/Schou (1985)
879	1972–82	+	—	NS	NS	NS	NS	NS	—	NS	Kopf (1987)
714	1964–82	+	+	+	+	NS	NS	NS	NS	—	Drzewiecki et al. (1990)
832	1972–82	+	—	+	NS	NS	NS	—	—	—	Vossaert et al. (1992)
4568	1955–86	+	+	+	+	+	—	+	—	NS	Balch et al. (1992)
3323	1971–91	+	—	+	+	+	—	+	—	—	Morton et al. (1993)
2004	1978–85	+	—	+	NS	+	—	—	—	NS	Gamel et al. (1993)
476	1960–84	+	+	+	+	+	+	NS	NS	NS	Thörn et al. (1994)
1978	1979–86	+	+	+	+	+	—	+	NS	+	MacKie et al. (1995)
675	1976–88	+	—	+	+	+	—	—	—	—	Karakousis/Driscoll (1995)
629	1980–85	+	—	+	+	+	+	—	—	—	Helfenstein et al. (1996)
548	1987–89	+	NS	NS	NS	NS	—	NS	NS	NS	Barnhill et al. (1996)
488	1972–79	+	—	+	+	+	—	NS	—	NS	Schuchter et al. (1996)
620	1970–96	+	+	NS	NS	+	—	—	—	NS	Averbook et al. (1998)
1229	1980–94	+	—	+	+	+	+	—	—	—	Levi et al. (1998)
691	1985–91	+	NS	+	NS	NS	—	—	NS	—	Ostmeier et al. (1999)
727	1965–89	+	+	+	+	+	—	—	—	NS	Måsbäck et al. (2001)
Number (%) of studies with effect on prognosis		18 (100%)	7 (78%)	14 (78%)	11 (61%)	11 (61%)	4 (57%)	4 (40%)	1 (17%)	1 (8%)	

Source: Adapted from Måsbäck et al. (2001) (207), with permission.

[a] +, significant effect on prognosis; NS, no significant effect; —, not examined.

TABLE 12-8 Prognostic factors for clinical stage III melanoma (regional lymph node involvement).

Factor	Effect on prognosis
Nodal Factors	
Number of positive nodes	Worse prognosis with increasing number of positive nodes
Percentage of positive nodes (< 20% vs. > 20%)	Worse prognosis with increasing percent positive nodes
Micro vs. macrometastases	Worse prognosis with macrometastases
Extent of nodal metastasis (limited by, or invasion through, capsule)	Worse prognosis with invasion through capsule
Total tumor diameter as percentage of total node diameter (≤ 15% vs. ≥ 15%)	Worse prognosis with total tumor diameter ≥ 15%
DNA-ploidy	Worse prognosis with DNA aneuploidy
Clonality (monoclonal versus polyclonal)	Worse prognosis with monoclonality
Primary melanoma factors	
Tumor thickness (especially for minimal nodal disease)	Worse prognosis with increasing tumor thickness
Ulceration	Worse prognosis with ulceration
Clinical factors	
Anatomic site (axial versus extremity)	Worse prognosis with axial site
Age	Worse prognosis with increasing age

were number of metastatic nodes, whether the nodes were clinically occult or apparent, and the presence or absence of primary tumor ulceration. Ulceration was the only primary tumor feature that predicted an adverse outcome in stage III disease, being associated with a χ^2 value of > 23 ($p < .00001$) and reducing the 5-year survival rate of patients with one involved lymph node from 65 to 45% ($p < .0001$) (16). Extracapsular extension of nodal metastases on microscopic examination can be an additional adverse prognostic factor on multivariate analysis (177).

The advent of sentinel lymphatic mapping has considerably stimulated interest in the prognostic effects of tumor characteristics within the nodes draining primary melanomas. The number of positive sentinel lymph nodes correlates significantly with overall and disease-free survival, such that the 5-year survival with negative nodes was 97.9% in one study (182). Tumor thickness > 1.5 mm, ulceration, and lymphatic invasion are the independent variables by multivariate logistic regression that significantly predict the presence of micrometastasis in the sentinel node (183). The hazard of positive micrometastasis to the sentinel node correlates directly with Breslow thickness of the primary tumor, with the frequency of involvement ranging from 1% for lesions ≤ 0.75 mm in thickness to 35.5% for tumors > 4.0 mm (184).

In regard to survival, the presence or absence of lymph node metastasis as determined by sentinel mapping, along with other parameters such as Breslow thickness and ulceration constitute the major, independent prognostic factors in some analyses (185,186). The 5-year disease-free survival in sentinel node negative and positive patients was 91% and 49%, respectively, in the report of Statius Muller et al. (186). Extracapsular spread of tumor within a sentinel node is an adverse prognostic factor (75).

RT-PCR for tyrosinase and related melanocytic markers (e.g., Mart-1, MAGE-3) within sentinel nodes has been applied to increase the sensitivity of detection of occult metastases over that achievable by routine histologic staining or immunostaining alone. From ~20 to 35% of histologically negative sentinel nodes will be positive for melanocytic markers by RT-PCR (187,188). Moreover, positive signal for tyrosinase by this method of amplification has correlated with significantly higher tumor thickness compared to patients without evidence for a tyrosinase signal (187) and has been associated with a significantly increased risk of disease relapse on multivariate analysis in more than one study (188,189). Patients with histologically melanoma-free sentinel nodes who are positive for melanoma signals by RT-PCR analysis are at significantly increased risk of relapse by multivariate analysis (183). In patients with truncal melanomas, the presence of multiple draining lymph node basins by sentinel lymphatic mapping is another independent prognostic factor predicting increased likelihood of regional lymphatic metastasis (190).

PROGNOSTIC FACTORS FOR STAGE IV MELANOMA

With the development of distant metastasis, the median survival drops precipitously to approximately 6 or 7 months (191–194), with an estimated 5-year survival rate of 6–7% (192,193). There has been no improvement in this dismal statistic within recent decades. In one database covering the period from 1971 to 1993, the survival rates of stage IV metastatic disease did not change over the 22-year period of observation (192). The principal variables determining the median survival in stage IV disease are the number of metastatic sites, initial site of metastasis, surgical resectability of the metastatic deposits, duration of remission before relapse, and size of the metastases (Table 12-9). In addition to the adverse effect of high numbers of metastatic sites and male gender (in some datasets), metastases to the brain, gastrointestinal tract, liver, and lung are adverse prognostic indicators (190–194). Nonvisceral metastasis (skin, subcutaneous tissue, distant lymph nodes) is associated with a better prognosis than visceral metastasis (16,195). Within a large dataset ($n = 217$) of late (> 10 years) recurrences from melanoma, the site of initial relapse (declining prognosis: local $>$ nodal/intransit $>$ distant) and type of initial surgical treatment (wide local excision plus elective lymph node dissection more favorable than wide local excision alone) significantly correlated with overall survival (196).

When metastatic deposits are surgically resectable, prolonged survival is possible (191). Metastatectomy at various visceral sites is an independent, favorable prognostic factor in multivariate analyses (197). In collated databases from Australia and California, median overall survival was improved in univariate analysis by total macroscopic resection of liver metastasis (198). Complete pulmonary metastatectomy improves survival significantly more than incomplete metastatectomy (199,200). Multiple resections of sequential lung metastases can also be effective in prolonging survival (201).

Histologic parameters within the metastatic tumors have been correlated with prognosis. High blood vessel density by PECAM-1 (CD-31) and VEGF immunolabeling of metastatic tumors was found to be a significant independent predictor of shortened survival in one database (202,203).

PROGNOSTIC MODELS

The purpose of multifactorial prognostic models is to identify the major variables most closely linked to outcome, thereby facilitating the prediction of survival for individual patients. Several investigators have developed mathematical models that best fit their databases. Using a large (4568) collated dataset from the University of Alabama and the Sydney Melanoma Unit, Soong et al. (204) integrated clinical with pathologic variables into an algorithm that predicts 5- and 10-year survival rates, as depicted in Table 12-10.

Similar efforts by Clark et al. (2) were founded on stage of tumor progression, dichotomized as radial and vertical growth phase, and modified by 8 prognostic variables. In their dataset, patients with melanomas restricted to the radial growth phase, irrespective of Breslow thickness, have 100% survival at 8 years. Of the 23 variables analyzed in their study, the major clinicopathologic factors were mitotic rate (worse prognosis with higher rates), tumor infiltrating lymphocytes (the more dense the infiltrate, the higher the survival), thickness, anatomic site (extremity melanomas associated with better survival than axial lesions), sex (better prognosis for females), and regression (absence of regression associated with better prognosis). Other variables with no prognostic value in their model were ulceration, microscopic satellites, levels of invasion, and pathologic stage of lymph nodes. This is surprising because multiple later studies have identified ulceration and lymph node status as potent prognostic indicators. Thus intrinsic biases in their dataset, the definition or implementation of VGP, or the limitations of extrapolation from small sets of subjects, could account for the discrepancies with other studies. Their model remains to be independently validated as a prognostic algorithm more predictive than that of thickness alone.

In an update of the multifactorial prognostic model of Clark et al., a validation group was incorporated in the analyses to better establish the predictive value of the model (7). Their dataset included 488 patients followed for more than 10 years. The major independent prognostic factors in this "four-variable model," along with odds ratios in declining order, were tumor thickness (50.8), site (4.4), age (3.0), and gender (2.0). (Table 12-11). An independent

TABLE 12-9 Prognostic factors for clinical stage IV melanoma.

Prognostic variable	Effect on prognosis
Number of metastatic sites	Worse prognosis with increasing number of sites
Location of metastases	Worse prognosis for visceral sites (lung, liver, brain, bone) versus nonvisceral sites (skin, subcutaneous tissue, distant lymph nodes)
Disease-free interval and stage of disease before distant metastasis	Worse prognosis for shortened disease-free interval and higher stage of disease before distant metastasis[a]
Presence of "resectable" metastases	Better prognosis for solitary respectable metastases
Sex	Worse outcome for males
Duration of remission	Shorter duration of remission associated with worse prognosis

[a]From Ref. 192.

TABLE 12-10 Predicted 5-year and 10-year survival rates from initial diagnosis for patients with localized melanoma.

Tumor thickness (mm)	Anatomic site	Ulceration	Clark's level	Sex	5-Year survival rate[a] (%)	10-Year survival rate[a,b] (%)
< 0.76	Extremity	—	II	—	99	97
	Extremity	—	Other	—	97	94
	Axial	—	II	—	96	92
	Axial	—	Other	—	91	84
0.76–1.49	Extremity	No	II	—	98	97
	Extremity	No	Other	—	93	89
	Extremity	Yes	II	—	94	91
	Extremity	Yes	Other	—	82	72
	Axial	No	II	—	95	93
	Axial	No	Other	—	85	77
	Axial	Yes	II	—	88	81
	Axial	Yes	Other	—	64	49
1.50–2.49	Extremity	No	—	—	86	81
	Extremity	Yes	—	—	76	69
	Axial	No	—	—	76	67
	Axial	Yes	—	—	61	49
2.50–3.99	Extremity	No	—	F	80	72
	Extremity	No	—	M	73	62
	Extremity	Yes	—	F	74	64
	Extremity	Yes	—	M	64	51
	Axial	No	—	F	73	63
	Axial	No	—	M	63	51
	Axial	Yes	—	F	65	52
	Axial	Yes	—	M	53	39
4.00–7.99	—	No	II/III	—	80	73
	—	No	IV/V	—	68	58
	—	Yes	II/III	—	67	57
	—	Yes	IV/V	—	51	38
> 8.00	—	—	—	—	43	25

Source: Soong and Weiss (1998) (204).
[a]The projected survival rates were adjusted for the effects of surgical treatment in those subgroups in which it was a significant factor.
[b]The projected 10-year survival rate for an individual patient is considered this patient's clinical score.

TABLE 12-11 Probabilities of 10-year survival in patients with primary cutaneous melanoma.

	Probability of 10-year survival (95% CI)			
	Extremity location		Axial location	
Variable	Females	Males	Females	Males
Thickness < 0.76 mm				
Age ≤ 60 years	0.99 (0.98–1.0)	0.98 (0.96–0.99)	0.97 (0.93–0.99)	0.94 (0.88–0.97)
Age > 60 years	0.98 (0.95–0.99)	0.96 (0.89–0.98)	0.92 (0.82–0.96)	0.84 (0.70–0.93)
Thickness 0.76–1.69 mm				
Age ≤ 60 years	0.96 (0.92–0.98)	0.93 (0.85–0.97)	0.86 (0.76–0.92)	0.75 (0.62–0.84)
Age > 60 years	0.90 (0.80–0.95)	0.81 (0.64–0.91)	0.67 (0.50–0.81)	0.50 (0.33–0.67)
Thickness 1.70–3.60 mm				
Age ≤ 60 years	0.89 (0.80–0.94)	0.80 (0.65–0.89)	0.65 (0.50–0.77)	0.48 (0.35–0.61)
Age > 60 years	0.73 (0.57–0.85)	0.57 (0.38–0.75)	0.38 (0.24–0.55)	0.24 (0.14–0.37)
Thickness > 3.60 mm				
Age ≤ 60 years	0.74 (0.53–0.87)	0.58 (0.36–0.77)	0.39 (0.21–0.60)	0.24 (0.13–0.40)
Age > 60 years	0.48 (0.28–0.69)	0.32 (0.16–0.53)	0.18 (0.08–0.35)	0.10 (0.04–0.20)

Source: From Schuchter et al. (1996) (7), with permission.

group at New York University validated the prognostic model of Schuchter et al. (7) with their dataset, confirming the prognostic power for predicting 10-year survival of the above criteria, except for gender (205).

REFERENCES

1. Sondergaard K, Schou G. Survival with primary cutaneous malignant melanoma, evaluated from 2012 cases. A multivariate regression analysis. Virchows Arch A Pathol Anat Histopathol 1985;406:179–95.
2. Clark WH Jr, Elder DE, Guerry D, et al. Model predicting survival in stage I melanoma based on tumor progression. J Natl Cancer Inst 1989;81:1893–904.
3. Vollmer RT. Malignant melanoma. A multivariate analysis of prognostic factors. Pathol Annu 1989;24:383–407.
4. Balch CM, Buzaid AC, Soong SJ, et al. Final version of the American Joint Committee on Cancer staging system for cutaneous melanoma. J Clin Oncol 2001;19:3635–48.
5. Rigel DS, Friedman RJ, Kopf AW, Silverman MK. Factors influencing survival in melanoma. Dermatol Clin 1991;9: 631–42.
6. Garbe C, Buttner P, Bertz J, et al. Primary cutaneous melanoma. Identification of prognostic groups and estimation of individual prognosis for 5093 patients. Cancer 1995;75:2484–91.
7. Schuchter L, Schultz DJ, Synnestvedt M, et al. A prognostic model for predicting 10-year survival in patients with primary melanoma. The Pigmented Lesion Group. Ann Intern Med 1996;125:369–75.
8. Retsas S, Henry K, Mohammed MQ, MacRae K. Prognostic factors of cutaneous melanoma and a new staging system proposed by the American Joint Committee on Cancer (AJCC): validation in a cohort of 1284 patients. Eur J Cancer 2002;38:511–6.
9. Merkel S, Meyer T, Papadopoulos T, et al. Testing a new staging system for cutaneous melanoma proposed by the American Joint Committee on Cancer. Eur J Cancer 2002; 38:517–26.
10. Breslow A. Thickness, cross-sectional areas and depth of invasion in the prognosis of cutaneous melanoma. Ann Surg 1970;172:902–8.
11. Balch CM, Murad TM, Soong SJ, et al. A multifactorial analysis of melanoma: prognostic histopathological features comparing Clark's and Breslow's staging methods. Ann Surg 1978;188:732–42.
12. Cascinelli N, Morabito A, Bufalino R. Prognosis of stage I melanoma of the skin. Int J Cancer 1980;26:733–9.
13. Balch CM, Soong SJ, Murad TM, et al. A multifactorial analysis of melanoma. II. Prognostic factors in patients with stage I (localized) melanoma. Surgery 1979;86:343–51.
14. Thorn M, Ponten F, Bergstrom R, et al. Clinical and histopathologic predictors of survival in patients with malignant melanoma: a population-based study in Sweden. J Natl Cancer Inst 1994;86:761–9.
15. Barnhill RL, Fine JA, Roush GC, Berwick M. Predicting five-year outcome for patients with cutaneous melanoma in a population-based study. Cancer 1996;78:427–32.
16. Balch CM, Soong SJ, Gershenwald JE, et al. Prognostic factors analysis of 17,600 melanoma patients: validation of the American Joint Committee on Cancer melanoma staging system. J Clin Oncol 2001;19:3622–34.
17. Allen AC, Spitz S. Melanomas: diagnosis and prognosis. Cancer 1953;6:1–45.
18. Lund RH, Ihnen M. Malignant melanoma. Clinical and pahtologic analysis of 93 cases. Is prophylactic lymph node dissection indicated? Surgery 1955;38:652–9.
19. Lane N, Lattes R, Malm J. Clinicopathological correlations in a series of 117 malignant melanomas of the skin of adults. Cancer 1958;11:1025–143.
20. Petersen NC, Bodenham DC, Lloyd OC. Malignant melanomas of the skin. Br J Plast Surg 1962;15:49–94.
21. Mehnert JH, Heard JL. Staging of malignant melanoma by depth of invasion. Am J Surg 1965;110:168–176.
22. Green MS, Ackerman AB. Thickness is not an accurate gauge of prognosis of primary cutaneous melanoma. Am J Dermatopathol 1993;15:461–73.
23. Day CL Jr, Lew RA, Mihm MC Jr, et al. The natural break points for primary-tumor thickness in clinical Stage I melanoma. N Engl J Med 1981;305:1155.
24. Buettner P, Garbe C, Guggenmoos-Holzmann I. Problems in defining cutoff points of continuous prognostic factors: example of tumor thickness in primary cutaneous melanoma. J Clin Epidemiol 1997;50:1201–10.
25. Buttner P, Garbe C, Bertz J, et al. Primary cutaneous melanoma. Optimized cutoff points of tumor thickness and importance of Clark's level for prognostic classification. Cancer 1995;75:2499–506.
26. Keefe M, Mackie RM. The relationship between risk of death from clinical stage 1 cutaneous melanoma and thickness of primary tumour: no evidence for steps in risk. Scottish Melanoma Group. Br J Cancer 1991;64:598–602.
27. Gershenwald JE, Mansfield PF, Lee JE, Ross MI. Role for lymphatic mapping and sentinel lymph node biopsy in patients with thick (> or = 4 mm) primary melanoma. Ann Surg Oncol 2000;7:160–5.
28. Zettersten E, Sagebiel RW, Miller JR III, et al. Prognostic factors in patients with thick cutaneous melanoma (> 4 mm). Cancer 2002;94:1049–56.
29. Cherpelis BS, Haddad F, Messina J, et al. Sentinel lymph node micrometastasis and other histologic factors that predict outcome in patients with thicker melanomas. J Am Acad Dermatol 2001;44:762–6.
30. Massi D, Borgognoni L, Franchi A, et al. Thick cutaneous

malignant melanoma: a reappraisal of prognostic factors. Melanoma Res 2000;10:153–64.
31. Kim SH, Garcia C, Rodriguez J, Coit DG. Prognosis of thick cutaneous melanoma. J Am Coll Surg 1999;188: 241–7.
32. Stidham KR, Johnson JL, Seigler HF. Survival superiority of females with melanoma. A multivariate analysis of 6383 patients exploring the significance of gender in prognostic outcome. Arch Surg 1994;129:316–24.
33. Balch CM, Soong S, Ross MI, et al. Long-term results of a multi-institutional randomized trial comparing prognostic factors and surgical results for intermediate thickness melanomas (1.0 to 4.0 mm). Intergroup Melanoma Surgical Trial. Ann Surg Oncol 2000;7:87–97.
34. Clark WH Jr, From L, Bernardino EA, Mihm MC. The histogenesis and biologic behavior of primary human malignant melanomas of the skin. Cancer Res 1969;29: 705–27.
35. Vilmer C, Bailly C, Le Doussal V, et al. Thin melanomas with unusual aggressive behavior: a report on nine cases. Melanoma Group of French Federation of Cancer Centers. J Am Acad Dermatol 1996;34:439–44.
36. Mansson-Brahme E, Carstensen J, Erhardt K, et al. Prognostic factors in thin cutaneous malignant melanoma. Cancer 1994;73:2324–32.
37. Marghoob AA, Koenig K, Bittencourt FV, et al. Breslow thickness and Clark level in melanoma: support for including level in pathology reports and in American Joint Committee on cancer staging. Cancer 2000;88:589–95.
38. Ronan SG, Han MC, Das Gupta TK. Histologic prognostic indicators in cutaneous malignant melanoma. Semin Oncol 1988;15:558–65.
39. Larsen TE, Grude TH. A retrospective histological study of 669 cases of primary cutaneous malignant melanoma in clinical stage I. The consequences of a reclassification of the original group of lentigo maligna melanomas. Acta Pathol Microbiol Scand A 1979;87A:255–60.
40. Lock-Andersen J, Hou-Jensen K, Hansen JP, et al. Observer variation in histological classification of cutaneous malignant melanoma. Scand J Plast Reconstr Surg Hand Surg 1995;29:141–8.
41. Balch CM, Wilkerson JA, Murad TM, et al. The prognostic significance of ulceration of cutaneous melanoma. Cancer 1980;45:3012–7.
42. Vossaert KA, Silverman MK, Kopf AW, et al. Influence of gender on survival in patients with stage I malignant melanoma. J Am Acad Dermatol 1992;26:429–40.
43. Eldh J, Boeryd B, Peterson LE. Prognostic factors in cutaneous malignant melanoma in stage I. A clinical, morphological and multivariate analysis. Scand J Plast Reconstr Surg 1978;12:243–55.
44. Schmoeckel C, Braun-Falco O. Prognostic index in malignant melanoma. Arch Dermatol 1978;114:871–3.
45. Kopf AW, Gross DF, Rogers GS, et al. Prognostic index for malignant melanoma. Cancer 1987;59:1236–41.
46. Boni R, Doguoglu A, Burg G, et al. MIB-1 immunoreactivity correlates with metastatic dissemination in primary thick cutaneous melanoma. J Am Acad Dermatol 1996;35: 416–8.
47. Talve LA, Collan YU, Ekfors TO. Nuclear morphometry, immunohistochemical staining with Ki-67 antibody and mitotic index in the assessment of proliferative activity and prognosis of primary malignant melanomas of the skin. J Cutan Pathol 1996;23:335–43.
48. Clark WH Jr, Elder DE, Guerry D, et al. A study of tumor progression: the precursor lesions of superficial spreading and nodular melanoma. Hum Pathol 1984;15:1147–65.
49. Guitart J, Lowe L, Piepkorn M, et al. Histological characteristics of metastasizing thin melanomas: a case-control study of 43 cases. Arch Dermatol 2002;138:603–8.
50. Cook MG, Spatz A, Brocker EB, Ruiter DJ. Identification of histological features associated with metastatic potential in thin ($<$ 1.0 mm) cutaneous melanoma with metastases. A study on behalf of the EORTC Melanoma Group. J Pathol 2002;197:188–93.
51. Abramova L, Slingluff CL Jr, Patterson JW. Problems in the interpretation of apparent "radial growth phase" malignant melanomas that metastasize. J Cutan Pathol 2002; 29:407–14.
52. Smith JL Jr, Stehlin JS Jr. Spontaneous regression of primary malignant melanomas with regional metastases. Cancer 1965;18:1399–415.
53. Gromet MA, Epstein WL, Blois MS. The regressing thin malignant melanoma: a distinctive lesion with metastatic potential. Cancer 1978;42:2282–92.
54. Paladagu RR, Yonemeto RH. Biologic behavior of thin malignant melanomas with regressive changes. Arch Surg 1983;118:41–4.
55. Trau H, Rigel DS, Harris MN, et al. Metastases of thin melanomas. Cancer 1983;51:553–6.
56. McGovern VJ, Shaw HM, Milton GW. Prognosis in patients with thin malignant melanoma: influence of regression. Histopathology 1983;7:673–80.
57. Briggs JC, Ibrahim NB, Hastings AG, Griffiths RW. Experience of thin cutaneous melanomas (less than 0.76 mm and less than 0.85 mm thick) in a large plastic surgery unit: a 5- to 17-year follow-up. Br J Plast Surg 1984;37:501–6.
58. Cooper PH, Wanebo HJ, Hagar RW. Regression in thin malignant melanoma. Microscopic diagnosis and prognostic importance. Arch Dermatol 1985;121:1127–31.
59. Kelly JW, Sagebiel RW, Blois MS. Regression in malignant melanoma. A histologic feature without independent prognostic significance. Cancer 1985;56:2287–91.
60. Sagebiel R. Regression and other factors of prognostic interest in malignant melanoma. Arch Dermatol 1985;121: 1125–6.

61. Sondergaard K, Hou-Jensen K. Partial regression in thin primary cutaneous malignant melanomas clinical stage I. A study of 486 cases. Virchows Arch A Pathol Anat Histopathol 1985;408:241–7.
62. Naruns PL, Nizze JA, Cochran AJ, et al. Recurrence potential of thin primary melanomas. Cancer 1986;57:545–8.
63. Ronan SG, Eng AM, Briele HA, et al. Thin malignant melanomas with regression and metastases. Arch Dermatol 1987;123:1326–30.
64. Shaw HM, McGovern VJ, Milton GW, et al. Malignant melanoma: influence of site of lesion and age of patient in the female superiority in survival. Cancer 1980;46:2731–5.
65. Slingluff CL Jr, Vollmer RT, Reintgen DS, Seigler HF. Lethal "thin" malignant melanoma. Identifying patients at risk. Ann Surg 1988;208:150–61.
66. Blessing K, McLaren KM, McLean A, Davidson P. Thin malignant melanomas (less than 1.5 mm) with metastasis: a histological study and survival analysis. Histopathology 1990;17:389–95.
67. Clemente CG, Mihm MC Jr, Bufalino R, et al. Prognostic value of tumor infiltrating lymphocytes in the vertical growth phase of primary cutaneous melanoma. Cancer 1996;77:1303–10.
68. Massi D, Franchi A, Borgognoni L, et al. Thin cutaneous malignant melanomas (< or = 1.5 mm): identification of risk factors indicative of progression. Cancer 1999;85:1067–76.
69. Kashani-Sabet M, Sagebiel RW, Ferreira CM, et al. Vascular involvement in the prognosis of primary cutaneous melanoma. Arch Dermatol 2001;137:1169–73.
70. Straume O, Akslen LA. Independent prognostic importance of vascular invasion in nodular melanomas. Cancer 1996;78:1211–9.
71. Barnhill R, Dy K, Lugassy C. Angiotropism in cutaneous melanoma: a prognostic factor strongly predicting risk for metastasis. J Invest Dermatol 2002;119:705–6.
72. Day CL Jr, Harrist TJ, Gorstein F, et al. Malignant melanoma. Prognostic significance of "microscopic satellites" in the reticular dermis and subcutaneous fat. Ann Surg 1981;194:108–12.
73. Harrist TJ, Rigel DS, Day CL Jr, et al. "Microscopic satellites" are more highly associated with regional lymph node metastases than is primary melanoma thickness. Cancer 1984;53:2183–7.
74. Leon P, Daly JM, Synnestvedt M, et al. The prognostic implications of microscopic satellites in patients with clinical stage I melanoma. Arch Surg 1991;126:1461–8.
75. Rao UN, Ibrahim J, Flaherty LE, et al. Implications of microscopic satellites of the primary and extracapsular lymph node spread in patients with high-risk melanoma: pathologic corollary of Eastern Cooperative Oncology Group Trial E1690. J Clin Oncol 2002;20:2053–7.
76. Breslow A, Macht SD. Evaluation of prognosis in stage I cutaneous melanoma. Plast Reconstr Surg 1978;61:342–6.
77. Hansen MG, McCarten AB. Tumor thickness and lymphocytic infiltration in malignant melanoma of the head and neck. Am J Surg 1974;128:557–61.
78. Elias EG, Didolkar MS, Goel IP, et al. A clinicopathologic study of prognostic factors in cutaneous malignant melanoma. Surg Gynecol Obstet 1977;144:327–34.
79. Day CL Jr, Lew RA, Mihm MC Jr, et al. A multivariate analysis of prognostic factors for melanoma patients with lesions greater than or equal to 3.65 mm in thickness. The importance of revealing alternative Cox models. Ann Surg 1982;195:44–9.
80. Schmoeckel C, Bockelbrink A, Bockelbrink H, et al. Low- and high-risk malignant melanoma—I. Evaluation of clinical and histological prognosticators in 585 cases. Eur J Cancer Clin Oncol 1983;19:227–35.
81. Drzewiecki KT, Andersen PK. Survival with malignant melanoma: a regression analysis of prognostic factors. Cancer 1982;49:2414–9.
82. Kopf AW, Welkovich B, Frankel RE, et al. Thickness of malignant melanoma: global analysis of related factors. J Dermatol Surg Oncol 1987;13:345–90, 401–20.
83. Pastorfide GC, Kibbi AG, de Roa AL, et al. Image analysis of stage 1 melanoma (1.00–2.50 mm): lymphocytic infiltrates related to metastasis and survival. J Cutan Pathol 1992;19:390–7.
84. Mascaro JM, Molgo M, Castel T, Castro J. Plasma cells within the infiltrate of primary cutaneous malignant melanoma of the skin. A confirmation of its histoprognostic value. Am J Dermatopathol 1987;9:497–9.
85. Brocker EB, Zwadlo G, Suter L, et al. Infiltration of primary and metastatic melanomas with macrophages of the 25F9-positive phenotype. Cancer Immunol Immunother 1987;25:81–6.
86. Koh HK, Michalik E, Sober AJ, et al. Lentigo maligna melanoma has no better prognosis than other types of melanoma. J Clin Oncol 1984;2:994–1001.
87. Cox NH, Aitchison TC, Sirel JM, MacKie RM. Comparison between lentigo maligna melanoma and other histogenetic types of malignant melanoma of the head and neck. Scottish Melanoma Group. Br J Cancer 1996;73:940–4.
88. Slingluff CL Jr, Vollmer R, Seigler HF. Acral melanoma: a review of 185 patients with identification of prognostic variables. J Surg Oncol 1990;45:91–8.
89. Schmoeckel C, Bockelbrink A, Bockelbrink H, Braun-Falco O. Low- and high-risk malignant melanoma—II. Multivariate analyses for a prognostic classification. Eur J Cancer Clin Oncol 1983;19:237–43.
90. Huvos AG, Shah AP, Mike V. Prognostic factors in cutaneous malignant melanoma. A comparative study of long

term and short term survivors. Hum Pathol 1974;5: 347–57.
91. Hacene K, Le Doussal V, Brunet M, et al. Prognostic index for clinical stage I cutaneous malignant melanoma. Cancer Res 1983;43:2991–6.
92. Shaw HM, Balch CM, Soong SJ, et al. Prognostic histopathological factors in malignant melanoma. Pathology 1985;17:271–4.
93. Van Der Esch EP, Cascinelli N, Preda F, et al. Stage I melanoma of the skin: evaluation of prognosis according to histologic characteristics. Cancer 1981;48:1668–73.
94. Heenan PJ, English DR, Holman CD, Armstrong BK. Survival among patients with clinical stage I cutaneous malignant melanoma diagnosed in Western Australia in 1975/1976 and 1980/1981. Cancer 1991;68:2079–87.
95. Baak JP, Tan GJ. The adjuvant prognostic value of nuclear morphometry in stage I malignant melanoma of the skin. A multivariate analysis. Anal Quant Cytol Histol 1986;8: 241–4.
96. Folkman J. What is the evidence that tumors are angiogenesis dependent? J Natl Cancer Inst 1990;82:4–6.
97. Srivastava A, Laidler P, Davies RP, et al. The prognostic significance of tumor vascularity in intermediate-thickness (0.76–4.0 mm thick) skin melanoma. A quantitative histologic study. Am J Pathol 1988;133:419–23.
98. Rongioletti F, Miracco C, Gambini C, et al. Tumor vascularity as a prognostic indicator in intermediate-thickness (0.76–4 mm) cutaneous melanoma. A quantitative assay. Am J Dermatopathol 1996;18:474–7.
99. Carnochan P, Briggs JC, Westbury G, Davies AJ. The vascularity of cutaneous melanoma: a quantitative histological study of lesions 0.85–1.25 mm in thickness. Br J Cancer 1991;64:102–7.
100. Ilmonen S, Kariniemi AL, Vlaykova T, et al. Prognostic value of tumour vascularity in primary melanoma. Melanoma Res 1999;9:273–8.
101. Straume O, Akslen LA. Expresson of vascular endothelial growth factor, its receptors (FLT-1, KDR) and TSP-1 related to microvessel density and patient outcome in vertical growth phase melanomas. Am J Pathol 2001;159: 223–35.
102. Friedman RJ, Rigel DS, Kopf AW, et al. Volume of malignant melanoma is superior to thickness as a prognostic indicator. Preliminary observation. Dermatol Clin 1991;9: 643–8.
103. McGovern VJ, Shaw HM, Milton GW. Prognostic significance of a polypoid configuration in malignant melanoma. Histopathology 1983;7:663–72.
104. Baer SC, Schultz D, Synnestvedt M, Elder DE. Desmoplasia and neurotropism. Prognostic variables in patients with stage I melanoma. Cancer 1995;76:2242–7.
105. Levine J, Kopf AW, Rigel DS, et al. Correlation of thicknesses of superficial spreading malignant melanomas and ages of patients. J Dermatol Surg Oncol 1981;7:311–6.
106. Cohen HJ, Cox E, Manton K, Woodbury M. Malignant melanoma in the elderly. J Clin Oncol 1987;5:100–6.
107. Austin PF, Cruse CW, Lyman G, et al. Age as a prognostic factor in the malignant melanoma population. Ann Surg Oncol 1994;1:487–94.
108. Garbe C, Buttner P, Bertz J, et al. Primary cutaneous melanoma. Prognostic classification of anatomic location. Cancer 1995;75:2492–8.
109. Reintgen DS, Vollmer R, Tso CY, Seigler HF. Prognosis for recurrent stage I malignant melanoma. Arch Surg 1987;122:338–42.
110. Karakousis CP, Driscoll DL. Prognostic parameters in localised melanoma: gender versus anatomical location. Eur J Cancer 1995;3:320–4.
111. Day CL Jr, Sober AJ, Lew RA, et al. Malignant melanoma patients with positive nodes and relatively good prognoses: microstaging retains prognostic significance in clinical stage I melanoma patients with metastases to regional nodes. Cancer 1981;47:955–62.
112. Callery C, Cochran AJ, Roe DJ, et al. Factors prognostic for survival in patients with malignant melanoma spread to the regional lymph nodes. Ann Surg 1982;196:69–75.
113. Roses DF, Provet JA, Harris MN, et al. Prognosis of patients with pathologic stage II cutaneous malignant melanoma. Ann Surg 1985;201:103–7.
114. Holly EA, Weiss NS, Liff JM. Cutaneous melanoma in relation to exogenous hormones and reproductive factors. J Natl Cancer Inst 1983;70:827–31.
115. Holly EA. Melanoma and pregnancy. Recent Results Cancer Res 1986;102:118–26.
116. Holly EA. Cutaneous melanoma and oral contraceptives: a review of case-control and cohort studies. Recent Results Cancer Res 1986;102:108–17.
117. Holly EA, Cress RD, Ahn DK. Cutaneous melanoma in women. III. Reproductive factors and oral contraceptive use. Am J Epidemiol 1995;141:943–50.
118. Reintgen DS, McCarty KS Jr, Vollmer R, et al. Malignant melanoma and pregnancy. Cancer 1985;55:1340–4.
119. Walker MJ, Ronan SG, Han MC, et al. Interrelationship between histopathologic characteristics of melanoma and estrogen receptor status. Cancer 1991;68:184–8.
120. Shiu MH, Schottenfeld D, Maclean B, Fortner JG. Adverse effect of pregnancy on melanoma: a reappraisal. Cancer 1976;37:181–7.
121. Wong JH, Sterns EE, Kopald KH, et al. Prognostic significance of pregnancy in stage I melanoma. Arch Surg 1989 124:1227–30; discussion 1230–1.
122. McManamny DS, Moss AL, Pocock PV, Briggs JC. Melanoma and pregnancy: a long-term follow-up. Br J Obstet Gynaecol 1989;96:1419–23.

123. Slingluff CL Jr, Reintgen DS, Vollmer RT, Seigler HF. Malignant melanoma arising during pregnancy. A study of 100 patients. Ann Surg 1990;211:552–7; discussion 558–9.
124. Slingluff CL Jr, Seigler HF. Malignant melanoma and pregnancy. Ann Plast Surg 1992;28:95–9.
125. MacKie RM, Bufalino R, Morabito A, et al. Lack of effect of pregnancy on outcome of melanoma. For the World Health Organisation Melanoma Programme. Lancet 1991;337:653–5.
126. Heaton KM, Sussman JJ, Gershenwald JE, et al. Surgical margins and prognostic factors in patients with thick (> 4mm) primary melanoma. Ann Surg Oncol 1998;5:322–8.
127. Lambe M, Thorn M, Sparen P, Bergstrom R, Adami HO. Malignant melanoma: reduced risk associated with early childbearing and multiparity. Melanoma Res 1996;6:147–53.
128. Travers RL, Sober AJ, Berwick M, et al. Increased thickness of pregnancy-associated melanoma. Br J Dermatol 1995;132:876–83.
129. Cohn-Cedermark G, Mansson-Brahme E, Rutqvist LE, et al. Outcomes of patients with local recurrence of cutaneous malignant melanoma: a population-based study. Cancer 1997;80:1418–25.
130. Dong XD, Tyler D, Johnson JL, et al. Analysis of prognosis and disease progression after local recurrence of melanoma. Cancer 2000;88:1063–71.
131. Balch CM, Soong SJ, Smith T, et al. Long-term results of a prospective surgical trial comparing 2 cm vs. 4 cm excision margins for 740 patients with 1–4 mm melanomas. Ann Surg Oncol 2001;8:101–8.
132. Ng AK, Jones WO, Shaw JH. Analysis of local recurrence and optimizing excision margins for cutaneous melanoma. Br J Surg 2001;88:137–42.
133. Sorensen FB, Kristensen IB, Grymer F, Jakobsen A. DNA level, tumor thickness, and stereological estimates of nuclear volume in stage I cutaneous malignant melanomas. A comparative study with analysis of prognostic impact. Am J Dermatopathol 1991;13:11–9.
134. Binder M, Dolezal I, Wolff K, Pehamberger H. Stereologic estimation of volume-weighted mean nuclear volume as a predictor of prognosis in "thin" malignant melanoma. J Invest Dermatol 1992;99:180–3.
135. Mauri MF, Boi S, Micciolo R, et al. Morphometric analysis in prognostic evaluation of stage I thick cutaneous melanomas. Anal Quant Cytol Histol 1997;19:311–5.
136. Kheir SM, Bines SD, Vonroenn JH, et al. Prognostic significance of DNA aneuploidy in stage I cutaneous melanoma. Ann Surg 1988;207:455–61.
137. Herzberg AJ, Kerns BJ, Borowitz MJ, et al. DNA ploidy of malignant melanoma determined by image cytometry of fresh frozen and paraffin-embedded tissue. J Cutan Pathol 1991;18:440–8.
138. Herzberg AJ. Significance of DNA ploidy in cutaneous lesions. Arch Dermatol 1992;128:663–72.
139. Karlsson M, Boeryd B, Carstensen J, et al. DNA ploidy and S-phase in primary malignant melanoma as prognostic factors for stage III disease. Br J Cancer 1993;67:134–8.
140. Martin G, Halwani F, Shibata H, Meterissian S. Value of DNA ploidy and S-phase fraction as prognostic factors in stage III cutaneous melanoma. Can J Surg 2000;43:29–34.
141. Karjalainen JM, Eskelinen MJ, Nordling S, et al. Mitotic rate and S-phase fraction as prognostic factors in stage I cutaneous malignant melanoma. Br J Cancer 1998;77:1917–25.
142. Skowronek J, Adamska K, Filipiak K, et al. DNA ploidy in malignant melanoma, skin cancer and pigmented nevi. Neoplasma 1997;44:282–8.
143. Friedman RJ, Grin CM, Heilman E, et al. Distinguishing benign and malignant melanocytic lesions with the AgNOR method. Dermatol Clin 1991;9:689–93.
144. Gambini C, Casazza S, Borgiani L, et al. Counting the nucleolar organizer region-associated proteins is a prognostic clue of malignant melanoma. Arch Dermatol 1992;128:487–90.
145. Smolle J, Smolle-Juettner FM, Stettner H, Kerl H. Relationship of tumor cell motility and morphologic patterns. Part 1. Melanocytic skin tumors. Am J Dermatopathol 1992;14:231–7.
146. Smolle J, Hofmann-Wellenhof R, Kerl H. Prognostic significance of proliferation and motility in primary malignant melanoma of the skin. J Cutan Pathol 1992;19:110–5.
147. Niezabitowski A, Czajecki K, Rys J, et al. Prognostic evaluation of cutaneous malignant melanoma: a clinicopathologic and immunohistochemical study. J Surg Oncol 1999;70:150–60.
148. Ostmeier H, Fuchs B, Otto F, et al. Prognostic immunohistochemical markers of primary human melanomas. Br J Dermatol 2001;145:203–9.
149. Smith B, Selby P, Southgate J, et al. Detection of melanoma cells in peripheral blood by means of reverse transcriptase and polymerase chain reaction. Lancet 1991;338:1227–9.
150. Battayani Z, Grob JJ, Xerri L, et al. Polymerase chain reaction detection of circulating melanocytes as a prognostic marker in patients with melanoma. Arch Dermatol 1995;131:443–7.
151. Palmieri G, Strazzullo M, Ascierto PA, et al. Polymerase chain reaction-based detection of circulating melanoma cells as an effective marker of tumor progression. Melanoma Cooperative Group. J Clin Oncol 1999;17:304–11.
152. Hoon DS, Bostick P, Kuo C, et al. Molecular markers in blood as surrogate prognostic indicators of melanoma recurrence. Cancer Res 2000;60:2253–7.
153. Proebstle TM, Jiang W, Hogel J, et al. Correlation of positive RT-PCR for tyrosinase in peripheral blood of malig-

nant melanoma patients with clinical stage, survival and other risk factors. Br J Cancer 2000;82:118–23.
154. Schittek B, Bodingbauer Y, Ellwanger U, et al. Amplification of MelanA messenger RNA in addition to tyrosinase increases sensitivity of melanoma cell detection in peripheral blood and is associated with the clinical stage and prognosis of malignant melanoma. Br J Dermatol 1999; 141:30–6.
155. Ghossein RA, Coit D, Brennan M, et al. Prognostic significance of peripheral blood and bone marrow tyrosinase messenger RNA in malignant melanoma. Clin Cancer Res 1998;4:419–28.
156. Schrader AJ, Probst-Kepper M, Grosse J, et al. Tumour microdissemination and survival in metastatic melanoma. Anticancer Res 2000;20:3619–24.
157. Glaser R, Rass K, Seiter S, et al. Detection of circulating melanoma cells by specific amplification of tyrosinase complementary DNA is not a reliable tumor marker in melanoma patients: a clinical two-center study. J Clin Oncol 1997;15:2818–25.
158. Reinhold U, Ludtke-Handjery HC, Schnautz S, et al. The analysis of tyrosinase-specific mRNA in blood samples of melanoma patients by RT-PCR is not a useful test for metastatic tumor progression. J Invest Dermatol 1997;108:166–9.
159. Farthmann B, Eberle J, Krasagakis K, et al. RT-PCR for tyrosinase-mRNA-positive cells in peripheral blood: evaluation strategy and correlation with known prognostic markers in 123 melanoma patients. J Invest Dermatol 1998;110:263–7.
160. Hanekom GS, Stubbings HM, Johnson CA, Kidson SH. The detection of circulating melanoma cells correlates with tumour thickness and ulceration but is not predictive of metastasis for patients with primary melanoma. Melanoma Res 1999;9:465–73.
161. Miliotes G, Lyman GH, Cruse CW, et al. Evaluation of new putative tumor markers for melanoma. Ann Surg Oncol 1996;3:558–63.
162. Buer J, Probst M, Franzke A, et al. Elevated serum levels of S100 and survival in metastatic malignant melanoma. Br J Cancer 1997;75:1373–6.
163. Schlagenhauff B, Schittek B, Ellwanger U, et al. Significance of serum protein S100 levels in screening for melanoma metastasis: does protein S100 enable early detection of melanoma recurrence? Melanoma Res 2000;10: 451–9.
164. Hauschild A, Michaelsen J, Brenner W, et al. Prognostic significance of serum S100B detection compared with routine blood parameters in advanced metastatic melanoma patients. Melanoma Res 1999;9:155–61.
165. Hauschild A, Engel G, Brenner W, et al. S100B protein detection in serum is a significant prognostic factor in metastatic melanoma. Oncology 1999;56:338–44.
166. Martenson ED, Hansson LO, Nilsson B, et al. Serum S-100b protein as a prognostic marker in malignant cutaneous melanoma. J Clin Oncol 2001;19:824–31.
167. Puig S, Castro J, Ventura PJ, et al. Large deletions of chromosome 9p in cutaneous malignant melanoma identify patients with a high risk of developing metastases. Hospital Clinic Malignant Melanoma Group, University of Barcelona. Melanoma Res 2000;10:231–6.
168. Piepkorn M. Melanoma genetics: an update with focus on the CDKN2A(p16)/ARF tumor suppressors. J Am Acad Dermatol 2000;42:705–22; quiz 723–6.
169. Florenes VA, Maelandsmo GM, Faye R, et al. Cyclin A expression in superficial spreading malignant melanomas correlates with clinical outcome. J Pathol 2001;195:530–6.
170. Salti GI, Manougian T, Farolan M, et al. Micropthalmia transcription factor: a new prognostic marker in intermediate-thickness cutaneous malignant melanoma. Cancer Res 2000 60:5012–6.
171. Berset M, Cerottini JP, Guggisberg D, et al. Expression of Melan-A/MART-1 antigen as a prognostic factor in primary cutaneous melanoma. Int J Cancer 2001;95:73–7.
172. Balch CM, Buzaid AC, Atkins MB, et al. A new American Joint Committee on Cancer staging system for cutaneous melanoma. Cancer 2000;88:1484–91.
173. Fusi S, Ariyan S, Sternlicht A. Data on first recurrence after treatment for malignant melanoma in a large patient population. Plast Reconstr Surg 1993;91:94–8.
174. Breslow A. Tumor thickness, level of invasion and node dissection in stage I cutaneous melanoma. Ann Surg 1975; 182:572–5.
175. Day CL Jr, Mihm MC Jr, Sober AJ, et al. Predictors of late deaths among patients with clinical stage I melanoma who have not had bony or visceral metastases within the first 5 years after diagnosis. J Am Acad Dermatol 1983;8:864–8.
176. Balch CM, Soong SJ, Murad TM, et al. A multifactorial analysis of melanoma: III. Prognostic factors in melanoma patients with lymph node metastases (stage II). Ann Surg 1981;193:377–88.
177. Hughes TM, A'Hern RP, Thomas JM. Prognosis and surgical management of patients with palpable inguinal lymph node metastases from melanoma. Br J Surg 2000; 87:892–901.
178. Messaris GE, Konstadoulakis MM, Ricaniadis N, et al. Prognostic variables for patients with stage III malignant melanoma. Eur J Surg 2000;166:233–9.
179. Cochran AJ, Lana AM, Wen DR. Histomorphometry in the assessment of prognosis in stage II malignant melanoma. Am J Surg Pathol 1989;13:600–4.
180. Buzaid AC, Tinoco LA, Jendiroba D, et al. Prognostic value of size of lymph node metastases in patients with cutaneous melanoma. J Clin Oncol 1995;13:2361–8.
181. Stroobe LJ, Jonk A, Hart AA, et al. Positive iliac and ob-

turator nodes in melanoma: survival and prognostic factors. Ann Surg Oncol 1999;6:255–62.
182. Ramnath EM, Kamath D, Brobeil A, et al. Lymphatic mapping for melanoma: long-term results of regional nodal sampling with radioguided surgery. Cancer Control 1997; 4:483–490.
183. Nguyen CL, McClay EF, Cole DJ, et al. Melanoma thickness and histology predict sentinel lymph node status. Am J Surg 2001;181:8–11.
184. Lens MB, Dawes M, Newton-Bishop JA, Goodacre T. Tumour thickness as a predictor of occult lymph node metastases in patients with stage I and II melanoma undergoing sentinel lymph node biopsy. Br J Surg 2002;89:1223–7.
185. Cascinelli N, Belli F, Santinami M, et al. Sentinel lymph node biopsy in cutaneous melanoma: the WHO Melanoma Program experience. Ann Surg Oncol 2000;7:469–74.
186. Statius Muller MG, van Leeuwen PA, de Lange-De Klerk ES, et al. The sentinel lymph node status is an important factor for predicting clinical outcome in patients with stage I or II cutaneous melanoma. Cancer 2001;91:2401–8.
187. Blaheta HJ, Schittek B, Breuninger H, et al. Lymph node micrometastases of cutaneous melanoma: increased sensitivity of molecular diagnosis in comparison to immunohistochemistry. Int J Cancer 1998;79:318–23.
188. Bostick PJ, Morton DL, Turner RR, et al. Prognostic significance of occult metastases detected by sentinel lymphadenectomy and reverse transcriptase-polymerase chain reaction in early-stage melanoma patients. J Clin Oncol 1999;17:3238–44.
189. Blaheta HJ, Ellwanger U, Schittek B, et al. Examination of regional lymph nodes by sentinel node biopsy and molecular analysis provides new staging facilities in primary cutaneous melanoma. J Invest Dermatol 2000;114:637–42.
190. Porter GA, Ross MI, Berman RS, et al. Significance of multiple nodal basin drainage in truncal melanoma patients undergoing sentinel lymph node biopsy. Ann Surg Oncol 2000;7:256–61.
191. Balch CM, Soong SJ, Murad TM, et al. A multifactorial analysis of melanoma. IV. Prognostic factors in 200 melanoma patients with distant metastases (stage III). J Clin Oncol 1983;1:126–34.
192. Barth A, Wanek LA, Morton DL. Prognostic factors in 1,521 melanoma patients with distant metastases. J Am Coll Surg 1995;181:193–201.
193. Brand CU, Ellwanger U, Stroebel W, et al. Prolonged survival of 2 years or longer for patients with disseminated melanoma. An analysis of related prognostic factors. Cancer 1997;79:2345–53.
194. Manola J, Atkins M, Ibrahim J, Kirkwood J. Prognostic factors in metastatic melanoma: a pooled analysis of Eastern Cooperative Oncology Group trials. J Clin Oncol 2000;18:3782–93.
195. Presant CA, Bartolucci AA. Prognostic factors in metastatic malignant melanoma: the Southeastern Cancer Study Group experience. Cancer 1982;49:2192–6.
196. Shen P, Guenther JM, Wanek LA, Morton DL. Can elective lymph node dissection decrease the frequency and mortality rate of late melanoma recurrences? Ann Surg Oncol 2000;7:114–9.
197. Ollila DW, Hsueh EC, Stern SL, Morton DL. Metastasectomy for recurrent stage IV melanoma. J Surg Oncol 1999; 71:209–13.
198. Rose DM, Essner R, Hughes TM, et al. Surgical resection for metastatic melanoma to the liver: the John Wayne Cancer Institute and Sydney Melanoma Unit experience. Arch Surg 2001;136:950–5.
199. Leo F, Cagini L, Rocmans P, et al. Lung metastases from melanoma: when is surgical treatment warranted? Br J Cancer 2000;83:569–72.
200. Meyer T, Merkel S, Goehl J, Hohenberger W. Surgical therapy for distant metastases of malignant melanoma. Cancer 2000;89:1983–91.
201. Groeger AM, Kandioler D, Mueller MR, et al. Survival after surgical treatment of recurrent pulmonary metastases. Eur J Cardiothorac Surg 1997;12:703–5.
202. Vlaykova T, Muhonen T, Hahka-Kemppinen M, et al. Vascularity and prognosis of metastatic melanoma. Int J Cancer 1997;74:326–9.
203. Vlaykova T, Laurila P, Muhonen T, et al. Prognostic value of tumour vascularity in metastatic melanoma and association of blood vessel density with vascular endothelial growth factor expression. Melanoma Res 1999;9:59–68.
204. Soong S-J, Weiss HL. Predicting outcome in patients with localized melanoma. In: Balch CM, Houghton A, Sober AJ, Soong S-J, eds. Cutaneous Melanoma. St. Louis: Quality Medical, 1998:51–61.
205. Sahin S, Rao B, Kopf AW, et al. Predicting ten-year survival of patients with primary cutaneous melanoma: corroboration of a prognostic model. Cancer 1997;80: 1426–31.
206. Brownbridge GG, Gold J, Edward M, MacKie RM. Evaluation of the use of tyrosinase-specific and melanA/MART-1-specific reverse transcriptase-coupled–polymerase chain reaction to detect melanoma cells in peripheral blood samples from 299 patients with malignant melanoma. Br J Dermatol 2001;144:279–87.
207. Masback A, Olsson H, Westerdahl J, Ingvar C, Jonsson N. Prognostic factors in invasive cutaneous malignant melanoma: a population-based study and review. Melanoma Res 2001;11:435–45.

INDEX

A

Abtropfung hypothesis
  of melanocyte histogenesis, 7
  of the origin of melanocytic nevi, 51
Acanthoma, large-cell, transition of solar lentigo to, 41
Acquired dermal melanocytosis, of the face and extremities, 201
Acquired melanocytic nevi, common, 55–64
Acral melanomas, 280–284
  defined, 241
  distribution of, by skin color, 248–249
Acral nevus, melanocytic, 89–90
Activating transcription factor 1 (STF-1) gene, on chromosome 12, translocation of, in clear-cell sarcoma, 327
Adipocytes, accumulation of, in some nevi, 66
Adnexal involvement, of Spitz nevi, 160
Age
  at diagnosis of melanoma associated with congenital melanocytic nevi, 113
  as a factor in differential diagnosis of Spitz nevus, 170
  and melanoma arising from small congenital melanocytic nevi, 131
  and occurrence
    of acral melanoma, 280
    of ancient melanocytic nevus, 65
    of balloon cell melanoma, 90
    of Becker's melanosis, 44–45
    of clonal nevi, 98
    of congenital nevi in the first year of life, 115
    of desmoplastic melanoma and desmoplastic-neurotropic melanoma, 290
  of halo nevi, 90
  of melanocytic nevi, 55
  of melanoma, 136–144
  of small cell melanomas, 314–315
  of solar lentigines, 40
  of solar melanoma, 248, 267–275
  of subungual melanoma, 284
  of vulvar melanoma, 98
  and prognosis, in malignant melanoma, 380
  and recurrence of Spitz nevi, 188–190
Agminate Spitz nevi, 150–151
AgNORs (silver-staining nucleolar organizer region)
  counts of, as a prognostic factor, 382
  of Spitz nevi, 171
Albright syndrome, melanotic macules associated with, 40
Alternative reading frame (ARF) tumor suppressor gene of CDKN2A
  identification of, 23
  penetrant melanoma locus, 21
Amelanotic blue nevus, 204–206
Amelanotic melanoma, 249, 330
American Joint Committee on Cancer (AJCC)
  classification of satellite and in-transit metastases of malignant melanoma, 357–358
  stage III disease, 383–385
  stage IV disease, 358
  staging of localized disease, 373
Anatomic level of tumor invasion in the dermis and subcutis, 375–376
Anatomic site
  importance of, in classifying melanomas, 242–243
  of malignant melanoma metastases, and prognosis, 386
  of the primary melanoma, and prognosis, 380
  of Spitz nevi, 149
    as a factor in differentiating melanoma from, 170
Ancient melanocytic nevi, 65–66
Ancillary studies, for evaluation
  of melanocytic lesions, 13–16
  of recurrent Spitz nevi, 193–194
Aneuploidy, and prognosis, 381
Angiogenesis
  and prognosis in cutaneous malignant melanoma, 379
  in zones of regression of melanomas, 339
Angiomatoid Spitz nevus, variant of desmoplastic Spitz nevi, 175
Angiotropic tumor aggregates, as microscopic satellites, 261
Angiotropism
  of desmoplastic melanoma and desmoplastic-neurotropic melanoma, 293
  of melanomas, 301–302
  of Spitz nevi, 160
Angio-tumoral complex, 302
Animal-type melanoma, 331–333
Architecture
  of atypical nevi, 75–76, 124–125
  of cellular blue nevi, 210
  general, of melanocytic nevi, 64
  of pigmented spindle cell nevi, 180–185
Atypical intraepidermal melanocytic proliferation, with indeterminate biologic potential, 345–346
Atypical melanocytic nevi (AMN), 263–265

A

Atypical nevi (dysplastic nevi), 66–89
architecture of, 124–125
cellular blue, 215–216
differentiating from atypical melanocytic cells in a fibrotic matrix, 346
melanocytic, Pagetoid spread in, 263–265
p16 protein levels in, 25
relationship with the number of nevi in children, 140
significance of, 69–75
Spitz tumors, 160–171

B

Balloon cell melanoma, 330
age at occurrence of, 90
Balloon cell nevus, 90
Balloon cells
changes within nevi, 65
morphology of, in metastatic melanoma, 362
Basilar epidermis
density of melanocytes along, in lentigo simplex, 54
proliferation of pigmented dendritic melanocytes, 209
Basilar melanocytes
circumscribed pigmented lesions composed of, 37–50
correlation of the number of and sun exposure, 278
in solar melanoma, 277–278
Bathing trunk nevus, 114
Bax, promotion of apoptosis by, 31
Bcl-2
as an antiapoptotic factor, 31
expression of, in Spitz nevus compared with melanoma, 172
Becker's melanosis (BM), 44–46
differentiating from café-au-lait macules, 40
Benign juvenile melanoma. See Spitz nevi
Benign nevus, residual, in a regressed melanoma, 343
Bilirubin, distinguishing from melanin, 2
Biologic course of Spitz nevi, 149–150
Biopsies, types of, 11–12
Biphasic pattern of cellular blue nevi, 214–215
Bleaching to remove melanin, in evaluation studies, 13
Bloom syndrome, association of café-au-lait macules with, 40
Blue nevi, 199–222
criteria for designation as, 223
differentiating from desmoplastic Spitz nevi, 178
HMB-45 marker for, 14–15
melanomas arising in, 322–327
plaque-type, 217–219
sclerosing, differentiating from desmoplastic melanoma and neurotropic melanoma, 300
See also Malignant blue nevus
Body skin, fetal, pigment synthesis in, 8–9
Borderline lesions, suggesting melanoma, diagnosis and management of, 343–346
Bowen's disease, differentiating junctional Spitz nevus from, 164

C

Café-au-lait macule (CALM)
distinguishing from Becker's nevus, 46
distinguishing from freckles, 37, 39–40
CAM 5.2 antibody, specificity of, for mammary Paget's disease, 265
Caspase-3,8,9 cascade, apoptosis via, 31
CDKN2A (p16)
association with melanoma, 73–74
identification of, 22
locus and homologs of, 21–26
mechanism of action of, 20, 25–26
target for germline mutation in familial melanoma, 32
upregulation of, by ultraviolet radiation, 28
CDKN2A-Leiden mutation, melanoma risk associated with, 29
CDKN2B (p15) melanoma cell line, 22
aberrations of, in melanoma, 24
regulation of cell-cycle progression involving the CDKN2A/RB pathway, 25–26
cDNA microarrays, for identifying control elements in evolution of metastatic melanoma, 30
Cell-division cycle, 25–26
melanoma genes acting within, 32
S phase, mutant cells expressing 14p^{ARF} protein followed by p53 activation, 26
Cellular blue nevus (CBN), 209–216, 223
nodal, 217
Cellular density, of conventional melanomas, 251
Cellular type, classification of melanocytic nevi by, 53–54
C-*erb* protein, reaction with 21N antibody of adenocarcinomas, 265
Childhood melanoma, 136–144
Children's Hospital, Boston, congenital melanocytic nevi study at, 115
Chromosomes
9p
deletions from, and adverse outcome in malignant melanoma, 383
loss of heterozygosity in Spitz nevi, 175
mapping of the p16 gene to, 20–22
9p21, inactivation in the germ cell line and melanoma development, 73–74
11p, study of alterations in Spitz nevi, 174–175, 193–194
12q13, mutational hot spot in the CDK4 locus of, 27
multiple gains and losses consistent with melanoma, 194
numerical aberrations of, in atypical melanocytic proliferation, 132–133
t(11;22) translocation in clear-cell sarcoma, 362, 368
t(12;22) translocation in melanoma of soft parts, 17, 327
Circulating melanoma cells, 382–383
Classification
of melanocytic lesions with phenotypic hererogeneity, 225
of melanocytic nevi, 52–53
of melanoma, criteria for, 239–244
of metastatic disease in malignant melanoma, 358
Clear-cell melanoma, 333–334
Clear-cell sarcoma, 327–328
differentiating from cellular blue nevi, 216
differentiating from a nodule derived from cutaneous melanoma, 362
Clinical atypia versus histologic atypia, for assessing risk of melanoma, 71–72
Clinical factors affecting prognosis in malignant melanoma, 380–381
Clinical features
of acral melanoma, 280–282
of acral nevi, 89
of angiotropic melanoma, 302
of atypical nevi, 74–75
of balloon cell lesions, 90
of balloon cell melanoma, 330
of blue nevi
common, 202–203
compound, 209
cellular, 209
malignant, 324
plaque-type, 217
target, 220
of café-au-lait macules, 39
of clear-cell sarcoma, 328
of clonal nevi, 98
of congenital melanocytic nevi, 114
of conventional melanomas, 244–249
invasive, with little adjacent intraepidermal component, 266
of deep penetrating nevi, 233
of dermal melanocytic tumor, 333

of desmoplastic melanoma and
desmoplastic-neurotropic
melanoma, 290–291
of desmoplastic Spitz nevi, 175
of ephelides, 37
of halo nevi, 92
of lentigo simplex, 54
of melanocytic nevi, 56–57
of the genital skin, 98
recurrent, 96
with phenotypic heterogeneity, 226
of melanoma associated with dermal
nevi, 319–320
of mucocutaneous melanotic macules
and lentigines, 47–48
of neurotropic melanoma, 295
of nevoid melanoma, 303–304
of nevus spilus, 94
of recurrent Spitz nevi, 188–190
of small cell melanoma, 313
of solar intraepidermal melanocytic
proliferations, 44
of solar lentigo, 41
of solar melanoma, 268–271
of spindle cell nevus
pigmented, 180
plexiform, 235
of Spitz nevi, 149–160
of Spitzoid melanomas, 317–319
of subungual melanoma, 284–286
of verrucous melanoma, 311
Clonal nevus, 98–100
Cohesion, loss of, in Spitz nevi, 160
Combined nevus, 98–100
published accounts of, summary, 225
Combined Spitz nevus, 178
Common acquired nevi, differences from
congenital melanocytic nevi, 111,
123–124
Common blue nevus, 202–204
Common nevus, combination with blue
nevus, in melanocytic nevi with
phenotypic heterogeneity, 226
Comparative genomic hybridization
(CGH), Spitz nevus studies using,
174
Competitive inhibition, of CDKN2A with
cyclin D1 for CDK4 binding sites,
26
Complexity of conventional melanomas,
251
Composition of cellular blue nevi, 210–214
Compound nevus
blue, 209
histopathologic features of, 61
Concentric fibroplasia
in atypical nevi, 85–86
in tissue affected by lentiginous nevi, 57

Congenital anomalies, association of, with
neuroid congenital melanocytic
nevi, 123
Congenital lesions
characteristic attributes of, 65
melanomas, 134–136
Congenital melanocytic nevi (CMN),
111–134
with atypical features, 124–125
differentiating from Becker's melanosis,
46
giant, small cell type melanomas arising
from, 129, 140
small, melanomas arising from, 140
Congenital nevi
blue nevi, 323
comparison with malignant blue nevi,
327
in the first year of life, 115
location of, in the skin, 53
punch biopsies of, 11
Spitz nevi, 149
See also Congenital melanocytic nevi
Congenital nevi tardive, 111
Connecticut Tumor Registry, data on
desmoplastic melanomas, 290
Continent melanocytes, defined, 2
Contours of growth, irregular, at deep
margins in Spitz nevi, 159
Conventional melanoma, 244–256
defined, 241
invasive, 260–266
with little adjacent intraepidermal
component, 266–269
microinvasive, 256–260
Criteria for diagnosis. *See* Diagnosis
Cross-genomic hybridization (CGH), for
studying recurrent Spitz nevi,
193–194
Cross-sectional profile, of tumors, and
prognosis, 379
Cultured cell lines, genetic alterations in,
reflecting adaptive change to in
vitro conditions, 24
Curettage biopsy, 12
Cutaneous melanoma
age at diagnosis of, 238–239
stratification of risk factors for, 69
Cutaneous nevus versus cutaneous
metastasis, 366
Cyclin-dependent kinases
CDK4
penetrant melanoma locus, 20–21
role of, in cell division, 22
role of, in familial melanoma, 27
interaction with retinoblastoma gene
product and D-type cyclins in early
G_1, 26

Cyclins
A, protein levels of, and stage or
melanoma, 383
D1, expression of, in Spitz nevi, 172
D-type, as rate-limiting growth sensors,
26
Cysteinyldopas, pheomelanin formed
from, 1
Cytogenetics, of human melanocytic
tumors, 17
Cytologic atypia
of basilar melanocytes, in solar lentigo,
41
of congenital melanocytic nevi, 115,
124–125
of melanocytes, in nevoid melanoma,
310
Cytology
of atypical nevi, 83–85
of nevoid melanomas, 307–310
of nevus cells, 61–64

D

Danish Birth Registry, melanoma risk
from, association with congenital
melanocytic nevi, 113
Deep-penetrating nevus, 233
morphological similarity to melanocytic
nevi with phenotypic heterogeneity,
226–227
Demarcation, sharp lateral, of Spitz nevi,
158
Dermal cohesive cellular nodules, 346
Dermal component, of Spitz nevus, atypical
features of, 164–165
Dermal epithelioid cell, melanocytic nevus
with components of, 226
Dermal fibroplasia, in atypical nevi, 85–86
Dermal melanocyte hamartoma, 202
Dermal melanocytic tumor, atypical, 331–333
Dermal melanocytoses, 199–222
Dermal nevi, melanoma associated with,
319–322
Dermal nodular proliferations, 125–127
Dermal nodules, 230–233
Dermal/subcutaneous tumoral pattern, in
recurrent Spitz nevi, 191–193
Dermal variations, of melanocytic nevi,
65–66
Dermoepidermal junction
appearance of spindle cells of Spitz nevi
at, 153
giant nevus cells at, in Spitz nevi, 159
Desmoplasia
in nevi, defined, 65
and prognosis, 379
Desmoplastic melanomas (DM), 289–293
defined, 290

Desmoplastic-neurotropic melanoma
(DNM), 290–293
Desmoplastic Spitz nevus, 171, 175–178
distinguishing from desmoplastic
melanoma, 300
similarity with recurrent Spitz nevus, 190
Developmental abnormalities
association with Becker's melanosis, 44
association with congenital melanocytic
nevi, 114
Diagnosis
of atypical nevi, 75–86
of melanoma, criteria for, 239–244
conventional microinvasive, 257–260
intraepidermal, 287
malignant, 358–370
of solar intraepithelial melanocytic
proliferation, 278–279
of Spitz nevus, 161–162
special techniques for, 171–175
Differential diagnosis
of acral melanoma, 287
of acral nevi, 89–90
of amelanotic blue nevi, 205–206
of atypical nevi, 86–88
of balloon cell lesions, 90
of balloon cell melanoma, 331
of Becker's melanosis, 46
of blue nevi
atypical cellular, 216
common, 204
compound, 209
epithelioid, 209
malignant, 327
sclerosing, 204
target, 220
of café-au-lait macules, 40
of clear-cell sarcoma, 328
of clonal nevi, 100–103
of conventional melanomas with
intraepithelial components, 261
of dermal melanocytic tumor, 333
of desmoplastic melanoma and
neurotropic melanoma, 300–301
of desmoplastic Spitz nevi, 175–178
of freckles, 37
of halo nevi, 92–94
of intraepidermal Spitz nevi, 163–171
of lentigo maligna, 274–275
of lentigo simplex, 54–55
of melanocytic nevi
of the genital skin, 98
with phenotypic heterogeneity,
232–233
recurrent, 96
of melanoma associated with dermal
nevi, 322
of melanoma with little adjacent
intraepidermal component, 267

of Mongolian spots, 200
of mucocutaneous melanotic macules
and lentigines, 49
of myxoid melanoma, 331
of nevoid melanoma, 309–311
of nevus spilus, 94–96
of recurrent Spitz nevi, 195–196
of regressed melanoma, 341
hypopigmented, 341
with residual benign nevus, 343
of regression in melanoma, 342–343
of small cell melanoma, 313
of small congenital melanocytic nevi, 131
of solar intraepidermal melanocytic
proliferations, 44
of solar lentigo, 41–42
of solar melanocytic hyperplasia, 279
of spindle cell nevi
pigmented, 185
plexiform, 236–237
of Spitz nevi, 150–151
with halo reaction, 180
of Spitzoid melanoma, 319
of verrucous melanoma, 312
5,6-Dihydroxyindole units, in
eumelanins, 1
DNA, abnormal content of
in congenital melanocytic nevi,
133–134
in Spitz nevus, 173
DNA mismatch repair genes, expression in
atypical nevi and melanomas, 74
DNA-ploidy, as a prognostic factor in
malignant melanoma, 381
DNA repair, defective, in solar melanomas,
267

E

Ectasia, in zones of regression of
melanomas, 339
Edema, in Spitz nevi, 160
Electron microscopy
of melanocytes
for differential diagnosis, 16–17
for observing morphology, 3–4
for observing the morphology of
desmoplastic melanoma, 299
Embryology, of melanocytes, 8–9
Enzyme histochemistry, for evaluating
melanocytic lesions, 13–14
Epidemiology
descriptive, of malignant melanoma,
238–239
of Spitz nevi, 149
Epidermal changes
atrophy in solar melanomas, 251
in congenital melanocytic nevi, 123–124
hyperplasia
in melanomas from acral skin, 251

in Spitz nevi, 160
in melanocytic nevi, 64–65
Epidermal growth factor (EGF) receptor,
73–74
Epidermal melanin unit, defined, 1
Epidermal nevus, differentiating from
Becker's melanosis, 46
Epithelioid cell
atypical nevus, 86
histiocytoma, differentiating from Spitz
nevus, 171
morphology of, 359–364
variant, of blue nevi, 206
Epithelioid-cell type melanomas in
childhood, 141–142
Epithelioid melanocytes (type A cells)
appearance of, 7
of Spitz nevi, 153–157
zonation of, 158–159
Epithelioid melanoma cells, 260–261
in desmoplastic melanoma and
desmoplastic-neurotropic
melanoma, 291
and Pagetoid scatter, 254
Epithelioid melanomas, diagnosis with
melanocyte differentiation
markers, 14
Etiology
of balloon cell melanoma, 330–331
of childhood melanoma, 140–141
of depigmentation in halo nevi,
92–94
Eumelanin, 1
production of, binding of -melanocytic-
stimulating hormone in, 28–29
Eumelanosomes, stages of formation of,
3–4
Evaluation, of melanoma, ancillary
techniques for, 13–16
Ewing sarcoma oncogene, translocation in
clear-cell sarcoma, 327
EWS-ATF1 fusion gene, in melanoma of
soft parts, 368
Excisional biopsies, 11
Extravascular migratory metastasis, 302
Eyelid, congenital divided nevus of,
113–114

F

Familial aggregation, of congenital
melanocytic nevi, 114
Familial melanoma susceptibility loci,
20–29
major melanoma genes of, 32
Fas (CD95), role in cellular homeostasis,
utilizing apoptosis, 30–31
FasL, upregulation of the soluble form,
interaction with membrane
FasL, 31

Feedback loops, integration of the p16/retinoblastoma and alternate reading frame/p53 path, 27
Fibrotic papillary dermis, of atypical melanocytic nevi, entrapment of atypical nevus cells in, 264
Fibrous histiocytoma, malignant, distinguishing from desmoplastic melanoma, 301
Fibroxanthoma, atypical, distinguishing from desmoplastic melanoma, 301
Field effect, from melanoma, 279
Fixation, of skin excisions, 11
  evaluation of, 13
Fluorescence in situ hybridization (FISH)
  for identification
    of clear-cell-sarcoma, 328
    of *HRAS* gene mutation in Spitz nevi, 175
  for study
    of acral melanomas, 279–280
    of recurrent Spitz nevi, 193–194
Fontana-Masson stain, 13
Freckles (ephelides), 37–38
  carriers of variant alleles of melanocortin 1 receptor genes, 29
Frozen sections, for assessment of margins, 12–13

G

Gender, and prognosis in melanomas, 380
Genes
  alterations at the CDKN2A locus, 23–24
  cancer, types of, 20
  melanoma, major, 21
  N-*ras*, association with congenital melanocytic nevi and melanoma, 133–134
  See also Chromosomes; Inheritance
Genetic basis, for growth and development of nevi, 51–52
Genetic control
  of development of nevi, 55–56
  of the risk for melanoma, 69
  of the type of melanin pigmentation, 1
Genetic pathology of melanoma, 20–36
Genital skin, melanocytic nevi of, 96–100
Genomic structure of CDKN2A/ARF, 23
Giant nevus cells
  intradermal, 61
  in Spitz nevi, 159
gp100
  antibody to, for recognizing metastatic tumor deposits in sentinel lymph nodes, 358
  premelanosomal glycoprotein, 14–15
Grading
  of architectural disorder in atypical nevi, 86
  of atypical nevi, 88–89
  See also Classification
Grenz zone, separation of epidermis from dermal infiltration of nevus cells, 120
Guidelines, for grading atypical nevi, 88–89

H

Hair
  human, melanins of, 1
  transfer of melanin from the hair matrix cells to the follicles, 1
Halo nevus, 90–94
  atypical, differentiating from nevoid melanoma, 310
  differentiating from Pagetoid melanoma, 264
  differentiation from hypopigmented regressed melanomas, 341
  variant of, 86
Halo reaction in a Spitz nevus variant, 180
Hamartoma
  dermal melanocyte, 202
  epidermal nevus as, 46
  melanocytic nevus as, 51
  neurocristic, 219–220
Hamartoma, Becker's pigmentary. *See* Becker's melanosis
HDM2 marker, prognostic significance of 16
Hemosiderin, distinguishing from melanin, 2
Histochemical evaluation of Pagetoid involvement of the epidermis, 265
Histogenesis
  of congenital melanocytic nevi, 113–114
  of dermal melanocytoses and blue nevi, 199–200
  of desmoplastic melanoma, 297–299
  of melanocytes, 4–7
  of melanocytic nevi, 51–52
  of nevus cells, 7–8
Histogenetic type, and prognosis in malignant melanoma, 378–379
Histologic criteria, for melanocytic lesions, 53–54
Histologic features
  of acral nevi, 89
  of balloon cell lesions, 90
  of blue nevi and variant blue nevi, 223–225
  of clonal nevi, 98–100
  of halo nevi, 92
  of melanocytic nevi
    of the genital skin, 98
    recurrent, 96
  of metastatic melanoma, 358
  of nevus spilus, 94

Histologic variations
  within atypical nevi, 86
  within common acquired melanocytic nevi, 64–66
Histomorphologic criteria, defining conventional invasive melanomas, 260–266
Histopathologic criteria
  for conventional invasive melanomas with little intraepidermal component, 266
  for diagnosis of melanoma, 240–241
  for identifying acral melanoma, 282–284, 287–288
  for identifying angiotropic melanoma, 302
  for identifying balloon cell melanoma, 330
  for identifying blue nevus
    amelanotic, 205
    cellular, 209–216
    common, 203–204
    compound, 209
    epithelioid, 206–208
    malignant, 324–326
    target, 220
  for identifying clear-cell sarcoma, 328
  for identifying congenital melanocytic nevi, 115–124
  for identifying conventional melanomas, 249–256
  for identifying dermal melanocytic tumor, 333
  for identifying dermal melanocytoses, 202
  for identifying desmoplastic melanoma and desmoplastic-neurotropic melanoma, 291–293
  for identifying desmoplastic Spitz nevi, 175
  for identifying melanoma associated with dermal nevi, 320–321
  for identifying Mongolian spots, 200
  for identifying neurotropic melanoma, 295
  for identifying nevoid melanoma, 304–309
  for identifying pigmented spindle cell nevi, 180–185
  for identifying pilar neurocristic hamartoma, 220
  for identifying plaque-type blue nevi, 218
  for identifying sclerosing blue nevi, 204
  for identifying small cell melanoma, 313
  for identifying solar melanoma, 271–274
  for identifying Spitz nevi, 151–158
    versus melanomas, 190–193
  for identifying Spitzoid melanomas, 319
  for identifying verrucous melanoma, 311–312
  of solar intraepidermal melanocytic proliferations, 44

Histopathologic features
  of atypical nevi, 75
  of Becker's melanosis, 46
  of café-au-lait macules, 39–40
  of deep penetrating nevi, 233
  of ephelides, 37
  of lentigo simplex, 54
  of melanocytic nevi, 57–61
    with phenotypic heterogeneity, 226–228
  of melanomas in childhood, 141–144
  of mucocutaneous melanotic macules and lentigines, 48–49
  of plexiform spindle cell nevi, 235–236
  of solar lentigo, 41
Histopathologic reporting
  of atypical nevi, 88–89
  of melanoma, 346
Historical perspectives, on classification of melanoma, 242–244
HMB-45 tumor marker
  for distinguishing desmoplastic melanoma from other lesions, 300
  for melanocytes, 14–15
  negative, in neurotropic melanoma, 295–296
Hochsteigerung hypothesis, of melanocyte histogenesis, 7
Homogentisic acid pigment, 2
Hormones
  association of androgen with Becker's melanosis, 44
  association of estrogen with papillomatous changes in nevi, 64–65
Host response
  in atypical nevi, 85
  in invasive melanoma, 261
  in malignant melanoma, effect on prognosis, 378
HRAS gene mutation, fluorescence in situ hybridization (FISH) for identifying, 175
Hutchinson melanotic freckle, melanoma associated with, 267–275
Hydroxyl radicals from irradiation of pheomelanin, 1
Hyperkeratosis in conventional melanomas, 251
Hyperpigmentation of the basilar epidermis, in lentigo simplex, 54
Hypopigmentation of completely regressed melanoma, 341

I

Id1 repressor, of the CDKN2A gene, 24
Immune systems
  association of responses with halo nevi, 92
  genes functioning to evade, 30–31

Immunohistochemistry
  for evaluating desmoplastic melanoma, 299
  for evaluating desmoplastic-neurotropic melanoma, 295–296
  for evaluating melanocytic lesions, 14–16
  of Kamino bodies in Spitz nevi, 159
  of metastatic melanoma
    distinguishing from nodal nevi, 368
    with epithelioid or spindle cell morphology, 362
  of sentinel lymph nodes, 358
  of Spitz nevi, 171–172
Immunolabeling, of metastatic tumors, PECAM-1 and VEGF, 386
Immunophenotype analysis, of infiltrating cells of halo nevi, 92
Immunostaining
  for melanocyte differentiation antigens, 199–200
  unusual results associated with melanomas, 16
Incidence
  of congenital melanocytic nevi, 111
  of Spitz nevi, 149
Inflammatory infiltrate, perivascular, in Spitz nevi, 160
Inflammatory patterns, of congenital nevi, 121–123
Inflammatory response, participation of melanocytes in, 1
Inheritance
  autosomal dominant
    of freckling, 37–38
    of neurofibromatosis, 40
  See also Genes; Genetic *entries*
INK4 gene family, 23
Ink-spot solar lentigo, clinical features of, 41. *See also* Solar lentigo
Institutional review board (IRB), consent of, to obtain tissue for research, 13
Interobserver concordance
  in judging clinical atypia of nevi, 70–71
  study of Spitz nevus criteria, 166–168
  in judging histologic diagnosis of atypia of nevi, 75
Intraepidermal component
  missing, in malignant blue nevus, 323
  of Spitz nevi, atypical features of, 163
Intraepidermal epithelioid cells, melanocytic proliferations of, 262–263
Intraepidermal melanocytic proliferation
  atypical, 343–346
  disordered, in atypical nevi, 78–82
  with intermediate biologic potential, 345–346
Intraepidermal Pagetoid spread, of melanocytes, 125

Intraepidermal pigmented spindle cell, differentiating from intraepidermal melanoma, 263
Intraepithelial melanoma, histopathologic features of, 249
In-transit metastases, defined, 357–358

J

Junctional cleavage, in Spitz nevi, 160
Junctional nests
  of the basal epidermal zone, 57
  of Spitz nevi, 155–157
Junctional nevus
  defined, 57–61
  lentiginous, defined, 55
  transition of melanocytes to, 52

K

Kamino bodies
  in pigmented spindle cell nevi, 183
  in Spitz nevi, 159
Keratinocytes, transfer of melanin pigment particles to, 1
Keratoses
  lichenoid, 341
    transition of solar lentigo to, 41
  melanomas resembling, 249
  reticulated seborrheic, transition of solar lentigo to, 41
Ki-67 nuclear antigen
  assessing melanocytic lesions using, 16
  immunolabeling of, to assess proliferation rate, 382
  levels of, and stage of melanoma, 383
Knockout models, CDKN2A deficient mice, 25

L

Lactate dehydrogenase (LDH) levels and prognosis in metastatic malignant melanoma, 358
Lamellar fibroplasia
  in atypical nevi, 86
  in melanocytic nevi of the genital skin, 98
Leiomyosarcoma, cutaneous, distinguishing from desmoplastic melanomas, 301
Lentigines, mucocutaneous, 46–49
Lentiginous compound nevi, atypical, differentiating from small cell melanoma, 313
Lentiginous melanocytic hyperplasia, defined, 3
Lentiginous melanocytic nevi, 275–280
Lentiginous melanocytic proliferation (LMP), 345
  falling short of melanoma in situ, 271–274
  of the sun-damaged skin, 254

Lentiginous melanomas
  association with desmoplastic melanoma and desmoplastic-neurotropic melanoma, 291
  overlap with Pagetoid melanomas, 265
Lentiginous nevi
  differentiating from atypical nevi, 86–88
  differentiating from solar lentigo, 41
  histopathologic features of, 57
Lentiginous pattern
  in conventional melanomas, 254
  differentiating variants of, 265
Lentigo maligna melanoma, 141–142, 254, 267–275
  definition of, 42–44
  differentiating from atypical nevi, 87
  punch biopsies of, 11
  similarities with pigmented spindle cell nevus, 185
  See also Solar melanoma
Lentigo malin des vieillards of Dubreuilh, 267–275
Lentigo senilis. See Solar lentigo
Lentigo simplex, 40–44, 54–55
  differentiating from Becker's melanosis, 46
Leptomeningeal melanoma, 130
Leukoderma acquisitum centrifugum. See Halo nevus
Lichen sclerosus, melanoma associated with, 140–141
Lichenoid keratosis, 341
  transition of solar lentigo to, 41
Lichenoid pattern, in regressed melanomas, 341–342
Light microscopy, to observe the morphology of melanocytes, 2–3
Lipofuscin (wear-and-tear pigment), 2
Liverspot. See Solar lentigo
Location, of melanocytes in the skin, defining melanocytic nevi in terms of, 53
Locoregional metastases, 357–358
Longitudinal melanonychia, 287–288
Loss of function, of CDKN2A and ARF loci, 25
Loss of heterozygosity
  bracketing the CDKN2A locus on chromosome 9p in atypical nevi, 25
  on chromosome 9p, in Spitz nevi, 175
  of the neurofibromatosis 1 gene, in neurotropic melanoma, 299
Lupus erythematosus, cutaneous, distinguishing from regression of melanomas, 341
Lymphatic invasion by Spitz nevi, 160
Lymph nodes
  benign metastasis to, in congenital blue nevus, 324
  involvement of, by blue nevi, 216–217
  metastasis to, and prognosis in malignant melanoma, 383–385
  See also Metastasis
Lymphocytes
  resemblance of type B melanocytes to, 7
  response to microinvasive melanomas, 260
Lymphocytoid cells (type B nevus), 61

M

M2–7C10 antibody, to the Mart-1 melanoma cell line, 15
Macroglobules, melanin, in café-au-lait macules, 39–40
Macromelanosomes, association with melanocytic lesions, 2
Macular phase, of acral melanoma development, 280–282
Major histocompatibility complex (MHC), role in apoptosis of melanoma cells, 31
Malignant blue nevus (MBN), 128, 322–327
  differentiating from cellular blue nevus, 216
Malignant degeneration of congenital melanocytic nevi, 114
Malignant epithelioid schwannoma, associated with congenital melanocytic nevi, 128
Malignant fibrous histiocytoma, distinguishing from desmoplastic melanoma, 301
Malignant melanoma, 238–356
  differentiating halo nevus from, 94
Malignant melanoma of soft parts, 327–328
Malignant neuroectodermal tumor, 289–301
Malignant Spitz nevus, defined, 162
Management of cohesive cellular nodules, 346
Mapping of melanoma genes, 21–26
Markers
  A-103, for identifying human melanoma cells, 15
  HDM2, prognostic significance of, 16
  Mart-1
    for recognizing metastatic tumor deposits in sentinel lymph nodes, 358
    for Spitz nevus, 171
  Melan A
    for identifying melanocytes, 15
    prediction of outcome from levels of, 383
    for recognizing metastatic tumor deposits in sentinel lymph nodes 358
  melanocyte differentiation, for evaluating sentinel lymph nodes, 357
  NKI/C3, for identifying melanocytic lesions, 15–16
  p75 neurotrophin receptor, 15, 291
  T311 antibody to tyrosinase, for melanocytes, 15
  tyrosinase-related protein 1, for melanocyte differentiation, 15
  See also HMB45; S-100 protein
Mart-1
  as a marker for Spitz nevus, 171
  for recognizing metastatic tumor deposits in sentinel lymph nodes, 358
Masson-Fontana stain, 13
Maturation
  of melanocytes, defined, 158
  in melanomas, 345–346
  of nevoid melanocytes, 61
  of pigmented spindle cell nevi, 181
  in Spitz nevi, 158–159
Mean nuclear volume, of Spitz nevi, 172
Mel-5 antibody, 15
Melan A
  for identifying melanocytes, 15
  prediction of outcome from levels of, 383
  for recognizing metastatic tumor deposits in sentinel lymph nodes, 358
Melanin pigment, 1–2
Melanin stains, 13
Melanin-stimulating hormone (MSH), 1
Melanocortin 1 receptor (MC1R), 28–29
  association with freckles, 37
  mediation of the response to ultraviolet light by, 21
  role in pheomelanin synthesis, versus eumelanin synthesis, 32
Melanocytes, 1–10
  in ephelides, size and appearance of, 37
  large epithelioid, in Spitz nevus, 151–158
  spindle-shaped, in Spitz nevus, 151–158
Melanocytic nevi
  acquired, 7–8, 51–110
  comparison with nevoid melanoma, 310
  congenital. See Congenital melanocytic nevi
  conventional melanomas associated with, 261
  differentiating from lentigo simplex, 55
  with focal dermal epithelioid cell components (MNFDECC), 230–233
  of the genital skin, 96–100
  with phenotypic heterogeneity, 223–237
    defined, 225–226
  recurrent, diagnosing, 345
  status of CDKN2A in, 25

Melanocytic nuclear volume, and prognosis, 381
Melanocytic proliferation, benign, pattern of, 3
Melanoma in dermis, distinction from dermal nevus cells, 345–346
Melanoma in situ
  criteria for defining, 271–274
  criteria for differentiating from solar intraepidermal melanocytic proliferations, 44
  histopathologic data for diagnosing, 249
  threshold for diagnosing, 254–256
Melanoma of soft parts (MMSP), t(12,22) chromosome translocation in, 17, 327
Melanoma of the nail apparatus, 284–289
Melanomas
  association with nevi, 66–89
  association with nevus of Ota involving the eye, 201
  childhood, and giant congenital nevi, 140–141
  criteria for differentiating from atypical nevi, 87
  development of, in congenital nevi, 126–134
  primary cutaneous, versus melanoma metastatic to the skin, 364
  primary mucosal, versus melanoma metastatic to the skin, 364–366
Melanoma with nodular component, 249
Melanonychia striata, 57, 287–289
Melanosis, in metastatic melanoma, 369–370
Melanosomes, enzymes of, 3–4
Melanotic macules
  of Albright, differentiating from freckles, 37
  mucocutaneous, 46–49
Melasma
  clinical appearance of, 40
  differentiating from freckles, 37
Melastatin
  control of metastasis by, 30
  inactivation of, and neoplastic progression, 21
Memorial Sloan-Kettering Cancer Center, data on satellite metastases, 357
Meningeal melanoma, neurocutaneous melanosis as a precursor to, 114–115
Merkel cell carcinoma, small cell melanoma mimicking, 312–314
Mesenchymal tumors, arising from giant congenital melanocytic nevi, 131
Metastasis
  of desmoplastic melanoma and desmoplastic-neurotropic melanoma, 300

distally acting melanoma loci involved in, 29–30
  of malignant melanoma, 357–371
  of melanoma
    distinguishing from nevoid melanoma, 310–311
    to a fetus, 134
    with unknown primary site, 368–369
  of radial and vertical growth phases, 242–243
  of Spitz tumors, 171
  visceral, sites in malignant melanoma, 358
  See also Lymph nodes
Metastatic malignant melanoma, 357–371
MIB-1 labeling index, for distinguishing melanomas and Spitz nevi, 16
Microinvasive melanoma
  conventional, 256–260
  regression in, 336–337
Micrometastatic disease, as a prognostic factor, 375
Microphthalmia transcription factor (MITF)
  expression of, and prognosis in malignant melanoma, 383
  as a marker for melanocytes, 15
Microsatellite instability near the CDKN2A locus, 74
Microscopic metastases, survival rate, 380
Microscopic satellites
  of invasive melanomas, 261
  prognosis predicted from, 377–378
Minimal deviation melanoma (MDM), 302–303, 379
Minor susceptibility melanoma loci, 32
Mitosis
  dermal, in nevoid melanoma, 309
  rate of, and prognosis in cutaneous malignant melanoma, 375–376
  in Spitz nevi, 159
Models
  of histogenesis of melanocytic nevi, 51–52
  prognostic, in malignant melanoma, 386–388
Mohs micrographic surgery, for basal cell and squamous cell carcinoma treatment, 12
Molecular pathology of melanoma, 20–36
Molecular pathways, and the development of melanoma, 31–32
Moles. See Common acquired nevi
Mongolian spot, 200
Monoclonal antibodies
  A-103, for identifying human melanoma cells, 15
  for identifying human melanoma cells, 16
  See also Markers

Morphologic features, of cellular blue nevi, 214–215
Morphology
  of melanocytes, 2–4
  of metastatic melanoma, 359
Mortality from cutaneous melanoma, among white populations, 238–239. See also Survival rate
Mucin, interstitial accumulation of, in nevi, 66
Mucosal blue nevi, 220
Mucosal melanoma, 335–336
Mulberry-type giant cells, 61
Multiple lentigines, syndromes associated with, 54
Multiple melanomas
  CDKN2A mutations in, 24
  primary, incidence of, 368
Multiple Spitz nevi, 150–151
Multiple tumor suppressor 1 (MTS1), identification with p16, 22
Mutagenic agents, expression of $14p^{ARF}$ protein by, 26
Mutation analysis, of CDKN2A/ARF, 23–25
Myxoid melanoma, 331
Myxoid stromal reaction, in metastatic malignant melanoma, 362–363
Myxomas, distinguishing from desmoplastic melanomas, 301

N
National Institutes of Health (NIH), definition of nevus with architectural disorder and cytologic atypia, 68
Natural history of desmoplastic melanoma and desmoplastic-neurotropic melanoma, 299–300
Neoplasms, melanocytic nevi as, 51
Nerve growth factor (NGF) receptor, association with melanoma, 73–74
Nerve sheath tumors, distinguishing desmoplastic-neurotropic melanoma from, 301
Nested intraepidermal melanocytic proliferation, in conventional melanomas, 256, 345
Nests/nested pattern
  distribution of, in atypical nevi, 82–83
  junctional
    of the basal epidermal zone, 57
    of Spitz nevi, 155–157
  in melanoma, distinguishing from melanocytic nevi, 265–266
  of nevocellular nevi, 7
Neural nevus, 94
Neurocristic hamartoma, 219–220

Neurocutaneous melanosis (NCM), 111, 126
  association with congenital melanocytic nevi, 114–115
Neuroectodermal tumors, 289–290
Neurofibromatosis (von Recklinghausen's disease), density of melanocytes in café-au-lait macules and normal skin, 39–40
Neurofibromatosis 1 gene, loss of heterozygosity of, in neurotropic melanoma, 299
Neuroid congenital melanocytic nevi, differentiation in, resembling neurofibroma histology, 123
Neuromelanin, accumulation of, in catcholaminergic neurons during aging, 2
Neurothekeoma
  cellular, differentiating from Spitz nevi, 171
  distinguishing from desmoplastic melanoma, 300–301
Neurotized nevus
  differentiating from a neurofibroma, 94
  melanocytic, 66
Neurotropic melanoma (NM), 290, 293–301
Neurotropic tumor aggregates, as microscopic satellites, 261
Neurotropism
  defined, 295
  and prognosis, 379
  of Spitz nevi, 160
Nevocellular nevi, nests of, 7. See also Common acquired nevi
Nevoid melanoma, 303–311
Nevoid melanosis. See Becker's melanosis
Nevus cells, morphology of, 7
  as the site for melanoma development, 239
Nevus fuscocaeruleus acromiodeltoideus, 201–202
Nevus fuscocaeruleus ophthalmomaxillaris, 200–201
Nevus fuscocaeruleus zygomaticus, 201
Nevus of Ito, 201–202
Nevus of Ota, 200–201
Nevus spilus (Speckled lentiginous nevus), 94–96
NKI/C3 monoclonal antibody, for identifying melanocytic lesions, 15–16
Nodal nevus versus metastasis, 366–368
Nodular melanoma, 243
  acral melanoma as, 282
  defined, 266

Nomenclature
  of borderline lesions, 343–346
  of p16, 22
  terminology for describing the Spitz nevus, 148–149
Nonmelanocytic tumor, differentiating from metastatic melanoma, 359–364
N-ras gene, association with congenital melanocytic nevi and melanoma, 133–134
Nuclear atypia
  and architectural disorder, 75
  continuum of, 83–85
Nuclei, of melanocytes, electron microscopic appearance of, 3
Nucleolar organizer regions (NORs)
  and prognosis, 382
  of Spitz nevi, 171
  See also AgNORs
Nucleus of melanocytes, appearance under light microscopy, 3

O

Oncogenes
  CDK4, 21
  metastasis promoted by, 29–30
Outcomes, in recurrent Spitz nevus, 196

P

p14^{ARF}, gene product of the alternate reading frame ARF, 23
p16 (CDKN2A). See CDKN2A (p16)
p53, activation of, by expression of p14^{ARF} in the S phase of cell division, 27
p75 neurotrophin receptor (p75NR)
  marker for desmoplastic melanoma and desmoplastic-neurotropic melanoma, 291
  marker for spindle cell melanomas, 15
Paget's disease, differentiating junctional Spitz nevus from, 164
Pagetoid melanocytosis
  in conventional melanomas, 253–254
  defined, 53
Pagetoid melanoma
  anatomic sites of, 247–248
  characteristics of, compared with pigmented spindle cell nevus, 189
Pagetoid pattern
  and diagnosis of conventional melanomas, 251–254
  and diagnosis of melanomas with intraepidermal components, 261–265
Pagetoid proliferation, defined, 3
Pagetoid scatter
  in acral nevi of the palms and soles, 89

defined, 53
  in melanocytic nevi, recurrent, 96
Pagetoid Spitz nevus, 163
Pagetoid spread
  association with melanomas of sun-exposed skin, 251
  in conventional melanomas, 251–254
  intraepidermal, of melanocytes, 125, 343–345
  in pigmented spindle cell nevi, 185
  in Spitz nevi, 157
    intraepidermal, 163
    of melanocytes, 159–160
Papillary dermis, invasion of, by in situ melanomas, 256
Parakeratosis, in conventional melanomas, 251
Patchlike blue nevus, 217
Pathologic factors, and prognosis, in malignant melanoma, 374–380
Penetrance
  of familial melanoma loci, 20
  of germline mutations in CDKN2A, 24–25
  minor, of familial melanoma genes, 27–29
Perinevoid leukoderma. See Halo nevus
Perinevoid vitiligo, See Halo nevus
Peutz-Jeghers syndrome, lentigines of the oral mucosa and vermillion border in, 47
Phaeomelanosomes, development of, stages in, 4
Phase, of tumor progression, and prognosis, 376
Phenotypes, histomorphologic, of neuroectodermal tumors, 290
Phenotypic heterogeneity, and nomenclature, 223–225
Pheomelanin, 1
  production of, in response to low-affinity binding of melanocortin ligands, 28–29
  synthesis of, promotion by melanocortin 1 receptor polymorphisms, 32
Photochemotherapy (PUVA), lentigo induced by, 41
Photoprotection, by eumelanin, 28
Pigmentation, of Spitz nevi, 160
Pigmented actinic keratosis, differentiating from solar lentigo, 41–42
Pigmented hairy epidermal nevus. See Becker's melanosis
Pigmented spindle cell nevus (PSCN), 180–185
  with atypical features, 183–185
  intraepidermal, differentiating from intraepidermal melanoma, 263

Pigmented spindle cell variant, of solar melanoma, 271–274
Pigment incontinence, in desmoplastic melanoma, 291
Pilar neurocristic hamartoma, clinical features of, 219–220
Plaque-type blue nevus, 217–219
Pleomorphism, of nevus cells, 61
Plexiform spindle cell nevus, 233–237
  pigmented, morphological similarity with melanocytic nevi with phenotypic heterogeneity, 227–228
Plexiform Spitz nevus, 178–179
Pmel 17 gene family, role in melanogenesis, 1
Point mutations, in CDKN2A inactivation in familial melanoma, 23
Polypoid configuration of melanoma, 329
Postinflammatory hyperpigmentation, distinguishing from café-au-lait macules, 40
Postzygotic inactivation, of the CDKN2A locus, cancers associated with, 24
Postzygotic mutations, at genomic loci, in melanomas, 20
Precursors, to melanoma, atypical nevi as, 72–74
Pregnancy status, and survival from melanoma, 380–381
Presentation, of Spitz nevi, 149
Primary melanoma, complete regression of, 341
Primary melanoma of soft parts versus metastatic melanoma to soft tissue, 368
Prognosis
  of balloon cell melanoma, 330
  of melanomas in children, 141
  in metastatic melanoma, correlation with increased soluble FasL levels, 31
  of mucosal melanomas, 336
  of subungual melanoma, 284
Prognostic factors
  in cutaneous malignant melanoma, 372–394
  in stage I and II malignant melanoma, 373–383
    table, 384
  in stage III malignant melanoma, table, 385
  in stage IV malignant melanoma, 385–386
Prognostic indicator, melastatin levels in metastatic melanomas, 30
Prognostic models, in malignant melanoma, 386–388
Proliferating cell nuclear antigen (PCNA), labeling for, in assessing outcome, 382

Proliferation index
  of nevi and melanomas, 74
  prognostic value of, 382
Proliferation rate of Spitz nevi, compared with melanomas, 171–172
Proto-oncogenes, 20
Pseudomelanosis coli, pigment of, 2
Punch biopsies of cutaneous pigmented lesions, 11

R
Radial growth phase (RGP) of melanoma, 242–243
Ras protein, upregulation of, 31
Recurrence
  of clear-cell sarcoma, 328
  of desmoplastic melanoma, 300
  local, and prognosis, 381
  of malignant melanoma, 357
  of melanotic nevi, 88, 96
  of Spitz nevi, 185–196
Red hair and freckle gene, and the risk of melanoma, 27–29
Regressing nevoid nail melanosis, 284–285
Regression
  effects of, on prognosis in melanoma, 376–377
  of halo nevi, 92
  of melanomas, 336–343
    invasive, 261
    leading to metastatic melanoma with unknown primary site, 368
    microinvasive, 260
    Pagetoid, 248
Regulation, of melanogenesis, 1
Relative risk of melanoma
  association with polymorphisms of the melanocortin 1 receptor, 29
  relationship with the numbers of nevi, 71
Research, tissue for, 13
Restriction points, in the cell-division cycle, result of loss of control at, 25–26
Rete ridges, epidermal
  in lentigo simplex, 54
  in solar lentigo, 41
Reticular dermis, invasion of, by melanomas, 261
Reticulohistiocytoma, differentiating from Spitz nevus, 171
Retinoblastoma (RB) gene product, as a gatekeeper of the G_1/S cell-division cycle, 25–26
Reverse transcriptase-polymerase chain reaction (RT-PCR)
  for identifying clear-cell sarcoma, 328
  for identifying melanoma markers, 385
  for identifying tyrosinase mRNA expression, 358, 382–383

Rhabdomyosarcoma, alveolar, by metastatic melanoma, 362
RhoC gene
  overexpression of, and metastatic propensity of melanomas, 30
  promotion of neoplastic progression by, 21
Risk factors, for melanoma
  associated with red hair and inability to tan, 29
  atypical nevi as markers for, 69–72
  in childhood, 140–141
  in congenital melanocytic nevi, 111–112, 131–132
  correlation of histologic melanocytic atypia with, 74
  malignant, 238–239
  melanocytic nevi, 51–52
  stratification of, 69

S
S-100 protein
  as a marker
    for desmoplastic melanoma and desmoplastic-neurotropic melanoma, 291
    for epithelioid melanomas, 14
    for Spitz nevus, 171
  serum levels of, and survival rates, 382–383
Satellite metastases, 357–358
Satellites, of congenital melanocytic nevi, 114, 139
Satellitosis, of lymphocytes, in invasive melanomas, 261
Schmorl stain, 13
Schwann cell, differentiating from a blue nevus, 199–200
Schwannomas, distinguishing from melanoma, 16
Sclerosing blue nevus, 204
  differentiating from desmoplastic melanoma and neurotropic melanoma, 300
Seborrheic keratosis, reticulated, transition of solar lentigo to, 41
Secretory melanocytes, defined, 1
Sentinel lymph node (SLN) biopsy
  to assess atypical Spitz-like tumors, 163
  in conjunction with excisional biopsy, 11
  prognosis indicated by the results of, 385
  for staging risk for regional melanoma metastases, 357–358
  status from, and prognosis, 375
Shave biopsy, 11–12
Shoulder phenomenon, in atypical nevus architecture, 75–76
Signaling pathway, for the melanocortin1 receptor, 28

Signet-ring cell melanoma, 334
Signet-ring cell morphology, in metastatic malignant melanoma, 362
Silver-Russell syndrome, association with café-au-lait macules, 40
Silver-staining nucleolar organizer region (AgNORs). See AgNORs
Simple lentigines, differentiating from freckles, 37–38
Size
    of conventional melanomas, 249–251
    and histopathology
        of giant congenital melanocytic nevi, 123
        of larger congenital melanocytic nevi, 119–123
        of small congenital melanocytic nevi, 115–119
Skin and Cancer Foundation, Sydney, Australia, 313
Skin color
    and incidence of acral melanoma, 280
    and incidence of subungual melanoma, 284
    and number of nevi in individuals, 55
    and prevalence of longitudinal melanonychia, 289
Skin excisions, routine handling of, 12
Small cell melanomas, 312–316
    in childhood, histopathologic features of, 142–143
Solar intraepidermal melanocytic neoplasia, differentiating from solar melanocytic hyperplasia, 278
Solar intraepidermal melanocytic proliferations (SIMPs)
    with atypia, differentiating from solar lentigo, 42–44
    differentiating from solar lentigo, 41
    progression to invasive melanoma, 267–268
    sampling or removing lesions with features of, 256
Solar lentigines
    association with melanocortin 1 receptor, 37
    differentiating from freckles, 37–38
Solar lentiginous melanocytic nevi, 275–276
Solar lentiginous melanomas (LMM), desmoplastic melanoma and desmoplastic-neurotropic melanoma associated with, 290
Solar lentigo, 40, 275–280
Solar melanocytic hyperplasia (SMH), 278–280
    defined, 278
Solar melanoma, 267–275
    age at development of, 248
    characteristics of, compared with pigmented spindle cell nevus, 189
    defined, 241
    differentiating from Pagetoid melanoma, 265
    lentiginous pattern in, 254
    similarities with pigmented spindle cell nevus, 185, 263
    See also Lentigo maligna melanoma
Solar melanoma in situ, differentiating from solar lentigo, 41
Spindle cell melanocytes of Spitz nevi, 153–158
Spindle cell melanomas
    desmoplastic, S-100 protein as a marker for, 14
    specificity of monoclonal p75 neurotrophin receptor antibody for, 15
Spindle cell morphology, of metastatic melanomas, 362
Spindle cell nevi, pigmented, 180–185
    differentiating from atypical nevi, 88
    differentiating from Spitz nevi, 171
    See also Spitz nevi
Spindle cells
    proliferation of, in desmoplastic melanoma and desmoplastic-neurotropic melanoma, 291
    in solar melanoma, differentiating from PSCNs, 276–277
Spindle cell squamous carcinoma, distinguishing from desmoplastic melanomas, 301
Spitz nevi, 148–198
    combined, 98–100
    continuum of histologic features with pigmented spindle cell nevus, 181
    differentiating from atypical nevi, 88
    hyalinizing, 178
    melanomas simulating, in children, 144
    Pagetoid variant, differentiating from conventional melanomas, 263
    relationship with ordinary nevi in melanocytic nevi with phenotypic heterogeneity, 227–228
Spitzoid melanoma, 313–319
Spitz tumors
    atypical, 160–171
    defined, 148–149
    differentiating from desmoplastic melanoma and neurotropic melanoma, 300
    differentiating from nodular melanomas, 267
Sporadic melanoma, gene changes in, 21
Squamous carcinoma, spindle cell, distinguishing from desmoplastic melanomas, 301
Squamous epithelium, organization patterns within, in conventional melanomas, 251
Stage III melanoma, prognostic factors for, 383–385
Staghorn-like vascular pattern, in metastatic melanomas, 363
Staging system, for melanoma, 373. See also American Joint Committee on Cancer
Standardized morbidity ratio (SMR), of patients with giant congenital melanocytic nevi, 113
Starburst cells, in solar melanomas, 271–274
Stroma, 53–54
Stromal fibrotic reaction, in vulvar nevi, 98
Subcutaneous fat, extension of nevus cells into, 120
    in congenital nevi, 118
Subungual melanoma (SUM), 249, 284–287
Sunlight, exposure to
    intermittent, and conventional melanomas, 244–248
    protection against the effects of, by melanin, 1
    as a risk factor for malignant melanoma, 239
    as a risk factor for small cell melanoma, 313
Superficial spreading melanoma, 243
Surgical margins, interpretation of, 279
Survival rate
    in clear-cell sarcoma, 327–328
    in desmoplastic melanoma, 300
    in locally recurrent melanoma, 381
    in metastatic malignant melanoma, 357
Sutton's nevus. See Halo nevus
Symmetry, of Spitz nevi, 157–158

T

T311 antibody to tyrosinase, as a marker for melanocytes, 15
Target blue nevus, 220
T-cells, mediation of antitumor immunity by, 31
Telangiectasia, in Spitz nevi, 160
Territorial behavior, of melanocytes of the human epidermis, 2–3
Theque. See Junctional nest
Thickness of a primary tumor, and prognosis, 373–375
Tisch nodules (pigmented hamartomas of the iris), diagnostic of neurofibromatosis, 40

Tissue processing, for biopsies of melanocytic lesions, 12–13
Tissue regeneration, proliferation of epidermal melanocytes in response to, 3
Tuberous sclerosis (epiloa), association with café-au-lait macules, 40
Tubular Spitz nevus, 180
Tumoral melanosis, regression in, 342–343
Tumor cells
  dissociation of, in metastatic melanoma mimicking other neoplasms, 362
  type of, and prognosis in malignant melanoma, 379
Tumor-infiltrating lymphocytes (TILs), 261
  presence of, and prognosis in malignant melanoma, 378
Tumor invasion, depth of, and prognosis, 374–375
Tumor necrosis factor (TNF) transmembrane family, role in apoptosis in melanoma cells, 30–31
Tumor-suppressor genes
  CDKN2A and ARF, 21
  control of metastasis by, 30
  loss-of-function mutation of, in melanomas, 20
  p14^{ARF}, structure and function of, 26
Tumor vascularity, and prognosis, in malignant melanoma, 379
Tumor volume, and prognosis, 379
21N antibody, specificity of, for mammary Paget's disease, 265
Twin data
  concordance of nevus phenotype between identical twins, 56
  indicating genetic control of growth of nevi, 52
Type A nevus ceoosk 61
  inverted, 98–100, 228–230

See also Epithelioid melanocytes
Type B nevus cells, 61
Type C nevus cells, 61
  in the dermal component, 66
Tyrosinase
  activity of, demonstration with the DOPA oxidase technique, 13–14
  blood levels of, measuring to predict clinical relapse, 382–383
  for recognizing metastatic tumor deposits in sentinel lymph nodes, 358
  role of, in melanogenesis, 1
  T311 antibody to, as a marker for melanocytes, 15
Tyrosinase-related protein 1 (TRP-1; gp75), as a melanocyte differentiation marker, 15
L-Tyrosine, substrate for the melanin pathway, 1

U

Ulceration of the primary tumor
  and prognosis, 375–376
  in stage III disease, 385
Ultraviolet light (UV light)
  effect of, on development of nevi, 52
  response to
    mediation by the melanocortin 1 receptor, 21
    proliferation of epidermal melanocytes, 3
    upregulation of melanocortins in the skin, 28
  See also Sunlight, exposure to
Ultraviolet radiation (UV radiation), signature mutations of, involving C to T transitions, 24
Uniformity, of cells and nuclei of Spitz nevi, 154–157

V

Variants
  cytologic, of melanocytes in nevi, 7, 89–102
  of melanomas, 241–242
    and histomorphologic alterations, 328–336
    morphological and cytological, 289–328
  morphologic, of nevoid melanoma, 304–305
  of Spitz nevus, 171, 178–180
  Pagetoid, 263
Vascular invasion, and prognosis in malignant melanoma, 377
Verrucous melanoma, 311–312
Vertical growth phase (VGP), of melanoma, 242–243
Vimentin, of melanocytes, electron micrographs of, 3
Visceral blue nevi, 220
Vulvar lentigo, 48

W

Warthin-Starry stain, 13
Watson syndrome, association with café-au-lait macules, 40
Westerhof syndrome, association of café-au-lait macules with, 40

X

Xanthogranuloma, differentiating from Spitz nevus, 171
Xeroderma pigmentosum (XP)
  lentiginous lesions associated with, 267
  melanomas diagnosed in patients with, 141–142
  solar lentigines in, 41

Z

Zonation, in Spitz nevi, 158–159

ISBN 0-387-40326-4